PROF. C
HISTOLC
ADDENB
HILLS ROAD, CAMBRIDGE

THE ESSENTIALS OF
FORENSIC MEDICINE

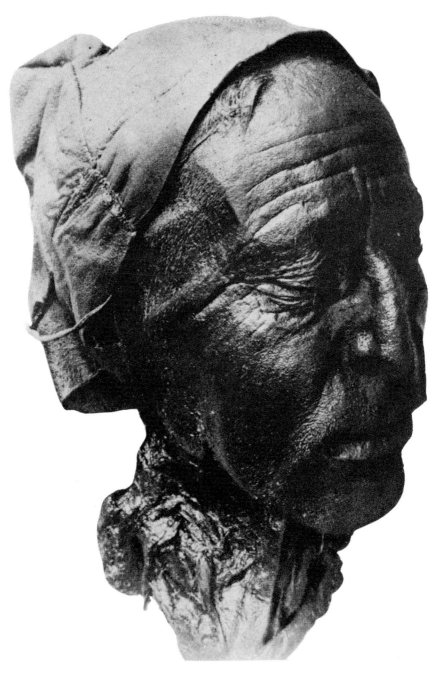

Frontispiece. The Tollund Man (Silkeborg Museum, Jutland).

THE ESSENTIALS OF FORENSIC MEDICINE

FOURTH EDITION

by

CYRIL JOHN POLSON

*M.D. (Birm.), F.R.C.P. (Lond.), F.R.C. Path., of The Inner Temple,
Emeritus Professor of Forensic Medicine, University of Leeds*

D. J. GEE

*M.B., B.S. (Lond.), F.R.C. Path., D.M.J., Professor of Forensic Medicine,
University of Leeds*

and

BERNARD KNIGHT

*M.D. (Wales), M.R.C.P. (Lond.), F.R.C. Path., D.M.J. (Path.), of
Gray's Inn, Professor of Forensic Pathology, University of Wales*

PERGAMON PRESS

OXFORD · NEW YORK · TORONTO · SYDNEY · PARIS · FRANKFURT

U.K.	Pergamon Press Ltd., Headington Hill Hall, Oxford OX3 0BW, England
U.S.A.	Pergamon Press Inc., Maxwell House, Fairview Park, Elmsford, New York 10523, U.S.A.
CANADA	Pergamon Press Canada Ltd., Suite 104, 150 Consumers Road, Willowdale, Ontario M2J 1P9, Canada
AUSTRALIA	Pergamon Press (Aust.) Pty. Ltd., P.O. Box 544, Potts Point, N.S.W. 2011, Australia
FRANCE	Pergamon Press SARL, 24 rue des Ecoles, 75240 Paris, Cedex 05, France
FEDERAL REPUBLIC OF GERMANY	Pergamon Press GmbH, Hammerweg 6, D-6242 Kronberg-Taunus, Federal Republic of Germany

First Edition 1960
Second Edition 1964
Third Edition 1973
Fourth Edition 1985

Library of Congress Cataloging in Publication Data
Polson, Cyril John, 1901–
   The essentials of forensic medicine.
   Includes index.
   1. Medicine jurisprudence. I. Gee, D. J. (David John)
II. Knight, Bernard. III. Title. [DNLM: 1. Forensic
medicine. W 700 P778e]
RA1051.P63   1984   614'.1   84–2867

British Library Cataloguing in Publication Data
Polson, C. J.
   The essentials of forensic medicine.—4th ed.
   1. Medical jurisprudence
   I. Title   II. Gee, D. J.   III. Knight,
Bernard, *1931–*
   614.1   RA1051

ISBN 0–08–028868–5

Typeset by Macmillan India Ltd, Bangalore
Printed in Great Britain by A. Wheaton & Co. Ltd, Exeter

Preface to the Fourth Edition

THE opportunity has been taken to subject the book to thorough revision. Pruning and re-casting has been extensive and several chapters have been re-written, e.g. Mechanical Asphyxia, Cruelty to Children, and Scenes of Crime. The basic material of Part I, Forensic Pathology, changes relatively little, but that of Part II has changed appreciably and rewriting, notably of the chapter on the General Medical Council, has been obligatory.

In this edition I am joined with Bernard Knight as the second co-author. David Gee and I welcome his participation and he, being a fellow barrister, is well qualified to undertake the responsibility for the chapters in Part II and, in particular, the chapter on the General Medical Council, since he is one of its elected members.

Harrogate   CYRIL JOHN POLSON

Preface to the Third Edition

This book began as an amplification of my lectures in the course of Forensic Medicine in the University of Leeds. During the years the ever-increasing scope of the medical curriculum allows medical students less and less time for the study of this subject; yet it plays a minor, but necessary, part in their instruction. Understandably, they turn to works of small compass, for example, the well-established book (8th ed., 1979) by Professor Keith Simpson, and the "Lecture Notes" by Dr. David Gee.

The publishers, therefore, suggested that this revision of the book should be undertaken with post-graduate students, pathologists, who include forensic pathology in their repertoire, and forensic pathologists, in mind. This suggestion was readily adopted, and I invited Dr. David Gee, who had been Acting-Head of the Department since I retired from the Chair, to become my co-author. He succeeded to the Chair in July 1972.

We have rearranged the text. Forensic Pathology is considered in Part I, and the Law relating to the Practice of Medicine forms Part II.

Certain topics have been eliminated, notably blood grouping and tests for blood, because these belong to the field of forensic science, and several monographs and other excellent publications by experts in this special field are readily accessible. This has afforded space for a more extensive consideration of Cruelty to Children, and Sudden Death, notably of children. ("Battered Babies" and "Cot Deaths" are terms we use with distinct reluctance.) Some chapters, notably the Signs of Death, and Electrical Injuries, have been expanded. We have added a few chapters, e.g. Scenes of Crime, and Anaesthetic Deaths. The recent work on the Age of Injuries has also received consideration. Our respective contributions are indicated in the Contents list.

Poisoning, in detail, is excluded from this work, since it is now dealt with in the companion volume, *Clinical Toxicology* by C. J. Polson Michael Green and Michael Lee. 3rd edition. 1983. London. Pitman Publishing Ltd.

The apparently mystic figures, e.g. F.M. 2090, are reference numbers which indicate that the case occurred in our practice. In the event that any reader wishes for more detailed information, a request, including the appropriate reference number, will allow prompt location of the relevant documents and photographs in the departmental files.

Harrogate   CYRIL JOHN POLSON

Preface to the Second Edition

REVISION has been considerable and certain chapters have been deleted to allow for expansion of others, notably that which deals with medical negligence. I have added several more summaries of cases from the practice of my Department.

Favourable comment on the bibliography has encouraged me to devote even more care to it; with few exceptions each reference has been personally examined.

Some of those who reviewed the first edition asked for pictures. These add appreciably to the cost of production, but, through the generosity of the publishers, the book is now illustrated. Every endeavour has been made to preclude the identification of the deceased and to avoid the sensational, etc. In consequence, the pictorial quality of some of the figures may have suffered, but, it is hoped, their instructional value has been retained.

I was taken to task by one reviewer, who has throughout been a generous friend of the book and, I hope I may claim, its author, because I had said it was intended, in the first instance, to meet the needs of the undergraduate. He protested at its length, particularly in view of a separate volume on clinical toxicology. Admittedly the chapter on identification is unduly detailed, but others, if somewhat long, deal with practical matters. The undergraduate will surely ignore the references and no harm will be done if he overlooks most of the small print. For the rest, I adhere to the view that this book has a claim on the attention of the undergraduate, to provide not only that which is of immediate practical value, but also to give information which should be a part of the general medical knowledge of an educated doctor. Even where less attention is given to some subjects, it is believed sufficient has been included to meet his requirements. I have deliberately excluded deaths related to anaesthesia because on most occasions the pathologist can only play a negative rôle. If the anaesthetic had played a part in the death, the only opinion worthy of consideration is that of the anaesthetist. Sexual offences, the examination of the victim apart, are for the psychiatrist to discuss.

Dr. Wiener honoured me with a letter in which he complained that blood grouping was inadequately considered. Even if I had the competence, to attempt more than I have done would overburden the text. I have indicated the better sources of information, including Dr. Wiener's own outstanding contributions, for those who require them.

The aim has been to provide reasonable coverage of the subject as a whole and to place on record, in the appropriate sections, experience gained in my Department. Inevitably some sections are therefore more comprehensive than others.

The University of Leeds   CYRIL JOHN POLSON

Preface to the First Edition

THIS book is an amplification of lectures delivered in the University of Leeds and it embodies experience gained through participation in a pathology service for the Home Office and for certain H. M. Coroners in Yorkshire.

It is intended, in the first instance, to meet the needs of undergraduates in medicine and in law. Resident hospital medical officers and general medical practitioners, however, are not rarely faced with duties and problems with which this book deals. Although the medico-legal expert may find its contents add nothing to his knowledge, the hospital pathologist, preoccupied with clinical problems, may turn to its pages for help when called upon to act as a medico-legal expert. Amongst the laity there are many who encounter medical evidence in the course of their duties. Coroners, magistrates, barristers, solicitors and police officers, therefore, are in mind and it is hoped that for them the present account of the subject has something to offer. It is also believed that much of the contents of the book is relevant in all civilised countries. The signs of death, modes of identification, a cut throat or a broken skull are not dependent on any particular system of law.

The information is in textual form, without pictorial aids or "classifications", because the aim is to focus attention on the text. Omission of the usual chapters on toxicology is also deliberate because that subject demands separate treatment and another book, on clinical toxicology, is in preparation.

The present endeavour has been to provide a reliable and up-to-date account of forensic medicine in readable form acceptable to medical and lay readers alike.

There has been no attempt to offer a complete or even a comprehensive bibliography. At the same time facts and opinions derived from others are duly acknowledged and the reader is also directed, as required, to authoritative sources which will provide a fuller account of the subject under consideration. Cases from my own Department's practice are indicated by the inclusion of their serial reference number in the text (e.g. F.M. 2056).

CYRIL JOHN POLSON

Acknowledgements

(FIRST EDITION)

WHEN the task of writing a book is done, it is a pleasure to recollect and acknowledge the help received during its preparation. In returning thanks I must make it clear that those I now mention are in no way responsible for what appears in the following pages. In one way or another, however, by encouragement, advice or criticism or by permission to use material, they have contributed to this book.

The necropsy practice at the Leeds City Mortuary has been the source of most of my personal cases and my thanks are due, therefore, to the late Dr. A. J. Swanton, formerly H. M. Coroner, City of Leeds, for the many kindnesses he has shown to me. I am indebted to him also for access to his records covering the past quarter of a century and for permission to use them for present purposes. I would like to record my sincere thanks to him for a pleasant relationship which has long existed between us. I am indebted also to my former colleague Professor I. G. Davies, who, in his capacity as Medical Officer of Health, ensured for me the best possible facilities at the City Mortuary.

Professor R. A. Willis gave freely of his time and patience to read and criticise many of the chapters, totalling over half of the book. Those who know him either personally or only through the medium of his own writings, will know how much I owe him for this help. I am indebted also to Mr. A. R. Taylor for criticism of the text.

The late Mr. Michael Heseltine, in his private capacity, subjected my chapters on the Medical Acts and the General Medical Council to detailed criticism. The Editor of the *Practitioner* permits me to reproduce my account of the Council which was published in that journal.

Professor Philip James revised certain of the chapters, notably that which deals with the Law Courts. I have also had the benefit of advice and criticism from Mr. Gilbert Leslie, Barrister-at-Law, on the chapters which deal with Consent to Medical Examination, Malpraxis and the Law of Abortion. The procedure of certification under the Lunacy and Mental Deficiency Acts has been based on their Manual and personal comments of Mr. J. S. Hoyle and Mr. T. S. Hawkesworth of the Mental Health Department of the City of Leeds.

The chapter on head injuries was read and criticised by Dr. A. F. J. Maloney. That on blood grouping was revised by Dr. R. R. Race, F.R.S. and Dr. J. A. V. Shone. My account of the determination of age, sex and stature was revised by Professor R. J. Harrison. Dr. G. R. Osborn checked and amplified my use of his published work. I have also had the benefit of criticism of the chapter on electrical injuries by an anonymous reader. I am indeed grateful to each of these experts for their generous help.

It has been my privilege, from time to time, to have had first-hand accounts of their cases from John Glaister, Keith Simpson and Francis Camps and the benefit of their views on many matters, in conversation, by letter or in published form. It is a pleasure to acknowledge this education.

My use of, or benefit from, copyright material has been sanctioned by Professor John Glaister and Messrs. E. Livingstone Ltd. in respect of his text-book and *The Medico-Legal Aspects of the Ruxton Case*, and Dr. Keith Simpson and the Editor of the *Police Journal* for his account of R. v. Donaghue, and Messrs. Jarrolds, who published the *Dobkin Case*, by the late Mr. Bechhofer Roberts, in their Old Bailey Trials Series. I am especially grateful to Mr. James H. Hodge, who not only gave his permission to draw freely upon the Notable British Trials Series but who also read and commented upon my summaries of notable cases, which form an appendix to the chapter on identification. If by mischance I have overlooked any other person to whom acknowledgement is due I can assure him it is inadvertent and wholly unintentional.

My thanks and those of my publishers are due to the Director of the National Museet, Copenhagen and to Professor P. V. Glob, of the Institute of Prehistoric Archaeology, University of Aarhus, for permission to reproduce their photograph of the Tollund man as a frontispiece.

The transcription of my manuscript has been undertaken by Miss Torfrida Maxwell Telling and Miss Rosemary Whiteley, who have ably performed a difficult and wearisome task. I am also indebted to the Hon. L. E. F. Zaidée Milner for her assistance with proof correction and Dr. T. K. Marshall, who prepared the index.

Additional Acknowledgements

IN RETURNING thanks to those now mentioned, it must be clear that none of them is in any way responsible for errors or opinions in the text.

The co-operation of several of H. M. Coroners has made it possible for the Department actively to engage in the practice of forensic pathology and thereby to acquire valuable experience and material. In this I am especially indebted to the late R. E. Nutt, Esquire, L.L.M., City of Leeds: Innes Ware, Esquire, O.B.E., City of York, Escrick District of the East Riding and York District of the North Riding, and S. E. Brown, Esquire, L.L.M., Craven District of the West Riding. I have received permission to refer to cases by B. W. Little, Esquire, O.B.E., Halifax District and Borough; R. Llewellyn Jones, Esquire, B.A., Flintshire County; G. Tudor, Esquire, Cardiff City, Roger E. L. Thomas, Esquire, Breconshire County, and E. Talog Davies, Esquire, County of Denbigh (Western Division).

I am also grateful for the ready co-operation of Professor D. B. Bradshaw, who, in his capacity as Medical Officer of Health, City of Leeds, provides facilities at the City Mortuary and, as Professor of Public Health and Preventive Medicine, congenial collaboration in the University.

I have been allowed to reproduce portions of articles already published. My thanks for this are due to Dr. Gavin Thurston, editor of the *Medico-Legal Journal*, Mr. S. S. Kind, editor of the *Journal of the Forensic Science Society*, and to Messrs. Butterworths, publishers of the *British Encyclopaedia of Medical Practice* (Medical Progress), edited by Lord Cohen of Birkenhead.

Mr. J. F. Fry, Director of the Fire Research Station, D.S.I.R., has permitted me to quote from "Fires Associated with Electrical Apparatus" by R. E. Lustig, F. R. Note No. 476/1961, and from a letter. Mr. L. A. Corney, Chief Safety Officer, The Electricity Council, has allowed me to quote from his statistics of electrical accidents 1960/61.

I am grateful to several others for material, by way of case reports, photographs and other information, supplied unstintingly and with full permission to use it. I would like to thank Mr. G. P. Arden for colour photographs and information concerning the lightning incident at Ascot in 1955, Dr. Lester James, the late Dr. Gerald Evans, Dr. Patrick Roche, Dr. A. C. Hunt, Dr. George Manning, Dr. A. S. Curry, Dr. Ian Barclay, Dr. J. G. Leopold, the late Dr. H. V. Phelon, Dr. William Goldie, Dr. H. Thompson, Dr. Denis Harriman, Dr. Keith Mant, Dr. D. G. Rushton, the late Dr. W. E. D. Evans and Dr. J. V. Wilson.

To Professor Harald Gormsen and Professor Dalgaard I express my special thanks for receiving me in their Departments and placing material at my disposal.

Our thanks are also due to Dr. Philip H. Addison, and the Medical Defence Union for permission to quote from their Annual Reports. Also to Dr. W. R. Lee for off-prints of his articles and other information relating to Electrical injuries.

We thank our publishers for their acceptance of the financial responsibility of publication and, not least, their generosity in the matter of illustrations.

The transcription of the revision of the manuscript was undertaken by Mrs. C. I. Sutton, S.R.N. and Miss Gillian Flather.

We also thank Miss E. M. Read, B.A., A.L.A., and Mr. Patrick Gaunt, H.N.C., L.R.I.C. for their help in checking references.

To Professor W. R. Lee for the gift of his more recent publications and statistics compiled by Miss McNamee of his Department staff.

To Mr. Whittlesone, Librarian; Mr. George Cappel of the Harrogate Library; Mr. Kenneth Harding, Barristers' Clerk to Magistrate, Harrogate District, and to Mr. Richard Irvine, Magistrates' Court Office, for tracing information.

To Miss Whitaker for assistance with preparing the manuscript.

Acknowledgement of the Sources of the Illustrations

IN ORDER to restrict, if not preclude, identification of the subjects, the precise sources of the illustrations are not stated. The majority, over eighty, of the illustrations were prepared under my direction and I am glad to acknowledge the expert assistance of Mr. A. L. Pegg, A.R.P.S. and Mr. J. Hainsworth, F.R.P.S., A.I.B.P.

I am particularly indebted to the Chief Constable of the West Yorkshire Constabulary for twenty and the Chief Constable of the City of Leeds for the majority of the illustrations. The Chief Constables of the following forces also contributed as follows: City of Cardiff and Borough of Halifax, two each; City of Glasgow, City of Bradford, City of York, Barnsley, Denbighshire, East Riding, Flintshire and Mid-Wales Constabularies, one each.

Dr. Ian Barclay, Dr. William Goldie, Dr. Dennis Harriman, Dr. J. G. Leopold, Mr. L. C. Nickolls and Dr. Patrick Roche each contributed an illustration.

The Editor of the *British Medical Journal* and Professor Chassar Moir allow the reproduction of their illustration of lightning burns. The Editor of the *Police Journal* and Mr. L. C. Nickolls allow the reproduction of their illustration of a bite mark in cheese. The publishers of the *Deutsche Zeitschrift für die gesamte gerichtliche Medizin*, Messrs. Springer-Verlag, and Professor Willie Munck allow the reproduction of their illustration of an electric mark.

(Information concerning the ownership of the copyright of any of these illustrations may be obtained from the Publishers.)

For new illustrations in the 4th Edition we are grateful to the Chief Constables of West Yorkshire, North Yorkshire and North Humberside Police Forces.

Contents

PART I   FORENSIC PATHOLOGY

1. *The Signs of Death*
   C. J. POLSON   3

2. *Identification*
   C. J. POLSON   40

3. *Injuries: General Features*
   C. J. POLSON and D. J. GEE   91

4. *Injuries of Specific Regions*
   C. J. POLSON and D. J. GEE   148

5. *Firearms and Injuries Caused by Firearms*
   C. J. POLSON   196

6. *Electrical Injuries and Lightning Stroke*
   C. J. POLSON   271

7. *Thermal Injuries*
   D. J. GEE   318

8. *Mechanical Asphyxia*
   C. J. POLSON   351

9. *Hanging*
   C. J. POLSON   357

10. *Strangulation*
    C. J. POLSON   389

11. *Drowning*
    D. J. GEE   421

12. *Suffocation*
    C. J. POLSON   449

13. *Sexual Offences*
    D. J. GEE   480

14. *Criminal Abortion*
    D. J. GEE   496

15.   *Infanticide and Child Destruction*
      D. J. GEE   514

16.   *Cruelty to Children: the "Battered Baby" (Non-Accidental
      Injury)*
      D. J. GEE   532

17.   *Sudden Natural Death*
      D. J. GEE   547

18.   *Scenes of Crime*
      C. J. POLSON and D. J. GEE   574

19.   *Anaesthetic Deaths*
      D. J. GEE   590

      PART II   THE LAW RELATING TO THE PRACTICE OF MEDICINE

20.   *The General Medical Council*
      B. KNIGHT   603

21.   *Consent to Medical Examination and Treatment*
      B. KNIGHT and C. J. POLSON   621

22.   *Medical Negligence*
      B. KNIGHT   638

23.   *Trauma and Disease*
      B. KNIGHT   659

24.   *Disposal of the Dead*
      C. J. POLSON and B. KNIGHT   677

25.   *The Medical Witness*
      C. J. POLSON and B. KNIGHT   696

26.   *The Abortion Act, 1967, and other Statutes which Relate to
      the Practice of Medicine*
      C. J. POLSON   705

      INDEX   721

PART I

Forensic Pathology

CHAPTER 1

The Signs of Death

Two phases of death are observed, namely, the extinction of personality, which is the immediate sign of cessation of the vital process, i.e. *somatic* death, and secondly, the progressive disintegration of the body tissues, or *molecular* death. The former is normally implied when we speak of death but the latter is of greater medico-legal importance.

Although the occurrence of somatic death is usually obvious, a knowledge of the signs of death is required by the doctor in order to distinguish death from suspended animation. The signs of death, moreover, permit an estimation of the time at which death occurred and this may be important in relation to homicide. The police will then wish to know not only that the victim is dead but also when he died.

The diagnosis of death is normally ascertained accurately by ordinary clinical methods but there are occasions when the distinction between death and suspended animation is one of special difficulty.

SUSPENDED ANIMATION

This death-like state can be induced voluntarily by practitioners of Yoga or it is the involuntary result of severe shock following an accident, electrical shock or poisoning by barbiturate or narcotic drugs. (Maupassant chose suspended animation as the subject of his short story "Family Life".)

The distinction between suspended animation and death is not certain when based on ordinary clinical methods and mistakes can occur unless additional tests are made with special instruments, e.g. the oscilloscope, ECG or EEG.

The occasions on which persons show signs of life after removal to a mortuary in the belief they are dead are uncommon, if not rare. Moreover, even when subjected without delay to "intensive care", resuscitation, when it occurs, is of short duration; death occurs within hours since, if not dead, the person was in fact moribund; post-mortem examination usually confirms that they were also suffering from incurable disease, or overdosage with drugs, etc.

But not always so, and, therefore, it should never be assumed that attempted resuscitation is pointless and need be but perfunctory. On the contrary, the attempt should always be continued for at least half an hour. This should be obligatory when the person has sustained an electric shock or has taken an overdose of a barbiturate or narcotic drug. On these occasions the treatment should continue until either death has occurred or, as in the following unusual case, it succeeds.

A young woman, aged 23, was found by two lorry drivers at 8.10 a.m. on 31 October 1969, lying on a beach near Liverpool, apparently dead. The police were informed and they summoned a local doctor. Details of his examination are not available, but he was reported to have said that although the body was still warm she appeared to be dead; he failed to see any sign of movement during 15 minutes, and certified her as dead. A pathologist arrived later on and agreed with this diagnosis. The body was then taken to a mortuary and at about 10.40 a.m., when the post-mortem was due to begin, one of the persons present noticed flickering of the lids of the right eye and the formation of a tear. The body was promptly covered with clothing and arrangements were made for its immediate transfer to an intensive-care unit. This treatment was successful, but she remained critically ill for several hours. Her condition then improved and she was transferred to a mental hospital as an informal patient. She had taken an overdose of a barbiturate. On Friday, 7 November, she took her own discharge and was presumed to have returned home. (*Sunday Times*, 2 and 9 Nov.; *Yorkshire Post*, 1 Nov. 1969.) Her recovery appears to have been complete because she was later reported to have accompanied a television unit which was filming the installation of an oscilloscope at the City Mortuary at Sheffield in February 1970.

While filming was in progress a woman, believed dead from an overdose of a drug, was admitted to the Mortuary. The oscilloscope detected activity of her heart muscle and she was immediately transferred to an intensive-care unit. Unfortunately the treatment was unsuccessful (*Yorkshire Post*, 27 Feb. 1970).

The diagnosis of death should be confirmed on all occasions by a doctor; the opinion of the laity alone can lead to distressing mistakes, although they may not make any material difference to the patient's condition. For example, a man was gravely ill and the relatives were told that his death was imminent. He lapsed into coma and his wife thought he had died. She had been told by a male nurse that when this happened she should send for the funeral director and, next day, call on the doctor for the death certificate. The funeral director removed the body to his premises and signs of breathing were then noticed. The patient was promptly taken to hospital but survived only a few hours. Post-mortem examination showed that the immediate cause of death was broncho-pneumonia and the patient had an incurable cancer of the kidney. He was moribund when removed by the funeral director and this premature removal had not accelerated his death. (*Yorkshire Post*, 21 and 26 Nov. 1969.)

On yet another occasion, in February 1971, a doctor, relying on information from a farmer, believed that an old man had died and reported the death to the Coroner. Inquiry by the police showed that the patient, aged 88, was ill but alive. He was taken to hospital and 3 days later he was reported to be slowly recovering and his condition was "fair". (*Yorkshire Post*, 5 Feb. 1971.)

These cases emphasise the importance of examination of the body by a doctor before death is certified and before a medical certificate of cause of death is issued. At present the doctor in attendance during the last illness is not required by law to examine the body before issuing a valid certificate, if he had last seen the patient alive within 14 days of the death.

The occasions which call for special care are those, like the Liverpool case, when a person is found dead in suspicious or unusual circumstances. Failure to detect a heart-beat or respiratory sounds after adequate auscultation must be accompanied by the demonstration of a rectal temperature at or below 75°F (23.9°C). Ophthalmoscopic detection of segmentation of the retinal blood columns lends further confirmation of the fact of death. If any doubt then remains, the patient should be transferred at once to an intensive-care unit for further attempts at resuscitation and examination by instruments which can detect heart and brain activity.

Estimating the Time of Death

For some time it has been realised that precise estimation of the time of death is, to say the least, difficult. Reliance can no longer be placed on visual or manual examination nor on the relatively more exact instrumental determination of body temperature. Even elaborate biochemical methods fail to yield reliable results. At best, it must be admitted, as Lyle *et al.* (1959) said, that the time of death can only be estimated within broad limits. There are several possible variable factors. Obviously the fewer there are and the greater number of signs observed, the greater is the accuracy of the estimate. The search for more reliable methods rightly continues but none is as yet capable of the degree of accuracy sometimes claimed. Morgan (1945) reported misleading evidence in estimating the time of death.

The hopes raised by biochemical investigations of the cerebro-spinal fluid after death (Schourup, 1950–1), have not been fulfilled. The researches by de Saram *et al.* (1955–6), by Fiddes and Patten (1958) and by Marshall (1959, 1962, 1965, 1969, 1979, 1981) on the cooling of the body after death serve, in the main, to remind us of the many variables which can influence estimates of the time of death based on determinations of the body temperature.

Of chemical methods proposed for estimating the time interval there are plenty. Attention was recently directed to the chemical composition of the vitreous or aqueous humour. It was first studied by Naumann in 1959, and since then Jaffe (1962), Gantner *et al.* (1962), Adelson *et al.* (1963), Sturner and Gantner (1964) and Hughes (1965) have attempted to correlate chemical changes in the vitreous with the time interval since death. For example, there appeared to be an increase in the potassium content after death but no accurate estimate of the time interval could be made since the results were inconsistent. The ascorbic acid level of the aqueous humour yielded no better guide (Gantner *et al.*, 1962). Many of these methods involve the use of expensive equipment and skilled technique, and it is profitless to embark on them as a general practice until it is clear that the results are reliable.

Nanikawa and Janssen (1965) determined the succinodehydrogenase activity after death and they considered further study of this might provide a reliable estimation of the time interval since death. This has yet to be confirmed.

Caution is imperative, and the more necessary when the time interval lengthens. Mann (1960) has instanced a case where the post-mortem changes in a half-submerged body indicated death at 3 to 4 weeks previously, whereas it was subsequently proved that the interval must have been less than 14 days. There is also the possible intervention of some wholly unexpected factor as in the case reported by Majoska (1960). An infant's body, enclosed in a plastic bag, was recovered from Pearl Harbour. The appearances were those seen after submersion for 2 to 3 weeks, except that there was no odour of putrefaction and the brain was well preserved. It was subsequently established that after its death by accident the child's body had been immersed in concentrated lye, and then thrown into the sea. The body was found within 24 hours of death.

Dating of skeletal remains is considered in Chapter 2 (see pp. 57–60).

The Traditional Signs of Death: Immediate

Within a few minutes of death, the changes which will be noted are as follows:

(i) *Pallor and loss of elasticity of the skin.*
(ii) *Ocular signs*: these include absence of the corneal and light reflexes of the eyes, cessation of circulation (segmentation) in the retinal vessels, reduction in intra-ocular tension, and clouding of the cornea.

(a) Segmentation of the retinal blood columns after death was first described by Albrand (1904) and Salisbury and Melvin (1936) first studied its experimental development. The stream in the blood vessels was seen to become irregular and "lumpy"; fragmentation of the columns followed and masses of red cells moved towards the optic disc and dropped over the edge of the cup. Motion of the blood was progressively reduced as fragmentation became more definite. When all movement ceased interruption of the columns remained unchanged during the time the media remained transparent. Segmentation was apparent within the first 15 minutes after apparent death and, when established, no further sign of life occurred. Segmentation was absent in profound shock until the moment of death.

Kervokkian (1961a, b) confirmed the occurrence of retinal segmentation and slowing of the blood flow as a sign of death in man. Standstill was demonstrated by pressure on the globe. He also described colour changes in the retina after death and claimed that they could be correlated with the post-mortem interval; they could serve as a "post-mortem" clock. These observations were practicable over a period of up to 15 hours because the cornea was kept clear by repeated applications of water or saline. The retina then had a grey or light-grey colour and the macula alone remained detectable. His claim that these colour changes had a high degree of accuracy in estimating the time of death has yet to be confirmed.

Tomlin (1967a, b) considered segmentation of the retinal blood columns had a grave prognostic significance when seen in patients subjected to modern methods of resuscitation. Segmentation was then accompanied by "rail-roading"; groups of red cells moved "in either direction along the vessel at random and may collide with each other". The movement was likened to that of movement of unbraked wagons of a goods train when it stops. He also noticed a widening and narrowing of the blood vessels. In his view segmentation was indicative of cerebral death, rather than cessation of circulation. Even if circulation be restored, the occurrence of retinal segmentation indicated that, if the patient survived, severe irreparable brain damage had occurred.

He illustrated this by the report of the case of a girl aged 10 years who "collapsed" at home during an asthmatic attack. She was subjected to cardiac massage and intermittent positive pressure ventilation within 15 minutes of her collapse. "Rail-roading" was widespread. She had ventricular fibrillation and this was relieved by a single shock which restored the circulation. The retinal vessels were now normal, but there was widespread oedema of the fundi. The patient survived for 14 days and then died of pneumonia. The post-mortem examination disclosed widespread infarction of the cerebral cortex, hypothalamus, right caudate nucleus and pons. Had she survived, she would have been decerebrate. This patient was the only one of a series of fourteen, in whom "rail-roading" had been observed, to have survived; resuscitation, sustained for up to half an hour, failed to restore the circulation of the others. Tomlin (1967b) added another six examples of failure of resuscitation when "rail-roading" had occurred.

John (1967) rejected "rail-roading" as an indication of cessation of the circulation and a sign of death. He had twice been called to a patient during the night and on each occasion he saw retinal segmentation. "The fragments were moving along in one direction in a faintly pulsatile fashion." The patient was suffering from an incurable intra-cranial lesion, she was in deep coma and "life" was sustained by continuous positive pressure respiration. The special circumstances of this case and the fact that she was moribund—she died within 24 hours of the ophthalmoscopic examination—does not negate the grave prognostic value of segmentation in the retinal vessels.

Wróblewski and Ellis (1970) submitted 300 patients, admitted to the Casualty Department of the General Infirmary at Leeds for the purpose of certification of death, to ophthalmoscopic examination. Attention was given not only to the occurrence of segmentation but the condition of the cornea was also noted. Whenever practicable the known or stated time of death and that of the examination were recorded. This interval ranged from less than 15 minutes to 3 days; in 68 per cent of the series the interval was within 12 hours of death. The fundi could be examined in 204 of the subjects; segmentation was present in one or both eyes in 115 and absent in the other eighty-nine. Although this sign was observed in only one-third of the total series it was present within 2 hours of death and, indeed, in the majority of that group, i.e. 80 per cent, the interval was within an hour of death.

Clouding, or haziness, of the cornea was observed by them at 2 hours in three-fourths of their subjects.

They concluded that static segmentation is a post-mortem change, for there was never any doubt that these patients had died. On the other hand, any obvious movement in the columns might be due to persistence of circulation. It was reasonable to assume that when static, resuscitation could be suspended, since there was then no hope of survival.

Static segmentation and clouding of the cornea were each indicative of death within the previous 2 hours.

(b) *Loss of intra-ocular tension* has long been recognised as a sign of death. Nicati (1894) invented an instrument to measure intra-ocular tension. He estimated that during life the tension could vary between 14 g and 25 g, but when the heart ceased to beat the tension fell, and did not exceed 12 g. Within $^1/_2$ hour of death the tension was reduced to 3 g or less, and at the end of 2 hours it was nil. Reduction in intra-ocular tension permits distortion of the pupillary margin by gentle pressure on the globe; this is impossible during life but may be demonstrated within 24 hours after death (Joll, 1881; cited Tonelli, 1932).

(c) *Tache noire de la sclérotique* is also an ocular sign of death, but it is rarely apparent until at least a few hours have elapsed, and may not appear until 2 days after death, but we have seen it within a few hours. It is seen only when the eyelids have remained open after death. The spots may be round or oval but are usually triangular, based directly on the cornea and more often on the outer than the inner side of the globe; that on the inner side develops, as a rule after the appearance of the outer one. At the outset the spots are usually yellowish in tint, becoming brown and, later, black in colour. The spots are due, possibly, to desiccation of the tissues but not, as was originally believed, to thinning of the sclera whereby the choroid becomes visible. There may be, however, some change which renders the sclera translucent.

> Niderkorn (1872) refers to Larcher's account of this phenomenon published in 1862 but points out that these observations were not the first since the change had been described by Sommer (1843) and even if Larcher had not seen or read this earlier account, in Latin, he could have read its translation by Jourdan, in Burdach's *Traité de physiologie.*

(iii) *Flaccidity (primary) of the muscles*. The limbs become flaccid after death and the body flattens over areas which are in contact with the surface on which it rests. Contact flattening, as it is termed, is usually seen over the shoulder blades, buttocks and calves. Since, at this stage, death is still only *"somatic"* response of muscles to electrical stimuli can occur and may persist until *"molecular"* death, i.e. of the individual tissues or cells, takes place.

(iv) *Cessation of circulation*. Pulselessness is an unsafe indication of death for the apparently dead may be pulseless for $^1/_2$ hour.

Absence of heart sounds, as determined by repeated auscultation, during a period of not less than 5 minutes, is normally sufficient proof of death. Care is necessary to exclude error occasioned by obesity, feeble heart action and slow rhythm, which may be reduced to only 12 beats per minute. When in doubt, tests with the ECG or oscillometer, if available, should be made.

Subsidiary tests, which are rarely used, include the ligature test, fingernail test, finger web inspection by transmitted light and the injection of fluorescin. It should be recalled that the yellow green tint of the skin produced by fluorescin in the living is to be detected only in daylight. Testators sometimes direct that one of their arteries shall be opened after death. None of these tests is necessary if auscultation is repeated by an experienced person.

Cardiac arrest causing reduction of the cerebral circulation will result in death if an adequate flow is not restored before the end of 10 minutes; the prospects of recovery of the patient without some neurological damage are remote when this interval exceeds 5 minutes.

(v) *Cessation of respiration*. The demonstration of this also calls for repeated auscultation during a period of not less than 5 minutes. Apnoeic intervals, as in Cheyne–Stokes breathing, are limited to about 20 seconds.

A number of subsidiary tests are known, for example the mirror, feather and candle tests, but these are unlikely to be used except by the laity.

Other Changes which Appear During the First 12 Hours after Death

(i) COOLING OF THE BODY

The determination of the rectal temperature is often an obligatory step in the investigation of any death which occurs in suspicious circumstances. Exceptions are usually those where the external appearances indicate that death took place more than 24–36 hours previously, when the body will of necessity have already cooled to the temperature of the environment. It must also be noted that much of the importance of temperature estimations apply only to cold and temperate climates—in tropical zones, the post-mortem fall in temperature may be minimal or absent and in some torrid climates, the dead body may even warm up after death.

In the usual forensic context, temperature measurement is required only as an index of time since death. In the still-living body, it is also vital to detect or prove the presence of hypothermia; suspended animation is now such a rare event that the use of temperature measurement to differentiate it from death is a mere curiosity, as better methods are available.

The Measurement of Body Temperature

The normal body temperature is not a fixed point, but varies both with the site of measurement and with physiological changes, there being a diurnal variation and cycles of longer change, such as those associated with the menstrual cycle.

Whereas clinical measurements are usually taken in the mouth, medico-legal temperature estimations are made in the rectum. If 37°C is taken as the accepted mouth temperature, the rectal temperature is commonly at least 1°C higher, but many calculations devised for forensic use have been based on the 37°C base-line and as the level of accuracy of time-since-death estimations is so poor, the difference is of little practical significance.

Estimations in the dead body should be made deep in the rectum to ensure uniformity, as there is a temperature gradient from the central body core to the surface. The tip of the measuring device should be inserted for at least 3–4 inches into the rectum and arranged so that the reading can be taken without further disturbing either the body or the instrument.

Until recently, the usual means of measurement was a long, straight chemical thermometer, the mercury column being visible at ambient temperature well up the stem of the instrument.

Though a 0–100° range is most readily available, a maximum scale reading of 50°C is more easily read, though the increased accuracy of the larger scale is of no great importance.

Recently, electronic thermometers have appeared on the market at a reasonable price. These are small battery-powered devices with a digital read-out, the temperature being monitored via a metal probe on a flexible lead. They are very accurate, settle to a constant reading quickly and are much easier to handle, as the observer is not confined to an awkward view of a mercury column placed between the thighs.

For research purposes, such thermometers can be attached to a constant-recording device which automatically traces the fall in temperature.

Whatever device is used, the important points are the insertion to a constant and sufficiently deep position and the maintenance of the thermometer in position for long enough to attain a constant reading—which may be up to 5 minutes in the case of some mercury instruments.

Some difference of opinion exists over the use of a thermometer at the scene of a suspicious death. Considerable caution must be employed when considering the taking of a rectal temperature with the body *in situ*. If there is any possibility at all of some sexual interference, whether homosexual or heterosexual, no interference with the clothing or perineum must be made until all forensic examinations have been completed. Certainly no instrument should be inserted into the rectum before trace evidence has been sought, which includes swabs, hair and fibre search, etc. The clothing must be kept intact, as the material in contact with the perineal area may be the most important from the point of view of seminal stains and other trace evidence.

Unfortunately these circumstances may not be known at the time of examination at the scene and only in the few cases where such an aspect can confidently be excluded, is it permissible to disarrange the clothing or even make a deliberate hole in the garments for the introduction of the thermometer.

In actual practice, where a body is to be removed to the mortuary for examination within a relatively short time, little is lost by this brief delay; only if some protracted interval is expected before a pathologist conducts his examination, is on-scene interference with the clothing justified, merely to take a temperature.

The Rectal Temperature as a Sign of Death

A low body temperature is a sign of either death or hypothermia. The finding of a rectal temperature of 27°C (80°F) or lower in an unconscious person indicates substantial hypothermia, which is usually accidental in nature, though this can hardly be applied to the victim of an assault who is left to die from exposure, a not uncommon event.

In a series of 23 patients suffering from hypothermia, the rectal temperatures ranged from 32°C (89°F) to 22°C (72°F). All the 6 patients whose rectal temperature was below 27°C (80°F) were unconscious and all but one died without regaining consciousness—the exception died soon afterwards (Duguid, *et al.* 1961).

A unique recovery from grave hypothermia was made by a negress aged 23 years who was found comatose in an alley. When in hospital, 90 minutes later, her rectal temperature was only 18°C (64°F). Owing to extensive frostbite, she suffered permanent mutilation of her extremities (Laufman 1951).

Despite this case, an as yet unique observation, it is reasonable to assume that a rectal temperature of 21°C (70°F) is presumptive evidence of death or a *moribund state*.

The Rectal Temperature and the Time since Death

In view of the obvious practical and sometimes vital importance of establishing the time since death, it is not surprising that a large forensic literature exists on this problem, much of it centred upon the fall in body temperature as an index of the interval since death. Many other factors which have been used to determine this interval, such as body chemistry, rigor, electrical activity, etc., are themselves at least partly temperature-related.

Though the problem continues to attract research in an attempt to provide a perfect formula, so many factors exist in the cooling of a body that errors continue to be large and quite unpredictable.

With perhaps touching faith, it was for long assumed that the rectal temperature at death was 37°C (99°F) and that it fell after death by 1.5°F per hour. Thus dividing the fall in temperature in degrees F by 1.5 was thought to give the time since death in hours.

Following this rather naive view, numerous research projects and papers appeared over a long period, which though recognising the pitfalls and permutations of modifying factors, did not greatly improve the accuracy of the estimation of the time since death. What was important was the realisation that accuracy was lacking, therefore limiting the rash and over-optimistic opinions of doctors. These opinions did the investigating officers—and possibly justice—a disservice by offering dogmatic and misleading precise times of death.

To survey the very extensive literature is not possible, but excellent summaries are contained in the publications of Marshall (1957, 1962, 1969, 1979, 1981). Together with Hoare (1962), he showed that the human body does not cool in accordance with Newton's law, a view previously widely accepted. They went on to devise a formula which takes into account some of the variables which beset this problem and preclude an accurate estimation of the time since death.

Marshall also constructed cooling curves based upon serial measurements of the body temperature, a method investigated by several researchers, including Nokes and Knight, who reworked Marshall's data using a simple computer program. However, these methods applied only to bodies lying in a constant environment and not in the variable and often unknown conditions of field work. James and Knight (1965) devised a simple method in which the fall in temperature in degrees centigrade was multiplied by a factor of 1, $1^1/_4$, $1^1/_2$, $1^3/_4$ or 2 for air temperatures of 0, 5, 10, 15 or 20°C respectively. This calculation tended to give an underestimate of the time since death, though it aimed only to give the centre of a time bracket during which death was thought to have occurred, modified by other factors detailed below.

All methods suffer from the variability of multiple modifying factors and thus attempts have been made, such as those by Marshall and by Nokes, to construct a *cooling curve* in each case by taking multiple measurements in order to discover the slope or angle of that particular cooling gradient. Even this manoeuvre can be frustrated by both the unpredictable behaviour of the curves and by changes in the environment and other factors during the period of cooling.

The following factors introduce variables into the cooling process:

(a) *The external environment.* Actual temperature changes, which may vary considerably during the interval between death and examination: winds and draughts: humidity affecting evaporation and cooling from damp clothing.

(b) *The posture of the body.* An extended or spread-eagled body will cool faster than one with reduced surface area due to a curled-up foetal posture.

(c) *Body physique.* An obese corpse will retain heat longer, both because of the insulation of the core by subcutaneous fat and because the surface area/mass ratio will be less.

(d) *Clothing.* The insulating effect is self-evident, a naked body cooling far faster than one heavily clothed, beneath bed covers or otherwise concealed.

(e) *Infants and children* tend to have a larger surface area available for heat loss relative to body mass, compared with adults.

(f) *Oedema.* Due to high specific heat of water, bodies who die with oedematous tissues, such as those in congestive cardiac failure, have been found to cool more slowly. This factor is more potent than body fat.

(g) *Body temperature at death.* Most calculations assume that the zero point at death is at 37°C. This may not be the case, one quite common example being where an assault occurs which does not cause immediate death. The victim may lie exposed for some hours, becoming hypothermic before life is extinguished. In these cases, the core temperature at the time of death may be many degrees below normal.

Similarly, some types of death are associated with raised body temperature. Pontine haemorrhage or other lesions affecting the heat-regulating centres and severe infections, such as septic wounds or abortions, may cause the individual to be above 40°C at death.

It has been said that an asphyxial death leads to a raised agonal temperature, but there is no convincing proof of this and in the usual circumstances of strangulation etc., the time factor would make this highly unlikely. The similar claim that severe agonal bleeding lowers the body temperature is equally without foundation.

Whatever method is used to calculate the estimated time since death from body temperature, all the variable factors must be taken into account to modify any basic formula, though this adjustment is very arbitrary and can only be attempted in the light of previous experience. When a "favoured" time of death is decided upon this should never be offered to the investigating authorities as a singular point in time. It must be used to construct a "bracket of probability", giving an earliest and latest time between which the doctor feels that death must have occurred. The width of this time bracket will depend upon the number and uncertainty of the variable factors known to the doctor and is likely to be longer the more remote the death was from the time of examination of the corpse.

It is futile mentioning any time in units of less than an hour, even when the death was quite recent. A medical witness who attempts to determine the time of death from temperature estimation in minutes or fractions of hours is exposing himself to a severe challenge to his expertise which may well amount to near-ridicule, thus denigrating the rest of his evidence.

The illustrative case of the use of the Marshall-Hoare (1962) formula (Marshall, 1981) is indeed impressive but it is made clear that its value is investigational, enabling the police to draw up lists of suspects for interview; it is not intended to cite the results in evidence. Those who, like myself, are incompetent mathematicians may take comfort from the recorded opinion of the late Milton Helpern: "Estimating the time of death is notoriously one of the most difficult and inaccurate techniques in forensic pathology—no one test is dependable, and all the possible evidence must be correlated to try to arrive at some sensible time bracket within which the death could have occurred" (Helpern and Knight, 1982).

Modern computing methods have furthered the undertaking of the manner in which various body sites (e.g., rectal, liver) cool under even varying environmental conditions. The post-mortem interval estimation by body temperatures, however, has not been significantly improved by these studies, (Joseph and Schickele 1970, Hiraiwa *et al.* 1980, 1981). At the Department of Forensic Medicine, University of Leeds, research has been carried out on some 150 bodies. Green and Wright (in press) recognised the essential validity of the method devised by Marshall and Hoare. However, they were unable to determine the constants of the two terms of the equation in the manner proposed by Marshall and Hoare's work. A method was devised whereby all the necessary information could be gained from just two or three temperature measurements over a period of about

1 hour. A time of death estimation can then be made with reference to a single reference curve. The method has been tested on data from some 50 bodies, of varying build, naked or clothed, with reasonable success even in the first 6 hours post-mortem. However, the results have clarified the errors due to the unknown body temperature at death, and have further shown that even the ambient temperature is difficult to measure with the required accuracy. The evidence is now strongly in favour of the conclusion that post-mortem interval estimation by these methods is open to significant errors. It should not be overlooked that no matter how accurate the measuring instrument may be, or how elaborate the procedure for ascertaining the body temperature, the precise rectal temperature at the moment of death is never known or ascertainable.

(ii) POST-MORTEM HYPOSTASIS (Lividity or Suggilation)

When *somatic* death occurs, circulation of the blood ceases and subsequent movement of the blood is by gravitation. In consequence, blood tends to accumulate in the capillaries and small veins in the dependent parts of the body. Filling of the subcutaneous capillaries in this manner imparts a purple or reddish-purple colour to the adjacent skin, a change to which the term "post-mortem hypostasis", lividity or suggilation, is applied.

Pressure of even mild degree is sufficient to prevent gravitation of blood into the compressed areas of "contact flattening". When laid on the back, the body has pale areas over the shoulder blades, buttocks and calves. Corresponding areas are present when the body lies face-down. Contact flattening also occurs at the site of garters, a belt or collar when worn at the time of death.

Hypostasis in bodies exposed to the air may acquire a pink colour, due to oxygenation of the blood, e.g. at the sides but not, as a rule, at the back or other areas which are close to the ground. This colour of the hypostasis might suggest a death from carbon monoxide poisoning but the distinction is readily made by inspecting the dependent areas, i.e. at the back, or front of the body, according to its position, for these also will be pink when death is due to carbon monoxide poisoning. Refrigeration may also produce pink hypostasis.

The external appearances receive the major attention but hypostasis occurs also in the viscera and provides some confirmation of the external observations. More important, there is need to remember its occurrence in the viscera, lest the appearances be regarded as pathological changes, which may thus be simulated. Hypostasis in the heart can simulate the effects of coronary occlusion and in the lungs it may suggest pneumonia; dependent coils of intestine might seem to have been strangulated.

The practical value of hypostasis is threefold; it is, firstly, a sign of death; secondly, its extent is a subsidiary means of estimating the time of death; and, thirdly, the most important feature, it indicates the posture of the body at the time of death and any movement of the body after death. The occurrence of hypostasis shows that attempted resuscitation is pointless.

Hypostasis, although it varies in its time of onset, is ordinarily apparent within $^1/_2$ to 2 hours after death, and its complete development is attained in from 6 to 12 hours. It is said sometimes to occur shortly before death, e.g. when due to cholera or typhus; it may also occur when the death is lingering, as in the debilitated and those who die of uraemia. Its onset is hastened in the tuberculous body, i.e. in lingering death, and delayed when death is due to anaemia. It is present in all bodies, although it may be inconspicuous in some and thus escape notice.

The initial change is a patchy mottling of the skin; the areas then enlarge and coalesce to produce extensive discoloration. The whole of the back of the body, except in areas of contact flattening, may be discoloured, with further extension of the change to the sides and the front.

Certain poisons, notably carbon monoxide, impart a distinctive colour to the hypostatic areas, which may then be bright red; they may be red also in cyanide poisoning although we have not seen this in our cases. Nitrates, potassium chlorate and aniline also yield distinctive hypostasis; i.e. red-brown, brown or deep blue. Bodies removed from the scene of a fire may appear pink in the unburnt areas when, as is not uncommon, the inhalation of carbon monoxide present in the fumes of the fire is a factor in the death; the blood may then be from 30, 40 or even 80 per cent saturated by carbon monoxide.

Sufficient has already been said to show how hypostasis indicates whether the body was laid on its back or face after death. If suspended after death, hypostasis will be most pronounced in the lower parts of each limb, particularly the legs, and, if suspension be prolonged for a few hours, the accumulation of blood may create sufficient pressure to rupture subcutaneous capillaries and produce petechial haemorrhages in the skin. In the rare event of suspension by the feet, the development of these haemorrhages in the face and eyes, post-mortem, might create difficulty by simulating haemorrhages of asphyxial origin. Occasionally, in a full-blooded person, these haemorrhages may accompany hypostasis, e.g. at the back of the body.

Once hypostasis has occurred, it is unlikely that movement of the body will completely displace the blood even though it is still fluid. Hypostasis may become less intense but evidence of its initial distribution remains. This is due, in part, to staining of the tissues by haemolysis. Meantime there is a secondary distribution, in the then dependent parts. Duality of distribution is important since it shows that the body had been moved shortly after death, i.e. within 8 to 12 hours. This is sometimes of importance in the elucidation of a death due to a criminal act.

The distinction between hypostasis and bruising. A recent external bruise, of faint purple-red colour, may be simulated by hypostasis, but, fortunately, this important distinction is readily made.

The bruise, due to blunt force, is the result of escape of blood during life through the walls of ruptured capillaries into the tissues, whereas hypostatic blood, save in the exception of suspended bodies already described, is retained within the capillaries. In bruising, moreover, accumulation of blood in the area often causes local swelling of the part, in no way simulated by hypostasis.

A bruise is usually deep to the skin, whereas hypostasis is always superficial. The bruise has ill-defined margins, whereas the margins of hypostatic areas, especially those adjacent to areas of contact flattening, are sharply defined.

Hypostasis occurs principally in dependent parts, whereas a bruise may occur anywhere on the body, most often in relation to prominent parts. The bruised area is usually raised above its surroundings, whereas hypostatic areas are always flush with the surface. Bruising in an area of contact flattening remains red.

The principal test, and one which should not be omitted in the examination of any body which may become the subject of criminal proceedings, concerns the appearances of the area when sectioned. The cut surface of a bruise shows that bleeding has occurred into the tissues to produce a uniform discoloration, whereas, in hypostasis, the blood is obviously lying within capillaries and oozes from them. When naked-eye inspection leaves this distinction uncertain, and reliance on colour alone is unsound, an appropriate piece should be taken from the area and subjected to microscopy. This step is advisable, even when the naked-eye appearances are clear, if the evidence will be material at a later stage. It is imperative when tiny faint bruises, alleged to be finger-marks, are the only external sign of murder by throttling.

(iii) RIGOR MORTIS

The initial flaccidity of the body after death is soon followed by stiffening or rigor mortis. (The first investigation of stiffening after death is attributed to Nysten (1811), cited by Forster (1963a).)

The time of its onset is varied by several factors, e.g. atmospheric temperature, humidity and movement of air around the body but, in general, it is likely to be apparent at about 4 hours, and complete in about 6 hours, after death; it may be complete at the end of 4 or even only 2 hours; its completion may be delayed until the end of 10 or even 13 hours. It is but a rough guide to the time of death but a better one than hypostasis because its progress can be determined.

Niderkorn's (1872) observations on 113 bodies continue to be cited as an index of the range of time which rigor mortis requires for its completion. In that series it was complete in from 4 to 7 hours in seventy-six (or 67 per cent) of the bodies, i.e. thirty-one at 4, fourteen at 5, twenty at 6, and eleven at 7 hours. In two cases it was complete in 2 hours but it was not complete until 13 hours in another two bodies.

Violent exertion shortly before death, and death in surroundings of moist heat, or when caused by convulsant poisons, or violent death as by cut-throat, firearms or by electrocution hasten the onset and passing of rigor mortis. Poisoning by alkaloids was said to hasten rigor mortis (Yamase, 1941). Rigor mortis is early, and its passing rapid, in deaths from septicaemia or from wasting diseases. Delay in its appearance occurs when the body is exposed to cold and in any other circumstances which delay putrefaction, for example, poisoning by arsenic or mercuric chloride. Rigor mortis is delayed also in asphyxial deaths, notably by hanging or carbon dioxide poisoning. It is delayed when the death has been immediately preceded by severe haemorrhage.

Rigor mortis is reported first to appear in the eyelids, face, lower jaw and neck. Subsequently it involves the trunk and limbs. It passes off in the same order and the body again becomes flaccid. It is usually established in 6 hours and lasts about 36 hours but it may persist for a much longer period. James and Knight (1965) observed strong rigor in subjects whose deaths had occurred from $43^1/_2$ to 60 hours earlier.

The order of onset and passing of rigor mortis may be determined by the quantum and kind of muscle involved; the smaller the muscle, the earlier the onset and passing of rigor mortis. Shapiro (1950) considered that this would explain fixation of the elbow or knee joints at an earlier stage than the shoulder or hip joints. It would also explain why rigor is first seen in the small tempero-mandibular joint. He considered that the traditional progress of rigor mortis, as given above, requires revision. If, as he contended, rigor mortis is a physico-chemical process simultaneously affecting all muscles, the course of rigor mortis is not from the upper to the lower end of the body, but one which involves joints according to their control by muscle mass. This would produce an approximate proximodistal progression, jaw, hands and feet, elbows and knees, shoulders and hips being involved in that order. Eyelids would be involved at an early stage and presumably the cervical before the dorsal or lumbar spine.

Rigor mortis also involves involuntary muscles; a left ventricle, contracted by rigor mortis, should not be deemed hypertrophied. (This warning to the inexperienced was originally given by Mascka in 1851 (cited Forster, 1964).)

Except when the body is frozen, rigor mortis is strongly presumptive of death. It is but a poor index of the time of death but may provide some confirmation of the other findings.

The underlying changes in rigor mortis. The precise changes which lead to stiffening, shortening and opacity of the muscles in rigor mortis have still to be determined. Although the changes are not unlike those which occur during physiological contraction of muscles, they differ in the important respect that those of rigor mortis are irreversible.

Rigor mortis may depend on the conversion of glycogen to lactic acid, the only reaction apparently to be detected to account for the gelation or coagulation of sarcoplasm. Smith (1930–1) confirmed that fatigued muscle passed more rapidly than resting muscle into rigor. He found that the lactic acid content of muscle, which when resting, was 0.03 per cent, rose to 0.5 per cent when rigor mortis occurred.

Szent-Györgyi (1947) described the contractile muscle fibre as "the loveliest toy ever provided by nature for the biochemist" and "Like most children the biochemist when he finds a toy, usually pulls it to pieces . . .". Attempts to pull myosin to pieces in his laboratory resulted in the discovery that this globulin-like protein was in fact an undefined mixture of two proteins; the properties of each were quite different from those of their mixture. As a tribute to pioneers in this field, he retained the name "myosin" for one of the new proteins but the other he named "actin". Their mixture or compound he called "acto-myosin". Neither of its components is of itself contractile but, when mixed in proper amounts to form acto-myosin, the resulting compound acquires contractility, which can be induced *in vitro* by the addition of adenosine triphosphate (ATP) and ion constituents, notably KCl of the muscle fibre.

The suppleness and plasticity of muscle depends on a union, by adsorption, between acto-myosin and ATP. This "contributes to the charge and hydration of the protein and herewith to the suppleness and plasticity of muscle". If ATP be removed, there follows dehydration and the formation of a stiff acto-myosin gel. In consequence the muscle contracts and stiffens, i.e. it passes into the state of rigor mortis. Under experimental conditions, and during life, this process is reversible by the addition of ATP. After death, however, destruction of ATP becomes permanent and the muscles then remain in rigor until putrefaction sets in and they disintegrate.

Decomposition of ATP begins immediately after somatic death but it is a gradual process and, therefore, sufficient remains to permit contraction of muscle to electrical stimuli during a brief period after death. Response steadily decreases *pari passu* with the decomposition of ATP. When all of it has been destroyed and exhausted, rigor mortis is complete.

Forster (1963a, b, and 1964) devised experiments to elucidate the physical changes in the musculature in rigor mortis. He found that there was a decrease of elastic and plastic deformation; decrease in elasticity was regular until a minimum was reached, but plastic deformation at first increased and then decreased to a minimum. Increase in plastic deformation, which occurred during the first 2 hours after death, was attributed to a corresponding increase in the ATP content of muscle at about this time. He found that the load required to tear fresh muscle, one of 8 kg/cm^2, was reduced to between 4 to 6 kg/cm^2, to tear muscle in rigor.

He also examined the shortening of muscle after death. A completely unloaded muscle did not shorten during rigor, but loading and increase of temperature caused shortening. This maximum shortening depended in the main on the loading. Shortening increased to a maximum and then decreased. These experiments were instigated by the alleged movements of the body by rigor, due to the belief that in rigor the muscles not only grew rigid but were also shortened. (A view attributed to Sommer, in about 1833, and the movements became known as "Sommer's Movements".)

It does appear that spontaneous movements of the feet and legs can occur after death. Badonnel *et al.* (1936) observed such movements at 13 hours after death; they are also said to occur after death from cholera or yellow fever. These authors suggest that the movements are due to accumulation of carbon dioxide in the blood and, possibly, the muscles.

Forster concluded that movements of a corpse, due to rigor mortis, could occur only in special circumstances, e.g. high temperature, extreme positions of the body at the moment of death or increased tonus induced by one of a small number of poisons.

Forster (1963b) tested the effects of parathion. This poison increased muscle tonus, which his former experiments showed to have an important influence on muscle shortening, which augmented rigor mortis.

Shortening of muscle will occur when the muscle is in a state of extension or strain and Forster, for the first time, demonstrated the absolute dependence of the magnitude of muscle shortening during rigor mortis on weight or muscle tension.

Forster (1964) also investigated the observation by Mascka (1851; cited without reference) that the heart muscle was stiffened and contracted by rigor mortis, so as to simulate concentric hypertrophy. The experimental animals were either stunned or exposed to carbon monoxide at the conclusion of the experiments.

He found that the heart had strongly reduced extensibility during rigor mortis; the fresh and rigor curves were dependent on the weight of the heart; in both, the curves were exponential.

There was a notable difference in the time of onset of rigor in the hearts of the two groups of animals. It was apparent at 3 to 5 minutes after the last heart-beat when the animals were sacrificed by CO poisoning but appreciably delayed in those which were stunned. Likewise, shortening occurred earlier in the CO group; in them it was completed, at a pressure of 10 cm of water, in 15 to 30 minutes, whereas it was not completed until 70 to 80 minutes after the death by stunning.

These experiments also demonstrated that the passing of rigor mortis depended, *inter alia*, on pressure; the higher the initial pressure the more rapid the passing off of rigor mortis.

INSTANTANEOUS RIGOR: CADAVERIC SPASM

Instant rigor mortis, involving a hand, a limb or even the whole body at the moment of death is a well-recognised but rare phenomenon. One expert of long experience had never seen an example and there have been only two in over 20 years in our practice at Leeds. It occurred in suicide by cut-throat and in suicide by shooting with a revolver (F. M. 13,222A).

The majority of the cases are those where an agent, e.g. a knife, razor or firearm, is *firmly* held and its removal requires far more force than is needed to break down ordinary rigor mortis.

It is a sign of distinct medico-legal importance when the death has been due to cut-throat, stabbing or shooting. It is then a "hallmark", tantamount to proof, of self-infliction, when the agent which caused fatal injury is held firmly by instant rigor. It cannot be reproduced after death by placing a weapon in the hand. Taylor (1965) deemed it probable that any such attempt would be detected not only by the light grip on the agent but also by error in the mode of its positioning in the hand; the blade could be facing the wrong way round, as in *R. v. Gardner*, or placed in the right hand of a left-handed person, who had sustained injuries which, if self-inflicted, must have been made by one who was right-handed. Taylor (1965) adds an important caution. It does not follow that if the weapon be lightly held, suicide is excluded; instant rigor is not an invariable consequence of violent death.

On the question of the ability to simulate a firm grip of a weapon during life by placing it in the hand post-mortem in rigor mortis, Forster (1936b) said there could be different answers. "In so far as an object (which effects some tension on the musculature) is placed in the hand, it may be taken into consideration that contraction occurs during rigor mortis and the object may be grasped firmly. If, however, the weapon or some other instrument has not effected tension of the musculature, rigor setting in later will not cause firm grasping."

There are examples of instant rigor which caused the deceased to clutch material, e.g., hair, from the assailant (*R. v. Ellison*, Bodmin Assizes, 1845). The hands, therefore, should be examined for hair, fibres or buttons, etc., which may be important clues in the detection of a murderer.

Instant rigor may occur in death by drowning. The victim may clutch, in a hand or foot, gravel or sand, weeds or grass of the kind in or near the water from which the body was recovered. (An example of grass, clutched by an old woman who was drowned when she fell into a well in her garden, is depicted by Taylor (1965, Vol. 1, fig. 5, p. 97) and another of grass in the left hand of an infant who died from exposure in the open (Glaister and Rentoul, 1966, fig. 24, p. 115, see also Littlejohn (1925); a table knife held by suicide—cut-throat).

When Miss Burnham, one of George Joseph Smith's victims, one of the "Brides in a Bath", was found dead in her bath it was said that she gripped a piece of soap in her hand. In Spilsbury's view this could have been due to instant rigor. Under pressure in cross-examination, he agreed that she might have clutched it during an epileptic fit; "it was not impossible; it is not very likely". He did not think it could have been placed in her hand so as to simulate clutching during the act of death (Watson, 1922, pp. 218, 221).

When several persons had been suddenly precipitated into water instant rigor fixed some of the bodies of the victims in postures indicative of attempts to save themselves from drowning (Tidy, 1882). In such circumstances emotion and, even more important, violent muscular exertion can produce instant rigor. This is in accordance with the results of Forster's (1963) experiments.

The importance of instant rigor in relation to drowning is that it is proof of life at the time of submersion. It is not proof of drowning but important corroboration of this cause of death.

Certain poisons may predispose to instant rigor. Tidy (1882) described a couple who were found dead rigidly locked in each other's arms after taking cyanide. Experiments by Brown-Séquard (1861) with strychnine produced instant rigor. Steer (1951) recorded rapid, if not instant, rigor, within 45 minutes after death, from poisoning by dinitro-ortho-cresol (DNOC). This poison hastens metabolism and its effects are the equivalent of violent exercise immediately preceding death. Forster (1963b) found that para-thion increased muscle tonus, which governs muscle shortening and augments rigor mortis.

Spilsbury (1944) recorded instant rigor in a person who died of cerebral haemorrhage. The late Dr. Grace told me of a man who was found dead in a kneeling posture, fixed by instant rigor. He had been about to light his fire. The cause of death was acute perforation of a duodenal ulcer. Dr. Grace attributed instant rigor to intense pain.

Extensive instant rigor involving the whole body is probably the rarest form. Tidy (1882) recalled the soldier whose body remained mounted on his horse after he had been killed by a shell at Balaclava. When several soldiers were killed by a shell at Sedan, the decapitated body of one of them remained rigid in a sitting position and his hand was firmly holding a cup (Rossbach, 1870; also depicted by Martin, 1950).

A warning is given to those who are first to arrive at the scene of death. Stupid interference caused an innocent person to come under suspicion and much unnecessary investigation, when a young married woman was found dead in bed with a revolver firmly held in her right hand. Her extended body lay back on the bed. It was apparent she had bled from a head wound but none was visible; it was presumed to be at the back of her head. The police also learnt that the domestic circumstances were unhappy and the house contained several other firearms. By the time the team of experts arrived at the scene, the revolver had been forcibly removed from the woman's hand and, to add to this, the person responsible had taken out the spent cartridges. Two bullets were found, one embedded in the wall, at about 6 ft above the floor to the left of the bed; the other had passed at about the level of the bed, in line with it, through the bedroom wall into that of the adjacent bathroom.

She had a thick head of dark hair but palpation detected a wound in the right temple and a second in the left parietal bone. Later, when the scalp was shaved, these were confirmed, respectively, as a contact, entrance bullet wound in the temple and an exit wound in the left parietal bone. The direction of aim, assuming there had been no deflection of the bullet, was consistent with her having shot herself in a sitting posture; she had collapsed into the posture in which the body was found.

Questioning the person who had interfered with the revolver elicited that it had been firmly gripped in her hand and he had had difficulty in removing it. There seemed little doubt that it had been held by instant rigor. (What was said to him by his superiors is not recorded but there were some pointed observations by the pathologist denied personal observation and photographic record of the original position of the weapon). The investigation left no doubt that this was a case of suicide. The second shot had killed her; the first might have been an unintentional discharge of the weapon or a trial shot (F. M. 13,222A).

Although instantaneous rigor mortis merits separate consideration because of the circumstances in which it occurs and its practical significance, the essential changes, which are physico-chemical, are those also of ordinary rigor mortis. The difference is one of speed of onset and degree of effect. In instantaneous rigor the changes are appreciably accelerated so that the normal flaccid state of the musculature at death does not occur or is of such short duration that it escapes observation. The contraction of the musculature is also most pronounced, possibly because of appreciable increase in tonus at the moment of death.

PUTREFACTION

Putrefaction of the body is the normal final sign of death. The process begins immediately after death in the cellular structures but visible evidence is delayed for several hours. Under normal conditions it is visible in from 48 to 72 hours but its onset may be hastened or delayed by one or more of several factors, notably atmospheric temperature and humidity.

Putrefaction is the result of bacterial and enzyme activity. The bacteria, for the most part, are derived from within the body and invade the tissues from the intestines, but other bacteria come from the atmosphere. They include streptococci, staphylococci, *B. Proteus, Ent. coli* and *Cl. welchii* (Burn, 1934); the latter, anaerobic bacteria, invade from the intestine, surrounding air or soil. Intrinsic lipases hydrolyse the body fat and this activity probably begins within minutes of death (Evans, 1963a); an even more important part is played by the enzyme lecithinase produced by *Cl. welchii* (Mant, 1957). In humid conditions fungi also contribute to the dissolution of the body tissues but their action is restricted to the surface and it occurs only in aerobic conditions. Fungi were not found by Evans in sealed coffins; they were absent from the sealed coffins examined at Huddersfield in 1970.

Putrefactive activities are optimal at temperatures which range between 70–100°F (21.1–37.8°C); they are retarded when the temperature falls below 50°F (10.0°C) or when it exceeds 100°F (37.8°C). Putrefaction is hastened after death from pyrexial illness, especially septicaemia.

The first visible sign of putrefaction is green or greenish-red discoloration of the skin of the anterior abdominal wall, normally beginning in the right iliac fossa. The discoloration, due to the formation of sulph-haemoglobin, spreads to involve the whole of the abdominal wall, chest, thighs and, in due course, the skin of the whole of the body. By that time about a week has elapsed since death.

In the next phase there is gas formation and the appearance of blisters in the skin, of up to 3 to 4 in. diameter; the blisters contain reddish watery fluid. They are distinguished from ante-mortem thermal injuries by the absence of "vital reaction" in the floor and vicinity; the fluid contains only a trace of protein whereas the thermal blister fluid contains much protein and may contain white blood cells.

Owing to gas formation, the body cavities swell and there is general tumefaction of the subcutaneous tissues. The interval since death is now about weeks. The rise of pressure in the body cavities can cause the escape of red fluid from the natural orifices and this fluid may be ascribed by the inexperienced to bleeding following ante-mortem injury.

This error brought a highly respectable professional man under unwarranted grave suspicion. His wife was found dead in her bed and blood-stained fluid had escaped from her mouth. It was known that there had been a quarrel and that the husband had left the house in a violent temper on the previous day. It was thought he had injured her and caused her death. It was during a hot summer and conditions favoured early putrefaction. Examination of the body in the bedroom showed that putrefaction was advanced and this had caused the escape of haemolysed blood from her mouth. There was no sign of injury and none of disorder; an empty bottle, which had contained tablets, was on the bedside table. Post-mortem examination excluded all signs of injury and disease. Analysis demonstrated that she had taken an overdose of amylo-barbitone; the dose was estimated to have been of the order of 60 tablets (F.M. 4366A).

Evans (1963a) recalled the legend that the body of Queen Elizabeth I swelled and burst her coffin. Lewis, in the mid-nineteenth century, failed to find burst coffins nor did he find evidence of explosive gases in them. Evans (1963a), who examined many coffins removed from vaults, never saw one to have been burst open. When some forty coffins were removed from a vault in Huddersfield in 1970, one or two of them, notably one of a child, bulged and contained gas under pressure. This was demonstrated by Dr. Brierley who used a manometer connected to a needle which he inserted into the coffin. Other coffins were not distorted because the lead lining had corroded and they were no longer gas-tight. Putrefaction was not advanced in these bodies at Huddersfield despite interment for over a hundred years; the last had been interred prior to 1850. The grave clothes had rotted but the remains were preserved by adipocere formation. Wood shavings but not sawdust had been used as packing.

(The exhumations at Huddersfield were carried out under the personal supervision of Dr. J. S. W Brierley, the Medical Officer of Health, who invited a team of experts to assist him; it included dental surgeons, bacteriologists and members of the Department of Forensic Medicine, University of Leeds. A complete record was made and each stage of the procedure was photographed.

Post-mortem luminescence is a legendary supernatural phenomenon but Evans (1963b) said it is commonly due to contamination by bacteria, e.g. *Photobacterium fischeri*, and the light emanates from them and not putrefying material. He also mentioned luminescent fungi as another source of light. *Armillaria mellea* (Ramsbottom) grows on damp wood and the young mycelia are especially luminescent. (Fungal luminescence was studied by Airth and Foester, 1963, cited by Evans, 1963b. In his *Mushrooms and Toadstools*, Ramsbottom (1953) gives a detailed account of the luminosity of fungi and says that *Armillaria mellea* are responsible for most, if not all, luminous wood in this country.)

The body neutral fat is changed during putrefaction into oleic, palmitic and stearic acids. Palmitic acid increases and oleic acid decreases as the process develops. Intrinsic enzymes effect this slowly but the enzymes produced by *Cl. welchii* are much more effective, when the temperature is between 70°F and 100°F (21.1–37.8°C). Water is also essential but there is normally enough of it in the body tissues. If the process be arrested the fatty acids remain as adipocere (see pp. 23–27) for an indefinite period. Fat is also changed by oxidation due to the action of bacteria, fungi and air. Exposure of the body hastens the process; in sealed coffins hydrolysis is the dominant process (Evans, 1963a).

The body proteins are also broken down to proteoses, polypeptides and, ultimately, amino acids. The rate of this process is modified by humidity, temperature and bacterial activity. Drying by air retards at also unduly low or high temperatures; moisture hastens the process. The by-products include phenolic substances, skatol, indole and gases, which include carbon dioxide, hydrogen sulphide, methane and ammonia (Evans, 1963a).

Proteolysis is not a uniform process in the body. On the contrary it occurs much earlier in some tissues than others. The brain and epithelial tissues are normally the first affected although skin is relatively resistant. The liver and kidneys disintegrate at an early stage but if they contained an excess of fat at the time of death they may be preserved by the formation of adipocere. Muscular organs, e.g. the heart and more especially the resting uterus and prostate, may survive for long periods. It will be recalled that it was possible to identify a fibroid of the uterus in the remains of Mrs. Dobkin at 15 months after death (*R. v. Dobkin*, 1942). Thrombosis of the left coronary artery was demonstrated in one of the Huddersfield bodies. A gravid uterus, on the other hand, especially if infected, disintegrates at an early stage.

At about the third week the skin, hair and nails are loosened and can be readily detached. It is also at about this time that the body cavities rupture.

Eventually all the organs and soft parts are destroyed, connective tissue and cartilage are resistant for some time. There then remains only the skeleton.

There are as yet no means of ascertaining the precise age of a skeleton but the researches of Knight (see Dating of skeletons, pp. 57–61) enable distinction to be made between a modern, i.e. less than 50 years old, and an ancient one. The introduction of the radioactive carbon technique by Libby (1961) permits a remarkably near estimate of the age of prehistoric remains, e.g. turf found in the interior of Silbury Hill was dated at between 2300 B.C. and 2000 B.C. (Atkinson, 1969) and the bodies in the Danish bogs at a date of 100 years on either side of A.D. 310 (Glob, 1965, 1971).

Putrefaction is traditionally held to be delayed by poisoning, notably arsenic, mercuric chloride and possibly antimony, zinc and thallium. It is probable that preservation of the body of one who died of arsenical poisoning is fortuitous since the amount required to kill is infinitely less than the amount required to embalm a body. At the same time, in the event of an exhumation, remains which are in good preservation some months after burial should bring to mind the possibility of a death from poisoning by arsenic (Polson, Green and Lee, 1983).

Putrefaction of bodies which have been submerged is rapid and therefore the post-mortem examination must be prompt unless there are adequate facilities for refrigeration in the mortuary.

Although putrefaction can render the features unrecognisable at an early stage, identification is possible by the dental characteristics and finger-prints. Dermal impressions, i.e. of the digits denuded of epithelium, are also valuable, as shown by the Ruxton case. Dermal impressions from the maid tallied with impressions at Ruxton's house (*R. v. Ruxton*, 1936). Mrs. Manton was identified by her dental characteristics as well as a finger-print, although her features were no longer recognisable (*R. v. Manton*, 1943).

Miliary Plaques

This term was applied by Gonzales *et al.* (1954) to small white granules, of post-mortem origin, which may be seen on the outer surface of the heart and on the endocardium. In my experience they are rare. The granules in my case appear rather larger than those depicted by Gonzales *et al.* They measured from 0.5 mm to 1.5 mm, in diameter and were seen only on the endocardium of the left ventricle (Fig. 1). Microscopy showed that they were amorphous structures but Gonzales *et al.* found bacteria and calcium salts in their plaques. The Leeds subject was a woman aged 57 who died of an overdose of Soneryl. She was last seen alive on 23 October but her body was not found, in her own home, until 19 November 1958. Putrefactive changes were general and at an advanced stage (F.M. 6159).

It is improbable that anyone with experience of morbid anatomy would confuse this appearance with miliary tuberculosis. The mechanism of the production of the plaques

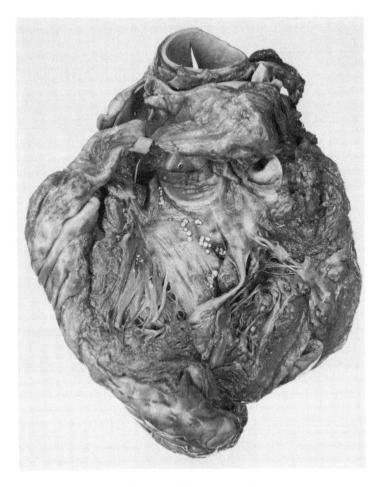

FIG. 1. "Miliary plaques."

(or spheres) is as yet obscure; superficially they resemble colonies of bacterial growth on media but, in our case, no bacteria were demonstrated in these structures.

ADIPOCERE

Adipocere is a variant of putrefaction by which post-mortem dissolution can be delayed, if not arrested, for many years, owing to changes in the body fat by hydrolysis and hydrogenation. It is a spontaneous form of preservation without mummification, although the distinction between these two changes, as Evans (1963[a]) suggested, may not be as precise as formerly believed.

It was long held that adipocere formation was restricted to subcutaneous fat, e.g. of the cheeks, breasts of the female, and buttocks. It is now established that the change can also occur in internal organs, notably the liver, kidneys and heart. This is especially probable if owing to disease they contained an excess of fat at the time of death. The liver, heart and kidney were affected in the woman aged 93, buried for 100 years (F.M. 6205A). Mant (1957) found a quantity of palmitic acid in the liver of one of his subjects.

When relatively recent, adipocere is a soft greasy material which may be white or stained reddish brown, as seen in the bodies exhumed at Huddersfield in 1970. Old adipocere is white or grey. Depending on its age or dryness it is a waxy material which has been likened to suet or cheese. It may be dry and brittle (F.M. 6205A). Evans (1963a) said it had an odour "in which earthy, cheesy and ammoniacal constituents blended, the smell of ammonia being the most persistent". This was apparent in the Huddersfield bodies. It is inflammable and burns with a faint yellow flame. When distilled it yields a dense oily vapour. It is a mixture of stearic, oleic and palmic acids with a proportion of calcium soaps. Glycerol, a by-product of the hydrolisation of fats, may also be present but in most of the bodies, by the time they come to examination, it has been dissolved out of the tissues. This is especially the case when the body has been lying in damp surroundings.

It is a traditional belief that adipocere forms in a damp environment, either after submersion or interment in damp or waterlogged ground. Although these are the usual circumstances, there is ample evidence that adipocere formed in bodies which had been interred in dry vaults; the intrinsic water content of the body was then the adjunct to the formation of adipocere.

Macleod (1946) examined the bodies of 335 males who had been shot and their clothed bodies had been stacked in caves. Bodies in the lower tiers presented adipocere formation in the anterior abdominal wall and lower limbs. Mant (1953, 1957) observed adipocere formation in bodies exhumed from a variety of graves when they were relatively dry. The extent of the change was related to the degree of nourishment.

Wood shavings or sawdust used as packing can hasten decomposition, because, when damp, the shavings ferment and generate heat. This is not invariable because the majority of the bodies in the Huddersfield vault, although their coffins contained wood shavings, were almost all well preserved by adipocere. The bodies were in triple coffins, the middle one being of sealed lead, and the coffins were then enclosed within stone slabs.

Mant (1957) also found adipocere in bodies buried in lead-sealed coffins which were water-tight.

Evans (1960, 1063a, b) examined bodies exhumed from vaults in order to permit interment in new coffins elsewhere. These, like the vault at Huddersfield, were constructed with bricks and were dry; none of the bodies had been interred in earth. In over 50 per cent of 109 bodies he found extensive adipocere formation: it was present in 62.7 per cent of females and 45.4 per cent of males. This is to be anticipated since, normally, the female body contains a higher proportion of fat than that of a male.

In 1950, when a number of bodies were disinterred from a burial place in order to allow road widening, the majority had been reduced to skeletons. One, however, an old lady of 93, who had been buried for over a hundred years, was remarkably well preserved (Fig. 2). Opportunity was provided to examine the body and extensive, dry adipocere formation, involving the internal organs as well as the subcutaneous fat, was widespread. It seemed probable that in this case intrinsic water had aided hydrolysis of fat (F.M. 6205A).

The optimum conditions for the formation of adipocere are a damp, warm environment, but bacterial activity, and especially by *Clostridium welchii* is even more important. Providing cooling of the body after death is not too rapid, activity by *Cl. welchii* an invader from the intestinal tract, will produce lecithinase, a powerful enzyme, which aids hydrolysis and hydrogenation of fat. This activity ceases when the temperature falls below about 70°F and the fat then remains as adipocere (Mant, 1957).

Although it is probable that fat hydrolysis begins within a few days of death, visible (macroscopic) adipocere is delayed for weeks or months. Matzdorff (1935) found that when bodies of newly born infants were exposed to a stream of running water he detected the formation of crystals of fatty acids in their body fat towards the end of the 7th day.

The rate of adipocere formation is modified by humidity, temperature, the fat content of the body, clothing or lack of it, and bacterial activity. It is probable that several weeks, if not months, must elapse before adipocere is apparent to the naked eye; no precise time can be stated.

Devergie (1840) estimated that it required 3 to 4 months but extensive changes required not less than a year after submersion, or upwards of 3 years after burial. Casper (1861) estimated the minimum time at 6 months, but recognised that it could be seen much earlier. He found extensive adipocere in the body of an infant at 13 months after burial and this interval is more in accord with modern reports. Mant (1953) observed advanced adipocere in an adult body which had been buried for a year, but in his experience this was exceptional; the time interval in other bodies was much longer.

The medico-legal importance of adipocere lies in its ability to preserve the body to an extent which can permit identification long after death. Had there been any survivors who knew the deceased, they could have identified the old lady of 93 (Fig. 2) even at a hundred

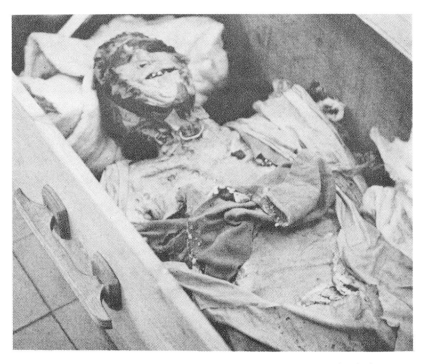

FIG. 2. Adipocere: generalised (burial 105 years prior to examination).

years after her death. It is also probable that several of those interred in the Huddersfield vault for upwards of 150 years could also have been identified by their features.

Preservation by adipocere can also permit at least tentative conclusions as to the cause of death. Coronary atheroma with a clot was demonstrated by M. A. Green in one of the Huddersfield bodies. When the body of a murdered child had been thrown into a river, adipocere formation of the facial fat preserved the features, and by these, hair and the clothing, the father was able to identify the body 5 months after her death. The mark of a ligature was also identified (*R. v. Nodder*, 1937). The mother of Leslie Anne Downey was able to identify the face of this child whose body had been buried for 10 months in wet peat (*R. v. Brady and Hindley*: Chester Assizes, 1966, the "Moors" case: autopsies by Gee and Polson).

Adipocere is a positive sign of death, which indicates that the time interval since death was at least weeks and probably several months. The resulting preservation of the body can permit identification long after death.

MUMMIFICATION

Putrefactive changes may be inhibited and replaced by mummification, which is characterised by drying and shrivelling of the tissues. Mummification of the bodies of adults occurs in countries, notably Egypt, where the climate is dry and warm. Mummification is likely to be seen in England when the body is that of a newly-born infant and it has been kept in a warm, dry place. It may be a drawer, a trunk, the underdrawing of a house, beneath the floorboards or in a recess beside a fireplace. Once the change is complete the body will remain in that condition indefinitely (Fig. 3), unless attacked by the brown house moth.

Although mummification occurs most readily when conditions favour evaporation Evans believed that environment was not the only factor. Fatty acids had been detected in the subcutaneous tissues of natural and embalmed mummies and he had little doubt that adipocere had formed in some of these bodies. The differentiation between mummification and adipocere formation can be less easily made than has been implied in the past.

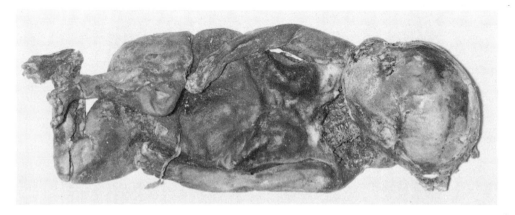

Fig. 3. Mummification: and post-mortem injury by rodents, simulating cut-throat

The occurrence of hydrolysis in a drying environment, as distinct from a dry one, is a possibility but the process is halted by the continuing and relatively rapid loss of water by evaporation (Evans, 1963b).

Mummified tissues may be sufficiently preserved to permit identification and the determination of the probable cause of death. Elliot Smith (1912) described and depicted a mummy of the seventeenth dynasty (*ca.* 1650 B.C.) where, even after over 3000 years, it was still possible to demonstrate that the death was by violence. Wounds consistent with blows by an axe or sword, by a spear and handle of a spear, were recognised. Some of them are apparent in the photograph of the head of the victim. Elliot Smith believed that the victim had been attacked when asleep, lying on his right side, and that there were two or more assailants and their approach had been from the left. The distribution of the injuries, notably two on top of the head, led Elliot Smith to the belief that the victim could not have been erect when struck. The absence of injuries elsewhere on the body suggested that no attempt at defence had been made. It was appreciated, however, that the first blow might have felled the victim and the remainder had been inflicted when he lay on the ground. Whether the interpretation has value or not, the photograph clearly depicts injuries which could only have resulted from a determined attack.

The time required for complete mummification of a body cannot be precisely stated. It is influenced by the size of the body, bodily habit, atmospheric conditions and the place of disposal. In Egypt mummification of an adult body may be advanced by the end of a few weeks. There is insufficient evidence to assess the period likely to be required in this country but it is probably a matter of several weeks, if not months.

Mummification of the bodies of adults in this country is unusual if not rare. In May 1960 the mummified body of a woman was found in a large wooden cupboard in a house at Rhyl, North Wales. It had been there for a considerable time, probably 20 years. The late Gerald Evans found a distinct groove round the neck and the remains of a stocking, tied in a reef knot, in relation to the groove. It was alleged that she had been strangled but Evans could not show that the ligature had been applied to the neck during life. The accused accepted the identification of the body as that of her lodger. It was suggested by the Defence that the stocking might have been applied by the deceased for the relief of a sore throat. The accused said she had found the woman on the floor in pain; she died shortly afterwards and her body was dragged into the cupboard and the door locked. This occurred shortly after the deceased had come to live in the house, i.e. about 20 years earlier. Although closed there was free access of air into the cupboard. Mummification of this body was deemed a natural process; no poison was detected in the remains. (R. Harvey, Ruthin Assizes, 1960: Evans, 1961).

Our Department in Leeds, so far, since its foundation in Oct. 1947, has examined only two mummified adults. One was a man who committed suicide by hanging from a bough of a tree. He was last seen alive on 17 June, 1956 and his body was found on 22 Oct., 1956. The head, neck, chest and parts of the limbs were mummified (F.M. 4987A).

The second subject was a man aged 31 who had intended to enter office premises to steal and who chose to enter by one of its chimneys. His body was discovered in the chimney by workmen engaged in repair of the building. When viewed from above the hands and arms were seen to be about 5 or 6 feet below. The interior of the flue of the chimney measured only $14 \times 14\frac{1}{2}$ inches (35×36 cm) and the front and back of the body touched the brick margins of the flue. The body was erect, with its arms extended and the hands rested on top of the head. The feet rested on the bottom portion of the flue where it turned sharply, almost at right angles, to reach the back of the building. Identification was established by dental examination, by Mr. F. F. Ayton, dental surgeon. The body was fully dressed and heavily soiled by dust. It was very dry and mummification was advanced; the tissues were hard and dry (Figs. 4a, b). Most of the body surface was intact but some damage by insects had occurred. Beetles, identified as *Dermestes lardarius* and *Necrobia rufipes*, emerged through holes in the body surface. No missile nor other foreign body was found inside the

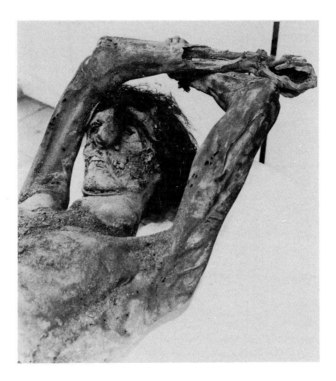

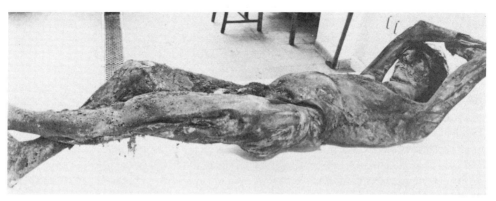

Figs. 4a, b. Mummification; concealed in central heating duct for several years (F.M. 21059A).

body. No skeletal injury, neither recent nor old, was detected by X-Ray examination. There was no evidence of natural disease. There was no ligature round the neck. The body had been inside the chimney for about two years (F.M. 21,059).

Mummification of the body of a newlyborn infant in this country is likely to take several weeks, even when it is that of a non-viable infant.

A male foetus, one of triplets, born at about the 20th to 24th week of gestation, which weighed 455 g (16 ounces), and was 11¼ in. long, was used in a test. The body was wrapped in a single layer of lint and placed in a perforated cardboard box, filled with sawdust. The box was placed in a dry cellar, near the boiler of a central heating system, where the atmospheric temperature was at approximately 122° F. The experiment was begun on 22 November 1951 and concluded on 21 April 1952, when mummification appeared to be complete. There had been periodic inspections during these 5 months. At the end of that time the body weighed only 325 g (11¼ ounces) and was then only 9 in. long. Thereafter, as up to March 1954, no further change took place and the body is likely thus to remain as a museum exhibit for an indefinite period.

Although the examination of small pieces of mummified tissue may be facilitated by immersion in sodium carbonate or a mixture of alcohol, formalin and sodium carbonate, chemical analysis is likely to be vitiated by these methods. The body of the North Wales mummy was therefore immersed in a 15 per cent, solution of glycerine. Adequate softening, to permit an internal examination, occurred in 42½ hours (Evans, 1961).

Preservation in Peat Bogs

Some remarkable photographs were published (Glob, 1951), one of which I am privileged to reproduce as the frontispiece of this book, of the body of a man, discovered during peat cutting in a Danish bog, the Tollund bog in central Jutland, in May 1950. The excellent preservation of this body and the presence of a rope noose around his neck led the police to believe that this was the victim of murder. Dr. Glob, however, formed the opinion that this was the victim of a ritual sacrifice, made some 2000 years previously. Despite this distance of time,

His face (was) so well-preserved and as expressive as though he had but a moment ago fallen asleep . . . only the dark, brown leather colour showed his age . . . It is obvious that this man, clothed only in a cap and belt, had been hanged and then deposited in the bog . . . About one hundred bodies of men, women and children have, in the course of the last two centuries, been recovered from peat bogs in the area covering Jutland, north-west Germany and Holland . . . Many, like the Tollund man, are practically naked and many have only a leather cape over their shoulders. Very many have a noose of rope or leather around their necks, while others have crushed heads, broken limbs or mortal wounds in their body. Some are bound hand and foot, and others are pinned down in the bogs by a wooden stake or hook, this last being a precaution against haunting.

In these ancient, pre-Christian times hanging was not considered a dishonourable death; on the contrary, such victims were sacred to Odin. This hanging was possibly part of a rite intended to bring fertility and fortune to his fellow-men.

The body of a girl, whose age was estimated to be 14 years, was discovered by peat cutters in a bog in Schleswig-Holstein; it was well preserved although death had occurred some 2000 years ago. It was removed in a huge block of peat and transported to the museum in Gottorp Castle for examination.

The girl's body was naked except for a collar of hairy ox-hide and the left side of the scalp had been shorn presumably with a shaving knife—and the state of growth indicates that this was done about 3 days before death . . . "Round the eyes a cord-like bandage had been tied—still fully preserved, with its technique of weaving still quite clear". It was

The Essentials of Forensic Medicine

believed that death was by drowning and a large stone behind the body may have been used to weight it down (Schlabow, 1953).

The explanation of the circumstances of her death is a matter of conjecture but attention was drawn to the ancient punishment of adultery, described by Tacitus. "After the cutting off of her hair, the husband draws her forth from his home naked in the presence of the neighbours." There are also circumstances of the case which resemble those described by Glob; this girl may have been another victim of a ritual sacrifice.

In April 1952 yet another well-preserved body was discovered in a peat bog near Grauballe, in Denmark. It was removed intact in the surrounding peat and submitted to detailed examination by Professor Glob and his colleagues (Glob *et al.*, 1956).

The body was that of a male of over 30 years of age and deposition in the bog was estimated, by pollen analysis and Carbon-14 test, to have occurred about 2000 years previously. The dating was A.D. 310 ± 100, i.e. in the Roman Iron Age.

The body was naked and no trace of any clothing was found in the bog. It was remarkably well preserved and lay prone, with the left arm and leg extended and the right arm and leg flexed. This posture had been noted on two earlier occasions. The appearances of the skin resembled those of tanning.

The hair and skin had a dark red colour, due to staining by the peat fluids. Preservation of the skin was such that, when first seen, the ridge pattern of the fingers was clearer than that of the observer (Vogelius Andersen, 1956). The viscera had perished. The skeleton was now extensively decalcified. The long bones and skull were soft and flattened; they bent almost as easily as if they had been cartilaginous. The skull and some of the bones had been flattened by pressure of the peat. The teeth were worn as in advanced age. Those in another body, preserved in the Medico-legal Institute at Copenhagen, had a dark mahogany colour. I noticed that while some were well worn by food attrition, others presented sharp points round the occlusal surface. This unusual feature was discussed with Professor Jackson of the Leeds Dental School and he attributed this change to decalcification; the enamel had been removed to expose the dentine. He treated some teeth with acid and when these were subsequently coloured with iodine, they were a replica of the teeth at Copenhagen.

The Grauballe man had a large incised wound extending from ear to ear, apparently produced by two or more cuts. It was deemed to have been inflicted by another during life and not self-inflicted or inflicted after death.

The natural preservation by humic and tannic acid in the peat was continued in the laboratory by artificial tanning with a solution of fresh oak bark. The body was then treated with Turkish red oil and, finally, with a mixture of glycerine, lanoline and cod-liver oil, equal parts. It has been mounted for permanent preservation in a teak and steel case (Glob, 1956; with Jorgensen, Munck, Krebs and Ratjen, Vogelius Andersen, Lange-Kornback and Tauber, see *Kuml*, 1956). Professor Glob also gives a detailed account of these Iron Age burials in his *Mosefolket* (1965); English translation *The Bog People* (1971).

Bodies long buried in peat have been recovered on occasion in Ireland and Scotland, but none appear to have been well preserved. Portions of such bodies are to be seen in the museum of the Department of Forensic Medicine in Edinburgh.

Preservation in peat bogs is explained by the fact that the surroundings are cold, airless and acid, whereby bacterial growth is inhibited. It is likely also that humic and tannic acids operate to tan the remains.

MACERATION

Maceration is the term applied to the aseptic autolytic changes which occur in the body of a child which has died *in utero*; they are not apparent unless the death has occurred at least 5 days prior to delivery, and, normally, they take about a week to develop. Examination of the body must be prompt since exposure to air permits the occurrence of putrefactive changes, an entirely different process, to be superimposed. When present, maceration is conclusive evidence of still birth.

The body has a rancid odour and the skin has a red-brown colour; peeling of the skin and blister formation occur. The blisters contain red-brown watery fluid. There is no gas formation. An outstanding feature is an abnormal flaccidity of the body and undue mobility of the skull which gives the head a flattened appearance; the limbs are readily separated from the body.

Rarely, restricted maceration, e.g. of the skin of the legs, may occur in a live born child, e.g. that of a colleague, which survived only for a few days.

BIOCHEMICAL INVESTIGATION OF THE CEREBROSPINAL FLUID AFTER DEATH

The investigations by Schourup (1950–1) led him to the belief that chemical analysis of the cerebrospinal fluid after death, coupled with the determination of body temperature, would provide a satisfactory estimate of the time of death. The findings, applied to a somewhat elaborate formula, yielded estimates of the time of death which, in fifty cases, were claimed to be accurate to within $\pm 1^1/_2$ hours and, indeed to within ± 1 hour in forty-two or 84 per cent of the experiments.

This mode of estimating the time of death requires the determination of the amino-acid content and, where practicable, that of lactic acid and nonprotein nitrogen content of the cerebrospinal fluid.

The adoption of Schourup's methods calls for better determination of body temperature than the measurement of the axillary temperature. To rely on the latter in conjunction with the performance of elaborate biochemical procedures is a waste of valuable time and material. The initial hopes raised by his research have not been fulfilled.

The potassium content of the cerebrospinal fluid rises rapidly after death and the increase is in proportion to the log of the time since death but the variations which occur preclude its practical application (Mason *et al.*, 1951). Murray and Hordynsky (1958) also observed a correlation between the potassium content of cisternal fluid and the time interval since death. Their observations were confirmed by Breazeale and Suarez (1961) who claimed accuracy for this method over an even longer range, i.e. for up to 38 or 40 hours after death. They found that the potassium concentration was in the form of a "straight line" increase as the time interval lengthened.

These methods, if they are to have any value, demand samples of cerebrospinal fluid without contamination by blood. Moreover, when used for the determination of potassium content, the samples must be refrigerated to 4–5°C soon after collection.

BIOCHEMICAL INVESTIGATION OF CADAVER BLOOD

Biochemical changes in cadaver blood have been studied by Jetter and McLean (1943), by Enticknap (1960) and Laves (1960), but the results are as yet without practical application.

HEAT STIFFENING

The body proteins, notably albumens and globulins, are coagulated by heat when exposed to temperatures above 50° C (122° F), and in consequence there is stiffening of the body. The usual appearance is one of flexion, especially of the upper limbs, described, with good reason, as the pugilistic attitude; it is an exaggeration of the flexion, due to shortening of the muscle fibres, which occurs in less degree in rigor mortis (Fig. 5, F.M. 749).

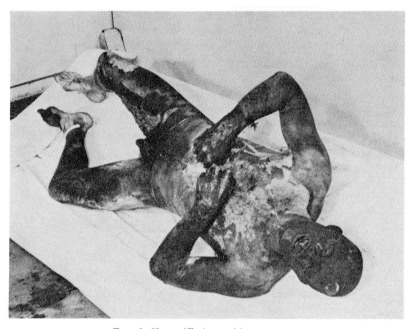

FIG. 5. Heat stiffening and heat ruptures.

COLD STIFFENING OR FREEZING

Bodies when exposed, especially on mountains or moorland, may become frozen and thus appear to be in a state of rigor mortis. Manipulation of the joints will yield crepitation due to fracture of the frozen joint fluid. If the body is allowed to thaw, true rigor ensues.

THE STOMACH CONTENTS AND THE TIME OF DEATH

Examination of the stomach contents after death may indicate the nature of the last meal before death and provide an approximate estimate of the probable time interval since death.

When the contents include recognisable food material, even part-digested, their accurate identification can confirm the stated composition of the last meal. Thus, in the Truscott case (1966), white meat, part-digested, recognisable as of poultry, portions of potato and of undigested peas, together with red meat, part-digested, were identified in the stomach contents. The last meal known to have been given to the girl was stated to include skin of turkey, a portion of breast of turkey, potatoes and peas. The deceased also had had access to ham, which was kept in a refrigerator. If these were the facts, then there is no doubt that the last meal taken by the deceased was that eaten at approximately 5.45 p.m., 9 June 1963, on the day she was last seen alive. The state of the stomach contents, scarcely digested, was also consistent with scanty, hurried mastication and completion of the meal in about 15 minutes. This evidence, however, confirmed only the time of the last meal and its composition. It could corroborate other evidence bearing on the probable time interval since death. Attempts to fix this time based solely on an examination of the stomach contents are unsatisfactory even when allowance is made for factors which either hasten or retard digestion; allowance must also be made for individual variation.

As a rough guide to preliminary police investigations, it may well be that, in a healthy person, the presence of a pint or more of undigested or part-digested food in the stomach indicates the partaking of a meal shortly before death, probably less than 2 hours. Conversely, an empty stomach suggests that nothing had been eaten for not less than 2 hours before death.

The foregoing, however, cannot be relied upon, nor should it be relied upon, as crucial evidence which purports to fix the time of death within narrow limits, especially when the estimated time happens to coincide with a period of time during which the movements of an accused are not satisfactorily ascertained. It was alleged in the Truscott case that the appearances and amount of the stomach contents indicated that death occurred between 7.15 p.m. and 7.45 p.m. on 9 June 1963. Estimates of this precision demand full confirmation by evidence from other sources. There was no unanimity in the views of the expert witnesses in the Truscott case (1966).

We agree with Helpern and Knight (1982) that the account of this case by Mrs. Le Bourdais (1966) is well written and extremely persuasive but it is entirely biased in favour of Truscott. Helpern's recorded account is to be noted.

This concept of a 2 hour emptying time appears to be based on the results of test meals given to healthy persons. In these tests an emptying time exceeding 2 hours is presumptive evidence of abnormality. But this relates to a *standard* meal of gruel. Even then some allowance must be made for individual variations. There are no comparable results for the emptying time after a mixed meal of turkey and ham or duck and green peas. It is, however, well recognised that several factors can delay emptying of the stomach and by an appreciable time. In other circumstances it can be hastened when, for example, a person swallowed her denture and it reached the jejunum in 15 minutes (Morgan, 1945).

Most elaborate tables have been prepared of the time taken by the stomach to digest certain articles of diet, but they are wholly unreliable (Taylor, 1965).

The examination of stomach contents is a necessary part of the post-mortem examination, but the conclusions drawn are at best only of minor value in ascertaining the time interval since death. The examination can confirm the stated contents of the last known meal.

The presence of tablets, whole or partially disintegrated, has obvious importance.

Objects which resemble grape skins or red berries should at once excite interest since they may prove to be capsules which contained a barbiturate. A boy aged 5 months was murdered in 1955 by the administration of seconal. Capsules found in his stomach at the first post-mortem were then thought to have been red berries but, after exhumation, death was proved to have been due to poisoning by seconal (*R. v. J. Armstrong and J. Armstrong*, Winchester Assizes, December (1956).)

THE ENTOMOLOGY OF THE DEAD

Occasions arise when the study of insects or their maggots infesting a dead body may be a means of ascertaining the probable time of death or the date on which the body was placed where it is discovered.

This ingenious application of entomology was first reported by Bergeret (1855). The body of a newly born infant was found in a triangular space near the chimney in a house where two bricks had been removed to allow the insertion of the body. Mummification had occurred and the body became the breeding ground of moths. A study of their nymphae and larvae led Bergeret to fix the date of the deposit of the body at a time which exculpated three recent tenants of the house and suggested that the offender was a woman who had previously lived there. Although she was known to have been pregnant at that time and was brought to trial, the charge of infanticide failed because the death of the infant could have been due to natural causes. It is of interest to note that the body was discovered on 22 March 1850, and the date of its deposit near the chimney was estimated to have been during the summer of 1848.

Lichtenstein *et al.* (1885) examined the mummified body of a foetus which was discovered by workmen when they lifted the floorboards in a house during its demolition. On this occasion it was estimated by a study of the larvae that at least 4 years had elapsed since the body had been hidden.

The interest of Mégnin, an entomologist, in this kind of investigation was aroused by Brouardel who consulted him in connection with an alleged infanticide in 1883. His studies continued and he published the results in *La Faune des Cadavres* in 1894; this monograph is still a principal reference.

The Ruxton case, in 1936, included entomological investigations by Mearns (1937, 1939), who examined the eggs and maggots present on the decomposing remains found at Moffat. He identified them as the larvae of the common bluebottle and estimated that the largest of the larvae could not have been more than 12 days old. Since this fly normally lays its eggs on fresh meat, it was probable that the remains could not have been left in the ravine more than a fortnight previously. The possibility that the maggots were a second generation was excluded because that would have required a time interval of a month, i.e. at a date when the deceased persons were known to have been alive. The remains were found on 1 October and it was believed they had been placed in the ravine on or about 6 September 1935. The entomological investigation, therefore, lent confirmation.

Lopatenok *et al.* (1964) studied the larvae of flies and beetles as a guide to the post-mortem interval but it is doubtful if their results add value to those of Mégnin (1894), Mearns (1937, 1939) and of Lothe (1964).

Lothe emphasised the need for caution when making any estimate of the interval. Thus, it must not be assumed that the eggs were deposited on the body at or near the time of death. It is also important correctly to identify the species, since the life cycle varies from species to species. When the larvae are correctly identified it is possible to determine the *minimum* post-mortem interval.

The entomologist should be provided not only with larvae killed with boiling absolute alcohol and stored in 50 per cent alcohol (Glaister and Rentoul, 1966) but also live larvae. These should be placed in a container together with a small piece of raw meat or a portion of muscle from the corpse. This food should not be too plentiful lest the larvae die from drowning in an excess of moisture. Whenever practicable it is much better for the entomologist to attend the scene and collect the material; it also enables him to study the environment (Easton and Smith, 1970).

Voigt (1965) examined a body extensively damaged by larder beetles (*Dermestis lardius* and *D. haemorrhoidalis*). These insects are common in Denmark and normally feed on carcases and butcher's refuse. They are prevalent in the spring and summer. They begin their attack on a body at about 3 to 6 months after death, i.e., when the body fat has been converted into fatty acids and the fat is rancid (Mégnin, 1894).

From the extent of the damage Voigt estimated that death had occurred about 6 months prior to the spring of 1961; there had been a severe pest of these beetles during that year. The deceased, a male, was believed to have died over 18 months prior to the discovery of his body in April 1962. Papers on the body showed that he had been released from prison on 19 August 1960; he went to live in the flat of a friend. It appeared he had died on a settee but his friend, instead of reporting the death, stored the body in a wardrobe, where it was found. Post-mortem examination and other investigations led to the conclusion that death had been due to natural causes.

These beetles had transformed the soft tissues into material with resembled horse hair; it took the form of coils of slender, dry brownish or whitish, fairly long fibres. They were composed of collagenous connective tissue, covered with a thin layer of mucin. The fibres were accompanied by larval skin and pupal cases but no adult beetles remained amongst the fibres. The fibres were larval excrement and the mucinous covering had been formed in the intestinal tract to protect the intestine against the mechanical action of the excrement during its escape from the body of the beetle (Voigt, 1965).

The brown house moth will attack hair, skin and internal organs (Forbes, 1942). The activity of their larvae was responsible for the curious appearance of the head hair of the North Wales mummy; it was reduced to a stubble, 1–3 mm long, and microscopical examination showed that the hairs had clean-cut ends (Evans, 1961). Attack by moths produced the simulation of cut-throat in the mummified body of a newly born infant (Fig. 3).

A body lying in the open may be invaded by no less than eight successive waves of attack by insects. This commences with the arrival of calliphora (blue bottles) and ends with an attack by coleoptera (beetles). Although in theory this is an orderly progression and identification of the insects present should result in a satisfactory estimate of the time interval since death, Smith warned that the factors involved make assessment a complex one. Easton also pointed out that the appearances and abundance of fauna are more related to the season than the stage of decay. In many instances the reverse obtains. More research is needed in this field and, in Easton's opinion, a study of coleoptera would be of special value (Easton and Smith, 1970).

Erzinclioglu (1983) has reviewed the literature, and indicates the nature of the insect succession on corpses. He recommends that insect larvae should be taken from as many different parts of the body as possible, and their position on the corpse recorded. He draws attention to the range of insects involved, beyond the common "blow-flies", and emphasises the importance for the forensic scientist of access to entymological expertise.

POST-MORTEM INJURIES BY ANIMALS

Animals, rats or dogs may attack a dead body and cause mutilation, which may simulate the effect of violence inflicted during life. Our departmental file of photographs includes an example of mutilation of the body of a dead woman by cats. The body was found several days after death in a room where there were five cats. The famished animals had attacked the head, neck and front of the chest and had removed almost the whole of the soft parts, after her death.

The body of one of the victims of the "Moors Murders" in 1965, that of the girl Leslie Ann Downey, bore certain external injuries, which, at first sight, suggested that she had been stabbed and her external genitalia had been excised. Dissection promptly excluded stabbing, since the two eliptical wounds in her chest wall, each of which measured over an inch on their long axes, were wholly superficial, involving only the skin and subcutaneous tissues. A long curved wound at the lower part of the abdomen, when examined under low magnification, was proved to be slightly irregular throughout and not clean cut as by a knife. It was also found that in the intact skin, close to the margins of the injury, there were superficial punctures of small size at intervals along the margin of the injury. None of the injuries was accompanied by bruising or other evidence of bleeding in the vicinity. These were deemed injuries by the teeth, or possibly the claws, of an animal. As a control, a portion of meat was fed to a dog, and when this was examined the dog had produced changes which tallied with those found in the skin of the child. It was concluded that the injuries had been inflicted by a fox or dog, which had found the body.

The child was last seen alive on 26 December 1964 and her body was found buried in the moor in 15 October 1965, i.e. 10 months later. Owing to post-mortem changes and damage by an animal it was impossible to ascertain the cause of death. A second body, that of a boy who had been missing for 23 months, was found within 500 yards of that of the girl 6 days later, at a place which coincided with that being viewed by Myra Hindley and photographed by her friend Brady. This body had not been attacked by animals but, unfortunately, post-mortem changes were advanced and the cause of death could not be established. (Gee and Polson, witnesses at the trial of *R. v. Brady and Hindley*, 1966. Both of the accused were convicted.)

The absence of vital reaction, a careful study of the wounds and a knowledge of the circumstances will furnish a correct interpretation.

Bodies submerged in water may be nibbled by fish or gnawed by rats. When exposed in a woodland area, the body may be attacked by insects. These usually produce injuries near unprotected, moist parts, e.g. the eyelids, nose and mouth. The injuries produced by insects may resemble abrasions, but they are not accompanied by bruising.

References

ADELSON, L., SUNSHINE, I., RUSHFORTH, N. B. and MANKOFF, M. (1963) *J. Forens. Sci.*, **8**, 503.
AIRTH, R. L. and FOESTER, G. E. (1960) *J. Cell. Comp. Physiol.*, **56** (3), 173.
ALBRAND, W. (1904) *Arch. Augenheilk.*, **50**, 145–66.
ANDERSEN, VOGELIUS (1956) *Kuml*, ed. P. V. Glob, pp. 151–4.
ATKINSON, R. (1969) *Silbury Hill.* London: British Broadcasting Corp.
BADONNEL, M., FORTINEAU, E. and NEVEU, P. (1936) *Ann. Méd. lég.* **16**, 491–6; also abstr. *Med.-leg. Rev.* (1937), **5**, 102.
BERGERET (of Arbois) (1855) *Ann. Hyg. Publ. (Paris)*, 2nd ed., **4**, 442–52.
BIRDWOOD, G. (1968) *World Medicine*, **3**, 6.
BREAZEALE, E. L. and SUAREZ, E. F. (1961) *Police*, **6**, 49–51.
BROUARDEL, P. (1883) *Gaz. Hôp. (Paris)*, **56**, 212–13.
BROWN-SÉQUARD, C. E. (1861) *Proc. Roy. Soc.*, **11**, 204–14.
BURN, E. G. (1934) *J. Infect. Dis.*, **54**, 388–94.
CASPER, J. L. (1861) *Handbook of Forensic Medicine*, 3rd ed., vol. 1, English trans. G. W. Balfour, London: New Sydenham Soc,
DE SARAM, G. S. W., WEBSTER, G. and KATHIRAGAMATAMBY, N. (1955–6). *J. Crim. Law and Criminol.*, **46**, 526–77.
DEVERGIE, A. (1840). *Médicine Légale*, 2nd ed., Paris; Bailliere.
DUKE, W. (Ed.) (1950) *Trials of Frederick Nodder*, Vol. 72. *Notable British Trials.* London: Hodge.
DUGUID, H., SIMPSON, R. G. and STOWERS, J. M. (1961) *Lancet*, ii, 1213–19.
EASTON, A. M. and SMITH, K. G. V. (1970) *Med. Sci. Law*, **10**, 208.
ETICKNAP, J. B. (1960). *J. Forens. Med.*, **7**, 135–46.
ERZINCLIOGLU, Y. Z. (1983) *Med. Sci. Law*, **23**, 57–63.
EVANS, E. G. (1961) *Med. Sci. Law*, **1**, 33.
EVANS, W. E. D. (1960) 2nd Internat. Meeting on For. Path. and Medicine, New York. *Program and Abstracts*, p. 41.
EVANS, W. E. D. (1963a) *The Chemistry of Death.* American lecture series. Illinois: Charles C. Thomas.
EVANS, W. E. D. (1963b) *Med. Sci. Law*, **3**, 145.
FIDDES, F. S. and PATTEN, T. D. (1958) *J. Forens. Med.*, **5**, 2–15.
FORBES, G. (1942) *Police J.*, **15**, 141.
FORSTER, B. (1963a) *J. Forens. Med.*, **10**, 91.
FORSTER, B. (1963b) *J. Forens. Med.*, **10**, 133.
FORSTER, B. (1964) *J. Forens. Med.*, **11**, 148.
GANTNER, G. E., Jnr., CAFFREY, P. R. and STURNER, W. Q. (1962) *J. Forens. Med.*, **9**, 156.
GLAISTER, J. and RENTOUL, E. (1966) *Medical Jurisprudence and Toxicology*, 12th ed. Edinburgh: Livingstone.
GLOB, P. V. (1951) *Illustrated London News*, 4 Nov.
GLOB, P. V. (1956) *Kuml*, pp. 99–110; English summary pp. 111–13.
GLOB, P. V. (1965) *Mosefolket*: Copenhagen; Gyldendal. English translation by Rupert Bruce-Mitford, 1971: *The Bog People*, London: Faber & Faber. Paladin paper-back edition.
GONZALES, T. A., VANCE, M., HELPERN, M. and UMBERGER, C. T. (1954) *Legal Medicine*, 2nd ed., p. 64. New York: Appleton-Century.
GREEN, M. A. and WRIGHT, J. (1982) in the Press.
HELPERN, M. and KNIGHT, B. (1982) *Autopsy.* pp. 116: 148–152 London: W. H. Allen. A "Star" paperback.
HIRAIWA K., OHNO, Y., KURODA, F., SEBETAN, I. S. and OSHIDA, S., (1980) *Science and the Law*, **20**, 2.
HIRAIWA, K., KUDO, T., KURODA, F., OHNO, Y., SEBATAN, I. M. and OSHIDA, S. (1981) *Medicine, Science and the Law*, **21**, 1.
HUGHES, W. M. H. (1965) *Med. Sci. Law*, **5**, 150.
JAFFE, F. A. (1962) *J. Forens. Sci.*, **8**, 231.
JAMES, W. R. L. and KNIGHT, B. H. (1965), *Med. Sci. Law*, **5**, 111.
JETTER, W. W. and McLEAN, R. (1943) *Amer. J. Clin. Path.*, **13**, 178–85.
JOHN, P. P. L. (1967) *Brit. Med. J.*, **4**, 357.
JOLL, (1881) Cited in abstr. of Tonelli (1932) and cited by Albrand. Orig. ref. not traced.
JOSEPH, A. E. A. and SCHICKELE, M. S. (1970) *Journal of Forensic Sciences*, **15**, 3.
KAHN, M. H. (1913) *Med. Rec.*, **83**, 801–3.
KEVORKIAN, J. (1961a) *J. Forens. Sci.*, **6**, 261–72.
KEVORKIAN, J. (1961b) *Clin. Symposia*, **13**, 51–62.
LeBOURDAIS, I. (1966) *The Trial of Steven Truscott*, London: Gollancz.
LAUFMAN, H. (1951) *J. Amer. Med. Ass.*, **147**, 1201–12.
LAVES, W. (1960) *J. Forens. Med.*, **7**, 70–72.

LIBBY, W. F. (1961) *Science*, **133**, 621; cited Evans, 1963a.

LICHTENSTEIN, J., MORTESSIER, A. and JAUMES, A. (1885) *Ann. Hyg. Publ.* (*Paris*), **13**, 121–7.

LITILEJOHN, HARVEY (1925) *Forensic Medicine*. London: Churchill.

LOPATENOK, A. A., BOIKO, L. P. and BUDYAKOV, O. S. (1964) *Sud.-Med. Ekspert*, **7**, 47; abstr. *Dtsch. Z.g. gerichtl. Med.* (1965) **56**, 89.

LOTHE, F. (1964) *Med. Sci. Law*, **4**, 113.

LYLE, H. P., STEMMER, K. L. and CLEVELAND, F. P. (1959) *J. Forens. Sci.*, **4**, 167–75.

MACLEOD, W. (1946) *J. Roy. Army Med. Corps.*, **87**, 10.

MAJOSKA, A. V. (1960) *J. Forens. Sci.*, **5**, 33–39.

MANN, G. T. (1960) *J. Forens. Sci.*, **5**, 346–55.

MANT, A. K. (1953) *Modern Trends in Forensic Medicine*, ed. K. Simpson. London: Butterworths.

MANT, A. K. (1957) *J. Forens. Med.*, **4**, 18–350.

MARSHALL, T. K. (1959) Thesis, M. D. Leeds. (Available on application to the Librarian of the University of Leeds.) (Extracts have been published; see also Marshall and Hoare, 1962, and Marshall, 1962).

MARSHALL, T. K. (1962) *J. Forens. Sci.*, **7**, 189–210; *ibid.*, pt. 211–21.

MARSHALL, T. K. (1965) *Med. Sci. Law*, **5**, 224.

MARSHALL, T. K. (1969) *Med. Sci. Law.* **9**, 178–182.

MARSHALL, T. K. (1979) *Police Surgeon*. No. 16. 21–28.

MARSHALL, T. K. (1981) *Police Surgeon*. No.

MARSHALL, T. K. and HOARE, F. E. (1962) *J. Forens. Sci.*, **7**, 56–81.

MARTIN, É. (1950). *Précis de Médecine Légale*, 3rd ed., p. 209, Paris: Doin.

MASON, J. K., KLYNE, W. and LENNOX, B. (1951). *J. clin. Path.*, **4**, 231–3.

MATZDORFF, (1935). *Dtsch. Z. ges. gerichtl. Med.*, **24**, 246–9.

MEARNS, A. G. (1937). In Glaister and Brash's *Medico-Legal Aspects of the Ruxton Case*, pp. 261–3 Edinburgh: Livingstone.

MEARNS, A. G. (1939) in Sydney Smith and Glaister's *Recent Advances in Forensic Medicine* 2nd. ed., pp. 250–5, London; Churchill.

MEDICO-LEGAL (1971) *Brit. Med. J.*, **3**, 716.

MÉGNIN, P. (1883) *Gaz. Hop.* (*Paris*), **56**, 212–13.

MÉGNIN, P. (1894) *La Faune des Cadavres*. Paris: Masson.

MORGAN, A. D. (1945) *Brit. Med. J.*, **ii**, 25.

MURRAY, E. F. and HORDYNSKY, W. (1958) *J. Forens. Sci.*, **31**, 480–5.

NANIKAWA, R. and JANSSEN, W. (1965) *Dtsch. Z. ges. gerichtl. Med.*, **56**, 44 (English summary).

NAUMANN, H. N. (1959) *Arch. Ophthal. Chicago*, **62**, 356.

NICATI, (1894). *Med. Rec.*, **45**, 480. (Medical item.)

NIDERKORN, P. F. (1872) in Melanges's *Anatomie et Physiologie*; cited *Brit. med. J.*, 1874, **i**, 303–4; also by TIDY (1882).

NOKES, L. D. M., BROWN, A. and KNIGHT, B. A self contained method for Determining Time Since Death from Temperature Measurements, *Med. Sci. Law* (1983) Vol. 23 No. 3.

POLSON, C. J. GREEN, M. A. and LEE, M. R. (1983) *Clinical Toxicology*, 3rd ed. London: Pitman Books.

R. v. JOHN ARMSTRONG and JANET ARMSTRONG (Winchester Assizes, Dec. 1956) Reported by Simpson, C. K. and Molony, J. T., *Med.-leg. J.* (*Camb.*) (1957) **25**, 53.

R. v. BRADY and HINDLEY (1966) Chester Assizes; Fenton Atkinson, J., *The Times*, 19 April–6 May.

R. v. DOBKIN (1942) *Trial of Harry Dobkin*, C. E. Bechhofer Roberts, 1944, Old Bailey Trials Series, No. 1, London, New York, Melbourne; Jarrolds: also Simpson, K. (1943) *Police J.*, **16**, 270–80, and (1943) *Med.-leg. Rev.*, **11**, 132–44.

R. v. ELLISON (1845) *Bodmin Assizes*; cited TIDY (1882).

R. v. MANTON (1943) The Luton Sack Murder, see Simpson (1945).

R. v. NODDER (1937) *Trials of Frederick Nodder*, *Notable British Trials*, vol. **72**, editor, Winifred Duke, 1950, Edinburgh: Hodge.

R. v. RUXTON (1936) Manchester Winter Assizes, *Trial of Buck Ruxton*; *Notable British Trials*, editors, R. H. Blundell and G. H. Wilson, 1937, Edinburgh, etc.: Hodge.

RAMSBOTTOM, J. (1953) *Mushrooms and Toadstools* (New Naturalist Series), London: Collins.

ROSSBACH, J. M. (1870) *Virchow's Arch.*, **51**, 558–68.

SALISBURY, C. R. and MELVIN, G. S. (1936) *Brit. Med. J.*, **i**, 1249–51.

SCHLABOW, K. (1953) *Illustrated London News*, 19 Dec.

SCHOURUP, K. (1950–1) *Dodstidsbestemmelse*, Copenhagen: Dansk Videnskabs Forlag.

SHAPIRO, H. A. (1950) *Brit. Med. J.*, **ii**, 304.

SIMPSON, K. (1945) *Police J.*, **18**, 263–73.

SMITH, E. C. (1930–31) *Proc. Roy. Soc.*, series *B*, **107**, 214–22.

SMITH, G. ELLIOT (1921) *The Royal Mummies*, Cairo: Inst. Franc. d'Archéol. Orientale; Cat. Gén. du Musée du Caire.

SMITH, SIR SYDNEY and FIDDES, F. S. (1955) *Forensic Medicine*, 10th ed., pp. 14, 19, London: Churchill.

SPILSBURY, SIR BERNARD (1944) *Med.-leg. Rev.*, **12**, 194.

STEER, C. (1951) *Lancet*, I, 1419.

STURNER, W. Q. and GANTNER, G. E., Jnr. (1964) *Amer. J. Clin. Path.*, **42**, 137.

SZENT-GYÖRGYI, A. (1947) *Chemistry of Muscular Contraction*, New York: Academic Press.

TAYLOR, A. S. (1965) *Principles and Practise of Medical Jurisprudence*, 12th ed., ed. K. Simpson. London: Churchill.

TIDY, C. M. (1882) *Legal Medicine*, vol. 1, pp. 62–69. London: Smith Elder.

TOMLIN, P. J. (1967a) *Brit. Med. J.*, **3**, 722.

TOMLIN, P. J. (1967b) *Brit. Med. J.*, **4**, 110.

TONELLI, L. (1932) *Il Policlin.*, **39**, 205; abstr. *Med.-leg. Rev.* (1933), **1**, 132.

TRUSCOTT Case (1966) *The Trial of Steven Truscott*: I. Le Bourdais, London: Gollancz; Editorial Review: *Med. Sci. Law* (1966) **6**, 5; condemned by Prof. K. Simpson as "inaccurate". See also *Toronto Globe and Mail*, 2–13 Oct. 1966 for full report. *Ibid.*, 8 May 1967: comment by editor.

VOIGT, J. (1965) *J. Forens. Med.* **12**, 76.

WATSON, E. R. (Ed.) (1922) *The Trial of George Joseph Smith*: London: Hodge.

WROBLEWSKI, B. and ELLIS, M. (1970) *Brit. J. Surg.*, **57**, 69.

YAMASE, Y. (1941) *Far East Sci. Bull.*, **1**, 52 (abstr.).

CHAPTER 2

Identification

IDENTIFICATION of the living is primarily a matter for police investigation and therefore it requires but brief mention here. Identification of the dead, on the other hand, may create a medico-legal problem of first magnitude, likely to tax the resources of the most experienced examiner.

Collaboration with an anatomist is often of first importance, as in the investigation of the Ruxton murders, and the identification of two of Christie's victims. The procedure of Glaister and Brash (1937), of Harrison (1953) and of Krogman (1962a, b) should be familiar to those called upon to undertake this task.

The value of good dental records cannot be over-stressed. When the victim's dental surgeon has been traced, his or her records can provide unequivocal evidence of identity. This is well illustrated by the Dobkin case (Mr. Kopkin), the Haigh case (Miss Helen Mayo), the Manton (Luton sack) case (Mr. Jacob Rackham) and the Christie case (Miles and Fearnhead).

When a body is found, one of the first steps is to establish its identity. If death is due to some criminal act, it has been said with truth the major problem is half solved when the victim has been identified, because the police have a firm foundation on which to base their investigations. So long as the body remains unidentified, loss of time and profitless expenditure of valuable police services may ensue, since it is then necessary to explore many possibilities which would be immediately excluded by a knowledge of the identity of the victim. That knowledge, moreover, often serves to narrow the search for the culprit.

Identification of the living

Until the value of fingerprints was recognised as a means of identification and fingerprint bureaux were instituted, identification of the living depended almost exclusively upon recognition by personal impressions, i.e. recognition by sight or hearing.

It is still necessary as part of the investigation of crime to hold identification parades. The suspect or accused is included in a group of persons of approximately similar build, age and appearance, and witnesses are invited to point out one of them as the alleged criminal. Alternatively, a witness in court may be asked to look round and see whether there is any person present whom he can identify as the offender.

The unsatisfactory nature of identification by personal impressions has long been stressed and is a matter of common knowledge. Few of us, relying upon personal impressions, have never mistaken a complete stranger for an acquaintance. Beyond momentary embarassment and the necessity to offer polite apology, these errors in private rarely have importance. It is otherwise if they give rise to what proves to be a false accusation, e.g. robbery with violence. Mistakes will inevitably continue to occur so long as this method of identification has a place, as it still must do, in the investigation of crime. It is easy to understand why in certain quarters there is a desire to record the fingerprints of the whole nation; this would have distinct advantages, which, on balance, would be appreciably greater than the alleged disadvantages or possible dangers.

Notable instances of mistaken identity include the cases of Adolf Beck (1877–1904) and Oscar Slater (1909), wrongly convicted of serious crimes, and those of Martin Guerre (1593) and the Tichborne Claimant (1874), examples of the assumption of a false identity for personal gain. [Summaries of these cases were given by Polson (1955).]

The wrongful conviction of Mr. Luke Dougherty in 1972 and Mr. Lazlo Virag in 1969, mainly on visual identification, led the Home Secretary to set up a committee, under the Chairmanship of Lord Devlin (1976). Its terms of reference were to enquire into the law and procedure of identification in criminal cases; special attention was given to identification parades, dock identification and the showing of photographs. The Committee first met on 1st May 1974 and its report was published on 26 April, 1976. It contains a detailed account of the trials of these two men. Mr. Dougherty had his conviction quashed by the Court of Appeal. It was established by the police that the crime for which Mr. Virag was convicted was probably committed by another man. Mr. Virag was granted a free pardon and £17,500 compensation. It is outwith the scope of this book to detail the matter further.

The Committee warned that there was a special risk of wrong conviction when a case depends wholly or mainly on eye-witness identification. An entirely sincere witness can be mistaken and there was no forensically practicable way of detecting this sort of mistake. Recommendations were made and it was suggested that a booklet be published for guidance especially of magistrates and police officers.

The living may also be identified by handwriting, and, although this is surer ground than personal impressions of appearance, gait or voice, it always calls for expert opinion.

The conviction of Adolf Beck depended in no small measure upon his handwriting, and upon an expert's opinion, which was subsequently retracted. At the same time, the method has value, as witness the innumerable occasions on which bank cashiers identify signatures on cheques often by a mere glance, and how rarely they find it necessary to confirm their authenticity. The investigation of handwriting in relation to criminal matters, and of disputed documents, is a complex and highly skilled procedure, which has been detailed by others, e.g. Osborn (1929), Ainsworth Mitchell (1944), Lucas (1946) and Harrison (1958). It must suffice here to say that the formation of the written characters is accompanied by certain peculiarities which are guides to the identity of the writer. These peculiarities can be forged, but their consistent reproduction is difficult to achieve. It may be possible to deceive the inexperienced, but few forgers can succeed in misleading the expert, who can demonstrate, by photographic enlargement and other means, discrepancies in a forged document, or can show that a given document is in all probability authentic.

It is also possible to identify, if not the operator, the machine used to prepare typescript, because each has its own peculiarities which are produced during its manufacture and in the course of wear and tear. Each machine, therefore, imparts its "signature" to typescript.

The police, notably in Glasgow, maintain files which record examples of typescript by most, if not all, of the new and obsolete makes of typewriter. It is possible, therefore, to narrow the search in the first instance to a particular make, and thereafter to limit the examination to that of typescript by selected machines.

Fingerprints, palmprints and sole- or toeprints are unique as a means of identification, both of the living and the dead. Although theoretically subject to error, the possibility of mistakes with this method is infinitely remote. The demonstration that when two separate impressions contain even eight points of similarity—although in practice sixteen are proved—is tantamount to strict proof of the fact that they must have been made by one and the same person. Attempts to discredit fingerprint evidence are occasionally made, notably by reference to dissimilarities between the two impressions. This defence is likely to fail, as in *R. v. Hoyle* (York Assizes, 1953), because proof depends on coincidence of similarities. Where this is unequivocal, there can be no reasonable doubt about an identification which is based upon them.

There are two subsidiary tests of identification of the living which, for obvious reasons, cannot be applied to the dead. It is possible to question the living in order to test their *mental calibre* and educational standard. On this ground, the illiterate Orton should have been readily exposed as an impostor when he pretended to be Sir Roger Tichborne. It is also possible to test the *knowledge* and recollection of the living in relation to specific matters. Here the impostor, as in the case of Martin Guerre, may prime himself with a close and intimate knowledge of sufficient detail and accuracy to permit him to mislead even near relatives of the person whose identity he has assumed.

Photography is a valuable aid in the identification of the living but may be useless in the identification of the dead. The family of the victim of the Luton sack murder, *R. v. Manton* (1943) failed to recognise photographs of the deceased's body. Appreciable change, exaggerated by putrefaction, can occur in the features after death. It would be wrong also to assume that excellent photographs never lead to error in the identification of the living. When one Will West, a negro, was admitted to jail, the records officer thought he recognised him as an ex-convict. The negro denied that he had even been in prison. When the officer produced the record of a convict named William West, the prisoner at once accepted the photograph in it as that of himself but could not understand how it had been obtained. Indeed, the reproductions of the photographs of the two negroes are indistinguishable and their anthropometric measurements were almost identical. A comparison of the finger-prints of Will West and those on the record of William West, however, at once proved that they were two distinct persons (Wilder and Wentworth, 1918).

Pulse rate has been reported as a means of identifying suspects ("Identification", *Medicine, Science and Law*, 1963). Two men ran away after breaking into a café at Scarborough. Shortly afterwards they were seen by a constable when they were then seated in deck chairs. He felt their pulses and, because the rate was fast, he arrested them; they were later convicted and sentenced. It is doubtful whether he had had valid consent. Many, faced with a policeman and alleged to have committed an offence, however innocent, might well react by an increase in pulse rate. It is also possible that the officer was in fact recording his own pulse, raised by chasing the offenders.

Identification of the dead

The problem of identification of the dead, as in the case of *R*. v. *Ruxton* (1936), is especially difficult when the murderer has not only dismembered the body, but has also mutilated it in ways calculated to obscure its identity. Although these are matters outside the scope of a pathologist, some knowledge of the procedure is part of his professional equipment.

The first problem is to decide whether the remains are human or animal. Next, if human, it is necessary to determine whether they are the remains of one or more bodies. Thereafter, the primary and secondary characteristics of each call for detailed investigation. When the remains are skeletal, their dating must be undertaken (see pp. 57–61).

The primary characteristics are those of sex, age and stature, and they may at once serve to disprove a supposed identity. *Secondary characteristics* include the eyes, teeth, hair, scars, tattooing, finger-prints, external peculiarities, deformities, whether natural or due to disease, clothing and objects on or near the body, etc. Although not classed as a primary characteristic, the teeth can furnish nearly strict proof of identity.

The examination of the clothing is normally undertaken by the police and forensic scientists, but, notably with wounds of the trunk or limbs, inspection of the clothing by the medical examiner is essential for his interpretation. Identity may often be established by laundry marks, tailor's labels, tears, or missing buttons. It is also possible that a button firmly grasped by a victim may lead to the detection of the assailant as in *R*. v. *Greenwood* (1918) where wire used to fasten it to his coat was of a peculiar kind (Humphries, 1953). Pocket books and papers, an identity card, watches, rings, etc., all aid in identification. When the body is incinerated metal objects amongst the ashes may be significant, e.g. a gold denture in the Parkman case (1850).

The primary and secondary characteristics are next considered separately in detail.

The Determination of Sex

The determination of sex, even in the living, is not always simple. It is important that the sex of an infant is correctly determined and recorded at birth, but mistakes can occur when as a result of congenital malformations (the "adreno-genital" syndrome in particular), a female infant may appear, externally, to be a male with hypospadias (F.M. 996). Young's monograph (1937) on *Genital Abnormalities, Hermaphroditism and Related Adrenal Diseases*, provides an exhaustive account of these matters, and, not least, an interesting chapter on their history.

In civil law the sex of a person has importance in relation to rights and duties reserved to one sex alone; it may also be relevant in causes which concern legitimacy, inheritance, divorce or nullity, etc.

When a mistake is discovered it is necessary for the birth to be re-registered. An application must be made to the Registrar General who, if satisfied by the information, will instruct the sub-district registrar to re-register the birth. Alternatively, statutory declarations by two persons, one of whom be a registered medical practitioner aware of the facts, may be accepted for the purpose of re-registration. This step was necessary when a child, believed to be a male with hypospadias, was proved by necropsy to be a female (F.M. 996). Her sister also had the adrenogenital syndrome and died, in infancy, about a year later.

Ordinarily, the determination of sex in the living depends upon presumptive evidence. The facial appearance, hair, bodily habit and clothing are normally distinctive, but there are males of feminine type and females of masculine type. The female, moreover, is not infrequently given to dressing in male fashion and males sometimes masquerade as females. Males may grow their hair long and submit to permanent waving, whereas females may find short hair styles fashionable and so forth.

Physical examination by a doctor will yield highly probable evidence of sex, namely the condition of the breasts and the external genitalia. It is normally sufficient, to prove sex, to have palpated a uterus or testis. In civil cases proof of sex by the production of operation or necropsy records, the authors of which are deceased, would be adequate. Certain proof is obtained by microscopical demonstration of ovarian, testicular or prostatic tissue, i.e. the demonstration of gonads or structures exclusive to one sex. Prostatic tissue can occur in the female but the amount and position distinguish it from that of the male (Young, 1937).

It should not be assumed, however, that this problem is simple and precise even when the scope of the examination includes microscopical studies of the gonads. There are very rare instances of an ovo-testis, and the absence of fully developed gonadal tissue is occasionally observed. It was the experience of Harrison (1954) that in a number of subjects examined by him sex was difficult to ascertain "even from histology of the reproductive tract, since there were remnants of both Müllerian and Wolffian tissue . . . examination of the pelvis gave the best guide on deciding the true sex". He had also found that "intersexuality can be associated with poorly developed sexual characteristics, not only in the soft tissue, but also in the skeleton".

The determination of sex in criminal proceedings is particularly important when the body has been dismembered and mutilated, as in *R. v. Ruxton* or *R. v. Dobkin*. In the former case the discovery of two vulvae amongst the remains and, in the latter, of a uterus which was affected by a "fibroid" were material observations.

The Determination of Sex by an Examination of the Skeleton

The determination of sex by an examination of the skeleton is based in the main upon the appearances of the pelvis, the sternum, the skull and the long bones. Additional information may be obtained from the scapula and metacarpal bones. Details of this subject, together with a review of the then recent information, were given by Harrison (1953) in his report on the examination of the skeletons of two of Christie's victims, namely Miss Eady and Miss Fuerst.

The sexing of skeletons was also studied by Thieme (1957), and by Iordanidis (1961, 1963). The latter concluded from his study that, given a skull and a femur, accurate sexing was of the order of 97.75 per cent; with the pelvis alone it was 97.18 per cent. In collaboration with Eliakis, he determined the sex of long bones on the basis of their medullary index; for this purpose the tibia, humerus, ulnar and radius were employed (Eliakis and Iordanidis, 1963a). They also found a correlation between this index and the age of the subject (Eliakis and Iordanidis, 1963b).

The present account is restricted to the principal criteria; the comprehensive account by Krogman (1962a), in his classic *The Human Skeleton in Forensic Medicine*, should be consulted for details.

The Pelvis

When available, the pelvis is a valuable guide to the sex of the subject, and it was estimated by Washburn (1948) and Krogman (1962a) that the pelvis alone was sufficient to establish the sex of not less than 90 per cent of subjects.

Washburn relied upon the ischium-pubis index because the older criteria, e.g. the subpubic angle, are dependent on, and are secondary to, elongation of the pubic bone. He argued that the measurement of its length is not only easier but also gives an estimate of the primary variable. He found that providing major racial groups are treated separately, the ischium-pubis index was higher by 15 per cent in over 90 per cent of females than in males. This index is determined by measurement of the length of the ischium and pubis from the point at which they meet in the acetabulum; the technique to be used is that of Schultz (1940; cited Washburn, 1948). The method is not simple, and Harrison stressed that "his criteria for measurement must be strictly followed", since the measurements are made in a particular manner.

Washburn also considered the shape of the greater sciatic notch to have value, since this may be a primary characteristic of the bone (Fig. 6). It was alone capable of determining sex in over 75 per cent of subjects. Hrdlička (1952) attached special importance to this feature and believed no other sex determinant had greater value. Harrison (1954) found the greater sciatic notch to be especially valuable in sexing the bone. It may be used also to sex late foetal material (Boucher, 1955).

A pre-auricular sulcus marking the attachment of the anterior sacroiliac ligament is

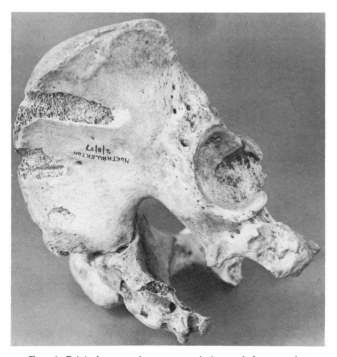

FIG. 6. Pelvic bone: male; narrow sciatic notch but see also
Fig. 7.

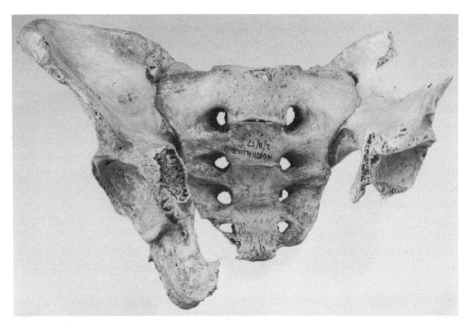

FIG. 7. Pelvic bone: Female; well marked pre-auricular sulci. (Same pelvis as that shown in Fig. 5.)

also of value as a sex determinant (Fig. 7). Recent investigators have found it well marked in female skeletons examined by them.

The value of the pelvis as a sex determinant, in skilled hands, is such that Harrison could say, "In fact, immediately the skeletons were received, examination of the pelvis allowed the deduction of the sex to be made confidently". Caution is necessary, however, because the features shown in Figs. 6 and 7 were those of the *same* pelvis.

The Skull

Determination of sex by an examination of the skull, which is the part most frequently presented, is essentially a task for the expert. There may be times when he can give a confident opinion without lengthy examination, but on most occasions, he will first prefer to examine several features before expressing any opinion. Harrison (1954) stressed that "the determination of the sex of the skull cannot be made from one characteristic alone, but must be assessed from the examination of a number of features taken together. The best characteristics are probably those of: the supra-orbital ridges, the mastoid processes, the dimensions of the palate, the outline of the orbit and the characteristics of the mandible." Furthermore, he pointed out, "it is only after the age of fourteen to sixteen years that the male characteristics begin to develop". It is his experience that up to that age it is often "exceedingly difficult, if not impossible, to sex the skull". Krogman (1962a) considered the examination of the adult skull, alone, yielded an accuracy of 90 per cent.

The Mastoid Process

Schmitt and Saternus (1970) in a study of 105 skulls, of which sixty-one were male and forty-four female, found a sex-linked difference in the surface area of the mastoid process. No significance was found in the mean values of the lateral and medical measurements but there was significant difference in the surface area, which was greater in males. This was probably accounted for by the insertion of stronger lateral neck muscles into the male process.

The Sternum

The ratio between the length of the manubrium and the body of the sternum should be determined. "The manubrium of the female sternum exceeds half the length of the body, while the body in the male sternum is at least twice as long as the manubrium" (Hyrtl, 1889). This rule was criticised by Dwight (1890) in whose opinion it was of no practical value; this is the modern view (Krogman, 1962a). On the other hand, Iordanidis (1961, 1963) claimed an accuracy of 80 per cent with the sternum alone.

The Long Bones

The determination of sex by an examination of the long bones is uncertain unless they have characteristics which are unmistakably either those of a male or of a female. They must be longer, heavier and show more pronounced ridges, impressions, articular surfaces, etc., than is possible in a female, before it is reasonable to assume they are those of a male.

The femur is probably the most valuable of the long bones for sex determination. Its percentage accuracy, with a single adult bone, is about 80 per cent, but the standards used should be those of the appropriate group of the population (Krogman, 1962a).

Harrison (1953) attached great importance to "the gross configuration, thickness, size of femoral head, compared with the rest of the bone" and also muscular and ligamentous markings and the X-ray appearances. These features, in his view, are as reliable as any series of measurements.

The Scapula

The height of the glenoid cavity is greater in the male. On the average it is as 3.92:3.36 cm in the female and the dividing line is 3.6 cm (Dwight, 1894; cited Harrison, 1953).

The Metacarpal Bones

These bones are shorter and narrower in the female, e.g. 41.6:47.4 (length) and 13.2:15.3 (breadth) for the index finger. Further details of Borovansky's results, compiled from girls and boys aged 18 years, and those of the Christie victims were tabulated by Harrison (1953).

Histological Determination of Sex

Barr and Bertram (1949) and Barr, Bertram and Lindsay (1950) demonstrated, with illustrations, a difference in the morphology of the nucleolus of nerve cells in the two sexes. Their studies of nerve cells of cats revealed that "In the female, a body about one μ in diameter appears as a small satellite to the large nucleolus in all types of nerve cells examined. In the male, nucleolar satellite is seldom seen distinctly. There is evidence that male nerve cells contain a nucleolar satellite so small that it lies at the limit of resolution with standard optical equipment." These authors believe that the nucleolar satellite may be a product of the X chromosome.

Similar findings were obtained with other tissues, e.g. human skin. Moore *et al.* (1953) found it a means of determining the chromosomal sex of pseudo-hermaphrodites. Barr (1954) and Barr and Hobbs (1954) used the method to determine chromosomal sex in transvestites. Hunter *et al.* (1954) found, given good fixation and staining, the examination of skin biopsies enabled them accurately to determine the sex of the patient. They recommend fixation in half-saturated mercuric chloride, in 15 per cent formol saline. The Feulgen reaction is better and easier than haemotoxylin stains. Killpack (1954) suggested that areas with thick epidermis or, alternatively, a wart or naevus or other blemish, should be selected for the purpose of sexing the skin. Emery and McMillan (1954) also demonstrated the value of skin biopsy in determining sex. The method is capable of application to medicolegal practice in the field of identification. A further development of yet greater practical importance is the demonstration of a morphological sex difference in the polymorphonuclear neutrophil leucocytes. Davidson and Smith (1954) described the occurrence of a solitary nuclear appendage of drumstick form in the white cells of females, where its incidence was about six in each 227 neutrophils but none was found in 500 neutrophils in the male. The examination requires experience in order to distinguish the "drumstick" from the appendages but a skilled observer made no error in the correct sex determination of each of fifty films from patients whose sex was not known to him. Age has no influence on this cell feature. Davidson (1960a) described these neutrophil drumsticks as structures with a dense chromatin head 1.5 $\pm$ in diameter, and characteristically, they are separated from the rest of the nucleus by a thread-like connecting neck. Nodules with a short thick neck and sessile nodules, although nearly diagnostic of the female neutrophils, also occur, but these are more difficult to distinguish from other nodules found in both sexes. Difficult or important cases call for the application of the Davidson and Smith test; six drumsticks are sought and in the normal female these are found in under 300 neutrophils whereas in normal males none are found in 500 or more neutrophils. Davidson recommends that the result be recorded as chromatin-positive or chromatin-negative rather than female and male. (See also Ashley (1957) on sex chromatin in blood and marrow, and Dixon and Torr (1956) on sex determination from cell morphology).

Cells of the buccal mucosa also exhibit sex differences. Moore and Barr (1955) applied the original method to smears of the buccal mucosa and provided a useful confirmatory test in the investigation of cases of doubtful anatomical sex. (See also Marberger *et al.*, 1955, and Greenblatt *et al.*, 1956.) The female "nodules" are also well defined in cells of cartilage and supra-renal cortex and in amniotic fluid (Davidson, 1960a).

It was claimed that microscopical examination of hairs may also permit the diagnosis of sex. Tovo and De Bernadi (1958) examined the whole bulbs of several hundred hairs obtained from thirty females and ten males. They found sex chromatin in 70 per cent of the female but only 7 per cent in male hairs. The test may have some confirmatory value but it is valueless unless a fair number of epithelial cells adhere to the hairs and an interval of less than 3 weeks has elapsed since the hairs were shed or torn from the subject. Another difficulty is created by super-imposition of nuclei in some specimens. A clear result is likely at best in only 80 per cent of cases.

These methods of sex determination are of considerable practical importance. In addition, however, the original discovery of Barr and Bertram has opened a field of research into the study of chromosomal structure. Davidson and Winn (1961) showed that the neutrophil drumstick and the nodule in the tissue cell are probable homologues and they represent a major part of the XX Chromosome mass.

Although Davidson considered that this work is only beginning, as indeed it may be, his article provides a valuable summary of the not inconsiderable advances already achieved.

The technique for demonstrating the sex of nuclei was described by Davidson (1960b); see also Moore *et al.* (1953).

An aceto-orcein staining method, devised by Sanderson and Stewart (1961), disclosed detail of nuclear structure permitting a high degree of accuracy in determining sex from an examination of oral smears. A correct diagnosis was made in 239 of 240 smears: the exception was an apparent example of triple-X syndrome. Only two false positives, (i.e. "female") were obtained with smears from males and these were cases of medullary dysgenesis. The test is claimed to have specific value when the female nodule is present. Error is more likely when, in its absence, the smear is diagnosed as one from a male.

Sexing based on the nuclear structure of white blood cells and those of skin, given satisfactory technique, could attain an accuracy of 100 per cent and even with post-mortem material it could be 85.5 per cent (Davidson, 1960a).

The Determination of Age

External inspection of the dead permits only an approximate estimate of age and it is liable to error by up to 10 years where the subject is an adult. Age, however, is a primary characteristic in identification, and its estimation is of importance; in infants, in relation to the crimes of child destruction and infanticide; in adults, murder, etc.

The skeleton and, when present, the teeth, are the principal sources of information upon which estimates of age are based. Some, like Krogman (1939, 1946, 1960, 1962a), are prepared to regard the study of the skeleton as an exact science which permits accurate determination of age, sex, and stature. There is no doubt that investigations of the kind made by Brash (1937) in the Ruxton case and those by Harrison (1953) in the Christie case narrow the issue of the nearest possible limits, and indeed, are almost exact as to age, sex and stature. There is danger, however, in the assumption that in any hands or on any occasion there will be the same degree of accuracy; there can be over-confidence in the scope of these investigations and the value of the results. Stewart (1948) warned against this and urged the need for caution.

Krogman (1960) reviewed the reliability of the identification of human skeletal remains. Where the age exceeds 20 years there is great variability, due to intrinsic and extrinsic factors, but it is possible to attain accuracy to ± 1 year in the first 2 decades. After

20 years reliability is only within a decade. Here the pubic symphysis is of best value and, with other parts of the skeleton, accuracy may be within about ±1 to 2 years. In sexing skeletons, accuracy is about 50 per cent with those of persons under 15 years but if the pelvis be available accuracy is then raised to 75–80 per cent. In the adult Krogman claimed 100 per cent accuracy if the entire skeleton is available; 98 per cent for skull and pelvis; 95 per cent for pelvis alone or 90 per cent for skull alone; the long bones alone permit accuracy to 80 per cent. Stature reconstruction formulae, of appropriate kind for sex and race, yield an accuracy of M ±2 S.E. or a 1:22 chance of being within ±2 in. to 3 in. of the true stature. Investigations of this kind demand the maximum amount of material available and Krogman stressed that great care should be exercised by the police to recover every fragment of bone.

In his *The Human Skeleton in Forensic Medicine* (1962a) Krogman said he had used the ten phases described by Todd for 30 years and found them to work "but they do tend to over-age, especially in the later decades of life". He found them more reliable in relation to the period of from 20–40 years than after that age. He considered the pubic symphysis as probably the best single criterion of the age of a skeleton and its study can register age in lustra of 5 years. In the third and fourth decades, the features of the pubic symphysis, with other skeletal criteria, would permit him to venture an accuracy of plus or minus 2 years.

For ordinary purposes, however, it is simpler, and no less accurate, to consider only three phases, namely (a) the new-born infant; (b) children and adults under the age of 30; and (c) adults over the age of 30 years. This division is adopted here.

(a) *The New-born Infant* The major problem with this group is to decide whether the child was viable, i.e. it was born after the 28th week of gestation; and if viable, if it was also mature and thus better able to overcome the hazards of delivery and the assumption of a separate existence.

These estimates are based upon the weight and length of the infant and the distribution of ossific centres in the skeleton.

The weight, although less important than the length, is easier to determine accurately than the length. At the 28th week the infant should not weigh less than $2^1/_2$ lb and, for practical purposes, if a single birth, any infant of less than 3 lb may be presumed to have been born before the end of the 28th week. Correction is necessary for sex, since the female infant normally weighs about 3 ounces (100 g) less than a male, and also for multiple birth.

The legal period of viability must not be confused with obstetric criteria, where a birth weight of below $5^1/_2$ lb is considered to show prematurity.

The crown-heel length is not easy to ascertain precisely but, when that is practicable, the result is probably the best single guide to the assessment of the age of an infant. The length in centimetres, divided by 5 or, if in inches divided by 2, represents the age in months of infants born after the 20th week of gestation.

Simpson (1969) relies, in the main, on the crown-heel measurement, which in his opinion permits assessment of attainment of the 28th week "with fair accuracy".

Appreciable reliance was placed in the past upon the distribution of *centres of ossification* (Fig. 8). It is now recognised that there is variation in the times of their appearance. With this in mind, however, their distribution has value in the assessment of

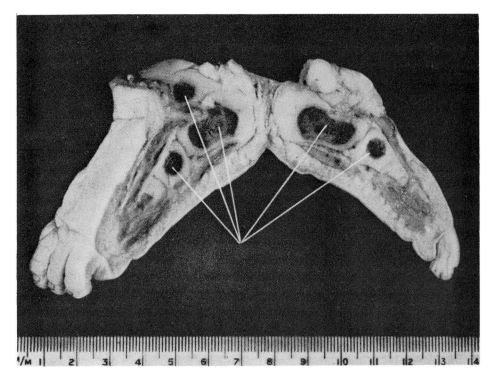

FIG. 8. Centres of ossification.

the age of an infant. When centres are found not only in the os calcis, the astragalus, lower end of the femur and in the cuboid bone, it is probable that the infant was mature at birth and had almost certainly attained the 28th week of gestation. These matters are considered in greater detail in Infanticide (see p. 514). Certain centres may be of value in assessing age up to about 5 years.

The time of appearance and fusion of ossification centres, as observed by rontgenographic methods, was the subject of a comprehensive survey by Flecker (1942). This, together with his earlier survey of the times of appearances of epiphyses and their fusion with diaphyses (Flecker, 1932) are standard references.

(b) *Children and Adults Under the Age of 30* The times of union of the epiphyses are only approximate because there is individual variation, but even so they have value in the assessment of age. The skeleton can be examined radiologically or the several bones may be directly inspected. A record of their condition, showing which epiphyses persist and which are united, is made. Reference is then made to tables, e.g. those of Flecker (1932) and of Krogman (1962a), which detail the ages at which union normally occurs.

Examination of the *spheno-occipital joint* may show that the subject is a young adult of an age between 17 and 25. In *females* this joint unites at about 17 and 20 and incomplete union at 25 years is exceptional. Glaister and Brash (1937), who found union, but with the line of union still recognisable in Body No. 1 of the Ruxton case, thus fixed the probable age at 20 to 22 years, and almost certainly between 18 and 25 years. The victim, Mary Rogerson, was aged 20 years.

The *clavicle* is the last of the long bones to become united. Union of the inner end (sternal) begins between the ages of 18–25 and may not be completed until 25–30 years; at 31 or over it is complete (see the table by McKern and Stewart, reproduced by Krogman, 1962a). It was the only long bone which remained incompletely united in the skeleton found in our area (F.M. 11,285B) and it provided corroborative evidence that the remains were those of Mrs. W . . . Her identification rested more certainly on a repaired upper denture (see p. 66).

Examination of the *vertebral bodies* can extend the period of assessment of age to about 30 years. Schmorl's studies showed that the immature vertebral body is characterised by "a series of deep radial furrows both on the upper and lower surfaces". This feature increases in prominence up to the age of 10, and then gradually fades at from 21 to 25 years. It may, however, persist to between the ages of 25 and 30, but there was no instance of vertebral furrows after the age of 30 in Schmorl's 8000 specimens (Beadle, 1931). This test was applied in the following case when Giese (1932) relied upon it to expose an attempted fraud on an insurance company:

Mr. A., aged 32, insured his life and disappeared. Later a body was found and identified by articles belonging to A. Determination of the age from the bones and, in particular, the vertebrae, proved that the dead person was less than 30 years of age because, in addition to persistence of epiphyseal lines at the lower ends of the radius, ulna and femur, there were distinct furrows on the vertebral surfaces, especially in the lower dorsal segment of the spine. The body, therefore, was not that of "A".

Assessment of the period 20–24 years also turns upon the condition of the pre-sacral vertebrae, at which age there is fusion of the secondary centres in epiphyseal plates with the upper and lower surfaces of the vertebral bodies (Krogman, 1946). Fusion of the sacral segments is usually complete by 25 years, but may be incomplete, in traces only, even until middle age (Harrison, 1953).

Further subdivision of this group is left to the expert. He may prefer seven or more groups.

(c) *Adults over 30 Years* Precise assessment of age is impossible but an estimate may be attempted by an examination of the condition of the skull sutures. These do not close at the same time but, on the contrary, there is a progression in the times of their closure. Some may remain open indefinitely. Closure at the inner table usually precedes that at the outer table of the skull.

The frontal suture is the first to close and this normally takes place early in life. Brash (1937) considered total absence of closure unlikely after the age of 30 years. The sagittal, coronal and lambdoid sutures normally begin to close at from 20 to 30, followed, about 5 years later, by the onset of closure of the parieto-mastoid and squamous sutures, which, however, may remain open or only incompletely closed at 60; the spheno-parietal suture does not usually close until the age of 70.

Franchini (1946) examined 629 skulls and found that there was no closure of sutures in four of them despite the fact that the subjects were aged, respectively, 45, 48, 55, and 74 years. A skull sent to me for examination had all sutures open but the jaw bone was clearly that of a middle-aged person (Figs. 9 and 10). In view of these observations and the lesser variations which occur, estimates of age based on the condition of the skull sutures must be guarded. Singer (1953) goes further and regards precise assessment of age on this evidence a hazardous and unreliable procedure.

The study of the cranial sutures as a guide to age seems to fascinate; there were no less than six reports, including that of Singer, 1953, during 1952–9, notwithstanding the extensive survey of Franchini (1946) which threw doubt on the value of the test. Perhaps the report by Dérobert and Fully (1960), based on a study of 480 skulls, will at last establish the unreliability of estimating the age by the condition of the cranial sutures. They considered it a criterion of value but one which must be interpreted " . . . avec la plus grande prudence". They said that they had examined skulls of over 60 years of age without finding a trace of obliteration of the sutures. Krogman (1962a) considered "estimation of age of the skull via suture closure is not reliable", but he would venture to place a skull in a decade, and if the skull is alone available that is the best one can do. Cave and Steel (1936) found that, contrary to previously held views, there was no evidence that the cranial vault thickened or thinned progressively with advancing years or that the diploic tissue disappeared in old age.

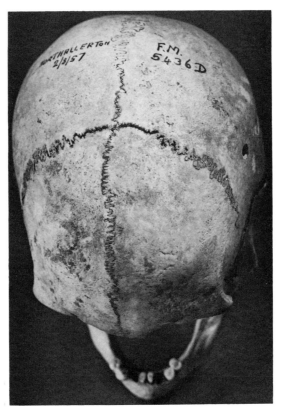

FIG. 9. Skull: Sutures as for a child but see jaw bone
on Fig. 10 (Side view of same skull.)

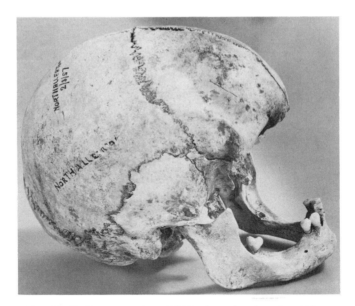

FIG. 10. Skull sutures as for a child but lower jaw that of a middle-
aged adult (same skull).

It does not appear that calcification of the larynx or ankylosis of the joints of the hyoid bone are better guides. It may be that these changes do not normally occur before the 40th year but our collection of hyoid bones shows much variation in the ages at which ankylosis has occurred.

Determination of age by inspection of the teeth: see Dental Identification, p. 61 *et seq.*

The Determination of Stature

The determination of stature is an important step in the identification of dismembered remains or when only the skeleton or part of a skeleton is available. It is possible to estimate, but it must be clearly appreciated only approximately, the probable stature of the deceased by assuming that the length of certain long bones represents a certain proportion of the total height. There are doubts about the validity of this assumption.

A simple means of estimating stature, which can go no further than to suggest whether the subject was short, tall or of medium height, assumes that the length of the humerus represents 20 per cent, the femur 27 per cent, the tibia 22 per cent and the spine 35 per cent of the subject's stature (Topmaid and Rollet, cited Ewing, 1923).

Those who embark upon this task must not only have the requisite knowledge and experience: " . . . The bones *must* be measured in a standard way and . . . an osteometric board must be used. Amateur calculations with tape-measures and calipers are useless" (Harrison, 1954). A modification of the Hepburn osteometric board has been designed by Dr. Trevor and this may prove to be a more accurate instrument.

Accurate, or apparently accurate, means of calculating stature from long bones were first devised by Rollet in 1888. His calculations were based upon the measurement of the cadaveric length of "fresh" long bones of fifty male and fifty female subjects in Lyons.

Ten years later Karl Pearson (1899) published tables for the estimation of stature, which were compiled by subjecting Rollet's material to mathematical analysis.

Pearson's formulae were deemed for many years the most satisfactory, superseding those of Rollet and of Manouvrier. In time, however, it was appreciated that Pearson's formulae yielded under-estimates. He had, however, recognised the need for separate tables for males and females and for fresh and dried bones. It has since been recognised that allowance is necessary also for ageing of the subject and racial differences.

It is clear that the estimation of stature by an examination of skeletal remains is a far more complex problem than it has been assumed in the past. It is now necessary to take into account not only the sex but also the race and age (growth in American whites is now no longer complete at 18 but appears to continue up to the age of 23). It is also important to use the same method of measurement of the bones as that used in the compilation of the tables to which the results are applied. More than one bone should be used and those of the leg yield more accurate estimates than those of the arm. Some allowance may have to be made for drying of the bones, but this is not a significant factor.

In the choice of the appropriate table for race, the skull or pelvis are better guides than the long bones, because their appearances are too variable to provide more than corroborative evidence of race (Krogman, 1962a).

In spite of the volume of research in this field it is doubtful if there is any material advance in accuracy, which was estimated by Pearson in 1899 as a minimum probable error of 2 cm. Krogman (1962) said that the calculated stature was correct within a certain range. "We may accept ± 2 S.E. (1:22) as a safe bet." He then gave an example of an estimated stature of 180 cm, one which lay between the range of 173.6–186.4 cm, a spread of 12.8 cm or a little over 5 in. The dogmatic witness, therefore, has been warned.

The problem received fresh attention during 1950–3 and, in particular, by Dupertuis and Hadden (1951), Trotter and Gleser (1952) and Harrison (1953). Although these considerable investigations have clarified the position, they have failed to provide a precise guide to the estimation of stature. Even careful measurement by skilled observers, as Keen (1953) said, will only yield estimates where the error "cannot be relied on to be less than $2^1/_2$ in. even in the most favourable circumstances. An estimate differing from a missing man's stature by $^1/_2$ in. therefore provides no greater proof of identity than one $2^1/_2$ in. different."

Dupertuis and Hadden (1951) based their calculations on the measurement of cadaver length and long bones of groups of 100 male and 100 female American whites and an equal number of both sexes of negroes. The stature of both groups averaged about 8.5 cm taller than for Pearson's series. As might be expected, the estimates from only one long bone were less reliable than from a combination of two or more. Estimates from bones of the lower limb were more accurate than those from bones of the upper limb. When race is not known, general formulae are used but, otherwise, formulae appropriate to race and sex yield more reliable estimates. Unlike Pearson, who allowed a standard amount, namely 2.5 cm, for lengthening of the body after death, these authors believed the cadaver length to be equivalent to living stature. Their formulae tend to yield results which over-estimate stature.

Trotter and Gleser (1952) compared the lengths of the long bones with the known living stature of the subject. Their comprehensive survey included, for example, a series of 710 white male subjects. In an earlier investigation (1951) they had also determined the correction for ageing, based on an examination of 855 bodies. It was found that after 30 years of age the loss was 1.2 cm per 20 years or an average annual loss of stature of 0.06 cm. They regarded the general formulae of Dupertuis and Hadden to have only apparent success because, by over-estimation, these tended to correct the under-estimates obtained with Pearson's formulae. They also disproved the assumption by Dupertuis and Hadden that the length of the cadaver represented the living stature; an increase by 2.5 cm was found to occur, thus confirming the older investigations.

In 1958 Trotter and Gleser reconsidered the problem and revised their calculations after a study of skeletons of victims of the Korean war; the subjects included negroes and whites, as well as mongoloid races. It is necessary, if approximation to precision is to be attained, to see the appropriate tables for race as well as sex. Although there was no material difference between the proportions for negroes and Puerto Ricans, they found it otherwise for white, negro and mongoloid skeletons. It was also found that the standard errors of estimates from the long bones of white subjects were larger than in their earlier studies. It had been assumed in the past that maximum stature had been attained at 21 years but it is apparent that maximum stature in American whites is now attained at 23; during World War II it had been attained at 18 years.

The review by Boyd and Trevor (1953), although valuable, had to be made without knowledge of the work of Trotter and Gleser. Reference should be made, in preference, to the observations of Harrison, who illustrated the relative value of these recent calculations by their application to the known measurements of five subjects. His analysis confirmed the systematic negative error yielded by Pearson's formulae. Although he found no evidence of a systematic positive error with the Dupertuis and Hadden formulae, he advised caution in assuming that such error does not exist. "The same reservation must be made in inferring that the scatter of the estimates is not significantly different as between the Trotter and Gleser and the Dupertuis and Hadden general formulae."

Harrison was more optimistic than Keen (1953) about the possibilities of these investigations. If it be correct to assume that the standard error of estimate from a single bone is the same for each used, then "the effect of averaging estimates based on several bones will be to reduce this standard error in proportion to the square root of the number of bones used. In this way the confidence limits for the presumed height may be considerably reduced in range". He finds no reason "to prefer the estimate based on any one bone to that based on any other; therefore the best estimate should include all the information available, and this involves either using a multiple regression equation based on all the available bones, or averaging the estimates obtained separately from all the bones".

Determination of stature from the height of the spine was first suggested by Dwight in 1878 in an essay on the "Identification of the Human Skeleton" (cited by Dwight, 1890) and elaborated by him in 1894 when he furnished tables for calculation of the stature by using a given coefficient by which to multiply the length of the spine of each of the sexes. In other tables he compared his results with those of Jopmaid, Rollet and Manouvrier. He concluded that his method was subject to an error within an inch in one-half of the cases but in a quarter of the cases it was likely to exceed 2 in.

Estimation of stature by combining the length of a long bone (femur or tibia) with the height of the spine was studied by Fully and Pineau (1960). They claimed that given a group of three vertebrae, estimates of stature were "assez bonne" and a group of six vertebrae, e.g. D 5–7 and L 1–3, yielded "la précision excellente". Their regression equation was:

Height of spine = 3.205 (height of D 5–7 + L 1–3) + 34.8 mm + K 9.6.

A reassessment of the estimations of stature from the length of long bones by Wells (1959) led him to the doubts about the accuracy of the results. He reviewed the tables of Pearson, of Dupertuis and those of Trotter and Gleser, including those revised by the latter in 1958. In his opinion there was need for further study in order to check the latest American formulae. This might show that the limits might prove even wider than the tables suggest. Estimates to be used in a criminal case, therefore, should allow a generous margin for possible error. Wells also commented on the uncertainties inherent in estimating stature from long bones.

Estimation of the Stature of Children

The tables for the calculation of stature all refer to adults. It is only recently that attention has been given to methods for the estimation of the stature of children.

(a) *Radiographic measurement.* This study by Telkka *et al.* (1962) was made on children under the age of 15 years of known height. The radiographic measurements of 3848 pairs of long bones were analysed. A regression formula, based on the length of the diaphyses, was devised and the results yielded errors somewhat higher than those obtained with adult formulae. Three groups of children were studied, i.e. those between 10–15, 1–9 years and the third of infants under the age of 1 year.

(b) *Measurement of the tibia.* This study was instigated by the need to assess the height of kyphoscoliotic patients and thus their pulmonary function, which is related to stature. What would their height have been but for the spinal deformity? Tables for adults were unsatisfactory. Zorab *et al.* (1963) obtained a regression equation based on the measurement of the length of the right tibia, from the inner condyle to the lower border of the internal malleolus. No significant difference was found in the two sexes.

Stature = (2.59 × tibial length) + 49.84 males.
(2.53 × tibial length) + 67.22 females.

The results were ±7.6 cm of the predicted height.

The dating of human bones

Whenever skeletal remains are discovered, for example in the course of excavation for building or road widening, they should be submitted to expert examination. It is normally a simple matter to distinguish between human and animal bones, but if human, their dating is difficult and the examination rarely, if ever, permits a precise estimate of the time interval since deposition in the ground. At the same time it is possible and important to decide whether they are "ancient" or "modern" bones, i.e. the interval is greater or less than 50 years. Obviously, if over 50 years, and certainly 75 years, and the death was due to some criminal act, there is little prospect of apprehending the culprit. The case of Mamie Stuart who disappeared in 1919 and whose remains were found and identified in 1961 is a good example of this limitation. The person believed to have been responsible for her death died in 1958 (Knight, 1971).

Until recently attempts to date bones were based in the main on their morphological appearances. From my own "sins" in this field I can agree with Knight and Lauder (1967) that the estimates were made with a confidence inversely proportional to experience.

It is indeed important, as Knight (1971) stressed, to have prior knowledge of the conditions of concealment. He had seen complete skeletonisation within 3 weeks, during a period of hot weather. We have seen it within a period of 18 months (the case of Mrs. W. F. M. 11,285B). At the other extreme, remarkable preservation of the bodies, but with decalcification of the bones, was observed in the remains of the Tollund and Grauballe men, whose deaths occurred some 2000 years prior to discovery of the remains. Dating by radiocarbon examination fixed the interval at between A.D. 210 and 410, and, allowing for error of 100 years on either side, the probable date was A.D. 310 (Glob, 1965).

Providing the environmental conditions of concealment be taken into account, it is possible to determine whether the bones be "ancient" or "modern", although precise dating is as yet impossible. This has practical value in that, if clearly "ancient", the police do not waste valuable time in identifying the deceased.

In recent years, a considerable amount of research has been carried out in an attempt to increase the accuracy of dating skeletal remains. Some of these depend on sophisticated laboratory techniques, such as radio-carbon analyses, which are difficult and expensive to perform. Radio-carbon is essentially a tool for archeologists, as its forensic use is limited because of the insignificant fall in the C-14 content of bones during the first century after death. This is the stumbling block for many physical and chemical methods for bone dating, as although old samples (in excess of 100–200 years) can fairly readily be differentiated from recent bones, discrimination between the dates of skeletal remains recent enough to be of interest to law enforcement agencies and coroners, is too poor to be of much practical use. However, some workers, such as Villeneueva (1980) claim that statistical analysis of several chemical parameters can give accurate results even in recent specimens.

Knight (1969 and 1971) and Knight and Lauder (1967) published details of a battery of physical and chemical tests which were helpful in discriminating between bones of recent enough age to be of medico-legal interest and those of greater antiquity. However, later (so far unpublished) work by Knight failed to confirm the reliability of these tests for bones less than 50 years since death—unfortunately the very period which holds the most forensic importance.

The environmental conditions are more potent than age in causing progressive degeneration of the bone: even different parts of the same skeleton (and even opposite ends of the same long bone) may be quite different in their chemical and physical properties, if local changes in inhumation such as drainage, are marked. Bones in wet peaty soil may be decalcified and crumble within two decades, yet bones in dry gravel or sand may remain almost pristine for millenia.

Naked-eye appearances can be very deceptive, but bones with remnants of periosteum, tags of ligament or soft tissue other than adipocere are likely to be less than 5 years old, unless kept in a dry protected place. A "soapy" texture of the surface, from residual fat, also indicates a date of less than a few decades.

Light, crumbling bones are likely to be in excess of a century since death, unless environmental conditions were severe.

Useful laboratory tests include the following: the results of each test should be interpreted in the light of the others and with due regard to the macroscopic appearances and the fullest information of the place of concealment and any circumstantial evidence.

(a) *Nitrogen content*: new bones contain 4.0–4.5 gm % of nitrogen, derived mostly from the collagenous stroma. After a variable interval following death, usually longer than 60–100 years, this declines. A value of 2.5 gm % usually indicates an age of at least 350 years.

(b) *Amino-acid content*: estimated by autoanalyser after acid hydrolysis of the residual protein. Up to 20 acids may be found in bones less than a century old. They then decline in number and concentration. Earlier work using thin-layer chromatography suggested that proline and hydroxyproline (constituents of collagen) vanished by about 50 years, but the more sensitive modern methods of analysis do not confirm this.

(c) *Blood pigments*: using the most sensitive, though nonspecific tests, blood remnants were found up to a century. Now that benzidine is proscribed as a laboratory reagent, due to its alleged carcinogenic activity, alternative tests such as phenolphthalein and leuco-malachite green fail to detect blood after 5–10 years, using either bone dust or the periosteal surface as the test area.

(d) *Fluorescence*: under ultra-violet light, fluorescence is seen across the whole freshly-sawn surface of a long bone for more than a century, but beyond that time, declining fluorescence is seen advancing from both the outer surface and the marrow cavity. The "sandwich" of fluorescence progressively narrows during the first 50 years and may vanish within 300–500 years, though it may persist in patches for a millenium.

(e) *Immunological activity:* eluted extracts of bone when tested against animal anti-human serum give a visible antibody-antigen reaction, either in cross-over electrophoresis or by passive diffusion in gel. Early work suggested that this persisted for 5–10 years, but recent repetition of the tests indicated that it ceases within months of death. Much depends on the efficiency of elution and the successful concentration of the extract.

Summary

A "modern" bone of potential medico-legal interest is one in which the nitrogen content is over 4.0 gm %: there should be at least 15 amino-acids discernible: it should fluoresce over the whole cut surface of a freshly-sawn diaphysis: if positive blood pigment and immunological activity tests are obtained, it must be within a very few years since death.

The demonstration that apatite crystals in bone increased in size in correlation with the age interval led to the proposal of their examination as a means of bone dating (Chatterji and Jeffrey, 1968). This method requires access to a stero-scan electron microscope, the skill to use it and to interpret its results.

Circumstantial evidence has importance. It could be, as at Arthington in Yorkshire, that the remains were those of a member of an ancient nunnery long since demolished. The site was consistent with that of its burial ground. Archeological assistance may help to decide whether the bones were ancient, as for example bones found in the vicinity of

Pontefract Castle on the site of the Battle of Marston Moor. In the event that articles accompany the bones, e.g. clothing or personal possessions, their design may indicate the period, e.g. prehistoric weapons or tools. Jewellery bearing a hallmark is also significant, if not precise, for dating. It could be, as near Leeds in 1950, an upper denture. This not only pointed to "modern" skeleton but it played an important part in the identification of the individual (F.M. 11,285в).

It is regretted that Knight's scheme was not available in 1950 when a skull and a pair of femora were found amongst rubbish on a hill-side at Knaresborough. Recollection of the case of Eugene Aram no doubt led the police to conduct a large-scale search, but no other parts of the skeleton were found. The bones were of normal weight and consistence; they had a smooth, somewhat polished surface, as by repeated handling. They were not tinted by iron. In the upshot, they were deemed to have been anatomical specimens which had belonged to a doctor long since departed from the district, and that they had been rejected, along with other rubbish cleared from an attic where he had resided. A second opinion was obtained from Professor Harrison who agreed that they were probably anatomical specimens. The appearances were those of negroid bones; there were pronounced femoral marks for the insertion of thigh muscles. Up to the date of finding these bones, coloured persons were unknown in the district. There was no report of a recently missing person whose characteristics coincided with those of the remains.

Dental identification*

Historical Note

With the exception of the alleged identification of the body of Charles the Bold, after the Battle of Nancy in 1477, by the absence of four front teeth from his lower jaw (Humble, 1933a), interest in dental identification appears to have been lacking until the early part of the nineteenth century.

Dental inspection was then used as a check on the age of children, either to ascertain whether they were under the age of 7 years—the then age of culpability—or under the age of 9 years, when, under the Factory Act, 1837, it was unlawful to employ them in a factory. A survey of some 338 children was the basis of the classic pamphlet "Teeth, a test of age", published by Saunders in 1837. His confidence in being able to assess the age of a child to within a year of the actual age was not shared by Spokes (1905) whose survey of over 600 children disclosed a distinct variation in the time of eruption of the second molar teeth.

Extensive and detailed study was made by Clements *et al.* (1953). Their observations on the mean time of eruption of the permanent teeth were based upon an examination of 1427 boys and 1365 girls aged 5 to 13 years. The mean times of eruption of the teeth in the pubescent of a superior socio-economic group tended to be earlier than those of other children. The mean time of eruption of the teeth of boys was, with the exception of the first molar, later than those in girls. The order in which the teeth erupt, as judged by investigation of the central incisor, canine, both pre-molars and the first and second molar teeth, showed considerable variation in both the upper and lower jaws. The most frequent

* Other contributions to this subject were by Thoma (1944), Bonnafoux (1960), Dechaume *et al.* (1960) and Fearnhead (1960).

order of eruption in the upper jaw was: first molar followed in succession by the central incisor, first pre-molar and second molar; in the lower jaw the central incisor was first to erupt, followed in succession by the first molar, the canine, first pre-molar, second molar and second premolar teeth. The third molar had not erupted in any of the children under examination.

The detailed findings of the authors cited are set out in a table in their report which should be consulted. It must suffice to say here that the first molar teeth of boys are likely to erupt at the age of from 73 to 74 months whereas, in girls, the age is from 70 to 72 months; the central incisors showed a wider range in time of eruption, which was 72 to 84 months in boys and 69 to 79 months in girls; similarly with the lateral incisors, of which the corresponding times of eruption were 88 to 98 months and 84 to 94 months, respectively.

The eruption of the third molar is especially liable to variation; moreover, these teeth are prone to be impacted. When they have erupted, the person's age may be not less than 17 years, but in some boys over 15 a third molar may be visible. Eruption of the third molars, although not usually delayed beyond the 21st year, may not occur until, say, the 23rd to 25th years, even when there is no impaction.

At about the same time (1837) dental identification of the person also received attention. Prior to the Anatomy Act, 1832, theft of bodies from churchyards to provide material for anatomical dissection became rife. The body of a woman alleged to have been stolen by the Resurrectionists was eventually found in a dissecting room. Although dissection was advanced, a dentist was able to identify the body because he found the condition of her teeth and jaws tallied with casts he had prepared for a patient (Ogston, 1878).

Identification by a dental chart of an unknown person and its circulation amongst dentists with a view to its recognition as that of one of their patients appears to have originated in Vienna. The police invited a professor of dentistry to prepare such a chart, and, in due course, a dentist to whom it had been circulated produced a record of one of his patients and the data coincided with the dental chart of the murdered woman. The dental identification was of special value because the assailant had worn gloves and had not left any fingerprints at the scene (Gollomb, 1931).

The composition of fillings can be important. One of the victims of the Stalheim Hotel fire was thus identified. At first sight he appeared to have amalgam fillings, but when one of them was treated with hydrochloric acid the blackening by fire was cleared to reveal a gold filling.

If some unusual compound be used as a filling, this can be of importance; Meyer (1933) suggested the chemical analysis of fillings as a means of identification.

The first detailed identification of the victim of murder by dental evidence was that of Dr. Parkman by Dr. Nathan C. Keep in 1850. The ashes in the laboratory furnace in Professor Webster's laboratory contained some mineral teeth and a gold denture. The denture was identified as one made for Dr. Parkman, in particular by marks of grinding on the gold— "the beauty of it was defaced by the grinding". Dr. Keep explained that grinding had been necessary to make more room for the tongue. (A verbatim record of the dental evidence is given in Dilnot's *The Trial of Professor John White Webster*, 1928).

Dental evidence, although of minor importance, provided corroboration of the probability that Ruxton had extracted teeth, in his attempt to conceal the identity of his victims. Dr. A. C. W. Hutchinson was of the opinion that the condition of the sockets was that of teeth extracted after death. The radiological appearances of the skull of one of the victims showed that except for the third molars, the second dentition had been complete. Calcification of the unerupted third molars permitted an estimate of age as between 18–20 years; Mary Rogerson, the maid, had been on the eve of her 20th birthday. The other victim might have worn a partial denture but no certain opinion was possible; no such denture was found (*R.* v. *Ruxton*, 1936).

The identification of Mrs. Dobkin was established by the crucial evidence of Mr. Kopkin, her dental surgeon. Having reason to believe the skeleton to have been the remains of Mrs. Dobkin, the police traced her dental surgeon and he was asked to examine a skull at Guy's Hospital, and to take with him his record of Mrs. Dobkin. He said in evidence: " . . . I picked up the skull when I first went into the laboratory itself, and recognised it immediately as being the skull of a patient I had once attended, because it corresponded in so much detail." He produced his record of the upper jaw of Mrs. Dobkin (the lower jaw of the body was missing). This was in the form of a mirror image, annotated sketch. The data, which included a note regarding two residual roots, corresponded precisely with the condition of the upper jaw of the skull. It was also shown by X-ray examination that there were two residual roots in the upper jaw. In his summing up Mr. Justice Wrottesley said that the evidence as to the sex, age and stature of the skeleton made it possible that the remains were those of Mrs. Dobkin, "but now you see, we come to something quite different, something definite and precise . . . The coincidence . . . is remarkable . . . you may think it has gone beyond coincidence, especially when linked up with all the other evidence . . . " (*R.* v. *Dobkin*, 1942).

In 1943 a body in a sack was found by two workmen in a stream. Post-mortem changes precluded identification by a photograph of the woman's face which was unrecognisable. Casts were made of her mouth and in due course they were recognised by Mr. Jacob Rackham, who produced his dental record of a Mrs. Manton whom he had last seen alive in May 1943. She was edentulous but had some residual roots, which produced swellings in the alveolar margins. Dentures which he had then prepared for her fitted the casts of the unknown woman's mouth (Simpson, 1945). It so happened that coincidentally the woman was identified by a fingerprint. In the course of a routine questioning of persons in the neighbourhood, the appearance of a young woman who opened the door to one of the officers resembled that of the dead woman. It was Mrs. Manton's daughter. A search of the house failed to yield any fingerprints which corresponded with those of the dead woman, until a disused pickle jar in the cellar was examined. This bore a single print which tallied with that of one of the dead woman's digits.

Dentures proved the identity of the last of Haigh's victims, Mrs. Durand Deacon. At the trial in 1949 Miss Helen Mayo, her dental surgeon, identified the set of dentures as those she had supplied to Mrs. Durand Deacon. She recognised them by certain peculiarities and could have described these dentures from her notes before she saw them. She was not cross-examined, since Haigh had decided to seek the special verdict of guilty, but insane (*R.* v. *Haigh*, 1949).

The detailed study by Professor Miles and Mr. Fearnhead, of the teeth and jaws of the two bodies buried in Christie's garden, provided valuable corroborative evidence that they were the bodies of Ruth Fuerst, an Austrian, and Muriel Eady (*R.* v. *Christie*, 1953). An unusual feature of special importance was a shell crown of the kind common in Central Europe but rare in England.

Several accounts of dental examination in the identification of the victims of mass disasters are now available. The importance of dental co-operation was recognised in 1878 when victims of a fire at the Vienna Opera House were identified by their teeth (Hofmann, 1882).

In more recent times it has become apparent that these complex investigations call for an elaborate plan, operated by a team of experts, of whom the dental surgeons are important members (Keiser-Nielsen, 1951). The magnitude of the task is well illustrated by the account of Grant *et al.* (1952) who identified several of the victims of the *Noronic* disaster. Fire broke out in this cruise ship while tied up in Toronto harbour. Fire spread rapidly and soon the ship was a blazing furnace. Passengers on board were trapped and when the fire was eventually quelled it was found that 118 passengers, forty-one male and seventy-seven female, had perished. After a matter of 5 months' intensive work all but three of the victims were identified. Owing to extensive damage of the features by fire dental evidence was of special importance. Of these 102 bodies examined, twenty were identified solely on dental evidence, it was a first lead in another twenty and assisted in identification in yet another nineteen bodies. Dental examination was impossible in nineteen and valueless in twenty-eight. The report embodied useful recommendations as to procedure and stressed the importance of accurate dental records.

The fire, which destroyed the Stalheim hotel near Voss in Norway in 1959, caused the death of twenty-four persons. The medical and dental investigations were conducted by Waaler and Ström. Six of the victims were identified by dental evidence and another nine by a combination of dental evidence and objects of value on or near the bodies. The victims included a number of Americans and, because their X-ray, as well as dental, records were available, their identification was appreciably simplified (Waaler, 1960).

[One woman was identified at first as a male by what appeared to be a gold watch case, engraved with a man's name. Information was received from America that a Miss R. C. possessed her father's watch case and had had it converted into a compact. It was then recognised that the object found near the body was, in fact, a compact, made from a watch case.]

Other circumstances in which dental examination played an important part in identification have included. the identification of Danish patriots who died in German concentration camps during World War II (Keiser-Nielsen, 1951) and victims of a railway accident in which a passenger train collided with a train of petrol waggons. Fire broke out and the engine and first coach of the passenger train were enveloped in flames for about 12 hours (Ström, 1946). Victims of aircraft accidents have also been identified by dental examination and there are a number of reports of these investigations (e.g. Stevens and Tarlton, 1963).

Another development in dental identification has been, in the main, due to Gustafson of Sweden, whose system of ageing teeth has attracted considerable attention. He first became interested in the macroscopic appearance of teeth as an index of the age of the person in 1947, when studying microscopical changes in teeth in relation to age. He devised a six-point system of macroscopic changes by which age can be estimated but even his expert use of the system appears to limit the estimate at best to ± 7 years of the actual age.

From time to time attempts have been made to include identification marks on dentures. During World War II the Canadian Dental Corps incorporated a piece of nylon, bearing the name of the patient, in acrylic dentures (Grant *et al.*, 1952). It has been suggested that the mark could be made in radio-opaque material (Warren Harvey, 1966). The problem is not as simple as it might seem and a search for a satisfactory solution continues.

The institution of a Public Dental Service and the provision of school dental officers has proved an important advance in the care of children's teeth. It has also resulted in the compilation of dental records which can be, and have been, valuable in the identification of the bodies of children. Two of the victims of Brady and Hindley had to be identified by other, less satisfactory methods because no dental records were available; both children were under school age (*R.* v. *Brady and Hindley*, April 1966, Chester Assizes). Brady did not appeal but Hindley's appeal, C. A., 17 Oct. 1966, was dismissed.

In a later case the child victim of homicide was positively identified by her school dental officer Mr. Graham Turner (see p. 65).

The case of Linda Agostini emphasised the importance of accuracy in the preparation of dental charts of "unknown" persons. When her partly burnt body, enclosed in pyjamas, was found in a sack at Albury in 1934, a dental chart was prepared and circulated. It was unrecognised by any of the dental surgeons. Ten years later, acting on information, the police reopened the case and an inquest was held. It was then apparent that the initial chart had omitted to mention the dental work on a first and second bicuspid.

The revised dental characteristics were then recognised by Mr. O'Brien, a dental surgeon in Sydney, as identical with those of his patient, Linda Agostini. Despite a disagreement between Mr. O'Brien and Mr. Bell concerning the filling of a molar tooth (Mr. O'Brien was confident it was one he had made in a first molar, and not a second molar tooth) the Coroner was advised to accept Mr. O'Brien's identification (Cleland, 1944).

Modes of Dental Identification

(i) DENTAL CHARTS

Inspection of the teeth is an obvious initial step in the identification of the dead, especially, in circumstances such as fire or aircraft disasters, when the features are destroyed. The value of this, however, depends first on a skilled and detailed examination and, second, on the existence of an accurate dental record of the person. There are two further requirements, namely a standard chart in general use for recording the condition of the mouth and, in the matter of dentures, a satisfactory mode of marking; the existence of an X-ray of a person's mouth is also of considerable importance.

The first step is to obtain the assistance of a competent dentist who prepares a detailed chart of the mouth. This is then circularised amongst dentists so that they can compare the data with records of their patients. Keiser-Nielsen (1963) made the important point that, in the identification of victims of mass disasters, the dental surgeon should attend the scene and personally select material for examination.

Identification by a dental chart has been and, in all probability, always will be the most important mode of dental identification. Unfortunately it has its limitations. In the *Noronic* disaster it became apparent that, at that time, there was "an appalling failure" on the part of dentists to keep any accurate records. The clear distinction between left and right was often lacking. Some records were in code intelligible only to the dentist himself. It also appeared to have been the practice of the dentist to record only the treatment personally given; the records failed to include details of treatment by other dentists. Marking of dentures was absent. These defects added greatly to the task of identifying the victims (Grant *et al.*, 1952).

Even accurate records have value directly proportional to the extent of the data available for comparison. It is possible, especially in children, for two patients to have similar charts (Gustafson, 1966). If there is only one filling, for example, it might well be in the same tooth in two or more children. On the other hand, extensive treatment, especially of a more unusual kind, can be conclusive evidence. A patient is in mind who has seven crowned teeth, several fillings and three extractions; her dental chart, if not unique, would readily permit her identification. Gold bridging was the outstanding feature which led to the identification of a skeleton (Knight, 1966). A crown of palladium–silver alloy was important corroborative evidence in the identification of the skeleton of an Austrian woman, murdered by Christie (Miles and Fearnhead, 1953). Evidence of an apicectomy was important in the identification of the body of a British officer killed in Egypt.

Under satisfactory conditions, the correspondence between the dental chart of the "unknown" and the record of a patient is capable of being proof of identity. This obtains if there are several points of similarity. The minimum number to constitute proof has not been decided. In fingerprint identification eight points of similarity are sufficient but, in practice, sixteen are the standard requirement. Half a dozen are probably sufficient for dental identification—the Dobkin case is a guide.

Whenever practicable the method should be used in conjunction with investigation by an anatomist or physical anthropologist and the best results are obtained by their combined efforts (Stewart, 1963). Anatomical examination, alone, cannot go further than the demonstration that the remains were possibly those of a particular person. It requires dental or digital evidence to prove it must have been that person. In the *Noronic* disaster, dental evidence alone provided proof of identity in twenty cases; it was the first lead in another twenty and provided corroboration in another nineteen of the 102 subjects examined.

The value of accurate school dental records was demonstrated by Mr. Graham Turner when he identified the skeleton of a child buried in the Yorkshire Moors. This child died at the house of a man accused of causing her death. He confessed he had buried the child and took the police to the place of burial. She had had several teeth filled and these, fortunately, still remained in the jaws. Their condition tallied precisely with the dental records of the child and within 15 minutes it was possible to confirm her identity (F.M. 13, 34417).

It is the practice of the Scandinavian Air Service to require all crew members to prove dental and fingerprint records (Keiser-Nielsen, 1963).

(ii) IDENTIFICATION BY DENTURES

No doubt when a satisfactory and universal system of marking dentures is at last established, dentures will be an invaluable aid to identification of unknown persons. Even without this aid, it is sometimes possible for a dental surgeon to identify dentures supplied to a patient. Miss Helen Mayo relied on certain peculiarities in her positive identification of dentures found on Haigh's premises as those she had supplied to Mrs. Durand-Deacon, one of Haigh's victims (*R.* v. *Haigh*, 1949).

An upper denture found beneath the skull of a young woman was recognised by a dentist as having the design his late father used in their practice. Their dentures had longitudinal ridges on the upper surface, as in this one, to give better adhesion. It was also their custom to preserve the canines; they were present in the skull. The denture had been repaired and a dental technician was confident that he had made this repair. The dental and anatomical evidence proved sufficient to satisfy the coroner of the dead woman's identity. Indeed, the only person who persisted in doubt and refusal to accept this, was the woman's husband (F.M. 11,285B).

(iii) TEETH, A TEST OF AGE

1. *The Foetus and Neonatal Infant* The determination of age in infancy was studied by Stack (1960), who devised a method based on gravimetric observations on the developing dentition. Growth status of the teeth was assessed by weight determination of dry mineralised tissue. It was thus possible to ascertain the age of the foetus between the 24th week and birth. The mean difference between the recorded and estimated ages was about 1 week during the period of 38th to 42nd weeks. Due allowance must be made for delay in development in cases of maternal toxaemia or placental deficiencies, which could cause delay of from 2 to 4 weeks. Delay also occurred in the presence of multiple pathological features, but less frequently where abnormalities of the circulatory or central nervous systems were disclosed. It is a complex method and requires study of the original text.

2. *The First Dentition* Assessment of the age of an infant between the age of 6 months to 2 years is practicable by observation of the condition of its first dentition. Any such assessment requires due allowance for individual variation. Whilst baby's first tooth should appear at about the 6th month, it may appear somewhat earlier or be delayed until the 8th month or later. Delay is likely in the severely subnormal child. In normal circumstances the first dentition is complete at the age of 2 years. [It is possible for a tooth or teeth to have erupted at the time of birth; instances were shown by Professor Hopper (Presidential address, 1971 Leeds and West Riding Medico-Legal Society).]
Tooth formation begins at the 3rd to 4th months and measurement of the width of the dentine provides an estimate of foetal age. Thus, at the 28th week, it is 2.9 mm wide in the central incisor and 2.4 mm wide in the canine and molar teeth. Longitudinal sections of the first molar of the newborn at term (36 weeks onwards) demonstrate a "neo-natal line", which forms at birth, when there is a temporary arrest of dentine formation for about 14 days. The width of the dentine, in relation to this line, provides an estimate of age; dentine is formed at the rate of about 4μ per day.

3. *The Second Dentition* The second dentition was first studied as a test of age by Saunders (1837), who examined some 300 boys aged 13. Spokes (1905) also examined boys (638 subjects) aged between 13 and 15 years and selected eruption of the 2nd molar teeth as his test material. Individual variation, apparently absent in the series of Saunders, was appreciable. Thus in boys aged 13–14 years all four second molars were erupted in 62 per cent, but in 4 per cent none had erupted. Although eruption of all four molars had

occurred in 82 per cent of boys aged 14–15, none had erupted in 2 per cent of this group. John Hunter (1835) recorded an instance of a third dentition.

4. *Age Determination by Inspection of Individual Teeth* Credit for the development of this method of age determination, however, is due to Gustafson (1947–66). He devised his well-known six point system which is based on an observation of the macroscopic appearances of teeth and the six features which are considered are: (a) attrition, (b) paradentosis, (c) secondary dentine formation, (d) cementum apposition, (e) root resorption and (f) root transparency. The observer notes the degree of each of these changes and scores points of up to a maximum of four for each.

Examples given by Gustafson (1966) include a case of slight attrition as the sole change. This was assessed at 1.5 and the total score was 1.5, indicative of an age between 14 and 22 years; the actual age was 18 years. In another test there were appreciable changes yielding a score of 12 points which indicated an age between 66 and 76 years; the actual age was 68 years.

It is an attractive method, not least because it calls for a minimum laboratory preparation of the material for study and leaves the specimens in a state which enables others to confirm or refute the observations. It is not surprising that it has attracted considerable attention, by way of approval, modification and condemnation.

Its principal weakness lies in the determination of the results by subjective examination. Only one of the six features is capable of precise measurement, namely, root transparency (Miles, 1963). The intuitive method by "visual guess", used by Miles and Fearnhead (1958, 1963), yielded results comparable in accuracy to those obtained with the Gustafson system.

Gustafson (1966) made it abundantly clear that his system is not for the inexperienced. The observer should not only have a knowledge of dental histology and pathology, but considerable experience. From time to time he should check his assessment against documented samples (Stewart, 1963). Moreover, the expert should ever be mindful of Gustafson's own statement that "after the age of 14 it is extremely difficult to estimate the age of any individual by the teeth". With great respect, it seems that the results of the expert, let alone the inexperienced, should be accepted with caution.

The possible degree of accuracy is indicated by the results of a control study of Gustafson's method conducted by Seifert (Pilz, 1959; cited by Gustafson, 1966). The average error by the Gustafson system was ±9 years; that with Seifert's method was ±8.9 years. It was also found that when front teeth were used by Seifert he reduced his error to ±7.4 years, whereas the pre-molars and molars increased the error to ±14.3 years.

Dalitz (1962) failed to confirm the accuracy claimed for the Gustafson system. He rejected root resorption and cementum formation as significant changes. With a four-point system, allotting a maximum of 5 for each change, he claimed an accuracy of ±6 years in 35 per cent of his tests. Given a single tooth he found the standard deviation of error was ±18 years.

In view of the standard of proof still required in criminal cases, the possible range of error of up to ±18 years, the method has little practical value. Even a result of ±6 years is not calculated to identify a person precisely, but it might have some corroborative value. Since these methods depend so much on subjective examination their results might be unable to withstand informed cross-examination.

At a meeting when this system was described to a group of dentists, a speaker in the discussion, a dentist of considerable experience, posed this question: "What allowance would the expert make for the possibility that the person from whom the teeth came was accustomed to grind his teeth when he played a round of golf?"

(iv) IDENTIFICATION BY BITE MARKS*

The alignment and occlusion of our teeth are specific characteristics which approximate in value to that of fingerprint impressions as signs of personal identity. Although reliable fingerprint identification requires expert opinion, identification of bite marks is even more complex. The material by which to gain experience is scanty and when received it may have been modified by interference or delay; the latter permits shrinkage due to drying (Fearnhead, 1961).

It is essential that the collection of material and its examination are undertaken only by dental surgeons and, preferably, by those who have special experience. Indeed, Ström (1963) goes further and considers that a positive opinion on a bite mark should always be agreed by at least two experts whenever practicable. He found the examination of bite marks simpler and of greater value as a means of *exclusion* of a suspect. Positive identification was more difficult and less certain. (His paper contains valuable practical advice.)

It is important to remember that in England it is still necessary to obtain valid consent before making a dental examination and taking a cast of a suspect's mouth. Ström wanted legislation in Norway to permit this without consent; compulsory examination is unlikely to be sanctioned in England, since the liberty of the subject and freedom from self-incrimination without consent still receive recognition.

Priority in the recognition of bite marks as veritable "signatures" is not clear, but the first practical techniques and analysis were described by Sörup (1924, 1926) who called it "Odentoscopie". He obtained plaster casts of the mouth of the suspect. After these were dried and varnished their incisal and occlusal surfaces were coated with printer's ink and pressed into moistened paper of good quality and a transparency of the bite was prepared. This was compared with the "unknown" mark. Precise coincidence is presumptive evidence of identity; lack of coincidence excludes the suspect.

In 1906 one of two men who had broken into a store left his bite marks in the side of a cheese. The man not only consented to the taking of a cast but did so with keen anticipation. He had taken the precaution to knock out the stump of one of his teeth subsequent to his arrest in the belief it would preclude identification. This seems to have been the first occasion on which identification was established by fitting a dental cast into bite marks in food (Annotation, *Brit. Med. J.*, 1906).

An early identification of bite marks in human material was reported by Reiss (1911). A murderer was identified by bite marks of his front teeth in his victim's breast.

The material in which bite marks have been identified include human skin, and a variety of food stuffs, e.g. cheese, chocolate, butter and fruit. The best marks for study are those in firm material, notably cheese. Those in fruit have value only if fresh, because bruising of the flesh extends rapidly and modifies the mark. Marks in human skin may be distorted

---

* See page 69: a subject fraught with difficulty.

since its elasticity may modify the mark as soon as the teeth are withdrawn. Modification is also likely if the specimen for examination is not collected with care. A breast bearing a bite mark should first be examined *in situ* and the breast then removed entire for detailed study, it being unsatisfactory to dissect off only the skin and subcutaneous tissues bearing the mark.

Bite marks may be evident only as patterned, elliptical bruises. An identification based on bruising alone should never be admitted in evidence (Fearnhead, 1961). These serve only to prove that the person has been bitten, or the part subjected to suction. Bleeding subsequent to the bite is likely to enlarge and distort the mark. It is otherwise when the skin has been punctured by teeth and the ellipse includes punctures and bruises, as in the case of Gorringe (*R. v. Gorringe*, 1948; Howe 1949). Punctures of the skin of his wife's right breast, corresponded in position with four lower and two upper teeth in the casts of Gorringe's mouth. (Illustrations of these marks are reproduced by Howe, 1949, Simpson, 1951, and Gustafson, 1966. A moulage was prepared by Cuthbert, 1958, and he presented a plaster cast copy to the Department of Forensic Medicine, University of Leeds.) Identification was established by demonstrating a precise coincidence between the mark on the breast and a bite mark with casts of Gorringe's teeth, using the Sörup technique or a modification of it, as described by Humble (1933a, b).

Other techniques have been devised for the identification of human bite marks. Ström (1963) substituted a layer of fatty lipstick for printer's ink in the Sörup technique. He considered the preparation of a phantom, as in the complicated technique of Buhtz and Erhardt, unnecessary.

The identification of bite marks in foodstuffs is well illustrated by the matching of a cast of the upper jaw of a suspect with marks in cheese at the scene of a warehouse break-in (Nickolls, 1950, Fig. 11). Identification was established not only by the fit of the cast in the

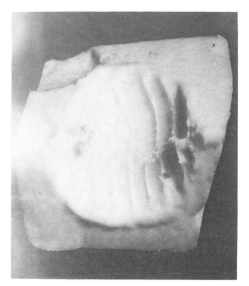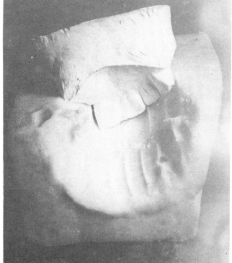

FIG. 11. Identification by bite-marks in cheese.

marks in the cheese, but also by scratches in the mark made by rough edges of the suspect's teeth.

Identification in this way should be established not only by the matching of the same number of teeth but by the demonstration of other coincident, minor features. Layton (1966) not only demonstrated the coincidence of the same number of the suspect's teeth and their marks in cheese, but, in all, twenty similar features. When confronted with this result, the suspect confessed.

Bite marks in cheese have also been reported by Anderson (1951) when the suspect, edentulous in his upper jaw, was not wearing his denture at the time, and by "West Sussex" (1954).

There are few reports of bite marks in fruit. Blench (1933) reported identification by a bite-mark on a part-eaten apple.

The identification of bite marks is further complicated by the fact that the mode of biting by the same jaws varies. The dynamics of the bite have to be taken into consideration. It is important, therefore, in identifying bite marks in foodstuffs that the test material is the same as that which bears the unknown bite mark. It must offer the same resistance and require the same force to bite it.

On all occasions, regardless of the material, the unknown marks must be examined and recorded with the minimum of delay.

Bite marks in human skin are modified by the circumstances. It may be the hurried, imprecise bite, as that of a"defence" bite, or a slow, deep bite by the sadist, as in sexual murder. The latter are likely to yield best material for identification. "Sadistic" sites include the breast, shoulder, neck, face and thigh. (We have seen an example of a "bruise" bite mark on a buttock (F.M., 594)). "Defence" bites are to be found on the hand or finger of an assailant (an example is depicted by Gonzales *et al.*, 1954).

Fortunately the majority of bite marks requiring identification occur in foodstuffs and these, as Ström said, are a much easier task to handle.

Changes in the Jaw due to Age

The lower jaw bone can give some indication, but only within wide limits, of the age of the subject; that is to say, it is possible to distinguish the jaw bones of an infant, an adult and an aged person. Thane (1899) described the jaw bone at birth as having a shallow body, and a very short ramus forming an oblique angle of about 140° with the body of the bone. Later, the body becomes thicker and longer and the angle between the ramus and the body less obtuse, until it is nearly a right angle. In old age, or after dental extraction, there is absorption of the alveolar margin, and the body again becomes shallow; the angle it forms with the ramus is increased to more than a right angle. In addition to this there may be, as a senile change, a distinct thinning of the bone, and, in consequence, the lower jaw may then be shattered by relatively mild violence. This is illustrated by my case of an old man who was found dead on the floor of his shop; he had not been seen for a few days. When he was examined, there was a gross deformity of the lower jaw, which led to the initial belief that he had been murdered. My examination of the mandible showed that, owing to senile atrophy, the cortext of its body had only the thickness of tissue-paper. While moving a packing case, he had accidentally tripped, and, in falling, he had struck his jaw on its edge. This caused comminution of the bone, and death was due, presumably, to shock.

Malocclusion

Malocclusion, if of an unusual kind, may aid identification, as happened when a decomposed body was found after prolonged immersion. The deceased had a malocclusion of uncommon kind, namely, Angel's Class III, i.e. protrusion of the lower jaw, with mesial occlusion of the lower teeth and the lower incisors inclined lingually. Angel found that it occurred in only thirty-four of the thousands of persons he examined (Angel, 1899).

The dental chart of an unknown person was valueless since it recorded only the extraction of a tooth. A photograph of the man was obtained, enlarged to life-size, and used in the manner of the Brash technique (Glaister and Brash, 1937). The result of this and the presence of an unusual malocclusion was accepted by the Coroner as sufficient evidence of identity (Berry and Hunt, 1967).

Forensic Odontology is now a recognised sub-specialty in dental practice. Recent research in this field was summarised by Whittaker (1982). The Gustafson's six-criteria method has received considerable attention and the current estimate of the degree of error lies somewhere between ± 3.7 years and ± 7 years., depending upon the experience of the observer.

The development of translucent dentine at the apex has been considered the most sensitive indicator of age. Bang and Ramm (1970), basing their estimates on 1013 teeth, claimed an accuracy of ± 4.7 years in 58 per cent and ± 10 per cent in 79 per cent.

Whittaker and Neale (1979), using a scanning electron microscope (SEM) techniques, found a rough correlation between tubules and age. They also showed that neonatal lines could be measured with the SEM techniques within hours or days of birth rather than the usual 2–3 weeks required when light microscopy was used.

Sex determination, heretofore, had been based on highly unreliable guesses but in 1973 Y chromosomes were demonstrated in pulpal tissue. Whittaker *et al* (1975) found the method less reliable than claimed, but were still able to detect sex in about 70 per cent of cases.

It had been suggested that blood group substances might be present in fragments of teeth. Whittaker says ABO systems have been demonstrated in bone and dentine and that exposure to heat destroys the ABO antigens.

Pink colouration of teeth some weeks after death is the product of breakdown of haem. Whittaker *et al* (1976) found that it was possible to produce the pigment in animal teeth but it was necessary that death was violent and some days or weeks passed before the pigment developed.

Lip prints might be used in the manner of fingerprints since it is claimed that no two persons have identical lip prints. It is also suggested that the pattern of the rugae of the palate might be unique. The situation in respect of bite marks is fraught with difficulty and can be extremely subjective. An elaborate technique using metal cast models of teeth, can relate the contours on a well-worn pipe stem with a particular dentition. It is clearly a highly specialised procedure and requires expert operation. Histological changes in bitten tissues may be indicative of the time since the bite.

Hair and Identification

Although only a secondary characteristic, the examination of hair can sometimes yield valuable evidence. It must be emphasised that this is essentially a task for the expert who, moreover, must have access to an adequate collection of standards, i.e. preparations of known hairs and fibres, for the purposes of comparison. Glaister's (1931) classical monograph, and his chapter in *Recent Advances in Forensic Medicine* (Smith and Glaister, 1939), where several of his former illustrations are reproduced with greater clarity, are the principal references.

The identification of a weapon responsible for murder may depend on the demonstration of hairs on it. In *R. v. Teague* (1851), for example, the victim had wounds on both eyebrows. The unsuccessful defence was that the hairs found on the hammer at the scene were goat hairs, the hammer having been used to beat a goat skin hanging on a hedge near the body. Examination proved, however, that they were human hairs, similar to those of the eyebrow of the victim. Hair on a hammer, used to destroy the victim, was one of the clues in the case of *R. v. Podmore* (1928).

In *R. v. Rouse* (1931) a mallet, found some 14ft from a burnt-out motor car, was soiled with mud in which three hairs were entangled. One of these was identified as a human hair of lightish colour; it had no root and appeared to have been broken. This evidence, however, played only a minor part at the trial.

The demonstration of hairs in a sack used to dispose of the body of a murdered child was important in another case because the hairs were identical with hairs from the head of the female prisoner (*R. v. Donald*, 1934; Glaister and Rentoul, 1966).

Motor vehicles responsible for injuries may be identified by the detection of hairs on the vehicle. This is of importance when someone is injured and the driver responsible fails to stop or to report the accident. Hairs found on a suspected vehicle are then compared with those of the injured person. The search should be directed to the parts below the chassis, as well as mudguards, radiator, etc.

Theft of furs has been proved by the demonstration of identical hairs on the clothing of a suspected person, or in a sack used for the removal of silver fox furs (Glaister and Rentoul, 1966).

Cattle maiming has been brought home to the offender by the demonstration of hairs, identical with those of the injured cattle, on the coat of a suspected person (*R. v. May*, 1926).

Charges of bestiality or of rape may also turn on the demonstration of hairs on the underclothing of the suspect. Hairs, identified as goat's hair, on a man's trousers led to a conviction of the former offence (Glaister and Rentoul, 1966). In a case of rape, hair removed from inside the prisoner's clothing was proved to be identical with the pubic hair of his victim (*R. v. Handley*, 1926; cited Glaister, 1931).

Fibres and hairs have a remarkable stability. Smith and Glaister (1939) demonstrated that fibres derived from the coverings of ancient Egyptian mummies retained their microscopical structure, and were readily identified as linen. They also found that hair from mummies belonging to the early Egyptian dynasties preserved clearly their taxonomic features and scarcely differed from fresh human hair.

Procedure

The examination is directed to the answers to the following questions:
    Is this hair, and, if so, is it human or animal hair?
    If human hair, from which part of the body was it derived?

What was the sex and age of the person?

Had the hair been altered by dyeing or bleaching?

Did it fall naturally, or was it forcibly removed?

If it had been cut, was the instrument blunt or sharp?

Glaister (1931) regards some of these questions as easy to answer, for example the first and second, but he admits that identification of the sex from a study of samples of hair may be impossible; he also cautions against any precise assessment of age. At best it may be suggested that the hair was from an infant, an adolescent, an adult, or an old person. Moreover, unless it is a representative sample which includes several hairs, grey hairs do not always mean old age; some become prematurely old and young persons may have localised patches of grey hair, a feature which may be inherited. A young acquaintance had dark hair, except for an almost white forelock present since early childhood.

The situation from which the hair came is best determined by the examination of transverse sections of hairs. Hairs of the head, which are soft, are round or oval, whereas the eyebrow hairs, which are stiff, are triangular or reniform in section.

Bleached hair is brittle and, in the mass, has a dry texture and a certain straw-yellow tint, unlike that of natural hair. Hydrogen peroxide or a bleach of nascent chlorine, produced by the mixture of bleaching powder and sodium carbonate, are the usual agents. Stoves (1943) says the agents attack the fibre as well as the pigments, and the shape of animal hairs may be modified.

Dyed hair, on macroscopic examination, may be detected by the presence of a segment of hair of natural colour near the scalp. If a body with dyed hair be exposed to rain, the dye, when water soluble, may run down and stain the clothing. Conversely, dye in the clothing may, in similar circumstances, colour the hair. Alteration of the colour of the hair with lampblack, flour, or chalk, may be detected by simple brushing and washing. Microscopic examination shows that even expert dyeing fails to produce a wholly uniform colouring; small undyed spots will be detected on the surface in the course of the hair. Glaister mentions that lack of uniformity of colour is to be found in undyed hair, but not to the same extent as in dyed hair. Modern dyes, e.g. "Inecto", are also detected by chemical examination (Green, 1920; Cox, 1929 and 1935).

The ends of a hair may tell of the mode of its removal. The hair bulb, if present, is normally rounded, but it forcibly extracted there will be rupture of the hair sheath and irregularity of the bulb; its surface may then appear undulated and show excrescenses. It is possible also to recognise crushing or bruising of the hair. The condition of the distal end may show whether it was cut by a blunt or a sharp instrument and whether this was recent or not.

Scars and Identification

Scars have long been accepted as a means of identification. St. Thomas was not convinced until he had examined the scars on the risen Christ (St. John xx, 25–28).

A single scar, when of unusual character, has significance of greater value than a tattooing, and the presence of two or more scars, corresponding in appearance and site with scars known to exist on the body of a missing person, raises a presumption of identity.

The mark of an alleged scar found on a piece of flesh amongst the scanty remains, believed to be of the body of Mrs. Crippen, was a prominent but strongly contested feature in *R.* v. *Crippen* (Filson Young, 1919). The medical witnesses agreed that the specimen of skin was from the lower abdomen and that it bore pubic hairs at one border, but the mark on it was held by the defence to be caused by folding whereas the prosecution maintained that it was a scar.

Single scars should be accepted with due caution as evidence of identity. In the old case of Lesurges (1794), a man, who was convicted and executed for murder, had been identified by a scar on his forehead. Some years later the real murderer was found to have an identical scar on his forehead.

The disappearance of scars was considered in *R. v. Orton*, alias Castro (1874). Sir Roger Tichborne was known to have had three distinct scars, namely, one of the eyelid, following a wound by a fish-hook, the scar of a seton in the arm, and a third, caused by venesection of a temporal vein. The absence of these scars from the body of Castro or Orton, the claimant to the Tichborne title, was unsuccessfully alleged to be due to their natural disappearance. It might be that one of the scars had become unrecognisable but it is improbable that all three had vanished. In two of my cases gunshot wounds were said to have been received some 30 years previously. No scar could be found on the first subject and only one small but quite distinct scar remained of two or more scars on the second subject. In the latter case the missile, or a part of it, had entered his chest and led to the formation of an arterio-venous aneurysm between the right internal mammary artery and the innominate vein (F.M. 321).

The Examination of Scars

Good lighting is essential when scars are sought for, and artificial daylight lamps are the only substitute for natural light.

The record should include the following details: their number, site, size (being accurately measured) and shape. Irregular scars should be sketched or, preferably, photographed. Of each scar there should also be noted: the level it bears to the body surface and its relation to the deeper tissues, whether fixed or free; smoothness or irregularity of the surface of the scar; its colour, and the presence or absence of glistening. The condition of the ends, whether tapering or otherwise, and the probable direction of the original wound should also be determined. In the living the presence or absence of tenderness is material to the assessment of the probable age of the scar.

When doubt exists about the presence of a scar in the living, the part should be rubbed briskly and re-examined. In this way scars over 35 years old become prominent because they remain as white areas (Taylor, 1956). Escaped galley slaves were detected by slapping the usual site of the brand, which, if present, soon became prominent as a pale area in the reddened skin (Devergie, cited Casper (1861)).

Suspected scars in the dead can be proved by microscopy, and, in particular, by sections stained to show elastic tissue. Scars invisible to the eye and indefinite by ordinary staining methods are then prominent because elastic tissue is not restored in the process of repair of a wound. An unstained gap occurs in the elastica at the site of the scar. Striae gravidarum, which superficially resemble scars, are recognised by the persistence of the elastica which, although stretched, preserves its continuity across the striae (Polson, 1962).

Wounds of organs or of the cornea are readily detected by the demonstration of scar tissue, which reveals their sites.

The Age of a Scar

In assessing the age of a scar due allowance must be made for the differences caused by one or more of several factors in the rate of repair. These include the site, size and nature of the wound, the vascularity of the part, the age and the subject and infection of the wound.

In spite of these difficulties, an attempt must be made to assess the age of a scar because the date of the infliction of the wound may be a material point in a criminal charge. The assailant may have been injured by the victim and, therefore, if the former bears a wound of an age which corresponds with the date of the attack, this may have value as circumstantial evidence. A bite, for example, is not excluded because the scar borne by the accused is not of a kind likely to be produced by teeth. The accused may have modified its pattern by applying caustics to it in order to escape detection (Smith and Fiddes, 1955).

The Erasure of Scars

The only satisfactory mode of erasure, as in the case of tattooing, is by excision and skin grafting, or, if the parts allow, suture of the edges of the excised area. Surgical treatment can improve appearance of a scarred area, but, inevitably, the result cannot be other than an exchange of scars, the new one being less obvious. Even when invisible to the naked eye, microscopy can still demonstrate the absence of elastic tissue in the scar.

The Medico-Legal Aspect of Scars

If, as the result of an accident, the injured person be disfigured, he cannot be compelled to submit to plastic surgery in order to lessen the defendant's responsibility. Nor may the defence attempt to mitigate the damages by reference to the possible benefits which the plaintiff might obtain from plastic surgery.

It may happen that an accused will attribute scars of wounds to disease or therapeutic procedures. In this event, it should be noted whether the site, size, etc., are of a kind likely to result from the alleged cause. Conversely, persons wrongly seeking redress for alleged injury may claim that scars, due to disease, are those of wounds. A jealous or vindictive woman, for example, may seek revenge by alleging that certain scars on her person, due to disease, were the result of an assault by the accused.

Identification by Tattooing

Tattooing, because it produces distinctive marks upon the individual, can be a means of identification and the more unusual the design, situation and extent, the greater is its value. At all times, however, there must be guarded reliance upon this means of identification since, as Henry Faulds (1911) pointed out, even the most elaborate tattooing, of which he depicted an excellent example, can be precisely reproduced on the bodies of two or more individuals, providing they are prepared to pay the price. The average kind of tattooing is never to be relied upon because it is likely to be reproduced in quantity and to be tattooed on approximately the same part of the bodies of several individuals, notably the back of a forearm or hand. Tattooing of the chest (Fig. 12) or lower limbs is occasionally seen.

Initials may have significance when on the body of a male since, on many occasions, they are likely to be those of the subject. It is otherwise if a woman's body bears initials since they are more likely to be those of an admirer. Brittain (1950) found that in the criminal population in the Los Angeles area there was over 60 per cent chance that two or more letters tattooed on a man were the initials of his name but that, with women, tattooed letters were infrequent and of less importance; when present they were often the initials of some male friend or relative. It has to be remembered, however, that the initial may be that of a diminutive form of the Christian name, e.g. "B" instead of "W" for William; it may also be that the initials are those of an alias, although it is more usual for the initials to be those of the original name.

Sexual proclivity may be indicated by a tattoo, e.g., "True Love", which we have seen with the separate letters on each digit; this is a sign manual of the homosexual. Designs adopted by prostitutes are intended to stimulate clients. The passive partner of a lesbian pair may bear the initials of her lover on the middle finger of the right hand. In France the tattoo of an eagle carrying a girl is restricted to pimps. Butterflies are the badge of burglars (a sign of their feelings when in action?) In the American West Coast it is said that a cross, tattooed between the index and thumb, surrounded by dots indicates the number of arrests they have experienced. (Post 1962). A "cobweb" pattern may be seen in drug addicts, at the sites of injections.

There have been "epidemics" of scarification and self-tattooing amongst school children, amongst girls as well as boys. They use either a needle or the point of scissors to inscribe the initials of boy or girl friend. One boy admitted dipping the needle in indian ink to make a more permanent mark (Polson, 1971). Tattooing of persons under the age of 16 was made illegal in 1969 (Tattooing of Minors Act, 1969).

Fading of tattooing, especially when the design has been executed with pigments other than carbon, is not unusual. Designs in red, green or blue pigments are likely to fade and even disappear within about 10 years. It is still possible, however, to say that a deceased person had been tattooed by the demonstration of the pigment in the lymphatic glands in his armpit. It will remain in that situation almost indefinitely. Tattooing with carbon pigment, which produces a blue or blue-black design, persists for remarkable periods and the design may remain clear for many years, especially if executed with gunpowder. The rate of fading depends not only on the composition of the pigment but also on the depth at which it penetrates the skin and the site which is tattooed. Parts protected by the clothing retain the designs for longer periods than exposed parts of the body. The influence of site is linked with that of its local lymphatic system by which route pigment particles pass from the tattooed area to the regional lymphatic glands. The degree of inflammatory repair, disrupting lymphatic paths, after the operation of tattooing, also affects the rate of fading.

Erasure of tattooing has for long been attempted by one or other of a variety of methods, some chemical, some electrolytic and others surgical. It has been claimed that the application of silver tannate, (a method introduced by Variot (1883–91); cited Shie (1928)) successfully removed tattooings in from 14 to 18 days. Irritants, for example Lysol, have been used, but this substance, which can be absorbed through intact skin and which can provoke an alarming inflammatory reaction, has its dangers. Small tattooings can be removed by the application of carbon dioxide snow; the resulting scar is slight. Unskilled attempts to erase tattooing, no matter what method be used, are calculated at best to result in the replacement of the design by a scar, which will call for adequate

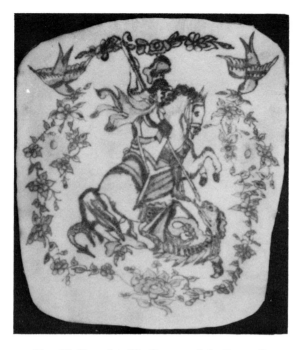

Fig. 12. Tattooing: "St. George and the Dragon."

explanation. The impostor Castro, who claimed to be Sir Roger Tichborne, erased the tell-tale initials of his true name, only to replace them by an ugly scar.

Surgical excision of the tattooed area, with or without skin grafting, as may be necessary, is the only certain and safe method of erasure. In skilled hands this may be eminently successful.

Females in a prison near York were being offered hospital treatment to have embarrassing tattoos, e.g., initials of former boy friends, removed from their arms. The treatment was free if advised by the prison medical officer. Acceptance was encouraged by the thought that removal gave them a better chance on their release. The treatment was probably by laser beam, under local anaesthetic (*Daily Telegraph*, Aug. 8, 1982).

The subject of tattooing is discussed more fully elsewhere (Polson, 1948).

Fingerprints, Palmprints and Footprints

The pattern of the friction skin of the body, whether of the fingerpads, palms or soles of the feet, is peculiar to the individual and affords the one mode of identification capable alone of establishing virtually strict proof of identity. The greater case of recording finger impressions and preserving their records has led to concentration on them, but it is not to be forgotten that a palm- or footprint affords an equally sure means of identification when fingerprints are not available for examination.

(My study of the history of fingerprint identification was published in the *J. Criminal Law and Criminology* (1950, 1951).

Although for obvious reasons fingerprints play the most important part in identification—and it is unfortunate that this is almost exclusively confined to the investigation of crime—palmprints, in the appropriate circumstances, have equal value. Footprints or toeprints likewise can be proof of identity. Although the late Colin Campbell, then of the Lancashire Constabulary, was the first to identify a criminal by a footprint, his claim to priority was denied because the culprit, when confronted by this evidence, pleaded guilty. The first occasion when a toeprint was admitted in evidence in a British court appears to have been the case of William Gourlay, who was convicted of a serious crime in a Glasgow court in 1952 (Wilton, 1953).

Mode of Production of Fingerprints, Palm- or Soleprints

The corium of the friction skin is folded and throws the overlying epidermis into ridges and furrows. Sweat glands open through small ducts, the mouths of which are distributed at points along the summits of the skin ridges. A constant stream of sweat from these glands bathes the skin and when the subject is excited, for example if engaged on safebreaking, the output of sweat increases. The sweat contains fat. If, then, any part of the friction skin is applied to a smooth surface, a greasy impression of its pattern is made on it. By adopting suitable techniques, it is possible to develop the impression and to record its pattern by photography. Simple but transient development is possible merely by breathing over a surface thought to bear an impression.

Principles of Identification by Impressions

The pattern of each person's impressions is unique. No two impressions have yet been found to coincide precisely unless both were made by one and the same area of friction skin. The accumulation of millions of records, over a hundred million in the U.S.A. alone, has as yet failed to disturb the validity of this observation. The chance that any two persons may have precisely the same fingerprints is as remote as at least one in 64,000 millions (Galton, 1892).

The pattern of an individual's friction skin remains unchanged throughout life. Herschel (1880: 1916), first demonstrated this. His own impressions taken when aged 28 and again at 82 were unchanged except for the addition of the coarse lines due to old age, and clearly recognisable as such.

Disease may temporarily modify or even obliterate fingerprint pattern (David *et al.*, 1970). They examined seventy-three patients suffering from coeliac disease and found that in sixty-three there was moderate epidermal ridge atrophy and even actual loss of fingerprint pattern. In a control series of 485 persons, ridge atrophy occurred in only three of them. The authors therefore considered ridge atrophy was a diagnostic sign of coeliac disease and there also appeared to be a correlation between its degree and the clinical condition of the patient.

Verbov (1971) described the occurrence of ridge distortion in dry or atrophic skin and he questioned their conclusions since, in his experience, incomplete atrophy of the ridges was not uncommon in dermatitis, including atopic dematitis. The change is seen in dry hands and those frequently immersed in water. The change is reversible.

Ridge alteration occurs in a number of skin disorders, e.g. eczema, acanthosis nigricans and scleroderma. Permanent impairment of the fingerprint pattern occurs in leprosy and after exposure to radiation. Jellinek (1932) observed loss of ridge pattern at the point of entry of an electrical current. It also occurred in the thumb of a photographer, who sustained a shock while manipulating a flash apparatus (Fig. 103); we obtained a series of photographs which, taken at subsequent intervals, showed the return of the pattern. We have also noted the flattening and broadening of the pattern in electric marks.

Mutilation of Fingerprints

Attempts have been made by self-inflicted wounds, by the application of corrosives or erosion against a hard surface, to destroy the finger skin pattern. In the latter event, if the subject is restrained from interfering with his hands, the pattern is restored in a few days. The other methods simply result in producing additional characteristics enhancing the value of the impressions; the attempt invariably leaves some part of the skin undamaged for the purposes of identification, unless skin grafts are made. These are taken from non-friction skin and yield smooth fingerpads which at once call for explanation as will the areas whence the grafts were derived, e.g. the sides of the chest, as in the following case from Texas. A man succeeded in removing completely the tell-tale skin pattern by undergoing skin-grafting of the pad of each digit. He became, however, a unique individual, possessed of smooth fingertips and ten oval scars, the site of the skin grafts, on his chest.

Forgery of Fingerprints

Impressions of single digits can be lifted and planted elsewhere, but the expert is unlikely to be deceived by their arrangement.

Forgery in other ways can be attempted and doubtless impressions used as signatures can be successfully forged, but practical difficulties lie in the way of the forger. Several ingenious methods have been devised.

It is reported from Singapore that hundreds of Indians have cut off and embalmed the thumbs of deceased relatives for use in continuing to draw pensions, after the lawful recipient is dead, when evidence of a thumb print is alone required to authorise payment. The director of Malaysia's pension division alleged that 567 persons had been "stamping" receipts with the severed thumbs of deceased lawful recipients, who had left the Malaysian service and retired to India. The Malaysian Government was estimated to have been losing a million Malaysian dollars annually because of these frauds. Up to that time the correct thumb print on a cheque was all that was required. The racket was discovered by "accident"; one of the Malaysian officers "stumbled" on it when on a visit to India. In future persons collecting pension money from the United Asian Bank are required to attend in person (*Daily Telegraph*, Jan. 4, 1982).

Practical Application of Fingerprints, Palm- and Footprints

1. The recognition of chance impressions left at a scene of crime. This is, of course, proof only that the suspect had been present, and is not proof of having committed the crime, but it raises a presumption of guilt, often sufficient to secure a confession.

2. The identification of suicides, deserters, persons suffering from loss of memory or those dead or unconscious after being involved in an accident.

3. Identification of decomposing bodies. Impressions from the separating skin or of the underlying derma are practicable and permit satisfactory identification. Similarly, with appropriate treatment, it is possible to obtain adequate impressions from the fingers of mummified bodies.

4. The solution of problems connected with accidental exchange of newlyborn infants. Footprinting of each infant shortly after birth provides an invaluable safeguard in institutions where an exchange might readily occur.

5. The prevention of personation.

6. Cheques, bank-notes and other legal documents, in addition to manual signature, can bear a fingerprint. (Herschel, 1880, 1894, 1916); see above.

Palm print of assailant in blood on the body of his victim: its preservation as a permanent exhibit

An elderly man was found dead and his body was heavily blood-stained; it was apparent that he had sustained severe injuries to his head and chest. Detective Chief Inspector Swann noted that, imprinted in blood on the man's right thigh, there was a hand mark, which included fingers and palm impressions. Ridge detail was absent in the finger marks but it was present in an area of the palm impression. Several ridge characteristics were seen and it appeared possible to obtain a positive identification. The deceased was at once excluded because he had had two fingers amputated from his right hand and he could have had difficulty in reaching the area with his left hand. The palm print of the suspect, a youth aged 16, was identical. He was later found guilty of murder and sentenced to be detained during Her Majesty's pleasure.

Preservation of the Specimen

The piece of skin bearing the print is now a permanent exhibit, embedded in transparent material. The technique whereby this was achieved was devised by Mr. Patrick Gaunt and Mr. Ian Newsome, technical officers in our Department.

The first problem was the fixation of the skin without dissolving the blood. Preliminary tests with pieces of skin bearing blood stains showed that ethyl alcohol 70 per cent (v/V) was satisfactory. During fixation the specimen was kept in a cardboard box at 4°C, pending further treatment. This ensured that any condensation would be absorbed and the stain remain undamaged. The next problem was to remove water from the specimen. This was done by passing it through several changes of acetone, each treatment lasting about 30 minutes. All fat had to be removed to prevent it soaking into the skin, thereby giving it an unnatural translucency. This was accomplished by passing the specimen through several changes of uncatalised resin. This not only removed the fat but also infiltrated the specimen with resin prior to the final stage of embedding. Care must be taken to avoid movement of the specimen while the monomer is still fluid. Mr. Gaunt said that the use of a rather larger mould than might be thought enough would allow for trimming to correct mal-alignment. They used the "Plasticraft" kit, a product of Turner

Research, Ltd. Leeds, L S 6 2 × H. Details of the identification and preservation of this blood impression were recorded by Detective Chief Inspector Swann in 1974.

Persistence of Impressions at a Scene of Crime

Impressions may persist for years, if undisturbed by cleaning. In the Ruxton case impressions found at his house, known to have been those of his maid, Mary Rogerson, were in agreement with impressions of the digits of Body No. 1. Even outside a house impressions may persist for weeks, e.g. on the window-sill or on a broken sheet of glass thrown into a water butt. Impressions on paper persist for a variable time according to the kind of paper. Thus impressions on blotting paper persist only for about 2 hours but if made on glazed paper, they have been developed and identified up to 3 years later. When describing a new method of detecting fingerprints, i.e. by the Ninhydrin reaction, Odén and von Hofsten (1954) depicted an excellent impression, made on a page of French grammar 12 years previously and developed by Ninhydrin.

Fingerprints and the Medical Practitioner

The practical importance of fingerprints to doctors is essentially of negative kind. Do not meddle with objects, especially weapons, at the scene lest careless handling blurs vitally important impressions on them. Medical examination of the apparently dead should be restricted to the steps essential to determine that death has occurred. The scene should be disturbed as little as possible until the police, if not already present, take charge. Until then the doctor should ensure that there is no interference by himself or others. If the patient still lives, obviously, the doctor must treat the victim and supervise the necessary arrangements for his removal to hospital. Removal should be effected with the minimum disturbance of the scene; the doctor should take note of it as found by him before any alteration was made.

Interference with weapons, by obscuring finger impressions on them, has more than once prevented the satisfactory interpretation of the circumstances of a death, e.g. as in *R. v. Barney* (1932).

A composite picture (Fig. 13), prepared by the City of Glasgow Police, shows the steps in identification: (a) print at scene, on a safe; (b) "developed" impression, found on the safe. (c) Accused's fingerprint record and (d) the comparison between the print on the safe and that of the corresponding digit of the accused. He was found guilty.

Identification by Occupational Marking

There are several occupations which may produce characteristic marking of the hands, by way of callosities, scars or tattooing. Examination of the hands, therefore, has a place in the identification of the dead. Even when the examiner has not had the requisite experience by which he can suggest the occupation of the subject, he should look for, and make an accurate record of, unusual markings. Proficiency with this mode of identification is attained only by those who have opportunity to study a large number of persons whose occupation is known. Without this, much may be learnt in particular from the publications by Ronchese (1951) and Gilbert Forbes (1946, 1947).

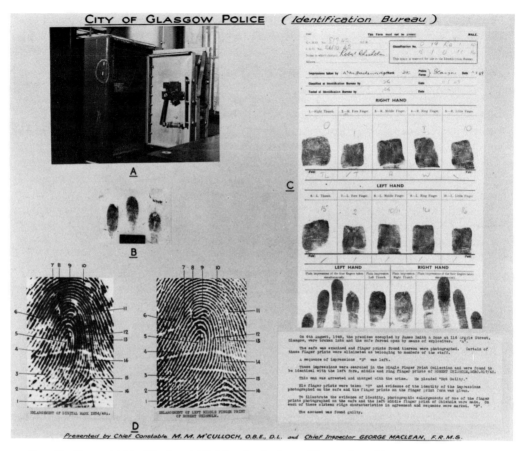

FIG. 13. Fingerprint Identification. (a) Safe bearing "unknown" impressions. (b) "Developed" unknown impressions. (c) C.R.O. record of the accused. (d) Comparison of the impressions and demonstration of sixteen points of similarity.

Occupational markings are to be expected and occur, in the main, amongst those who work in large industrial cities. Sheffield, for example, provided Forbes with a valuable field for investigation. It must suffice here to cite only a few examples of markings which, when well developed, should suggest the probable occupation of the subject. For instance, a callosity, when situated on the outer side of the distal phalanx of the middle finger of the right hand is likely to have been produced by the pen of a clerk; the more so, if his hands are otherwise soft and clean. Callosities also occur in a similar position on the hand of a draughtsman but, in addition, another callosity, produced by sliding the hand over the drawing board, is developed at the base of the hypothenar eminence and may be present on one or both hands. Thickening of the palmar skin of the fingers and of the palm at the roots of the fingers is seen on the right hands of butchers. Callosites of specific distribution may also be found on the hands of dental mechanics, glass cutters, bakers and others. Instrumentalists, notably violinists, guitar and saxophone players, may also have occupational markings of their hands.

Scars, produced by burns from hot fragments of scale, may be seen on the backs of the hands of blacksmiths.

Involuntary tattooing by particles of coal is most often seen on the hands of miners. This is probably the first occupational marking to have been recognised. Siderotic tattooing of the little and ring finger of millstone grinders was also one of the first occupational markings to be described (Moingeard, 1890).

Small cuts on the tips of the index finger and thumb of each hand are produced in the preparation of lenses by opticians, who are also likely to have particles of glass under and around their nails (Forbes, 1946, 1947).

Markings as by ring is also to be noted. The identification of Mary Rogerson included, as a minor point, evidence of a faint furrow on one of her fingers. She was known to have worn a ring on that finger (Glaister and Brash, 1937).

Occupational marks can be seen in window cleaners. They may develop a permanent radial deviation of the terminal joints of the index fingers, especially of the right hand. This is due to moving the fingertips along the margins of the window frame (Moir, 1954). A similar deformity may be produced by folding documents (Partington, 1954).

This mode of identification appears first to have been recognised by Esbach in 1876, in his monograph on "Modifications de la Phalangette" (cited by Ewing, 1923).

Forbes concluded from his study of 300 subjects that "in any industrial area there are so many different occupations that it would be the work of a lifetime to make a comprehensive survey. The results of the investigation were disappointing in that so many workers bore no characteristic marks at all. It follows from this that the condition of the hands as a means of identification is only of limited application." He was, however, of the opinion that this means of identification could have value in selected cases. This might well be true when the body of an unknown person is thought to be that of someone known to have been employed in an occupation likely to produce characteristic marking of the hands, and such marks were present.

Identification by Reconstruction of the Features

Several attempts to reconstruct the features of the dead for the purposes of identification have been made. These were based on limited material, for example a skull, a death mask or the recollection of relatives and acquaintances.

One of the earliest attempts was that of Welcker (1888); cited by Glaister and Brash, (1937), who was required to identify a skull as that of Schiller. In 1895 the method was developed by His, when he identified the skeleton of J. S. Bach from amongst a number of others in the burial ground where Bach was known to have been buried. The bodies of twenty-four male suicides, aged 17 to 72, chosen as subjects likely to be free from pathological changes in the face, were first studied. His determined the average thickness of the soft parts of the face at a series of fifteen, i.e. nine median and six lateral, predetermined points. He used a sewing needle, carrying a rubber disc, and thrust it vertically into the tissues until it reached the underlying bone. When the averaged results of these tests—individual variation being slight—were applied to a plaster cast of the skull, Seffner, the sculptor, was able to model a likeness which was considered the equal to any of the portraits of Bach. Although he was not told of the identity of the subject, it is possible that Seffner was influenced by reports of the disinterment and his success may have been in part due to his knowledge of the purpose of the task.

Williams and Pacini, using His's method, reproduced the likeness of a man whose skull was fractured in four places. The model was unhesitatingly identified by relatives.

Gerasimov, who died in 1970, specialised in the reconstruction of the features from skulls (Gerasimov, 1971). He had assisted the police in the reconstruction of unidentified bodies but he was more interested in historical and prehistorical personalities. He made outstanding documentary portraits of Ivan the Terrible and of Schiller, whose body had been interred at Weimar in a vault occupied by seventy-five other bodies. Nigel Dennis, in his review of the book (*Sunday Telegraph*, 28 Feb. 1971), "found it hard not to feel that at some stage in the reconstruction the scientist gives way to the artist and allows a certain amount of romance to seep into the plaster". Krogman (1962) regarded these skull-portraits as "a fascinating exercise in historicity but little else".

Gerasimov supported his claim to accuracy by depicting photographs of the known person beside those of his reconstructions. It may be that in skilled hands, such as those of a Gerasimov, who are rare birds, the method has practical value but the police are more likely to rely on Identikit or Photokit portraits; plastic reconstructions take time and the police need rapid identification.

In the case of Edith Wrathmell, found murdered in Leeds, the late Jacob Kramer painted a portrait of the dead woman based on descriptions given to the police; it was identified by acquaintances as a likeness.

When the body of a woman was found in the vicinity of Sutton Bank, near Thirsk, the Department of Medical Illustration, Manchester University, prepared a wax model of the head of the deceased. The method used was that which they had devised to restore the head of an ancient Egyptian girl. The result was interesting and perhaps a reasonable likeness. It was prepared in 1981 but so far, by October 1982, the deceased remains unidentified.

A novel use of photography, was invented by Brash in his identification of the bodies in the Ruxton case (Glaister and Brash, 1937); it was used by Simpson (1943a, b) in the Dobkin case.

Identification by Radiography

Following an air crash, and it was necessary to identify the bodies, it was known that one of the victims had been subjected to radiographic examination a year previously. The films were traced and they demonstrated certain abnormalities, which included scoliosis of the spine. Radiographic examination of one of the bodies showed corresponding abnormalities. [It was also known that his blood belonged to group B. Samples from muscle, kidney and liver of the deceased yielded a strong reaction for group B (Stevens, 1966).]

We were able to identify a body recovered from the sea because there was an unusual spinal deformity which tallied with that in the radiograph of a known patient.

In circumstances of this kind the teeth, identity discs, contents of the pockets, laundry marks and, if a service watch be worn, its number, all afford corroborative evidence (Mant, 1962).

The Eyes and Identification

The colour of the eyes in the living is readily determined but the colour of the eyes of the dead is an uncertain guide to their colour during life, because within a relatively short time of death the eyes of all persons tend to acquire a shade of greenish-brown.

It must be ascertained, also, before recording their colour, whether the eyes be natural or artificial, an easy trap to overlook.

Signs of disease, for example corneal opacities, deformity of the iris (including iridectomy) or of cataract may play a part in identification. Compression of the skin of the nose near the bridge may show that the person had been accustomed to wear spectacles.

Identification by Extraneous Means

Dust on the Clothing

Dust from trouser bottoms or pockets is another source of information, but only corroborative when of exceptional kind. Roche Lynch (1944) considered such evidence most dangerous unless the dust is of an outstanding kind. He accepted, as a good example of the latter, the demonstration of dust on the clothing of the accused and on the carpets of their homes, composed of sodium chlorate, iron oxide and aluminium powder. They were accused and convicted of having prepared and used thermite bombs, of a similar composition, during the I.R.A. disturbances. (The account of this trial, edited by Letitia Fairfield (1953), is now in the *Notable British Trials* series.) Ainsworth Mitchell (1944) instanced the detection of safe robbers by the presence of finely powdered furnace slag on their hands; it was similar to that used to pack the walls and door of a safe which had been broken into. Particles of glass on the accused's clothing may prove that he was concerned with breaking into premises when its composition resembles that of broken glass at the scene of the crime.

Dust in the Cerumen

Icard (1921), suggested that an examination of cerumen might provide information of value in identification. He found that in certain occupations some of the dust was mixed with cerumen. Examples include coal dust in miners, coffee dust in the ears of those who roast coffee beans, small pieces of hair in the cerumen of barbers, grains of starch in that of bakers, and asbestos fibres in the ears of those who work in this industry.

Dust, etc., in Nail Scrapings

It is now a routine procedure to collect material from beneath the finger-nails (with consent, from the living), for the purposes of criminal investigation. The victim of murder may have blood or fragments of flesh from the assailant beneath the nails and the same kind of material may be under the nails of the assailant. The drowned may have mud or sand beneath their nails and this may indicate they had struggled to save themselves, e.g. by clutching at the bank of the river.

Laundry Marks

The City of Glasgow Police established a registry of laundry marks in 1947 and have specimen marks used by all of the Scottish laundries, of which there were 205. The registry permits prompt recognition of any Scottish mark found on the clothing of a body, sheeting or other laundered cloth wrapped round a body or articles of clothing found at a scene of crime.

The first registry of this kind appears to have been established by Yulch (1941; cited Hamilton, 1952) of the Nassau Police Department, Minneola, New York. The Glasgow registry and the history of its institution was described by Hamilton (1952).

Articles on or near the Body

Pocket cases may contain documents which facilitate identification. Visiting cards, driving licences, watches, jewellery, etc., may also have value. A criminal may, however, plant documents and articles to mislead and to suggest the body is that of some other person, as once was done in attempted fraud upon an insurance company.

Typescript letters may afford a clue. The Glasgow police, for example, maintain a file of examples of typescript by all known makes of machine.

Manufacturer's Marks May also have Value in Identification.

Spectacles and Identification

Identification is possible by examination of spectacles found on the body or in a pocket of the clothing. An analysis should be made of the lenses and compared with a known prescription; the value of this test is, of course, enhanced if the person suffered from some unusual error of refraction. It has to be remembered that it is not unknown for a person to use glasses prescribed for another patient and to manage passably well.

Following a sexual assault by a man whom the victim had not seen, the police found a pair of horn-rimmed spectacles at the scene. The lenses were analysed and the result tallied with the prescription for a patient who had an unusual error of refraction. This provided corroborative evidence which led to the arrest and conviction of a young man, charged with rape (Spence, 1962).

References

ANDERSON, J. N. (1951) *Notes and News, Sheffield University*, p. 5.
ANGEL, E. H. (1899) *Dental Cosmos*, **41**, 248.
ANNOTATION (1906) *Brit. Med. J.*, **i**, Cumberland Assizes, Carlisle.
ASHLEY, D. J. (1957) *Nature* (Lond.), **179**, 969.
BANG, G. and RAMM, E. (1970) *Acta Odontol. Second.* **28**, 3–35.
BARR, M. L. (1954) *Lancet*, **i**, 779.
BARR, M. L. (1956) *Canad. Med. Ass. J.*, **74**, 419.
BARR, M. L. and BERTRAM, E. G. (1949) *Nature* (*Lond.*), **163**, 676–7.
BARR, M. L., BERTRAM, L. F. and LINDSAY, H. A. (1950) *Anat. Rec.*, **107**, 283–97.
BARR, M. L. and HOBBS, G. E. (1954) *Lancet*, **i**, 1109–10.

BEADLE, O. (1931) *The Intervertebral Discs*, Medical Research Council Special Report, No. 161, London; H.M.S.O.

BERRY, D. C. and HUNT, A. C. (1967) *Med. Sci. Law*, **7**, 67.

BLENCH, T. H. (1933) *Med.-leg. Rev.*, **1**, 280.

BONNAFOUX, H. (1960) *Annls. Méd. lég.*, **40**, 552.

BOUCHER, B. J. (1955) *J. Forens. Med.*, **2**, 51–54.

BOYD, J. D. and TREVOR, J. C. (1953) in *Modern Trends in Forensic Medicine*, edited K. Simpson, pp. 133–52, London; Butterworths.

BRASH, J. C. (1937) in Glaister and Brash's *Medico-legal Aspects of the Ruxton Case*, pp. 144–70. Edinburgh; Livingstone.

BRITTAIN, R. P. (1950) *J. Crim. Law and Criminol.* **40**, 787–90.

BUHTZ and ERHARDT (1938) *Dtsch. Z. ges. gerichtl. Med.*, **29**, 453.

CASPER, J. L. (1861) *A Handbook of the Practice of Forensic Medicine*, vol. **i**, translated by G. W. Balfour London; New Sydenham Soc.

CAVE, A. J. E. and STEEL, F. L. D. (1963) *Med. Sci. Law*, **3**, 83.

CHATTERJI, S. and JEFFREY, J. W. (1968) *Nature (Lond.)* **219**, 482; *Med. Sci. Law* (1969) **9**, 75.

CLELAND, J. B. (1944) *Austr. J. Dent.*, **48**, 107.

CLEMENTS, E. M. B., DAVIES-THOMAS, E. and PICKETT, K. G. (1953) *Brit. Med. J.*, **i**, 1421; 1425.

COX, H. E. (1929) *Analyst*, **54**, 649–701.

COX, H. E. (1935) *Analyst*, **60**, 793–800.

CUTHBERT, C. R. M. (1958) *Science and the Detection of Crime*. London; Hutchinson.

DALITZ, G. D. (1962) *J. Forens. Sci. Soc.*, **3**, 11.

DAVID, T. J., AJDUKIEWICZ, A. B. and READ, A. R. (1970) *Brit. Med. J.*, **4**, 594.

DAVIDSON, W. M. (1960a) *Brit. Med. J.*, **ii**, 1901–6.

DAVIDSON, W. M. (1960b) *J. Forens. Med.*, **7**, 14–17.

DAVIDSON, W. M. and SMITH, D. R. (1954) *Brit. Med. J.*, **ii**, 6–7; plate.

DAVIDSON, W. M. and WINN, S. (1961) cited Davidson (1960).

DECHAUME, M., DÉROBERT, L. and PAYEN, J. (1960) *Annls. Méd. lég. Crimin. Police Scient. et Toxicol.*, **40**, 165–8.

DÉROBERT, L. and FULLY, G. (1960) *Annls. Méd. lég.)n. Police Scient. et Toxicol.*, **40**, 154.

DEVLIN, LORD (1976). Report to the Secretary of State for the Home Department of the Departmental Committee on Evidence of Identification in Criminal Cases. Chairman: Rt. Hon. Lord Devlin London. H.M.S.O.

DILNOT, G. (1928) *The Trial of Professor Webster*. London: Bles.

DIXON, A. D. and TORR, J. B. D. (1956) *Nature (Lond.)*, **178**, 797.

DIXON, A. D. and TORR, J. B. D. (1957) *J. Forens. Med.*, **4**, 11–17.

DUPERTUIS, C. W. and HADDEN, J. A., Jnr. (1951) *Amer. J. Phys. Anthrop.*, N.S. **9**, 15–53.

DWIGHT, T. (1890) *J. Anat. (Lond.)*, **24**, 527.

DWIGHT, T. (1894) *Medical Record. N.Y.*, **46**, 293.

ELIAKIS, E. C. and IORDANIDIS, P. J. (1963a) *Annls. Méd. lég. Crimin. Police Scient. et Toxicol.*, **43**, 326.

ELIAKIS, E. C. and IORDANIDIS, P. J. (1963b) *Annls. Méd. lég. Crimin. Police Scient. et Toxicol.*, **43**, 520.

EMERY, J. L. and MCMILLAN, M. (1954) *J. Path. Bact.*, **68**, 17.

EWING, J. (1923) in Peterson, Haines and Webster's *Legal Medicine and Toxicology*, vol. **i**, pp. 146–7, 172–4.

FAIRFIELD, LETITIA (1953) *The I.R.A. Coventry Explosion, The Trial of Peter Barnes and others, Notable British Trials*, etc., London: Hodge.

FAULDS, H. (1911) *Knowledge*, **34**, 136–40.

FEARNHEAD, R. W. (1960) *J. Forens. Med.*, **7**, 11–13.

FEARNHEAD, R. W. (1961) *Med. Sci. Law*, **1**, 273.

FLECKER, H. (1932) *J. Anat. (Lond.)* **67**, 118.

FLECKER, H. (1932–33) *J. Anat. (Lond.)*, **67**, 118–24.

FLECKER, H. (1942) *Amer. J. Rontgenol.*, **47**, 97.

FORBES, G. (1946) *Police J.*, **19**, 266–74; reprinted in *J. Criminal Law and Criminology* (1947), **38**, 423–436.

FRANCHINI, A. (1946) *Boll. Soc. ital. Biol. sper.*, **22**, 151–4.

FULLY, G. (1956) *Annls. Méd. lég. Crimin. Police Scient. et Toxicol.*, **36**, 266.

FULLY, G. and PINEAU, H. (1960) *Ann. Méd. lég. Crimin. Police Scient. et Toxicol.*, **40**, 145.

GALTON, F. (1892) *Finger Prints*. London: Macmillan.

GERASIMOV, M. M. (1971) *The Face Finder*, trans. A. H. Brodrick. London: Hutchinson.

GIESE, E. (1932) *Dtsch. Z. ges. gerichtl. Med.*, **19**, 284–92; also abstr. *Méd.-lég. Rev.*, (1933), **1**, 129–31.

GLAISTER, JOHN (1931) *A Study of Hairs and Wools belonging to the Mammalian Group of Animals, including a special study of human hair considered from the medico-legal aspect*. Publication No. 2, Egyptian University Faculty of Med., Cairo: Misr. Press.

GLAISTER, JOHN (1953) in *Trial of Jeannie Donald*, Appendix ix, pp. 294–6; ed. J. C. Wilson, Edinburgh, Hodge.
GLAISTER, JOHN and BRASH, J. C. (1937) *Medico-Legal Aspects of the Ruxton Case*, Edinburgh: Livingstone.
GLAISTER, JOHN and RENTOUL, E. (1966) *Medical Jurisprudence and Toxicology*, 12th ed., p. 102. Edinburgh: Livingstone.
GLOB, P. V. (1965) *Mosefolket*. Copenhagen; Gyldendal; English translation R. Bruce-Mitford, *The Bog People* (1969), London; Faber; 1971. Paladin paper-back edition.
GOLLOMB, J. (1931) *Amer J. Police Sci.*, **2**, 266.
GONZALES, T. A. VANCE, M. and HELPERN, M. (1954) *Legal Medicine and Toxicology*. 2nd Ed. New York. Appleton-Century.
GRANT, E. A., PRENDERGAST, W. K. and WHITE, E. A. (1952) *J. Canad. Dental Ass.*, **18**, 3.
GREEN, A. G. (1920) *Analysis of Dyestuffs*, p. 55. London.
GREENBLATT, R. B., de ACOSTA, O., VASQUEZ, E. and MULLINS, D. F. JNR. (1956) *J. Amer. Med. Ass.*, **161**, 683.
GUERRE, The case of Martin (1593) *The Times* 12 Dec. 1871; and in Guy and Ferrier (1895) *Principles of Forensic Medicine*, 7th ed., pp. 48–51, ed. W. R. Smith. London; Renshaw.
GUSTAFSON, G. (1947) *J. Amer. Dent. Ass.*, **35**, 720.
GUSTAFSON, G. (1950) *J. Amer. Dent. Ass.*, **41**, 45.
GUSTAFSON, G. (1958) *Proc. Roy. Soc. Med.*, **51**, 1055–7.
GUSTAFSON, G. (1959) *Ann. Méd. lég.*, **39**, 5–25.
GUSTAFSON, G. (1966) *Forensic Odontology*. London: Staples.
HAMILTON, D. (1952) *Police J.*, **25**, 190–8.
HARRISON, R. J. (1953) in *Medical and Scientific Investigations in the Christie Case.* ed. F. E. Camps, pp. 56 to 99. London: Medical Publications.
HARRISON, R. J. (1954) Personal communication.
HARRISON, W. R. (1958) *Suspect Documents*. London: Sweet and Maxwell.
HARVEY, W. (1966) *Brit. Dent. J.*, **121**, 337.
HERSCHEL, W. J. (1880) *Nature (Lond.)*, **23**, 76.
HERSCHEL, W. J. (1894) *Nature (Lond.)*, **51**, 77.
HERSCHEL, W. J. (1916) *The Origin of Finger Printing*, O.U.P.
HOFMANN, E. VON (1882) *Wien. med. Wschr.*; cited Gustafson, 1966.
HOWE, R. M. (1949) (Hans Gross's) *Criminal Investigation*, 4th ed., p. 231, ed. R. M. Howe, London; Sweet and Maxwell.
HRDLIČKA, A. (1952) *Practical Anthropometry*, cited Harrison (1953).
HUMBLE, B. H. (1933a) *Brit. Dent. J.*, **54**, 528–36.
HUMBLE, B. H. (1933b) *Int. J. Orthod.*, **19**, 153–9.
HUMPHRIES, SIR TRAVERS (1953) *A Book of Trials*, pp. 99–105. London, etc.: Heinemann.
HUNT, E. E., JNR. and GLESER, G. (1955) *Amer. J. Phys. Anthrop.*, **13**, 479.
HUNTER, JOHN (1835) *The Works of John Hunter*, 2. *The Natural History of the Human Teeth*, p. 36, J. F. Palmerr London: Longman and others.
HUNTER, W. F., LENNOX, B. and PEARSON, A. G. (1954) *Lancet*, **i**, 372.
HYRTL, J. (1889) *Lehrbuch d. anatomie d. menschen*. Vienna: Braumuller; cited Harrison (1953) and Dwight (1890).
ICARD, S. (1921) *J. Amer. Med. Ass.*, **76**, 1693–4.
IDENTIFICATION (1963) *Med. Sci. Law*, **3**, 637.
IORDANIDIS, P. (1961) *Ann. Méd. lég.*, **41**, 23–34, 280–91, 347–58.
IORDANIDIS, P. (1963) *Annls Méd. lég. Crimin. Police Scient. et Toxicol.*, **42**, 117; *ibid.* 231.
JELLINEK, S. (1932) *Die Electrische Verletzungen*. Leipzig: Barth.
KEEN, E. N. (1953) *J. Forens. Med.*, **1**, 45–51.
KEISER–NIELSEN, S. (1951) *Odont. Tidskr.*, **59**, 57; cited Gustafson (1966).
KEISER–NIELSEN, S. (1963) *J. Dental Res.*, **42**, 303.
KILLPACK, W. S. (1954) *Lancet*, **1**, 417.
KNIGHT, B. (1966) *Med. Sci. Law*, **6**, 161.
KNIGHT, B. (1969) *Med. Sci. Law*, **9**, 247.
KNIGHT, B. (1971) *Criminologist*, **6**, 33.
KNIGHT, B. H. and LAUDER, I. (1967) *Med. Sci. Law*, **7**, 205.
KROGMAN, W. M. (1939) *F.B.I. Enforcement Bull.*, **8**, 3; cited Krogman (1946).
KROGMAN, W. M. (1946) *Proc. Inst. Med. Chicago*, **16**, 154–67.
KROGMAN, W. M. (1960) 2nd International Meeting on Forensic Path. and Med., New York, *Abstracts*, pp. 12–13.
KROGMAN, W. M. (1962a) *The Human Skeleton in Forensic Medicine*. Springfield, Illinois: C. Thomas.
KROGMAN, W. M. (1962b) *J. Forens. Sci.*, **7**, 253; an application of his methods.

"L.D.S." (1945) *Brit. Dent. J.*, **78**, 76.
LAYTON, J. J. (1966) *J. Forens. Sci. Soc.*, **6**, 76.
LESURGES, (1794) cited TAYLOR (1956), vol. **i**, p. 106.
LUCAS, A. (1946) *Forensic Chemistry*, 4th ed. London: Arnold.
LYNCH, ROCHE (1944) in discussion. *Med.-leg. Rev.*, **12**, 205–8 (207).
MANT, A. K. (1962) *Med. Sci. Law*, **2**, 134.
MARBERGER, E., BOCCABELLA, R. A. and NELSON, W. O. (1955) *Proc. Soc. exper. Biol. Med.*, **89**, 488.
MARJORIBANKS, E. (1930) *The Life of Sir Edward Marshall Hall*. London: Gollancz.
MEYER, H. (1933) *Dtsch. Z. ges. gerichtl. Med.*, **22**, 362–78.
MILES, A. E. W. (1963) *J. Dental Res.*, **42**, 255.
MILES, A. E. W. and FEARNHEAD, R. W. (1953) in *Medical and Scientific Investigations in the Christie Case*, ed. F. E. Camps, pp. 100–24. London: Medical Publications.
MILES, A. E. W. and FEARNHEAD, R. W. (1958) *Proc. Roy. Soc. Med.*, **51**, 1057–60.
MITCHELL, C. A. (1944) *Med.-leg. Rev.*, **12**, 195–205; discussion, 205.
MOINGEARD, A. (1890) *Ann. Hyg. publ.* (Paris), 3rd ed., **24**, 39–43.
MOIR, P. J. (1954) *Brit. Med. J.*, **ii**, 757.
MOORE, K. L. and BARR, M. L. (1955) Lancet, **ii**, 57–58.
MOORE, K. L., GRAHAM, M. A. and BARR, M. L. (1953) *Surg. Gynec. Obstet.*, **96**, 641–8.
NICKOLLS, L. C. (1950) *Police J.*, **23**, 263–4; and gift of prints of the exhibits.
ODÉN, S. and VON HOFSTEN, B. (1954) *Nature (Lond.)*, **173**, 449–50.
OGSTON, F. (1878) *Lectures on Medical Jurisprudence*, ed. F. Ogston, Jnr. London: Churchill.
OSBORN, A. S. (1929) *Questioned Documents*. New York: Boyd.
Parkman, the case of Dr. (1850) *The trial of Professor John White Webster*, ed. G. Dilnot, 1928. London: Bles.
PARRY, HIS HONOUR SIR EDWARD (1929) *The Drama of the Law*, pp. 43–51; 189–97. London: Benn.
PARTINGTON, M. W. (1954) *Brit. Med. J.*, **ii**, 1166.
PEARSON, KARL (1899). *Philos. Trans.*, Series A, **192**, 169–244.
POLSON, C. J. (1948). *Med.-leg. J.*, *(Camb.)* **16**, 96–102.
POLSON, C. J. (1950). *J. Crim. Law and Criminol.*, **41**, 495–517.
POLSON, C. J. (1951). *J. Crim. Law and Criminol.*, **41**, 690–704.
POLSON, C. J. (1962) *The Essentials of Forensic Medicine*, 2nd ed., Oxford: Pergamon.
POLSON, G. M. (1971) Personal communication.
POST, R. S. (1962) *J. Crim Law, Criminology and Police Science.*
R. v. BARNEY (1932) in Sir Patrick Hastings's *Cases in Court* (1949), pp. 249–62, London: Heinemann.
R. v. BECK (1877–1904) Adolf Beck (1877–1904) *Notable British Trials*, ed. E. R. Watson, 1924. Edinburgh and London: Hodge.
R. v. BRADY and HINDLEY (1966) Chester Assizes; *The Times*, 19 Apr., May 6th.
R. v. CHRISTIE (1953) *Medical and Scientific Investigations in the Christie Case*, ed. F. E. Camps. London: Medical Publications.
R. v. CRIPPEN (1910) *Trial of Hawley Harvey Crippen, Notable British Trials* (1919), ed. Filson Young. Edinburgh and London: Hodge; also Marjoribanks (1936).
R. v. DOBKIN (1942) *The Trial of Harry Dobkin, Old Bailey Trials Series*, No. I (1944), ed., C. E. Bechhofer Roberts, London, etc.: Jarrolds; also K. Simpson (1943a) and (1943b).
R. v. DONALD (1934). *Trial of Jeannie Donald, Notable British Trials*, No. 79, ed., J. G. Wilson, 1953. Edinburgh and London: Hodge.
R. v. GORRINGE (1948) *Maidstone Assizes*. See Howe (1949) and Simpson (1951).
R. v. GREENWOOD (1918) The Button and Badge Murder in *A Book of Trials*, Humphries (1953), pp. 99 to 105.
R. v. HAIGH (1949) *Trial of J. G. Haigh, Notable British Trials*, ed. Lord Dunboyne. Edinburgh and London: Hodge; also press reports of the trial.
R. v. MANTON (1943) The Luton Sack Murder; see Simpson (1945).
R. v. MAY (1926). *Reading Summer Assizes*, cited Glaister (1931) and Stoves (1943).
R. v. ORTON, alias Castro (1874). See *The Tichborne Case*.
R. v. PODMORE (1928) in *Bernard Spilsbury*, Browne & Tullett (1951), pp. 222–30. London: Harrap.
R. v. ROUSE (1931) *Trial of A. A. Rouse, Notable British Trials*, ed. Helena Normanton. Edinburgh and London: Hodge; also Hastings (1949) *Cases in Court*, pp. 263–78.
R. v. RUXTON (1936) Manchester March Assizes; *Notable British Trials*, 2nd ed. (1950), ed. R. H. Blundell and G. H. Wilson. Edinburgh and London: Hodge; also Glaister and Brash (1937).
R. v. SLATER (1909) *Trial of Oscar Slater, Notable Scottish Trials*, ed. W. Roughead (1910). Edinburgh and Glasgow: Hodge.
R. v. TEAGUE (1851) Cornwall Assizes, cited Tidy (1882) and Glaister (1931); also *Med. Times (Lond.)*, **48**, 731.
REISS, R. A. (1911) *Manuel de police scientifique technique*, vol. **1**, p. 515. Lausanne: Payot.

ROBERTS, C. E. B. (1944) *The Trial of Harry Dobkin.* London: Jarrold.

ROLLET, E. (1888) *De la mensuration des os longs des membres, etc.*, Lyons; cited Pearson (1899); also Stewart (1948) and Harrison (1953).

RONCHESE, F. (1951) *Proc. 35th Ann. Convention, Internat. Ass. Identification, July 25th,* 1950, pp. 151–4.

SANDERSON, Ann R. and STEWART, J. S. S. (1961) *Brit. Med. J.,* **2,** 1065.

SAUNDERS, E. (1837) *Teeth a Test of Age.* London: Renshaw.

SCHMITT, H. P. and SATERNUS, K. (1970) *Ztschr. Rechtsmedizin—J. Legal Med.,* **67,** 170.

SHIE, M. D. (1928) *J. Amer. Med. Ass.,* **90,** 94–99.

SIMPSON, K. (1943a) *Police J.,* **16,** 270–80 (R. v. DOBKIN.)

SIMPSON, K. (1943b) *Med.-leg. Rev.,* **11,** 132–44. (R. v. DOBKIN.)

SIMPSON, K. (1945) *Police J.,* **18,** 263–73. (R. v. MANTON.)

SIMPSON, K. (1951) *Internat. Police J.,* **6,** 312. (R. v. GORRINGE.)

SIMPSON, K. (1953) *Modern Trends in Forensic Medicine.* London: Butterworths.

SIMPSON, K. (1969) *Forensic Medicine,* 6th ed., London: Arnold.

SINGER, R. (1953) *J. Forens. Med.,* **1,** 52–59.

SMITH, Sir SYDNEY and FIDDES, F. S. (1955) *Forensic Medicine,* 10th ed., p. 95. London: Churchill.

SMITH, Sir SYDNEY and GLAISTER, JOHN (1939) *Recent Advances in Forensic Medicine,* 2nd ed. London: Churchill.

SÖRUP, A. (1924) *Vjschr. Zahnheilk.,* **40,** 385; cited Ström (1963).

SÖRUP, A. (1926) *Mschr. Zahnheilk.,* **21,** 277.

SPENCE, W. (1962) *Police J.,* **35,** 384.

SPOKES, S. (1905) *Brit. Med. J.,* **ii,** 568.

STACK, M. V. (1960) *J. Forens. Sci. Soc.,* **1,** 49.

STEVENS, P. J. (1966) *Med. Sci. Law,* **6,** 160.

STEVENS, P. J. and TARLTON, S. W. (1963) *Med. Sci. Law,* **3,** 154.

STEWART, T. D. (1948) *Amer. J. Phys. Anthrop.,* N.S. **6,** 315.

STEWART, T. D. (1963) *J. Dental Res.,* **42,** 264.

STOVES, J. L. (1943) *Med.-leg. Rev.,* **11,** 185.

STRÖM, F. (1946) *Norske Tannlaege foren. Tid.,* **56,** 153; cited Gustafson (1966).

STRÖM, F. (1963) *J. Dental Res.,* **42,** 312.

SWANN, P. M. (1974) The Identification and Preservation of a blood impression on skin. A report by Det. Ch. Insp. Swann. *Finger Prints & Scenes of Crime.* West Yorkshire Metropolitan Police. June 25 1974.

TAYLOR, A. S. (1956) *Principles and Practice of Medical Jurisprudence,* 11th ed., Vol. I, p. 104, ed. Smith, S. London: Churchill.

TELKKA, A., PALKAMA, A. and VIRTAMA, P. (1962) *J. Forens. Sci.,* **7,** 474.

THANE, G. D. (1899) in Quain's *Elements of Anatomy,* 10th ed., vol. **ii,** pt. **i,** p. 78. London: Longmans Green.

THIEME, F. P. (1957) *J. Forens. Med.,* **4,** 72–81.

THOMA, K. H. (1944) *Oral Pathology,* 2nd ed. St. Louis: C. V. Mosby.

TICHBORNE CASE (1874) Editor Lord Maugham (1936), London: Hodder & Stoughton; also Sir Edward Parry and R. v. Orton, [1873] 9 Q. B. 350.

TIDY, C. M. (1882) *Legal Medicine,* vol. pp. 256–78. London: Smith-Elder.

TOVO, S. and DE BERNADI, A. (1958) *Minerva Med.-leg.* (Torino), **78,** 233.

TROTTER, M. and GLESER, G. (1951) *Amer. J. Phys. Anthrop.,* N.S. **9,** 311–24.

TROTTER, M. and GLESER, G. (1952) *Amer. J. Phys. Anthrop.,* N.S. **10,** 463–514.

TROTTER, M. and GLESER, G. (1958) *Amer. J. Phys. Anthrop.,* N.S. **16,** 79.

VERBOV, J. (1971) *Brit. Med. J.,* **1,** 48.

VILLENEUEVA (1980).

WAALER, E. (1960) *Norske Tannlaege foren. Tid.,* **70,** 513, English trans. *Internat. Crim. Police Rev.* (1962), **161,** 242; photostat provided by the Librarian, Home Office.

WASHBURN, S. L. (1948) *Amer. J. Phys. Anthrop.,* N.S. **6,** 199–207.

WELLS, L. H. (1959) *J. Forens. Med.,* **6,** 171.

"WEST SUSSEX" (1954) *Police J.,* **27,** 131–4.

WHITTAKER, D. K. (1982) *Ann. Roy. Coll. Surgeons of England.* **64,** 175–179.

WHITTAKER, D. K., LLEWELLYN, D. R. and JONES, R. W. (1975) *Brit. Dent. J.* **139,** 403–05.

WHITTAKER, D. K. and KNEALE, M. J. (1979) *Brit. Dent. J.* **146,** 43–46.

WHITTAKER, D. K. THOMAS, V. C. and THOMAS, R. I. M. (1976) *Brit. Dent. J.* **140,** 100–102.

WILDER, H. H. and WENTWORTH, B. (1918) *Personal Identification.* Boston: Badger, Gorham Press.

WILTON, G. W. (1953) *Scots Law Times,* 14 Mar. 1953.

YOUNG, FILSON (1919) *Trial of Hawley Harvey Crippen, Notable British Trials.* Edinburgh: Hodge.

YOUNG, H. H. (1937) *Genital Abnormalities, Hermaphroditism and Related Adrenal Diseases.* Baltimore: Williams & Watkins.

ZORAB, P. A., PRIME, F. J. and HARRISON, A. (1963) *Lancet,* **1,** 195.

CHAPTER 3

Injuries: General Features

ACCURATE interpretation of the causation of wounds, particularly the distinction between incised and lacerated wounds, demands skilled examination at the earliest opportunity. Repair, whether natural or surgical, modifies the wound and can prevent a clear distinction which may be of paramount medico-legal importance. Even when the damaged tissues have been excised and preserved, examination of the specimen is rarely as satisfactory as the inspection of the wound *in situ* in its original state.

A detailed and accurate record should be made by the doctor at the time of the initial examination. This duty falls, as often as not, either to the general practitioner, resident hospital or casualty officer, rather than to the surgeon or medical jurist; even when a surgeon first sees the wound the record is not always as complete as it should be for medico-legal purposes.

Experience in New York was that "frequently hospital surgeons called upon to treat wounded persons, have neglected to describe accurately the patient's wounds, omitting mention of their exact nature, number, size and location. In many homicidal cases, not immediately fatal, the descriptions of the wounds in the hospital records are inadequate. It must be remembered that the original appearance of a fatal wound may be obliterated by a surgical operation, performed in the attempt to save the patient's life. . . . This information can be furnished only by the surgeon who first saw and treated the patient" (Helpern, 1946).

It is understandable that wounds in the living cause the clinician to be preoccupied with the breach of the tissues. How much damage is done and what steps are necessary to repair it? The circumstances in which it was inflicted, the agent responsible and other features of medico-legal importance are often overshadowed by this consideration. It is imperative, however, that whenever a wound is before him he takes thought of its possible medico-legal significance; and, if it appears likely that proceedings, especially criminal proceedings, will arise, he will immediately make an adequate record. Should some delay occur before he is called upon to give evidence, he is then well fortified because he is able to use his notes to refresh his memory and to regain a clear mental picture of the case.

Legal Definition of a Wound

There is no statutory definition of a wound but the Courts have decided that to constitute a wound, there must be a breach of the whole skin, involving both the epidermis and the cutis vera (*R.* v. *Wood,* 1830; *R.* v. *M'Loughlin,* 1838); it is also a wound if the inner lining of the lip be broken (*R.* v. *Smith,* 1837; *R.* v. *Warman,* 1846). In consequence, neither mere scratches (abrasions) nor fractures, without coincident breach of the skin, are wounds in law. This anomaly is unimportant in practice since there is an alternative charge of causing grievous bodily harm, for which offence a punishment of like severity can be imposed.

Medical Reports on Wounding

A medical report on wounding, whether prepared by the doctor who first sees the victim or the pathologist called upon to make a necropsy, is always likely to play an important part in any subsequent legal proceedings. The reports, therefore, must not only be adequate, but also couched in terms intelligible both to lay and medical persons. The arrangement, moreover, should provide a clear indication, when the wounds are multiple, of their relative importance and, when practicable, the order of infliction.

It is impracticable to devise a format which will suit every occasion since the circumstances vary a good deal. The report should take note of *every* injury observed, however trivial it may appear. When the case is complex, e.g. when there are lacerations, bruises and abrasions, which may be widely distributed, the drafting of the report is, admittedly, difficult. Prominence, obviously, must be given to the wound or wounds which play the major part, and trivial injuries may be relegated to a separate section. They are then in the report in a manner which permits reference to them, should the occasion arise, but they do not obtrude upon the principal injuries. It may be found convenient to deal with multiple injuries by grouping them according to their kind and severity. Alternatively, it may be better to group them anatomically, e.g. injuries of the head, of the trunk or of a limb. In the latter event, it may clarify the report if it includes a short summary of the injuries, grouped according to kind and severity.

There are certain features of wounds which are common to most and these are now briefly reviewed.

The size of the victim, i.e. stature, body weight and development, should be recorded.

The number and situation of the wounds must be recorded and each sited in relation to one or more easily identifiable landmarks, e.g. the middle line, a bony structure, a joint, the navel or the nipple. It will be remembered that the latter two are mobile landmarks.

The size and shape of each wound must be detailed. Precise measurement, with a ruler or tape measure, is a simple procedure and therefore there is no excuse for reference to plums, oranges, eggs, etc. The size should be stated in inches, and in metric terms. Irregular wounds, which are difficult to describe, should be sketched or photographed. A sketch should include a note of the measurements of the principal axes of the wound; a photograph should include a ruler, or other measure, arranged beside the wound.

The margins of the wound always require close inspection and for this purpose a hand lens is an invaluable aid; it is often wise to select tissue from the margin for microscopical examination. The margins of the wound may indicate (a) whether the wound was inflicted before or after death, (b) whether lacerated or incised, and (c) especially in relation to penetrating wounds, the direction of the weapon, as determined by shelving of the margins and the path or course of the wound. The depth indicates the probable length of the blade of the weapon, providing it be remembered that the blade may not be thrust home, or, alternatively, thrust home with force and the tissues compressed.

The floor of the wound may contain undivided, or irregularly divided structures; it may contain foreign material, e.g. soil, glass or part of a weapon. If over bone, especially the skull, inspection of the floor may reveal a fracture.

The condition of the wound in respect of haemorrhage, infection and repair is also to be noted.

Opinion

The points on which an opinion may be required will depend on the circumstances. In a fatal case it will have to be established that the wound was inflicted before death. It may be necessary to correlate the wound with the presence or absence of blood at the scene of wounding and on the assailant's clothing.

When there is more than one wound it may be necessary to determine which proved fatal, since the wounds may not have been made by the same assailant; nor at the same time. If the victim did not die at once, it may be necessary to assess the probable duration of survival and, especially with head injuries, the degree of mobility of the victim following the injury. Longer intervals of survival may have to be correlated with the stage of repair shown in the wounds.

When death is not directly due to wounds it may be necessary to determine how far, if at all, they accelerated death from some other cause.

Non-fatal injuries which result from accidents not infrequently lead to claims for compensation. On these occasions an opinion will be required not only as to present but also future disability. It must suffice here only to mention head and eye injuries. Head injuries which cause unconsciousness at the time of the accident call for great care when there appear to be no overt signs of permanent injury. It is then difficult to exclude psychological damage. If, however, the subject has been able to continue in his employment in a normal manner for several years, the head injuries cannot very well be a factor in his death from coronary disease. This may, however, be alleged and lead to an action for damages or compensation.

Penetrating wounds of the eyes, especially of young subjects, call for care in assessing future disability. Although a rare event, it appears that sympathetic ophthalmitis, which destroys the remaining eye, may set in at any time, months or even years after the accident.

Abrasions

These are superficial injuries, which involve only the outer layers of the skin, being trivial little scratches or grazes of no surgical importance. They are never too small or insignificant to ignore in medico-legal investigations; *they may be the only indication of severe internal injury*; e.g. head injury.

Their value derives from the fact that *they lie at the precise point of impact of blunt force*, an observation that most can confirm by personal experience of abraded knuckles or knees. Secondly, *they may exhibit a pattern*, which is sometimes an accurate reproduction of the surface, e.g. the radiator or other part of a motor car, which struck the victim. Or again, when they are crescentic and are seen on the neck or face the abrasion or scratch may well have been made by the fingernail of an assailant. Bite marks are also distinctive.

Pattern is the more likely to be imprinted by a crushing, as opposed to a tangential, scraping, of the cuticle. Parallel abrasions, in broken lines were produced by a piece of cycle chain, used as a knuckle duster or zip-fastener (Fig. 14).

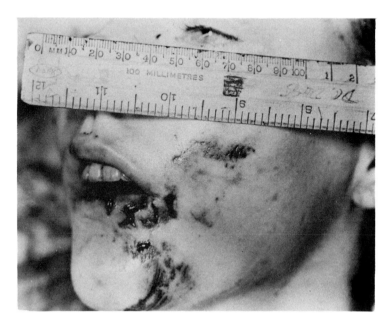

FIG. 14. Patterned abrasion on the cheek by a zip-fastener (F.M. 24574A).

Patterned abrasions are sometimes produced by the recoil of a firearm when discharged at contact range. The outline of the muzzle may be clearly reproduced or, in the case of a 12-bore shotgun, fired against the chest, there may be a pair of crescentic abrasions produced by part of the circumference of the barrels (F.M. 3744B).

Patterned abrasions which might be puzzling, unless the clothing be available for examination, can be produced by the metal hooks of corsets. Five circular abrasions, each $^1/_4$ in. in diameter, were set 1 in. apart over the course of a vertical right paramedian operation scar on the body of a female aged 77. The position of each abrasion corresponded with that of a hook on corsets she had worn at the time of her death (F.M. 6375).

In the case of road and other accidents, where the victim is dragged over the ground or against any resisting surface, there may be parallel grazes or brush marks. These lend corroboration to other evidence which suggests the victim had been injured in this manner.

Tyre marks: In some cases the passage of a wheel over the victim may leave a clear imprint of the tyre pattern, which, if unusual, can aid in the identification of the vehicle. When a boy aged 5 fell from a motor car he was run over by a following lorry. Tyre marks on the inside of his left thigh were a replica of the pattern on the tyre on the rear off-side wheel of the lorry (Fig. 15) (F.M. 6013A).

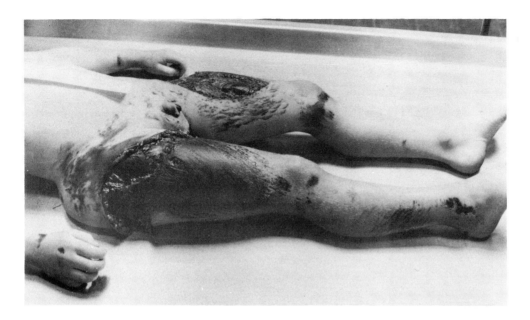

FIG. 15. Tyre marks on left thigh: lacerations and abrasions of both thighs and legs; parallel drag abrasions on right calf.

Scratches on the face of the accused were important in a case of murder by drowning because they indicated that the victim had made an attempt to defend herself (*R. v. Cook*, 1958, Fig. 16) (Dr. Gerald Evans, 1958). When they result from an impact, either forcible contact with part of a motor vehicle or the blow of a blunt object, the cuticle is crushed and the agent may impart a pattern to the abrasion. More often, abrasions result from dragging over a rough resisting surface or a tangential blow. In these circumstances broad abrasions without pattern, or sometimes with parallel scratches, will result. In drag or brush marks ruffling of the skin, a heaping up of the cuticle, may be observed at the distal end. This indicates the direction of the force applied to the skin.

When a man was found lying in the road, he was thought to have been knocked down by a motor car. The police suspected a particular vehicle but were puzzled by the absence of damage to its front. There was a patterned abrasion of the right side of his head; this was apparently a reproduction of the pattern of the car's tyre. There was a high level of alcohol in his blood. The findings indicated that he had been lying, drunk, in the road way and had been run over by a car (F.M. 14,607B).

Abrasions may be broader at the point of origin and this indicates the path of the agent. If a fingernail, it may be possible to say whether it was that of the victim or the assailant. In like manner it is sometimes possible to indicate the direction of dragging over a rough surface.

Nail marks and bites are conveniently included in the category of abrasions although they may, in fact, be incised or punctured wounds. Trivial though these injuries may be, they are of first importance on many occasions, notably in manual strangulation, rape or

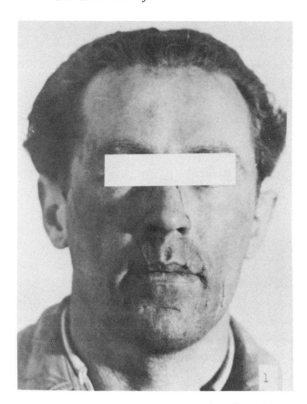

FIG. 16. Patterned abrasions: nail marks inflicted by
victim.

both. Nail marks are most often seen on the neck, as a result of throttling, or on the face following an assault. They may be seen on the inner aspect of the thighs in rape but violent intercourse with consent is equally capable of causing injury of this kind.

Appearances

Abrasions in the living may readily escape notice if the victim is examined in a poor light or if they are only slight; examination of selected areas under low magnification is sometimes necessary for their detection. The victim is well aware of their situation because they are sore or painful and moist.

In the dead, the circulation of the blood having ceased, plasma no longer exudes from an abrasion. In consequence its surface dries and becomes hard, acquiring the consistence of parchment; the abraded area is also brownish in colour. These areas, therefore, are not difficult to recognise; the need for caution turns rather upon the assessment of their severity, since the post-mortem changes tend to exaggerate the severity of abrasions. When there is some question of neglect of the deceased, care is necessary lest an adverse opinion is unduly weighted through an erroneous interpretation of the gravity of any abrasions present.

Abrasions sustained at or about the moment of death cannot with certainty be distinguished from those inflicted after death. If, however, by naked-eye examination or microscopy, bruising or other vital reaction be shown to co-exist, the wound was in all probability inflicted during life. Otherwise, any abrasion is to be considered *post-mortem* in origin.

Special attention should be paid to the nose, mouth and neck, especially of infants, where abrasions point to criminal violence. Abrasion and bruising of the thighs, especially on the inner side, of a female victim, at once raises the possibility of rape. If they are at the sides of the chest and have a more or less symmetrical distribution, inquiry should be made to discover whether artificial respiration had been practised. This operation in the hands of the unskilled can result in serious injury even to the extent of fracture of most of the ribs and the sternum (P.M. 117). This should be in mind now that extra-cardiac massage is not infrequently practised. Even in skilled hands, the patient may sustain fractures of the chest cage.

Differential Diagnosis

Abrasions must be distinguished from the following:

(a) *Marks produced by fish or insects*, after death. The latter injuries are without vital reaction, and may be seen at the angles of the mouth, the margins of the nose and eyelids or on the forehead.

(b) *Excoriation of the skin by excreta*. This is likely to be seen only in infants and its distribution is then usually self-explanatory. Care is necessary to avoid giving undue weight to it as a sign of neglect. Extensive excoriation, exaggerated by drying after death, may develop in a matter of hours, especially when plastic rompers or knickers are worn over a wet napkin.

(c) *Pressure sores*. These readily occur and the speed with which they may spread, especially when the patient has been nursed other than by professional nurses, must be borne in mind, otherwise an allegation of neglect may be unwise.

Bruises

A bruise is an escape of blood into the tissues of a living person, following the rupture of vessels, usually capillaries, by the application of blunt force.

Medico-Legal Significance

A bruise is evidence of the application of blunt force, and usually the circumstances are those of an accident or of homicide; it is unusual for the suicide to bruise himself by blows, since these occasion pain. This was important in the case of *R. v. Thorne* (1929). The victim, who had sustained several recent bruises of the scalp caused by blows, was alleged to have committed suicide by hanging; signs of hanging were stated to be present when the dismembered and decomposing body was examined, at a second necropsy, 3 months after her death.

A man, aged 75, was found dead with a cut throat and multiple lacerations of the scalp. The latter were all situated in position which were capable of self-infliction and there was no damage to the skull. The circumstances were those of suicide (F.M. 14,977A).

Unlike an abrasion, a bruise does not necessarily lie at the point of impact. The blood may travel for a distance in the deeper tissue planes before it reaches the surface; there may also be a delay in its appearance. On occasion, the bleeding may remain deep-seated, e.g. in relation to a fracture of the neck of the femur. Blows on the abdomen, although they may rupture internal organs and hollow viscera, may not produce an external bruise.

Situations of Special Importance

Bruises, in general, tend to be over prominent parts of the body but special attention is to be given to the neck where there may be bruising, which may be faint and in small areas, when made by the fingers in throttling, or by a ligature in strangulation and hanging. Bruises should also be sought for in the muscles of the neck where they are almost invariable in throttling, although none may be seen externally.

Bruising and abrasion of the shoulder blades indicates firm pressure on the body against the ground or other resisting surface, for example when an assailant kneels on his victim during strangulation or throttling. Bruising of the arms may indicate manual restraint.

Bruising of the thighs, especially the inner aspects, and of the genitalia, is common in rape, as are bruises on the arms or face sustained during a struggle. Kicks in the genitalia may cause severe bruising, with or without laceration.

Bruising of the scalp, with or without laceration, is easily overlooked. Careful search is necessary and there should be no hesitation to cut the hair or shave the suspected area, if it be thought necessary. These bruises may be apparent to the touch when invisible to the eye.

Bruising and the Agent: Patterned Bruising

In general, bruises are round or oval and are raised above the surface. When the victim lives, even if only for seconds after the blow, blood will continue to escape into the area during this time. In consequence the size of a bruise is likely to be larger than the surface of the agent which caused it. Bruises made by the fingers in throttling, although tending to be round or oval in shape, can be of larger area than the pads of the fingers of the assailant, but they may be only faint and of small size. Much depends on the time which elapses between the injury and the death of the victim. A patterned bruise may sometimes be relatively precise, for example those on the back of Heath's victim, which were replicas of the pattern of the leather riding whip, with which they were inflicted (*R. v. Heath*, 1946). On another occasion, a bruise reproduced the pattern of the wards of a key with which the victim was struck on the face. The exact point of contact with a motor car was determined by comparing the suspected part with a tracing of the pattern of bruising on a man's thigh (Spilsbury, 1939). Contact injuries from firearms may produce abrasion with bruising near the wound and its pattern may be a replica of the outline of the muzzle of the weapon.

The weapons most likely to leave distinctive bruising are whips, canes, knotted cords, belts or chains (Simonin, 1955; Martin, 1950). A ligature may sometimes produce a patterned bruise and, although the bruises produced by throttling are likely to be larger than the finger-pads, their round or oval shape and their position raise a strong presumption of their cause.

The skin of the trunk of a miner who died in an accident at the coal face was covered with patterned bruises in the form of parallel, zig-zag bruises. It was at first thought these were produced by the conveyor belt which had crushed him to the ground. The weave of the belt, however, clearly had a different pattern. The solution was provided by Mr. Ratcliffe, then technician in charge of the Leeds City Mortuary. He drew attention to the inside pattern of a woollen "pull-over" worn by the deceased at the time of the accident. Its pattern coincided with that of the bruising (F. M. 703).

A necklace (Lester James's case) or a rosary (the late Fyffe Dorward's case) may also leave their imprint on the skin of the neck in the form of abrasions, bruises or abraded bruises.

An old lady was found dead at the scene of a fire, which was clearly the result of arson. A bruise on her forehead bore the pattern shown to be an exact reproduction of the buckle of the belt of her assailant. (F.M. 25,947A, Figs. 17a, b).

Bruises caused by long rod-like objects produce a mark formed by two parallel lines of

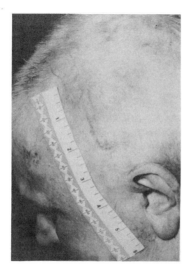

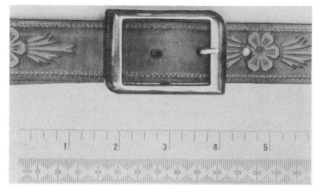

FIG. 17a, b. Patterned bruise on scalp caused by belt buckle (F.M. 25947B).

bruising—"tram lines". A man was found dead at home and it was suggested that he had fallen on the way back from a public house, striking his head and dying subsequently. He had two linear lacerations of the scalp, their axes at right angles to each other, one behind each ear. When the body was turned face down to reduce hypostatic staining, pairs of linear bruising were seen across his shoulders and chest, parallel to the wounds of his scalp. It was then clear that he had been struck by some rod-like agent across his back from both sides. He had then been strangled (F.M. 15,502B, Fig. 18b).

An unusual 'patterned" bruising was once seen widely distributed in the skin at the front of the chest. Pairs of close-set, linear bruises, each about $^1/_4$ in. long, were present between the collar bone and nipple on each side. The problem was promptly solved by the neurosurgeon in charge of the case. These were the result of pinching during life, to test the degree of loss of consciousness (F. M. 1950).

In the following case, a metal-studded belt produced distinctive bruising:

> The body of a boy aged 2 years had some small circular bruises, each $^1/_4$ in. in diameter, over the right hip joint and at the back of each knee joint. In the latter situation the purple-red circles were arranged in an equilateral triangle (Fig. 18a). A metal embossed belt bearing small brass cones each $^1/_4$ in. in diameter at their bases, arranged in equilateral triangles, had been used by the mother to chastise the child. She admitted this but maintained that she had struck the child with the belt several hours before it died of subdural haemorrhage. In my opinion the blows must have been inflicted shortly before death since the outline of the bruises was sharp (F.M. 7051; *R. v. Clark*; Leeds Spring Assizes, 1960).

Elliptical bruises, of up to an inch in their long axis and up to $^3/_4$ in. broad, are sometimes seen on the sides of the neck or the breasts. These are patterned bruises produced by suction or biting during erotic lovemaking or sexual intercourse (F.M. 14594, Fig. 19). A remarkable example was shown by Gormsen (1961); the bruises had been interpreted by the inexpert as evidence of manual strangulation; the distinction was made by the shape of the bruises and a total absence of any signs of asphyxia.

Bruising by Flexible Agents

Bruises produced by flexible agents have distinct characteristics. The whip or lash produces parallel, linear bruising which may encircle a limb or the trunk of the victim. The width between the marks represents the diameter of the agent. The terminal part of the

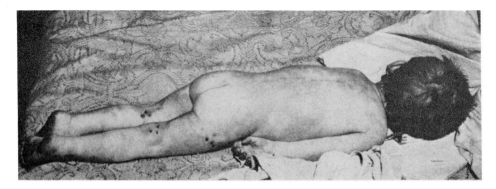

Fig. 18a. Patterned bruising: battered baby. Circular bruises, group in a triangle at the back of each knee; also at outer side of right thigh. Agent: a metal-studded belt applied by the mother.

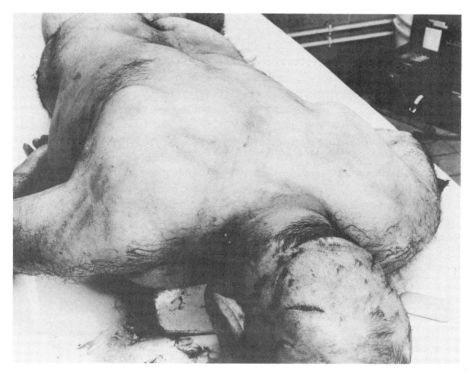

FIG. 18b. Patterned "tramline" bruising of back, caused by blows with rod-like agent (F.M. 15502B).

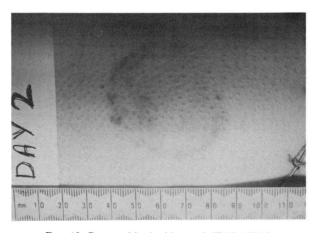

FIG. 19. Patterned bruise-bite mark (F.M. 18721).

mark, produced by the free end of the whip or lash, tends to be finer and may be abraded. Bruising by a cane also is in the form of parallel, linear bruising but, unlike the whip, the mark does not encircle the limb or trunk. If a strap be used and it has a pattern, the agent is then likely to leave its "signature", in the form of a patterned bruise. A riding whip, used by Heath, produced a notable "signed" bruising (*R. v. Heath*, 1946).

Bruising as a Measure of the Degree of Violence

Interpretation would indeed be easier if the size of a bruise were an accurate measure of the degree of violence which produced it. In general, it is true that a heavy blow is likely to produce a large bruise and a light blow, if it bruises at all, produces a small bruise. When bruising is slight it is right to assume, unless the contrary be clear from other findings, that the degree of violence was slight. Two men had an altercation and one received a blow to his mouth. He died from natural disease a day or so later and the blow was discounted as a factor in his death (F.M. 2141). A child's body bore several bruises of wide distribution but few exceeded $^2/_5$ in. in diameter. There were other children in the family and such bruises could have been produced by them in play or quarrels equally well as by the parent in chastising or alleged ill-treatment of the child. On the other hand, the rupture of the boy's liver and left kidney must have been due to violence greater than another small child could have exerted (F.M. 8143B).

In attempts to assess the degree of violence from the appearance of bruises several factors must be taken into consideration. The *situation* of the bruise is important because only mild violence is required to produce relatively large bruises of skin covering tissues which are loosely bound, e.g. the eyelids and the external genitalia. Conversely, where the tissues are closely applied to bone, e.g. the scalp, it normally requires substantial violence to produce a bruise.

The *age* and *sex* of the victim also play a part. The very young and the elderly bruise more readily than the young adult. The *obese* and those in *poor physical condition* are also prone to bruise unduly. A firm, playful grip of a well-nourished female arm can produce bruising which might suggest the application of substantial violence, as in an attempt forcibly to restrain. Those who suffer from a *disease of the blood* may also bruise readily, following the application of only mild force.

It is also possible for substantial violence to leave no trace of bruising. It is well recognised that grave internal abdominal injury, due to the application of substantial, i.e. moderately severe or severe, force, can be without any external sign of injury. Spilsbury (1939) said this occurred in 50 per cent of severe abdominal injuries. The liver and left kidney of a boy aged 3 years were ruptured without any external sign of injury; all bruising on his body was unrelated to these grave injuries (F.M. 8143B; *R.* v. *Wilson*, 1962).

If the head be free to move at the time of impact, a blow to the chin may not bruise the skin (Spilsbury, 1939).

Bruising may also be absent, notwithstanding the application of gross violence, if the pressure be continued until death occurred. Spilsbury instanced the continued pressure of the wheel of a vehicle on the chest. It is also accepted that external bruising may be absent when the grip in throttling is maintained until death occurs. This is possible if the immediate cause be vagal inhibition or, as Spilsbury mentioned, the victim had first been rendered unconscious by a blow or drug, thereby permitting prolonged retention of a grip.

Ante-mortem and Post-mortem Bruising

Bruising, as already defined, is essentially a vital phenomenon. For lack of a better term, the extrusion of blood from vessels into the tissues after death as a result of application of force to the cadaver, is here termed post-mortem "bruising".

There has been discussion from time to time about the possibility of producing "bruising" after death, and the distinction between such appearances from true bruises. Many, including myself (Polson, 1955), have given the impression that the distinction is simple and readily made. Robertson and Mansfield (1957) expressed their doubts about this and offered criteria which they believed to be of assistance on these occasions. A reconsideration of the matter (Polson, 1963) has left me in the firm belief that the occasions on which post-mortem "bruises" are likely to hinder interpretation, or to lead to false conclusions, are few. Where such "bruises" are small, i.e. of the order of $^1/_4$ in. or less, it may be impossible to distinguish them from bruises, by a consideration of the injury itself; any significance it may have is likely to be shown by a consideration of the findings as a whole. The quantitative differences are usually so great that a post-mortem "bruise" is not likely to be confused with an ante-mortem injury (Spilsbury, 1939; Moritz, 1954).

Experiments have shown me that the production of post-mortem "bruises" requires the application of considerable violence and the resulting "bruise" is almost always small or wholly disproportionate to the degree of force used. Although it is not true that such "bruises" are to be produced only in areas of hypostasis, it is only in these areas that a "bruise" of any size is likely to be produced. We did succeed on one occasion in producing a deep "bruise", $2^1/_2 \times 2 \times 1$ in., in a hypostatic area near the right posterior, superior iliac spine by administering three sharp blows with a wooden mallet (F.M. 7250).

The possibility of post-mortem "bruising" of the neck structures merits special consideration. On one occasion fracture of a great horn of the thyroid cartilage after death was accompanied by slight extrusion of blood into the adjacent tissues. This presented as a spindle-shaped haemorrhage at the root of the left great horn, $^1/_2$ in. long $\times$ $^1/_8$ in. at its maximum diameter (F.M. 736). No other "bruising" was produced. It is highly improbable that in throttling during life such a change would be alone present. Even in the absence of any bruising of the skin some muscular bruising, even if only slight, is likely to be coincident.

The question I posed (Polson, 1960) was whether post-mortem "bruising" of the skin of the neck was known or possible. I had examined a woman aged 72 who suffered from severe heart disease and who died after an assault upon her, the terminal phase being throttling. The nail marks on her face and neck could well have been produced near death, in the agonal phase, so that distinction between ante- and post-mortem infliction was impossible in respect of most of these marks. She had, however, a small recent red bruise below the right angle of the jaw and another smaller and fainter bruise at about the angle of the jaw. It is my opinion that bruises of this kind cannot be produced after death. It would involve a severe compression of the skin and there appears no way, other than by pinching, practicable, and the human hand is then unlikely to have sufficient power to succeed. Nearer to the middle line it is conceivable that gross compression of the skin against the spine might perhaps yield a small "bruise".

In general, post-mortem "bruising" is practicable only where the tissues can be forcibly compressed against bone and, preferably, also in an area of hypostasis.

Bruising of the occiput is, perhaps, an exception to the general conclusion that post-mortem "bruising" is unlikely to be confused with ante-mortem injury. Robertson and Mansfield (1957) instanced the production of a post-mortem "bruise" of the scalp, almost an inch in diameter, due to careless bumping of the head on a stretcher. I confess I was somewhat sceptical and it was outwith our experience in Leeds. We have now made some tests with a wooden mallet and find that a moderate blow to the occiput can produce a "bruise" which involves the whole thickness of the scalp in an area of up to an inch in diameter. The possibility of a head injury during life in our subjects was excluded by collateral evidence.

Clearly, therefore, bruising in the region of the occiput calls for care in interpretation. Before it is ascribed to injury during life, the possibility of a blow to the occiput after death must be excluded. Moderate force applied to the scalp, close to bone, in an area the site of hypostasis, can and does crush the vessels and drive blood into the tissue spaces, so as to simulate a bruise. There need be no accompanying breach of the skin; it was intact in our tests. The force used was moderated in order to avoid fracturing the skull.

Bruising in Relation to Poisoning by Carbon Monoxide

Where the bruise has a red-brown or brown colour, it is due to an injury prior to gassing, whereas a bruise sustained at that time is likely to have a bright red colour. Saturation of the blood by only 35 per cent is sufficient to impart this colour, yet the victim, unless gravely ill from some other cause, would not have had a lethal dose of carbon monoxide. Where the bruise is of reasonable size, even when enough to yield only a few drops of blood, it is practicable to estimate its content of CO. (Cf. the examination of blood in the track of a firearm injury, see pp. 218, 220.)

The Development of Bruising after Death

There are occasions when at his initial examination an observer has seen no bruising of a body, but bruising is apparent on re-examination, some hours later. In other circumstances the first to observe the body had seen no bruising but another, seeing the body some hours later, found obvious bruising. This is not necessarily due to faulty observation.

A bruise deep to the intact skin may extend after death so as to discolour the skin. This can be due to diffusion of blood pigment from the bruised area. Gravitation of blood may also occur. A bruise may thus become apparent externally for the first time, or bruises, already observed, may be intensified in colour and area, after death.

The examination of the whole body by ultra-violet light will sometimes show up otherwise undetectable areas of bruising (Cameron *et al.*, 1973; Hempling, 1981).

The Age of a Bruise

No precise estimate of the age of a bruise is practicable because the appearance of the colour changes which occur in an ageing bruise will depend upon one or more of several factors. The size and depth of the bruise are especially important; a large bruise or one which is deep-seated may remain red or dark red for days or weeks.

In general, a superficial bruise which is red, dark red or black is of recent origin and probably not more than 24 hours old. At the end of a week a greenish tinge may be apparent, succeeded, at the end of about 2 weeks, by yellowing of the area; bruises of small or moderate size may resolve completely by the end of a month. Some idea of the need for caution in expressing an opinion is shown by the fact that a greenish tinge is said by

Sydney Smith and Fiddes (1955) to appear in 4 to 5 days, whereas others give 7 to 12 days as the interval. Any attempt to distinguish a bruise sustained at the time of death and one which occurred a few minutes earlier is impracticable.

In regard to the age of bruises, Moritz (1954) says that diffusely extravasated erythrocytes disappear from tissues within a few days and that haemosiderin is detectable in phagocytes after 24 hours by means of the Prussian Blue reaction. However, the possibility must always be borne in mind that haemosiderin may be present in superficial tissues as a result of a previous injury in the same site. Robertson and Mansfield (1957) concluded that estimation of the age of a bruise is completely unreliable. Deep-seated bruises, or those where there is a considerable extravasation of blood with haematoma formation, may retain intact and apparently normal erythrocytes for a considerable period of time.

Proof of Bruising

The tissues in the suspected area should be incised and when the naked-eye appearances are equivocal, a portion must be taken for microscopy. This should be done in any event when the death may lead to criminal proceedings. Post-mortem hypostasis must be excluded as a cause of the changes seen, and if they are bruises, this must be proved. Microscopy will also exclude telangiectases of the skin (F.M. 2217A). This step would have been of great value in a case of alleged throttling. At the first necropsy, five faint, tiny bruises arranged in a line, one to the right, and four to the left of the middle line, in the skin of the neck, at the level of the upper border of the larynx were observed. These observations no doubt were accurate but, when a second necropsy (F.M. 3566A) was performed, 10 days later, these bruises were no longer apparent.

Lacerations

These common wounds are the result of tearing apart or splitting of the tissues; shearing or crushing of the skin until it splits is usually responsible. In the latter event the site of wound is likely to be near to bone, especially the skull. The mechanism responsible gives rise to wounds in which there is usually irregular and unequal division of the tissue planes; structures like arteries and nerves may be crushed or laid bare in the floor of the wound.

Lacerations are usually accidental; in homicide they are produced by a wide range of agents, some of which raise a presumption of premeditation and intent. Others, readily at hand, although they may be used with intent to injure, do not suggest premeditation. The suicide is rarely lacerated because the kind of injury responsible causes much pain; unless a mental patient, therefore, the suicide prefers other modes of self-destruction; falls from a height or suicide on the railway being excepted.

Examples of agents which produce lacerations may be grouped as follows:

(1) Passive agents; the ground, pavement edge, stairs or other parts of a building, or furniture; lacerations due to falls are especially common.

(2) Vehicles: especially motor cars and lorries.

(3) Weapons, indicative of premeditation and intent; these include a pistol butt, a knuckleduster, or bicycle chain adapted as a knuckleduster or used as a flail.

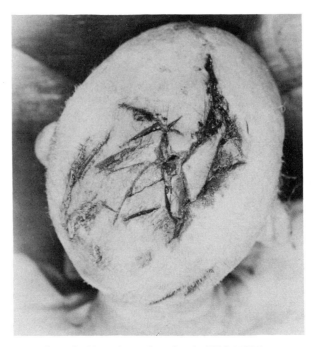

FIG. 20. Linear laceration of scalp (F.M. 27073).

Axes or heavy choppers, although cutting instruments, are often blunt and will then produce lacerations rather than incised wounds; the butt of such a weapon will always produce a laceration (Fig. 21).

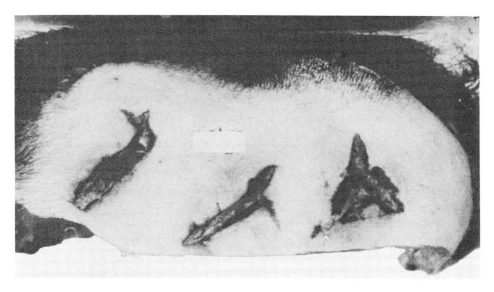

FIG. 21. Laceration of forehead by butt of an axe.

(4) Weapons indicative of intent but not usually premeditation: These include the fist, bare or covered with a boxing glove, or the booted foot; sticks, stones, hammers, pokers, shovels (Fig. 24) or bottles. The latter, if broken, may produce wounds which resemble both lacerations and stab or incised wounds; these variations may co-exist and complicate interpretation.

The Features of a Laceration

A laceration is usually situated over some prominent part of the body but grave lacerations elsewhere may be produced by a shearing force, as by a wheel passed over the body of someone laid on the ground.

These wounds vary in size from a fraction of an inch to several inches in length; they vary also in depth according to the thickness of the soft parts at the site of injury and the degree of force applied.

Characteristically, they are ragged wounds with an irregular division of the tissues; the skin is usually the more widely torn but, on occasion, the deeper tissues may also be forcibly torn apart to expose the underlying muscles which may or may not escape. Blood vessels and nerves are often spared and laid bare in the depths of the wound or the vessels may be partly torn or completely severed in irregular fashion. It is usual for the vessels to be damaged in such a manner that the torn ends are crushed and incompletely sealed. Bleeding, therefore, is relatively slight when compared with that due to an incised wound. On the other hand, the agents responsible are often heavily infected and the tissues, devitalised by the injury, are less able to resist infection; in consequence, inflammation is a common complication of the repair of these injuries.

The margins of lacerated wounds are bruised, an important feature, which may require

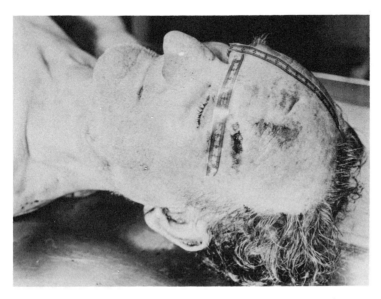

FIG. 22. Patterned "zig-zag" abrasion on forehead (F.M. 27073).

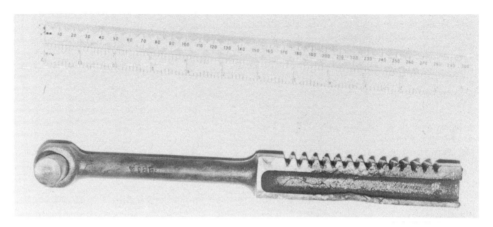

FIG. 23. Weapon responsible for wounds in Fig. 20 and 22.

low magnification for its recognition. If the wound is in a hairy part of the body it may also be found that the hair bulbs are exposed, uncut, in the margin of the wound (see p. 118).

The floor of the wound must be examined to determine the extent of the injury and for the presence of foreign material, e.g. soil, or particles of glass. Lacerations in the living, when contaminated with soil, etc., raise the possibility of tetanus, gas gangrene or other infection, and call for prophylactic measures. Failure to give appropriate treatment may result in action for negligence.

Lacerations of Tissue Applied to Bone

These wounds are in a distinct category because their recognition as lacerations often presents difficulty. Where skin is closely applied to bone and the subcutaneous tissues are scanty, blunt force may produce a wound which, by linear splitting of the tissues, simulates an incised wound. If, in addition, it is a hairy part, e.g. the scalp, even greater difficulty may be experienced in making the distinction.

The sites which call for special care are the scalp, the face and, in particular, the eyebrow, the iliac crests, the perineum, the vulva, and the shin. In general, it is a reasonable preliminary assumption that wounds in these areas are lacerations, until the contrary be proved. A definite opinion may be practicable only after microscopy and when there is an adequate knowledge of the circumstances. The wound must be examined in good lighting and with the aid of a hand lens, at the earliest opportunity, before repair has modified it. On all other occasions a guarded opinion is essential.

Kerr (1957) drew attention to parallel linear wounds one on each side of the anus caused by a kick in the perineum; they may simulate an injury produced by a cutting weapon, about an inch wide, driven into the perineum.

Homicidal blows with a shovel. Although the lacerations presented as splits in the scalp, in the following case, there was little doubt that these were lacerations produced by appreciable blunt force.

An old woman aged 86 was attacked by another woman aged 40. The principal injury was gross laceration of the scalp caused by blows with a shovel. Some were made with its edge, as judged by a linear bruise several inches long running across the right side of forehead. Seven lacerations of the scalp were linear splits with bruised margins, produced by swinging blows with the broad flat back of the shovel. They ranged from $2^1/_2$ in. to $4^1/_2$ in. in length and three lay parallel, between the occiput and the vertex; two more were to the right, one to the left and the seventh was at the front of the scalp (Fig. 24). There was no fracture of the skull, presumably because the force was widely dispersed. Slight subarachnoid haemorrhage was the sole intracranial change. Death was due to multiple injuries and scalding. The lower jaw and cervical spine were fractured (*R.* v. *Lloyd,* 1955; F.M. 4067A).

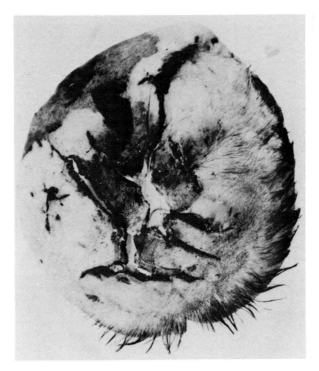

FIG. 24. Laceration of scalp by blows with a shovel (note parallel major splits on the scalp).

Laceration of an Eyebrow: single blow but two apparently separate wounds

The deceased had two apparently separate lacerations above his right eyebrow (Fig. 25a). He had been paying unwelcome attention to the assailant's wife. This led to an altercation during which the deceased received one blow from the clenched fist of the assailant. The police doubted this since they saw two separate splits; also there was a disused milk bottle at the scene and it was suggested that this had been the agent.

The man appeared to be telling the truth therefore a simple experiment was devised. A thick layer of Plasticine was applied to the head of our Fowler's Phrenology bust and the head was then forcibly struck with a closed fist. This produced indentations in the clay, following contact with the knuckles of the middle and ring fingers. The size and arrangement coincided with those of the injury. Examination of the accused disclosed an abrasion of the kunckle of his right hand, i.e., the middle finger, making the greater

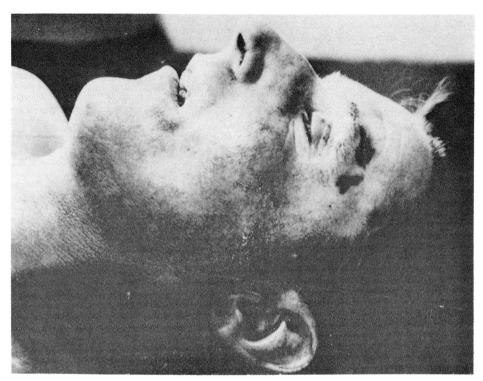

FIG. 25a. Laceration of eyebrow: allegedly by two blows but proved to have been by one; the separate lacerations by knuckles of the middle and ring finger.

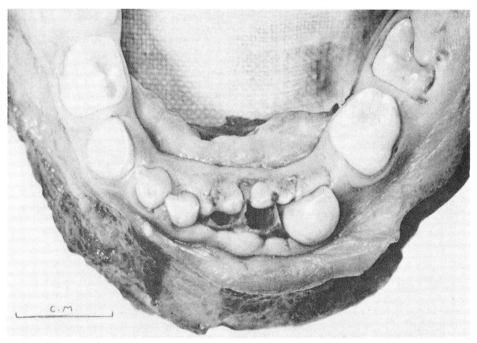

FIG. 25b. Loss of lower incisors and loosening of adjacent teeth. Sustained close to the moment of death but no bleeding from the sockets. (A case of battered baby: see Fig. 18a.)

contact with eyebrow of the deceased. The Court accepted his story and imposed a light sentence (F.M. 9604A).

Lacerations by the Shod Foot

Kicking is still in fashion and Teare (1961) provided useful criteria by which blows with the shod foot may be recognised.

The *site* of the injury is one relatively inaccessible to blunt agents normally used. Thus the lacerations are likely to be of the head and neck, especially beneath the chin, at the angle of the jaw or round or behind an ear but not on the vertex. They also occur at the sides of the chest or trunk. Teare (1961), reported five cases of which one is an excellent example of the results of a kick beneath the chin.

The *degree of external injury* depends on the point of impact. It is more severe where the skin is close to bone, e.g. below the chin, whereas on the cheek it may be trivial.

The *degree of internal injury* is proportionately greater than the external injury would suggest.

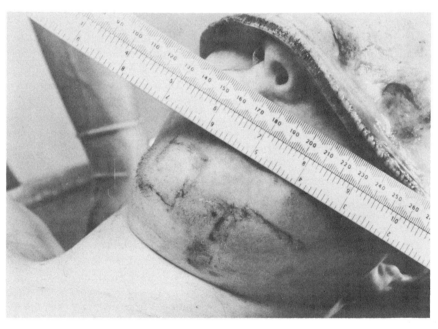

Fig. 26. Patterned abrasions on the chin caused by blows with the shod foot (F.M. 20951).

Lacerations Inflicted Before and After Death

The distinction between lacerations inflicted before and after death must depend on the presence or absence of vital reaction in the wound. Bleeding from the wound, and, more especially, bruising of its margins indicate infliction before death; total absence of bruising, proved by microscopy, is indicative of injury after death.

Occasionally, when the wound is sustained in circumstances which cause immediate death, or it is inflicted shortly after death, the distinction is well-nigh impossible.

In such circumstances the injury must be presumed to have occurred after death. A child aged 2 years had sustained multiple bruises, including patterned bruising by a metal-studded, leather belt. The cause of death was sub-dural haemorrhage. It was also found, however, that there was laceration of the gums and two lower incisor teeth had recently been dislodged. There were no signs of repair of the gums, of the sockets of the teeth, nor was there any trace of bleeding in relation to these injuries. Although it is possible that this injury of the mouth was caused by the last of a series of blows, it was impossible to prove that the child was then still alive. In consequence, this injury was promptly dismissed by the learned judge as irrelevant (F.M. 7051; Fig. 25b).

Eversion and gaping of the margins of the wound is usually seen only when it is inflicted during life, but in the thigh, for example, gaping may be seen in wounds inflicted after death because the weight of the tissues may then be sufficient to open the wound by gravitation.

The bodies of persons taken from navigable waters may bear gross wounds, usually lacerations, produced after death by contact with the bed of the sea, river or canal or with parts of ships, especially the propeller blades. The extent of the injuries and the absence of vital reaction in them is usually sufficient to establish their origin and time of infliction; nor do putrefactive changes, unless gross, necessarily preclude an opinion.

Lacerations following a street brawl may have special importance since a question to be determined is whether the wound was due to a blow or a fall. The site of the wound and the presence or absence of soil in it may be material on these occasions. Lacerations on the vertex of the scalp are the result of a fall from a height or of contact with a projection, e.g. when the victim suddenly stands erect from a stooping or kneeling posture and strikes his head against a corner of the mantelpiece or an open cupboard door above his head. In other circumstances wounds of the vertex are almost certainly inflicted by an assailant. The presence of soil, grit, etc., in the wound indicates a fall and usually excludes a blow as the cause. But an agent may bear grit or dust and thus soil the wounds, e.g. a coal hammer may bear coal dust and a blunt instrument may bear grit or coal dust.

Debris may indicate the possible nature of the agent. An elderly man, when found dead, had lacerations of his head and forearm, containing tiny black particles. These were fragments of coal dust. There was no coal in the room but the office was in the vicinity of a coal merchant's premises, the yard of which had a wooden fence. The agent was considered to have been a piece of wood, soiled with coal dust, taken from the fence (11,427A).

Blackish material soiled the margins of stab wounds. It was proved to be mineral oil and carborundum derived from its use to sharpen the weapon (25,904A).

Shelving of the margins of a laceration is common and its direction indicates that of the force responsible. This may be of special importance in head injuries as a means of distinguishing between the blow of a weapon and a laceration due to a fall.

Incised Wounds

The term "incised wound" is often loosely used by doctors, and it must be better appreciated that this loose terminology is indefensible when reference is made to a wound received in circumstances which may lead to criminal proceedings.

In such circumstances the term "incised wound" implies intent, because the weapon responsible, especially if it be an open razor or razor blade, is not of a kind commonly carried in the pocket; the assailant has taken steps to be armed. Incised wounds, when inflicted in criminal circumstances, are produced by a relatively limited range of weapons. The open razor was often used, but safety razor blades, which may be mounted to protect the assailant's hands and to give more control over the weapon, are now used. An assailant may embed one or more of these blades in the peak of a cloth cap and the weapon is then wielded, flail-like, in an attack. Not infrequently the motive is to disfigure rather than to kill. As already mentioned, axes and choppers, although cutting instruments, tend to produce lacerations rather than incised wounds because they are often blunt.

Appearances

The best examples of incised wounds are those made by a surgeon with a scalpel, which has a keen edge, and when the tissues are placed under tension to ensure a linear wound.

Although incised wounds, e.g. cut-throat injuries, may be deep, their length is greater than their depth. The sharper the blade, the more cleanly does it cut through the soft parts, including vessels, in the same vertical plane. Shelving occurs when the blade is at an angle to the surface.

Because the vessels are divided cleanly, profuse haemorrhage is invariably a feature of incised wounds. Common experience shows that even minor incisions of a vascular part, for example the finger tip, can give rise to troublesome bleeding. On the other hand, and probably because prompt bleeding washes out any bacteria carried into the wound by the weapon, septic complications are unusual. Prompt bleeding, even from a puncture wound with a septic needle, goes far to avert sepsis. It is therefore imperative that any wound sustained whilst performing a post-mortem examination is made to bleed at once; this may call for a swinging of the arm to drive blood into the wounded area.

The usual incised wound is linear but if the skin is loosely applied to the body, even if the cutting blade be sharp, the resulting wound may take a zig-zag (dentélé) course (Plate 2), because the skin is pushed in front of the blade before it is divided.

The margins of the incised wound, when unaltered by repair, are clean-cut and show no signs of bruising. Being produced, as a rule, by a sweep of a blade, such wounds are deeper at their origin and tail off, becoming more superficial, at their end.

Gaping is another feature of these wounds and, although usually of ante-mortem origin, this can be due to gravitation of tissues after death, especially when the wound involves the thigh.

Cut-throat Wounds

The situation and circumstances of incised wounds of the throat place them in a special category. They are rarely the result of an accident and the distinction of importance is between suicide and homicide. Rarely, accidental injury by glass may produce a wound of this kind but the distinction can be made by the presence of fragments of glass in the wound and by small side cuts in its margins and by the circumstances.

Suicidal Cut-throat

Incised wounds of the neck are a well-recognised mode of suicide, although their incidence has been less in recent years than formerly, when open razors were more often used for shaving.

The self-inflicted wound, when made by a right-handed person, normally begins high on the left side and passes downwards across the front, to end on the right side of the neck. It is deeper at its origin and tails off on the right. It can be, however, a wound which lies horizontally across the front of the neck (Fig. 27). It is normally a linear, clean-cut wound, since the skin is likely to be under tension when, as is usual, the victim throws back his head to clear a path for the weapon. Some stand before a mirror in order better to direct the hand. When present, separate, shallower incisions at the upper end of the wound are strongly indicative of self-infliction; these are the so-called "tentative" or "hesitant" incisions.

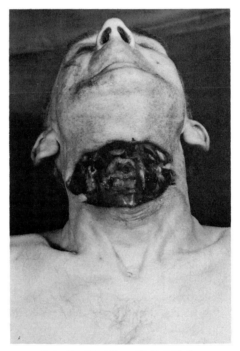

FIG. 27. "Cut-throat". (Suicide.)

The throat injury may be accompanied by incised wounds of the wrist (Fig. 28) or tentative incised wounds elsewhere (Fig. 29).

Cut-throat may be the act of an impatient suicide who had first chosen another mode, e.g. A man aged 33 ingested a quantity of aspirin. He was found dead in his garage with a superficial cut on his right wrist and a deep cut on his left wrist. There was an incised wound 3 in. long on the right side of his neck accompanied by tentative, superficial cuts. The major blood vessels were spared but he had severed the right anterior jugular vein. His stomach contained about 4 oz. of gritty, white, porridge-like material; bleeding had occurred into the summits of the folds of the stomach mucosa (acute gastritis). Analysis of the stomach contents: 130 grains of aspirin, the equivalent of 26 tablets, present. This overdose had been too slow to kill and he resorted to cut-throat. There had been appreciable blood loss before he died (F.M. 11,369A).

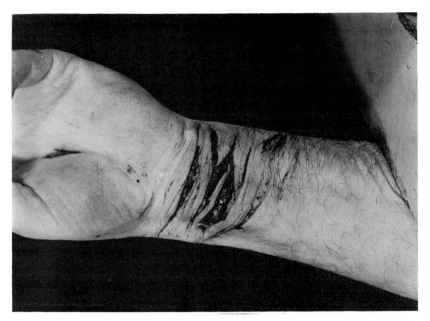

FIG. 28. Incised wounds of wrist: Suicide.

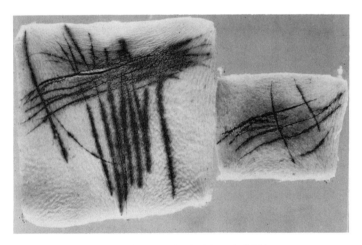

FIG. 29. Tentative incisions (suicide).

The homicidal wound lacks the planning of a self-inflicted wound and is unaccompanied by tentative incisions (Fig. 30). On the contrary, it may be accompanied by deep cuts elsewhere on the head and neck. It tends to lie lower in the neck and is, perhaps, more horizontal. There may be under-cutting or bevelling of its margins and they are likely to be toothed (dentélé) because the skin is not under tension as the blade traverses it and is thrown into folds before severance, even by a sharp blade. Homicidal cut-throat is likely to divide a jugular vein or a carotid artery, whereas these structures may be protected by

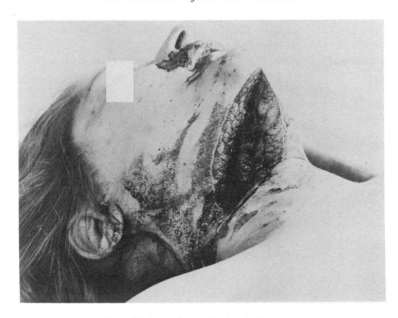

Fɪɢ. 30. Incised wound of neck: homicide.

the sternomastoid muscle, when the head is extended by the suicide. This protection, however is not general in suicide, since the vein and artery are by no means invariably spared.

The hands and forearms should be inspected, since they may bear incisions. They could be self-inflicted in a preliminary attempt at suicide. Not rarely the initial step is by horizontal incisions across the front of the wrists, presumably with a view to cutting the radial artery (Fig. 28). (A faulty knowledge of anatomy has led to horizontal cuts at the back of a wrist.) These incisions are normally multiple and parallel within the target area; they vary in severity, some being tentative wounds. Defence injuries, on the other hand, are not planned and are relatively severe. Their distribution is consistent with an attempt to grasp or ward off the weapon (Fig. 31). Cuts then occur on the palmar aspect of the hands or on the knuckles; there may be slashes on the forearms.

Rarely, the suicide may cut his neck from behind. A butcher, who had failed to commit suicide by the usual incision, succeeded on a later occasion by adopting the incision, at the back of the neck, which he was accustomed to use when slaughtering animals.

Suicidal cut-throat is one of the modes of death which may lead to instantaneous rigor. If the razor, carver or table knife is found thus firmly held in the victim's hand, there can be no doubt of the fact of suicide, even when other features are equivocal (F.M. 2964).

It is sometimes material to know what range of movement is practicable after the infliction of a cut-throat. Simpson (1962) related how one victim, who had nearly decapitated himself, was still able to kick his would-be rescuer downstairs with such force that this well-meaning person sustained a broken wrist.

The power of speech may be retained even when the wound is below the larynx (Littlejohn, 1925).

The absence of a cutting agent at the scene, and certainly its absence from premises, is a

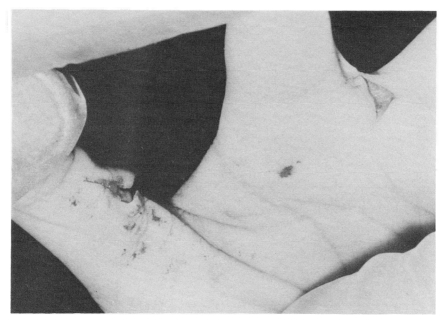

FIG. 31. Defence wounds of the hand caused by a plane blade (F.M. 21286).

strong indication of homicide. When present, the circumstances of the death may still require a thorough investigation in order to distinguish between homicidal and self-infliction. It is possible for the homicide, who finds, or renders, his victim incapacitated, to inflict an injury which resembles a self-inflicted cut-throat.

The Cause of Death

A cut-throat wound may cause death in one of several ways. When one or both carotid arteries are severed death is due to haemorrhage. If, as is usual, the trachea is also opened, blood may be inhaled and choking is then a contributory factor.

On rare occasions death may be due to air embolism. This is a possibility when the external jugular vein is incompletely divided. A man aged 53 died of air embolism when he cut his throat with a carving knife. The left external jugular vein was incompletely divided. Blood in the right ventricle and pulmonary arteries was foamy. Putrefaction had not occurred (F.M. 151).

In the event of complete division of the trachea, it is likely to be drawn down into the thorax; the soft parts of the neck then fall in and closure of the air way results, to cause death from mechanical asphyxia. In other subjects minor wounds, if complicated by sepsis, especially infection of the larynx, may cause death from secondary broncho-pneumonia, several days after the wounding.

Pseudo "Cut-throat" Injuries

Three unusual cases of injury to the throat, simulating cut-throat, merit record.

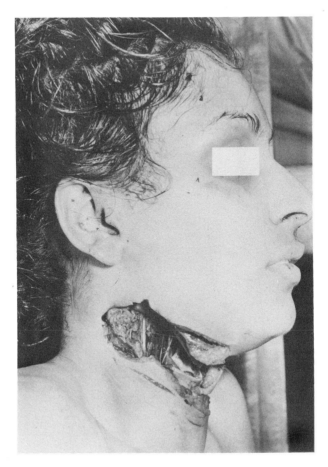

FIG. 32. Ragged incised wound caused by the blade of a
carpenter's plane (F.M. 21286).

The first concerned a male aged 40 whose body was found at the foot of Malham Cove.
A wound across the front of the neck led to the initial belief that he had cut his throat prior
to precipitating himself from the top of the cliff.

The wound is 13.5 cm long gaping by up to 1.5 cm. It is deeper at the left and fibres of
the sternomastoid muscle had been severed. The margins are irregular and obviously
bruised; hairs, exposed down to their bulbs, lie along the margins of the wound, uncut.
The deeper tissues were lacerated but not cleanly divided (Fig. 33).

The hyoid bone was fractured on each side at about the junction of the great horn with
the body of the bone and the horns were displaced outwards. There was a fracture 2 cm
long which separated the alae of the thyroid cartilage and the trachea had been avulsed at
a point 3 in. (7.5 cm) below the vocal cords.

Examination of the cliff showed that a branch of a tree growing from it had been
damaged. It appeared that during his fall the man's neck had struck this branch. The
impact had also fractured his lower jaw (F.M. 12/50, Dr. John Benstead).

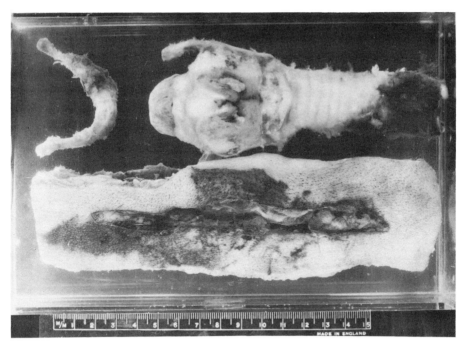

FIG. 33. Laceration of neck simulating cut-throat. Also broken hyoid bone and thyroid cartilage. Contact with bough of a tree during suicidal fall from a cliff.

The second case, details of which are given in the section on stab wounds (see p. 123), was one of apparent cut-throat due to injury by a hay fork. Slashing with it across the front of the neck had produced several lacerations, one of which was not unlike an incised wound (Figs. 34, 35). Close examination confirmed that it was a laceration, and experiments with a hay fork reproduced the appearances (F.M. 6128A).

The third case was one in which a man aged 50 was killed by an intruder, present with intention to rob him. The principal injuries, which included a broken nose and the dislodgement of teeth, were due to blunt force. It appeared that during the attack the accused had struck the deceased with a bread knife, inflicting superficial cuts on the left ear and temple and an incised wound of the neck. The deceased had atheroma of his left coronary artery and the right branch was unduly small (F.M. 7636; *R. v. Pankotai*).

Wounds by Glass

Wounds produced by glass may cause difficulty in interpretation in the absence of information concerning circumstances of the injury. They can mimic, at least superficially, lacerated, incised and stab wounds. Basically, they are all lacerated wounds but if the sharp edge of a sheet of glass comes into contact with the skin, the resulting wound closely resembles that produced by a sharp cutting instrument. If a spicule of glass enters by its point, the wound is then stab-like in appearance.

The usual wound by glass is an obvious laceration, often accompanied by multiple

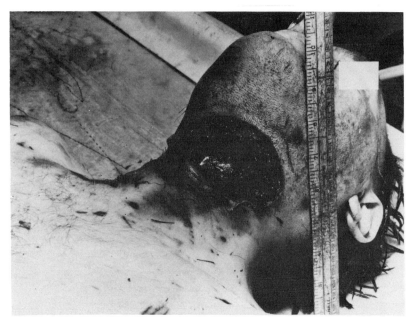

FIG. 34. Laceration of neck: Simulating an incised wound associated with stab wounds. Produced by the tine of a hay fork.

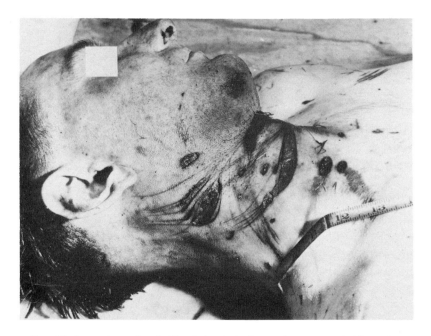

FIG. 35. Lacerations of neck: Simulating incised wounds; accompanied by stab wounds. (Injuries produced with a hay fork: see also Figs. 34, 44.)

scratches or abrasions, when, for example, the head of the injured person is forced through the windscreen of a motor-car. The appearances of the lesser injuries are somewhat reminiscent of the imprint of a bird's foot. Multiple angular abrasions accompany lacerations of varied severity. A good example (Fig. 36) is that of a woman who was thrown through the windscreen when her car was over-run by a horse van, which got out of control when descending a steep hill (F.M. 6064A).

When the wound simulates an incised wound examination with a hand lens at an early stage will probably detect slight bruising of the margins. Side-cuts are also likely to be seen and the latter, when present, are characteristic of a wound by glass. Search should be made for flakes or particles of glass in the wound.

Simulation of a cut-throat by a sharp weapon may be sufficiently close to permit distinction only by the demonstration of fragments of glass in the wound. Gonzales, *et al.* (1954), depict an example, where the victim, when drunk, fell down a flight of stairs and went headfirst through a heavy plate glass door, at the bottom. Another man fainted and his head went through a window, with the result that he sustained a deep laceration across the front of his neck (Smith and Fiddes, 1955) and yet other examples have been reported by Cathcart (1909–10) and Scott (1928).

Stab-like wounds by glass are unusual. The following are examples:

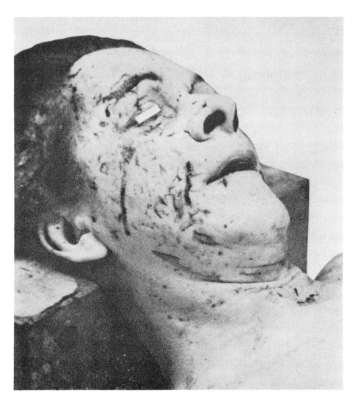

FIG. 36. Abrasion and laceration by glass: road accident; victim
thrown through windscreen.

A woman, who was carrying a box of ducklings covered by a sheet of plate glass, was seen to reach a fence and then suddenly collapse. Examination showed that the glass had shattered, presumably by contact with the fence; a dagger-like fragment had penetrated her chest and transfixed her heart. Professor Webster found puncture marks in her clothing and her chest. A dagger-shaped piece of glass near the body fitted the wound; a small recent cut on the woman's finger suggested that this was caused when she had withdrawn the glass from her chest (*Birmingham Mail*, June 4th, 1948; Webster, 1960). On another occasion a girl was killed in a similar fashion by a dagger-like fragment from the window of a swing door. As she was about to pass through, a person coming the other way banged the door against the girl and one of its opaque glass panels was shattered.

While the *Deblin*, a Polish ship, was sailing from Poland to Hull, then in international waters, a member of the crew was found lying injured on the starboard side; he lay in a space between the superstructure and deck cargo. Blood was freely distributed on the deck and adjacent parts of the ship in the form of pools and some splashes. The appearances were those of venous rather than arterial bleeding. He was carried below and laid in his bunk. The Captain summoned a doctor from Grimsby but by the time he boarded the ship the patient had died. Inspection of the body disclosed a stab wound in the left groin; it was deemed to have been homicidal. The police were summoned when the ship docked in Hull and the crew were submitted to interrogation. One member whom they wished to interview had locked himself in his cabin and refused to see them. In another cabin they found freshly washed outer garments and a red-brown stain on the cabin door. At this juncture the atmosphere was distinctly tense.

The post-mortem examination (F.M. 8618A) confirmed the presence of a punctured wound in the left groin 1 in. long, gaping by $^2/_3$ in. situated 1 in. below the fold of the groin, towards the inner side of the thigh. Its margin shelved upwards and its course was upwards and backwards. It was elliptical but had a small, secondary side cut at its inner end. Nearby, on the outer side of the wound there two superficial abrasions, each $^1/_{10}$ in. long. He also had a laceration, $^3/_4$ in. long, under his chin and a scratch above his left eyebrow. Dissection demonstrated a pointed fragment of glass, $^1/_4 \times ^1/_{12} \times ^1/_{12}$ in. deep in the thigh wound. The front of the femoral vein had been punctured and opened for a distance of one third of its circumference; the femoral artery was intact. The blood on the deck had come, in the main, from the injured femoral vein. Inspection of the clothing disclosed several fragments of glass in the left-hand trouser pocket. Some of these bore pieces of the label of a bottle of vodka. Several of the fragments were sharply pointed and dagger-like. There was a recent cut in the lining of the pocket, and trouser leg.

This was the result of an accident. He had been below drinking with friends and had gone on deck to get more drink for the party. He was not drunk but might have been under the influence of drink; his blood alcohol after death was 148.3 mg/100 ml. On his way back to the party he had put a bottle of vodka in the left hand pocket of his trousers. When on deck, either because of his condition or because the ship had suddenly pitched or rolled, he had fallen. In consequence the bottle of vodka was shattered and one of the fragments had punctured his thigh. He had also struck his chin during the fall.

A boy, aged 11, was found dead in the playground of his school. He had multiple stab wounds in his neck. These injuries were accidentally sustained when he broke a window in order, illegally, to enter his school and then after breaking a glazed door in the school. Pieces of glass on his clothing matched glass from the door (F.M. 14,033A).

Yet another example of these rare, but ever potential, accidents is that of an elderly obese woman who was transfixed by a sabre-like fragment of a broken mirror. She had fallen against a dresser on which it stood and the mirror was shattered (Gonzales *et al.*, 1954).

Stab or Punctured Wounds

These wounds are the result of a thrust with some pointed instrument. They are characterised by a depth which is normally greater than the dimensions of the external injury. They are especially dangerous because of the possibility of grave injury to internal organs or major blood vessels. The majority are homicidal injuries; suicide by stabbing, or accidental stabbing, is infrequent.

A wide range of agents, many readily to hand in the home, can produce stab wounds. Daggers, although the "type" agent, have been supplanted in this country by sheath knives or "flick" knives. The latter were "outlawed" by the Restriction of Offensive

Weapons Acts, 1959: 1961, but the purchase of sheath knives is still unrestricted. Pointed kitchen (bread or carving) knives, pocket knives, files, screwdrivers, butchers' steels and pointed sticks are other examples. Hat pins which, in the 1920s or thereabouts, were several inches in length had their place and may still be used. Accidental stabbing, as by hypodermic needles, post-mortem needles or spicules of bone, has its own special danger of infection.

Stabbing with an *umbrella* was the probable mode of injecting a victim with ricin. Mr. Georgi Markov, aged 45, was found to have died of ricin poisoning at an inquest held by the late Mr. Gavin Thurston on 31st., Dec. 1978. It was the first known instance in this country of its use and mode of administration. It appeared that, while waiting for a bus on 7th. Sept, he felt a jab in the back of his right thigh. He looked round and saw a man drop an umbrella and take a taxi. He returned home and within a few hours he was sick and feverish. High fever continued and he was admitted to hospital the next day. He now had an inflamed area with a central puncture approximately 2 mm. in diameter at the back of his right thigh. He died 3 days later.

At the post-mortem examination a metal sphere, 1.52 mm. in diameter composed of platinum, 90 per cent and iridium, 10 per cent, was recovered from his thigh. There were two minute holes, each 0.35 mm. in diameter, which had been bored through the sphere. Dr. David Gall examined the sphere at Porton Down; he was unable to isolate any specific poison but it was most likely to have been ricin. The exceptional toxicity of the poison, in such a small dose, made ricin virtually the only choice. The verdict was Death by ricin poisoning, administered unlawfully. (Knight, 1979).

The External Appearances of Stab Wounds

Characteristically, the external wound is elliptical, with clean-cut margins when the agent is a thin, sharp blade (F.M. 2181, 3737; 5452, Fig. 37). A pointed stick, on the other hand, is likely to produce an external wound which has bruised and lacerated margins. When the weapon has a sharp edge but a thick back, the wound meets at an acute angle at one end, but the other may be rounded or squared (F.M. 3729). If there is bevelling or under-cutting, this should be noted since it may indicate the direction of the thrust.

There is a wide range in the shape of these external injuries. Although the ellipse is the most characteristic, some are square, other diamond-shaped or cruciate. A thrust with an agent of which the cross-section is square yields a cruciate wound in the skin, e.g. a plumber's widener (Littlejohn, 1925). The prong of a hay fork produced small elliptical wounds (Fig. 34, F.M. 6128A).

Although the external wound may suggest the kind of agent, it is by no means conclusive evidence. The site of the wound in relation to the tissue planes may have a modifying effect on its pattern. Traction of the tissues may cause the wound to appear to have been made by a blade having a thick back, when it was in fact a thin sharp blade which would have produced an elliptical wound elsewhere (Rabinowitsch, 1959; Beddoe, 1958). Elastic recoil of the skin may also reduce the dimensions of the wound to suggest a smaller agent than that used; conversely, rocking of the blade in the wound or re-entry may enlarge the wound so as to appear greater than the width of the blade. The cross-section of the blade may be accurately reproduced when the blade enters the skull (Fig. 38).

It must be remembered that a weapon of varied shape, such as a screwdriver, according

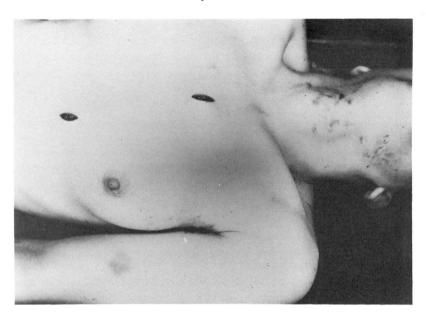

FIG. 37. Stab wounds of chest: homicidal: also marks of throttling.

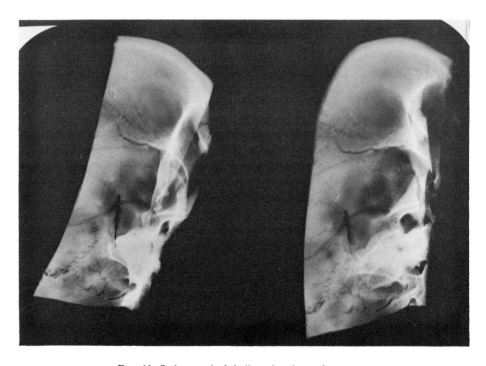

FIG. 38. Stab wound of skull: wedge shape: dagger agent.

to the depth to which it is thrust into the body, may affect the appearances of the wound in the skin. When a Phillips screwdriver was used to produce multiple stab wounds, most of the wounds of the skin were round or oval. Only a few bore the characteristic cruciate shape caused by the four blades at the tip of the weapon (F.M. 20,891).

Interpretation of the external wounds must therefore be guarded. Whenever practicable, experiments with a replica of the alleged agent should be made, in order to ascertain the appearances of wounds it can cause. These experiments are also of assistance in an attempt to assess the probable degree of force required to cause wounds of the kind found on the victim. Unless this is done, it is easy to err when expressing an opinion. Ostensibly, a thrust into the chest with a pointed kitchen knife, for example, calls for the exercise of substantial force. Tests showed how little force was in fact required; the skin offered a little resistance, but that being overcome, the blade went deep into the chest with alarming ease, even though a costal cartilage was severed. Whilst such experiments are best made on the cadaver, some assistance is given by thrusts of the blade into plastic material such as dental wax or plasticine.

Knight (1975) and Green (1978) have carried out tests using electronic recording devices.

The direction of the wound has importance. This is indicated not only by any under-cutting of the external wound but, more especially, by the track of injury by the blade. A track which passes downwards may be due to homicide or suicide, but an up-going track is normally indicative of homicide rather than suicide; it is easier to stab oneself by downward or horizontal thrusts. The latter are also consistent with accidental contacts, e.g., by falling against or rushing on to a knife. Lateral deviation should also be noted and it may be relevant to know whether the victim was left- or right-handed.

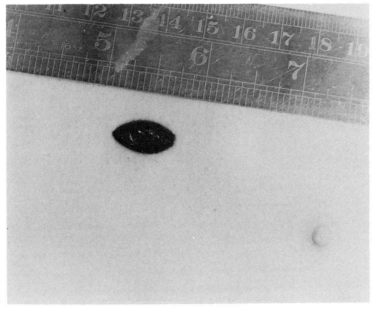

Fig. 39. Stab wound of the chest, caused by a knife with one sharp and one blunt edge (F.M. 17271A).

Care must be exercised in interpreting the circumstances from the direction of the wound alone. It may be suggested that the victim sustained a downward and inward stab because he rose from a sitting posture on to a blade held above him (F.M. 5452).

The depth of the wound, i.e. the length of the track, is a guide to the length of the agent, but this is not by any means infallible. It presupposes that the agent was thrust into the body to the limit of its length; a long table knife, having an 8-in. blade, need enter for less than half its length to cause fatal injury to the heart or major vessels (F.M. 5452). On other occasions the track may prove to be appreciably longer than the blade. Lester James (1961) examined a victim who sustained a fatal stab to the heart by a small pocket knife. When the thrust is forcible it can compress the body, e.g. the chest cage or epigastrium, so as to carry the point of the agent an inch or more beyond the length of the blade.

If thrust into the body in this manner the weapon may, rarely, leave an impression of the hilt on the skin surrounding the wound. A mark in greasy mud around a wound was the impression of the hilt of a home-made weapon (F.M. 25,350A).

The site of the wound has particular importance. Obviously if it lies in a position which is inaccessible to the victim, it is not self-inflicted. The homicide and the suicide often aim at the heart and, in consequence, wound the left side of the chest or upper abdomen. Homicidal thrusts tend to lie rather higher than self-inflicted ones.

The number of wounds: multiple stab wounds suggest homicide, especially when they are scattered and most, if not all, have penetrated deeply. Although homicide may be accomplished by a single stab (F.M. 5452; 3737) or only a couple of stabs (F.M. 2181), it is more usual to find many, e.g. forty (*R. v. Briggs*, Leeds Assizes, 1947; Leeds City Coroner: No. 147/47), or even sixty or more (Forensic Medicine Section, No. 55; Gordon Museum,

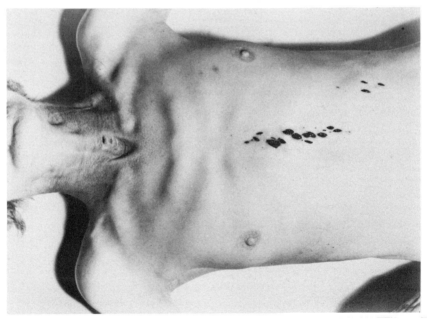

Fig. 40. Stab wounds of chest: suicide. Note tentative superficial punctures and the vertical arrangement of the injuries.

Guy's Hospital). It may be on these occasions that even after a lethal stab has been inflicted, the assailant continues to stab.

When the victim has sustained a single stab wound, the interpretation is much more difficult. Such a wound can be homicidal, suicidal or accidental. Accurate information concerning the circumstances and the antecedents of the deceased is of considerable importance in making the correct diagnosis. Were there any previous attempts at suicide? Was the room in which the body was found locked? Was there a suicide note? etc. The really difficult cases are those in which the injury is sustained during a fight. The usual defence is then that the deceased ran on to the knife. An interpretation must take into account such features as the presence or absence of "defence" injuries; the angle of the wound, the position of the clothing, etc. For example: a man was alleged to have died after running on to a knife during a brawl in the street. Examination of his clothing showed that the stab in his anorak was at a lower level than that in his shirt and that, in turn, was at a lower level than the stab in his vest and skin. Moreover, there were two stabs in the vest. This indicated that at the time the knife entered his body he had been gripped by the shoulder so as to cause displacement upwards of the outer clothing and a folding of the vest. In effect, a situation which was wholly inconsistent with running on to the knife (F.M. 18744B).

Multiplicity of wounds by no means excludes suicide, but on these occasions it is usual to find that a proportion of the wounds are superficial and, indeed, some may have failed to puncture the skin, i.e. the latter are "tentative" or "hesitation" injuries (F.M. 4939A, Fig. 40; 633/48, Fig. 42).

The homicide and the suicide, intending to injure the heart, may well choose the same target area, namely, the left lower quadrant of the front of the chest. Certain features, when present, permit the distinction. Thrusts by the homicide are all likely to penetrate the chest wall and more than one may be lethal. There may be a few outlying thrusts, beyond the target area. The suicide, on the other hand, is likely to confine thrusts to a smaller and more restricted area. There are likely to be fewer deep thrusts and only one or two lethal. The particular feature of suicidal stabbing, is the presence of "tentative" wounds. These are superficial, circular and unlikely to penetrate beyond the dermis (Figs. 40 and 42). The superficial injuries in Fig. 42 may have been "tentative" punctures but, since the agent was a pair of domestic scissors, used with the blades open, the major wounds were produced by the larger and wider blade and, coincidently, the narrower and sharply pointed blade had produced superficial punctures. (F.M. 4939A: L G I 633/48).

Another case of suicidal stabbing was also characterised by the co-existence of tentative injuries and planned deep thrusts. This was a woman aged 65 who stabbed herself with a small dagger. Twelve thrusts were made in an almost vertical line, $3^1/_2$ in. long, at about an inch to the left of the sternum; half were deep and half were superficial stabs; a small group of three more, all superficial and probably the initial stabs, lay near the costal margin in an area $^1/_2$ in. in diameter, 2 in. below the main group (Fig. 40, F.M. 4939A).

Suicide is occasionally attempted by transfixion of the neck. Provent and Simonin (1940) recorded the case of a chronic alcoholic aged 71 who thrust a pointed table knife into the front of his neck; he then drowned himself. Since beards are again in fashion, the case of Harvey Littlejohn (1925) is recalled. At first sight there was no injury to account for the blood beside the body on the floor and on his bed. A bloodstained bread knife was

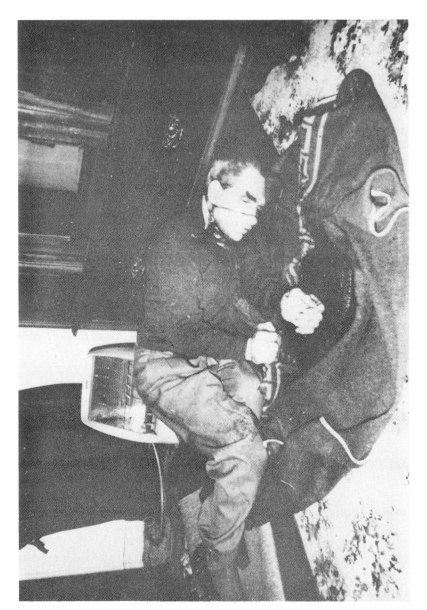

FIG. 41a. Scene of transfixion of the neck with a sheath knife: suicide.

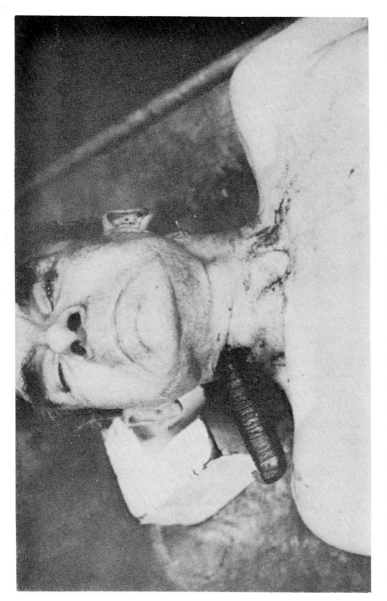

Fig. 41b. Transfixion of the neck with a sheath knife: self-inflicted. Death due to haemorrhage due to severance of the carotid artery.

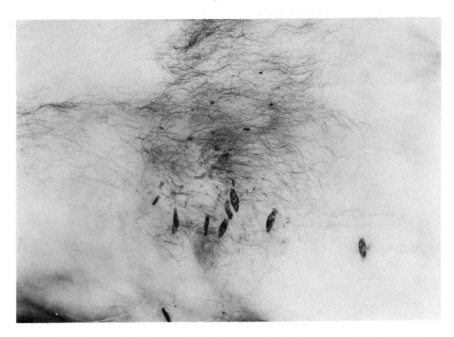

FIG. 42. Stab wounds of chest: suicidal. Agent: a pair of scissors—one blade of which produced the superficial punctures which were not "tentative" on this occasion.

on a table in the room. When the victim's beard was lifted, two wounds of the neck were found; one has passed behind the larynx to the left and had divided the left external and internal carotid arteries just above the bifurcation. . . . The wound on the left side passed backwards and communicated with the other wound. A transfixion from right to left or the result of two separate introductions of the knife? Harvey Littlejohn did not tell the reader. Assuming it was suicide, is not transfixion the more likely? Transfixion of a limb can be a species of "defence" injuries. The wound shown in Fig. 43 was sustained during an attack on a woman. The blade entered the leg just above the knee and emerged near the groin.

Two instances of suicidal transfixion of the neck have occurred in our practice at Leeds. The first was a labourer aged 58 who for 2 years had suffered from emphysema; during the 7 weeks prior to his death his condition had worsened and he had been unable to work; he slept downstairs. On the day of his death his wife had left the house to go shopping at 10.30 a.m. She left him in bed and locked both of the house doors. On her return, an hour later, he was not in his bed; she thought he had gone upstairs to dress. Since he did not appear and she heard no sounds of movement she went upstairs to find him. He lay dead on the floor of the bedroom and had fixed a "suicide note" on the door. (She identified the writing as that of her husband.)

The man lay on the floor fully clothed. The handle of a knife protruded from the right side of his neck and the point emerged by $1/_4$ in. on the left side. There had been no struggle and no one had entered the house. The knife was 9 in., and its blade was $4^3/_4$ in. long. It had entered the neck an inch below the lower jaw on the right side and emerged

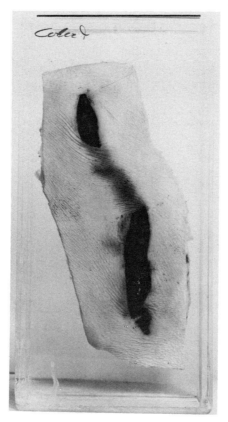

FIG. 43. Transfixion by stabbing, with dark band of bruising in the track between the wounds—direction from above knee towards groin.

$1^1/_2$ in. below the external opening of the left ear and $1^1/_2$ in. behind the angle of the lower jaw on the left side. The track was directed at an angle of approximately 30° above the horizontal and there was a slight backward inclination. Bleeding had occurred at the sides and front of his neck, on both hands and forearms and the front of his chest but there was none on his knees. The blade had severed the right sterno-mastoid muscle, right common carotid artery and internal jugular vein; it had passed behind the pharynx, left common carotid artery and internal jugular vein; the vagi were intact. The circumstances of this death were unequivocally those of self-infliction (Figs. 41a, b; F.M. 13,511).

The second subject was a man aged 68 who had been a heavy drinker for several years. He had been a widower for 2 years and during that time his drinking habits had worsened; he was rarely sober. When last seen alive he was leaving a public house when under the influence of drink. Three days later, because of an accumulation of milk bottles at his house, the police were informed. An officer called at the house, found the door unlocked, and entered. He found the man dead in the bedroom. Examination of the body showed that the handle of a knife protruded from the left side of the neck in front of the ear; the blade had been thrust in up to its hilt. The track passed downwards and to the right. The blade had severed both common carotid arteries and the oesophagus; its tip had reached the superficial muscles on the right side of the neck but had not penetrated the skin. A second, "tentative" wound was also present on the left side of his neck; it was a superficial incision at no point deeper than $^1/_4$ in.; it extended from behind the left ear to the left angle of the jaw. His urine contained 135 mg per cent of alcohol. There were no signs of a struggle; there were no defence injuries nor any other injuries. There was no suicide note. However, the distribution of blood at the scene was consistent with infliction of the injuries while seated before his dressing-table mirror; he had then slumped back on to the bed into the position in which his body was found. There was reason to believe that he was left-handed. His drinking companions had noticed that he always raised his glass with his left hand, as if his right hand was weak. The circumstances were consistent with self-infliction, notwithstanding that his house door was unlocked (F.M. 14,067A).

Stab wounds of the heart are at all times serious, but their gravity is appreciably modified by the site of the wound. If the blade traverses the wall of the right ventricle or that of one of the auricles, a fatal haemorrhage is to be expected, whereas injury to the wall of the left ventricle may not prove fatal; when the blade is withdrawn, muscular contraction can close the track. Sometimes a single thrust must prove lethal, if the blade severs a branch of the coronary artery.

> A youth aged 18 sustained a stab wound, inflicted with a clasp knife. The descending branch of the left coronary artery was divided at a point $1^1/_2$ in. above the apex of the left ventricle; the track passed through the ventricle just to the left of the interventricular septum and the point of the blade had gained the posterior wall at about its junction with the septum. Death was not immediate; he survived for about 8 hours. This may in part have been due to the administration of many pints of blood. It is just possible that had the precise nature of the injury been recognised, and the artery ligatured, he might have survived (F. M. 3626A).

Accidental Penetrating Injuries

Accidents with a circular saw may cause the sudden separation of a portion of wood, which is forcibly thrown off, so as to inflict serious injury to the operator. A splinter of wood, 7 in. long, thus caused fatal haemorrhage when it entered the right side of the neck; the pleura and innominate artery were penetrated (Forensic Medicine Section, No. 49; Gordon Museum, Guy's Hospital; Professor Keith Simpson). Similar accidents can occur in metal cutting. A rectangular piece of metal, 4×4.25 m 3.0 cm, having a chisel-like edge at its lower, narrower border, was jerked from a machine and penetrated the upper part of the chest. The left common carotid and subclavian arteries were severed at 0.5 cm above the aortic arch. The foreign body emerged from the chest beside the left shoulder blade (Department of Forensic Medicine, University of Copenhagen; Professor Gormsen). Another specimen in that department shows a metal rod firmly fixed in the body of a dorsal vertebra. The victim had been grinding a metal rod. When examined in hospital, a small perforation was found immediately to the right of the sternum at the level of the second rib. Post-mortem examination showed that a metal rod, 11 cm long and 0.4 cm in diameter, had traversed the pericardium and lodged in the spine.

A similar disaster occurred when a young research student was conducting experiments with gases. These were passed through a meter, which had to be cleared before a subsequent experiment. When he carried out this check there was a violent explosion and the meter was shattered. One of the metal pieces was driven into the right side of his chest and severed his innominate artery. Death from haemorrhage occurred within too short a time to permit any treatment (F.M. 11,990).

Dunkerley (1956) urged that penetrating agents should not be pulled out as the first step, but they should be left *in situ* until the patient is brought under favourable conditions for skilled treatment. He described a case of penetration of the external iliac vein by a splinter of wood which broke off from a projecting piece when the boy had been pushed against it.

Homicidal Stabbing with a Hay Fork

The victim, a male aged 33, was killed by a fellow mental patient. Multiple injuries caused death and there were other injuries inflicted after death. The two men had gone to a hay loft one afternoon and reclined on the hay. For some reason the deceased was attacked unexpectedly and throttled, probably to the point of unconsciousness but not death. He was then pitched off the hay stack to the ground, a distance of about 10 feet. His assailant followed and possibly by accident, jumped on the deceased. [This was the probable explanation of the crush injury of the right chest and rupture of the liver.] The assailant then armed himself with a two-pronged hay fork and attacked the dying man by thrusting and slashing at his body. The final stage, which probably occurred after death, since no vital reaction was detected in the damaged tissues, was a violent attack on the genitalia. The scrotum was torn open and the testicles were avulsed.

The injuries by the hay fork were of two kinds: (a) stab or puncture wounds (Fig. 44) and (b) pseudo-incised wounds; lacerations by slashing with the weapon (Figs. 34, 35).

The punctured wounds were widely distributed for the most part over the front of the body; six were on the right side of the neck, but many others were present on the chest, abdomen and thigh; about half a dozen were at the back of the body. All were elliptical, but they ranged in size from $^1/_{10}$ in. to $^3/_4$ in. in their longest axis; the average size was $^1/_4$ in. Variation in size was accounted for by depth of penetration; some were shallow punctures by the tip of the prong, e.g. in the neck; others were deep and the full thickness of the prong had punctured the skin, e.g. upper chest and pelvis. The direction varied considerably. Some were due to thrusts from right to left and others to thrusts from left to right.

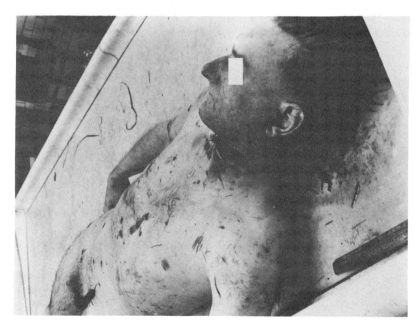

FIG. 44. Stab and lacerated wounds produced with a hay fork.

The majority showed no sign of vital reaction, but a few were associated with bleeding and had been inflicted during life.

The prongs or tynes of the hay fork had a maximum diameter of $^1/_4$ in. and on cross-section they were circular in the lower $^1/_2$ in., but above they were oval. Experiments confirmed that thrusts with a replica produced similar punctured wounds.

The pseudo-incised wounds were confined to the front of the neck. The initial impression was that they could have been caused by a razor. The major laceration had the appearances of a cut-throat; the wound extended from a point of approximately 2 in. below the left angle of the lower jaw and crossed the neck horizontally to a point 1 in. in front and 2 in. below the right angle of the lower jaw; it was 4 in. long and gaped by an inch. The larynx was exposed and had been fractured; the left sterno-mastoid muscle was apparently cut. There was no injury to the carotid arteries or jugular veins. Although the margins of this wound appeared to have been clean cut, slight irregularity was found under low magnification. It was also found that hair follicles were exposed as by splitting and not by cutting. The deeper tissues, e.g. muscle, were more obviously lacerated and not cut. There was no vital reaction in the skin or adjacent tissues. Other lacerations of like kind but less severity were present. A group of six, near the right angle of the jaw, took a course parallel to the lower border of the jaw bone; the lower arm of each had severed the skin, but the upper arm was only a superficial scratch. A number of long linear scratches were on the right side of the neck and one other group, arranged in parallel, was on the upper part of the left side of the chest.

These injuries were at first puzzling, but the possibility of slashing across the neck with the hay fork was considered. Experiments with a replica reproduced similar "incised" wounds. It was also noted that in spite of a relatively sharp point to the tyne, substantial force by a swinging stroke was required to lacerate the skin. Since all of the lacerations on the body showed no vital reaction, they were considered post-mortem injuries, slashing followed stabbing with the hay fork. The accused, acquitted of murder but found guilty of manslaughter, was sentenced to imprisonment for life. Diminished responsibility was accepted. (*R.* v. *Hamill*, 1958; F.M. 6128A.)

Similar bizarre stab wounds are likely to occur during the course of road accidents. We have seen a man's body impaled on a *piece of wood* which had transfixed his heart. The wood came from a fence into which his car had crashed. (F.M. 25, 609).

Homicidal Stabbing: an Attempt to Destroy the Body by Fire

A women aged 37 was found dead in a house which was on fire. She lay face down with her clothing disarranged. Examination of the body, at the scene, showed obvious injuries, for example, stab wounds of the neck and cheek and a cut on the left forearm. A blood-stained carving knife was near the body.

She had been killed by her nephew, a youth aged 18. He had deserted from the army and called at the house for shelter which was refused. He knew that his aunt kept money in a cash box and this was found empty at the scene. When he was apprehended his left hand was wrapped in a bloodstained handkerchief. He said he had cut it when sharpening a pencil with a razor. He was told that this clothing would be examined and he then confessed that he had killed his aunt and he showed the police where he had hidden the money.

The stab wounds included stabbing behind the left ear and on the neck at both sides; the latter had caused partial severance of each jugular vein. She had defence wounds on the palm of the left hand. There was no evidence of rape. The motive apparently was robbery. The elliptical stab wounds were produced by a carving knife, the blade of which was up to $^{11}/_{16}$ in. broad. (*R.* v. *Humphreys* (1940), Leeds Assizes, March 13th; Leeds City Coroner's No. 924/39.)

Accidental Stabbing

Accidental stabbing is an unusual event, and the probable circumstances are illustrated by the following cases.

A girl aged $5^1/_2$ years, who died from haemorrhage a few minutes after piercing her neck with a pencil. Her father had sharpened pencils for his two girls and this one, holding her pencil, then ran towards him and fell; the pencil entered the side of her neck and pierced the jugular vein.

A woman aged 52 who was found lying on the floor of her kitchen, near the foot of some stairs. There was a good deal of blood behind her head and shoulders (Fig. 45). A pair of household scissors lay on the floor to her right. She had a stab wound, 1.6 in. long, gaping up to 0.4 in., over the upper part of the right side of her chest (Fig. 46). The wound was directed obliquely downwards and inwards, at an angle of about 30°; its lower end was level with the angle of Louis and $1^1/_2$ in. to the right of the middle line. The wound was an elipse, which was somewhat constricted just below its middle point, in hour-glass fashion (Fig. 47).

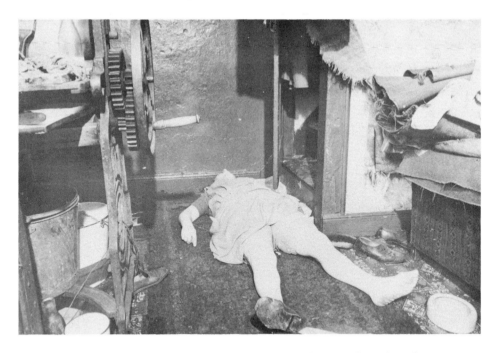

FIG. 45. Scene of accidental stabbing. Simulation of a scene of sexual murder.

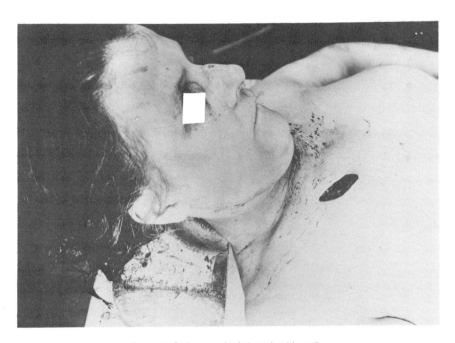

FIG. 46. Stab wound of chest (accidental).

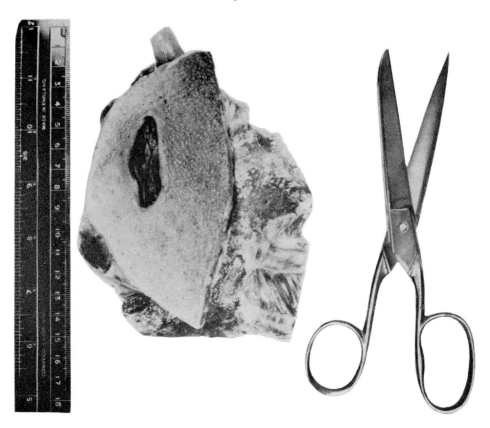

Fig. 47. Stab wound of chest: accidental following fall on to a pair of scissors.

At first sight the circumstances seemed to be those of murder; investigation showed, however, that the house had been under observation and no one had been seen to enter. She had been engaged in papering the wall of the staircase. Some of the paper was still wet and paste, which was still wet, was on her hand. There was also a bowl of paste on the table. It was concluded that she had slipped when about to cut the paper with pointed, household scissors, and lost her footing and fell downstairs on to the scissors; the blades entered the chest. There was a laceration of the middle finger of her right hand, consistent with injury sustained during her fall on to the scissors. There was a slight bruise on the left side of the scalp, a small laceration over the left eye and one or two abrasions on the face (F.M. 2659). [An experimental study of wounds with scissors was made by Obiglio (1939).]

Manslaughter by Stabbing: R. v. Donoghue (1950)

Two men friends, Donoghue and Meaney, went drinking and eventually returned to Donoghue's flat. When last seen, late that night, they were fuddled but friendly. Just before midnight one of the residents in the block of flats heard three thuds and then all was silent. At 7.30 a.m. next morning Meaney's body was found lying face down on the landing outside Donoghue's flat. It was fully clothed. Sixteen deep stab wounds were distributed over the left side of the neck and face. Rucking up of the overcoat suggested that the body had been dragged out of the flat by the shoulders; a trail of blood led from the body to the flat. The coat collar and the accused's hands were blood-stained. In Donoghue's room there was a blood-stained dagger, proved to have been used in the attack. There were no defence injuries on the hands of the victim.

The successful defence was that Donoghue, whilst drunk, had roused himself to find what he thought to be a dummy sharing his bed, put there for a practical joke. He proceeded to stab it with the bayonet at a time when, because of drink, he was too confused to know he was killing a man. It was not possible to determine the alcoholic content of the blood of the accused at that time but since the blood of the deceased contained no less than 347 mg. per cent and the urine contained 450 mg. per cent and, further, because Meaney was the more sober of the pair when they were last seen, it was inferred that the level in Donoghue's blood must have been at least equal to that of his companion. Meaney, in his drunken sleep, could have offered no resistance. In the opinion of the prison medical officer, the degree of drunkenness present at the time of the alleged offence was such that the accused could have mistakenly believed he was, in fact, stabbing a dummy and not a human being. Donoghue pleaded guilty to manslaughter and was sentenced to 3 years' imprisonment. (Simpson, 1954).

Surgical Intervention with Wounds

In so far as is practicable, surgical incisions, which have to be made in the course of the treatment of the victim of wounding, should be separate. In a case of stabbing, the stab wounds were obscured by their inclusion in the course of surgical incisions. In consequence the pathologist had only one intact stab wound for inspection in the interpretation of the circumstance of the attack upon the victim (F.M. 3626A).

Special Aspects of Wounding

1. *Grave Internal Injuries, without any External Wound* A practitioner who fails to find any external injury when the patient complains of severe internal pain, especially following a blow on the abdomen, and has, perhaps, other symptoms, should never dismiss the matter lightly. Although infrequent, a sufficient number of examples are on record to show that grave and fatal internal injuries may thus occur in the absence of any apparent external injury.

A youth, struck in the abdomen by the shaft of a cart, doubled up at once and thereafter complained of abdominal pain of increasing intensity, which persisted until he died some hours later. The autopsy showed that his duodenum had been ruptured by the blow. No external mark was found (P.M. 4425).

On other occasions external injury is found only by painstaking search. Étienne Martin (1950) tells of the girl who threw herself from a height on to the paving below and died an hour later. When she was found no external injury was at first apparent, but, later, a bluish discoloration of the skin, about $1^1/_2$ in. in diameter, was noted in the fold of her left buttock. Although this was the sole external sign of injury, she had a fracture of the lumbar spine, comminution of the pelvis, with rupture of the left lung, of the spleen and of one of the kidneys.

A man who was crushed by a steel plate and whose internal injuries were extensive, had external injury limited to a minor abrasion of his face (F.M. 548).

2. *Unusual Wounds* Burns inflicted by a red-hot iron bar or poker may simulate wounds caused by firearms but adequate examination will correct an erroneous impression based on external appearances.

Nails or chisels driven into the head are a rare finding and usually indicate suicide by a person of unsound mind. This is also a rare mode of murder, of which there is an example in the Old Testament. Jael, having lured Sisera into her tent. "took a nail of the tent, and took a hammer in her hand, and went softly unto him, and smote the nail into his temples, and fastened it into the ground: for he was fast asleep and weary. So he died" (*Judges* iv 21).

Head injuries of any kind are otherwise almost invariably the result of accident or homicide. Rarely, the suicide may attempt to kill himself by butting his head against a wall or by blows with a hatchet or hammer (see p. 163).

Suicide can be attempted in many unusual ways. A man detonated dynamite in his mouth. Another man fashioned a metal holder for the cartridge of a firearm; the holder was clipped to his braces and suicide was accomplished by striking the detonator of the cartridge with a spanner (Collins, 1948).

The cunning suicide, perhaps with the intention to defraud an insurance company, or to throw suspicion on an innocent person by way of revenge, may plan his death in a manner which suggests homicide. More often, attempts are made by a murderer to present the result of his crime as a suicide. This rarely deceives for long because homicidal injuries, for example laceration of the scalp or strangulation, are usually unmistakable. Suspension of the body after strangulation by a ligature, however, may give rise to difficulty in interpretation.

3. *Multiple Wounds of Unlike Gravity: which Wound Caused Death?* Occasionally a victim may die of wounds which were inflicted by two or more assailants. It may then be necessary to determine which of the wounds caused the death, if a distinction be practicable, in order to apportion the blame. The distinction must depend upon the circumstances of the particular case, and, in any event, a definite opinion is unlikely unless only one of the wounds was capable of causing death. A man who sustains a lacerated wound and dies of septicaemia will have died from that wound and not from a light blow on the abdomen, inflicted shortly before his death, by a second assailant. These problems require the consideration of each wound, separately, as the possible cause of death.

4. *Wounds Sustained in the Presence of Pre-existing Disease, or Poisoning* Three possible factors, namely the wound, disease, and death by poisoning, must be fully investigated. The following case is an example. A man had an altercation and received a blow of light or moderate severity on the chin. He left the scene apparently none the worse for his injury, but died within 24 hours; cerebral haemorrhage, accompanied by changes elsewhere indicative of essential hypertension, was demonstrated at necropsy. The effects of the blow were discounted (F.M. 2217A).

The first step is to determine whether the injury could have been the cause of the fatal changes. In the example it was clear the death was due to disease. The real difficulty is to determine whether the blow accelerated the death. When acceleration is material, it is relatively easy of demonstration, since this turns upon the presence or absence of substantial injury, i.e. something more than a small bruise. On the other hand, if acceleration is by but a matter of hours or less, obviously any assessment is distinctly speculative, the defendant is entitled to the benefit of doubt.

5. *Head Injuries and Intra-cranial Meningioma* The vexed question of the relationship between trauma and the development of tumours yields strongly conflicting answers. It does appear, however, that head injury may be so closely related to the genesis of an intra-cranial meningioma that its part as an aetiological factor is inescapable. Sir Francis

Walshe, in reporting three cases, drew attention to the earlier reports by Harvey Cushing (1922) and to the classical monograph by Cushing and Eisenhardt (1938), which should be consulted. In their experience the incidence of trauma was particularly high, i.e. in nearly 33 per cent. This aetiological relationship is especially important when injury involves a cranial suture and, later, the tumour is found immediately subjacent to the site of injury (Walshe, 1961).

In the latter circumstances the effects of the blow alone must first be considered to determine its possible consequences. In the example cited the only injury was a small bruise at the angle of the mouth, one which of itself could not have caused other than temporary discomfort. It was therefore disregarded as a factor in the death. A contrary view might have resulted in the assailant standing his trial for manslaughter.

It must be appreciated, however, that an assailant takes his victim as he finds him. It is no defence to plead that, had the victim been a healthy man, he would not have died of the injuries. If he has an abnormally thin skull and dies of a blow which would not have caused injury to a normal skull, the assailant cannot thus escape all blame, although it is a factor which no doubt would be taken into account in mitigation of punishment. On the other hand, surgical intervention has also to be taken into account; it may or may not be a *novus actus* which would then shift responsibility from the defendant.

It is not uncommon for a person to die in the course of an altercation and for the autopsy then to reveal only trivial injuries but also severe heart disease. It is our opinion that in these circumstances the exertion and stress occurring during the altercation were likely to have precipitated a heart attack and death. The precipitating factor would be the deceased's own exertions and not the activities of the other person, nor the result of any trivial injuries which may have been inflicted. The situation becomes more difficult, however, when an elderly person is set upon by another and dies at once or shortly afterwards. It is indeed hard to escape the conclusion that in these circumstances the fright or shock, with associated tachycardia etc. may have precipitated the death. But this is difficult, if not impossible, to prove pathologically. On the other hand, if the deceased had sustained injuries which, though non-fatal, were substantial, it is then reasonable to consider that they contributed to the death (See also "Trauma and Disease" at page 659).

6. *Self-inflicted Wounds which are not Suicidal: Fictitious Wounds* Occasionally wounds are self-inflicted in order to establish a false charge of attempted murder or unlawful wounding. This may be in furtherance of a desire for revenge or it may be an attempt to conceal personal guilt. The murderer may inflict wounds upon himself and then allege that he and his victim had been attacked by another. The wounds may be a manifestation of hysteria. Close attention to the wounds as well as to the story of their infliction will show that they are relatively harmless, being superficial and situated in an area readily accessible to the victim.

Another group of self-inflicted wounds may be seen amongst persons in the armed forces. The wounds are usually inflicted with a view to release from the service, or transfer from foreign to home service. The wound is usually in the hand, usually the left, when, for example, the index finger of the left hand is placed over the end of a rifle and shot away, or the man may send a bullet through his foot. They are nearly always injuries by firearms and of a kind which will disable only to the extent that the victims become unfit for full military duties. The man uses his own weapon, a revolver in preference to a rifle; the wound is, of course, a near or contact wound. Care is needed to counter his possible explanation that he had been shot by the enemy. Self-mutilation whilst on active service is, of necessity, a grave offence and, when it occurs, it may be imitated by others in the unit. Injection with lighter fuel to produce local injuries, it appears, has been practised in some American prisons.

The Age of Injuries

The pathologist has first to ascertain whether the injury was sustained before or after death. If sustained during life, he has then to estimate the probable age of the injury. There are occasions when injuries have been inflicted by two or more persons, and it is then necessary to attempt to distinguish the order and gravity of multiple injuries in order to apportion blame. When inflicted by one person alone, the order of infliction, when it can be established, may assist in a reconstruction of the circumstances. It may be material also to estimate the probable duration of life subsequent to injury.

Example; Multiple Deaths from Shotgun Injuries

A whole family, which included the parents and their two children, were found dead of shotgun injuries. The mother and one of the children lay close together on a bed. Both had been killed by "near", if not contact, head injuries; the second child, also on the bed but separated from his mother, had been shot twice; a near wound in the chest and a contact wound of the head via the mouth. The father was found in another room, dead of a contact shotgun injury to his head.

The appearances at the scene and of the injuries permitted the conclusion that the father had shot the mother and one child in her arms at close range while they slept. He then shot the second child in the chest at rather longer range, but still within a yard. This was not immediately fatal and the gun was then put into its mouth and the second discharge destroyed the brain. The man went into an adjacent room and shot himself in the head. He was heavily in debt and had been pressed to pay his debts (F.M. 15,916).

The Distinction Between Ante-Mortem & Post-Mortem Injuries

The distinction between injuries sustained at a substantial interval before death, and injuries sustained at corresponding periods after death, is usually comparatively simple.

The ante-mortem injury is characterised by changes which are often summarised by the convenient term "vital reaction".

(a) Bleeding; is the outstanding feature, not only free bleeding from the wound but into the adjacent tissues in the form of bruising (it has to be borne in mind that free bleeding can occur after death and, in certain circumstances and situations, it is possible to produce bruises, post-mortem).

(b) Inflammatory reaction; the invasion of the injured parts by leucocytes is essentially a vital phenomenon which begins within a few hours of injury. In the event of the victim's survival these changes go on to repair by first intention, or suppuration and subsequent repair by scar tissue.

Post-mortem injuries even if there be some free bleeding, are devoid of any leucocytic invasion or vascular or fibroblastic repair.

The difficulty arises when the injuries are sustained close to, or within minutes of, the time of death. For example, injury to the chest cage and organs can be caused by external cardiac massage performed shortly after the person's collapse. Sometimes these injuries may be associated with slight bleeding. It is then impossible to state with certainty whether this occurred during the last moments of life or within a short space of time following permanent arrest of circulation, i.e. death. Blood could leak from a liver ruptured after death, and a small amount of blood might then be found in the peritoneal cavity.

Nail marks inflicted during life but close to the time of death can be indistinguishable from those inflicted after death, unless associated with bruising.

Rupture of major blood vessels, with associated other injuries which caused immediate death, can be followed by appreciable escape of blood, post-mortem, into the body cavities (Shapiro and Robertson, 1962) or, if the wound communicates with the exterior, blood may collect beside the body at the scene. This is likely to be augmented by hypostasis if the wound is in a dependent part. It may be, as suggested by Mole (1948), that haemolysis also facilitates this blood loss. Conversely, in life, haemostasis, by clotting of blood and fibrin formation, may reduce the amount of blood loss.

Wounds sustained shortly before death, however, are not, in our experience, invariably associated with thrombosis or fibrin deposition. We submitted a number of bruises, including those sustained after death, to the technique for the demonstration of fibrin (Lendrum, 1962) but our results were inconsistent and we are unable to rely on this test for the detection of ante-mortem injury. Laiho and Uotila (1966), using fluorescent antibody techniques to demonstrate fibrin, were able to demonstrate a fibrin network in all the in vitro-coagula and in most of the tissue haemorrhages that had occurred both ante-mortem and shortly after death.

Raekallio (1966) rejected the presence of fibrin as a reliable vital reaction.

The only vital sign, detectable by conventional methods, is inflammatory reaction, but this is not apparent until several hours after injury. The interval which elapses before its first stage, the invasion of polymorphs, is not precisely established. Thus it could be within the first 24 hours, 8 hours (Fatteh, 1966), 6 hours (Malek, 1970) or only 1 hour (Ojala *et al.*, 1969).

The criteria for distinguishing ante-mortem and post-mortem bruises were reviewed by Robertson and and Mansfield (1957). Ante-mortem bruising was probable only when the bruise was a large one. Small escapes of blood into the tissues could occur from injury after death.

Swelling of the bruised area is consistent with injury during life but absence of swelling does not exclude ante-mortem injury.

Coagulation of blood in the area is not peculiar to ante-mortem injury.

Colour changes in a bruised area indicate ante-mortem injury but these changes do not appear until days after injury. (Incidentally precise estimation of the probable time interval based on the colour of the bruise is unreliable).

Robertson and Mansfield concluded that the appearances were similar in recent ante- and post-mortem bruises; a distinction could only be made when there had been an appreciable interval, one of days rather than hours, between the injury and death.

No significant differences were observed in the naked eye appearances of small recent ante- and post-mortem bruises. Their microscopical appearances were also similar. Swelling of small ante-mortem bruises (and many bruises of the scalp) is slight or absent, but, when present, it is indicative of infliction during life (Polson, 1963).

Careless dissection of the neck structures is notoriously liable to produce escape of blood into the tissue planes and simulate the results of ante-mortem injury. Gordon *et al.* (1953) stressed the importance of scrupulous care in these dissections.

The conventional histological methods of detecting vital reaction were reviewed by Raekallio (1961).

Suggestions have been made in the past that it is possible to distinguish between ante-mortem and post-mortem wounds by examination of the elastic fibres in the tissue. However Fatteh (1971) found no evidence of any such difference.

Various histochemical techniques have been devised by Raekallio and others as means of assessing age of injuries (see below). These may be used as methods of indicating the ante-mortem nature of an injury. The earliest enzyme reaction is reported to be detectable one hour after wounding (esterase).

Recently biochemical methods of detecting vital reaction have been studied. Serotonin was investigated (Raekallio and Makinen, 1969a; 1969b). They found a distinct increase in serotonin in the margins of wounds inflicted on mice. These authors (1970) also found increase in serotonin in the vicinity of ligature marks in hanging, abrasions and lacerations. The serotonin and free histamine content from tissues from ante-mortem wounds was appreciably greater than that of intact skin and of tissue from post-mortem injuries. The free histamine increase occurred within a few minutes of injury and was deemed characteristic of vital change. Fazekas and Kis (1971) also examined wounds from autopsy material of various kinds and found that the free histamine content of the vital skin injuries was considerably higher than that of the intact skin and post-mortem wounds. The free histamine surplus formed in the few minutes after the injuries, in the author's opinion, was characteristic of the vital injuries. In a recent review of the literature (Raekallio, 1973) the author mentions the relationship of the amounts of serotonin and histamine found. According to him a large increase in serotonin and a small one in histamine indicates an agonal wound. There is a greater increase in histamine than serotonin in wounds sustained 5 to 15 minutes before death, and the reverse in wounds occurring 15 to 60 minutes before death.

The simplest and most convenient method of detecting histamine in wounded tissue is by histochemical means. Sivaloganathan (1982) has described such a technique using o-phthalaldehyde to produce fluorescence of the histamine, detectable with ultraviolet light using a fluorescence microscope.

The Rate of Healing of Wounds: Estimation of their Age

When healing is by first intention, a wound which is still red and swollen is probably under 12 hours old. Vascular buds form by the end of 24 hours and a capillary network is in formation by the end of 36 hours. In from 36 to 48 hours new vessels are growing towards the skin surface and fibroblasts lie at right angles to the surface, and epithelium begins to migrate in from 24 to 48 hours (Lindsay and Birch, 1964). By the 3rd to 5th day, when repair is well advanced, fibroblasts are parallel to the surface.

Firm union should occur in from 5 to 6 days, yielding a reddish or bluish "angry" scar.

By the end of 14 days the scar becomes pale; it is still soft and sensitive; there may be little further change up to the end of 2 months. The scar will acquire a brown or copper-red tint during the 2nd to the 6th months, but it remains soft and shows no corrugation due to contraction of the fibrous tissue in it. After 6 months the scar becomes white and glistening; it is now tough and may be corrugated. Once this stage is reached no further change except, rarely, calcification or ossification may be found in it.

Infection or laceration of tissue, leading to repair by granulation, prolongs the process of repair appreciably. Signs of infection take about 24–48 hours to become apparent, and granulation tissue repair is rarely appreciable before the end of a week.

No precise time interval can be given because repair rate is influenced by the size of the injury and other factors, e.g. injury by thermal heat, corrosives and radiation, all of which delay healing. Bodily condition and certain diseases, e.g. of the endocrine system, may also delay healing. Any opinion on the date of infliction of a wound, therefore, must make due allowance for these modifying factors. Prolonged suppuration precludes precise estimation of the age of the injury.

According to McMinn (1969), epithelium begins to migrate across the wound surface in 24–48 hours and the rate of regeneration in animals is approximately 0.2 mm per day. Epithelial cells grow down the sides of the wound margins, as shown by Lindsay and Birch (1964). Robertson and Hodge (1972) studied the histopathology of healing abrasions. They found perivascular cellular infiltration at 4 to 6 hours. At 12 hours three layers were detectable; a surface zone of fibrin and red cells; a deeper zone of infiltrating polymorphs; and a deepest layer of abnormally staining collagen. At 48 hours the scab is well formed. By this time epithelial regeneration has commenced at the margins of the scab. Complete epithelial covering of small abrasions has occurred by 4 to 5 days. Sub-epithelial formation of granulation tissue is prominent at 5 to 8 days. Reticulum fibres are demonstrable at 8 days, and collagen fibres at 9 to 12 days.

In regard to the age of bruises, Moritz (1954) says that diffusely extravasated erythrocytes disappear from tissues within a few days and that haemosiderin is detectable in phagocytes after 24 hours by means of the Prussian Blue reaction. However, the possibility must always be borne in mind that haemosiderin may be present in superficial tissues as a result of a previous injury in the same site. Robertson and Mansfield (1957) concluded that estimation of the age of a bruise is completely unreliable. Deep-seated bruises, or those where there is a considerable extravasation of blood with haematoma formation, may retain intact and apparently normal erythrocytes for a considerable period of time.

A great deal of experimental work has been carried out over the past few years into the histochemical detection of changes, principally in enzymes, occurring around wounds. The principal author in this field is Raekallio and the reader in search of detail is advised to consult his recent reviews (1972, 1973). In summary, for most injuries, histological changes, notably cellular infiltration, are not apparent for 6 to 8 hours. Altered enzyme reactions are detectable from 1 hour, for esterases, for 8 hours for alkaline phosphatase; iso-electric focusing may demonstrate enzyme changes after 30 minutes. Changes in mucopolysaccharides occur at about 30 hours, and in nucleic acids at 32 to 64 hours. Changes appear later in bruises than in other forms of injury.

Raekallio demonstrated two zones of altered enzyme activity in relation to wounds: (a) a central zone in the immediate vicinity of the wound, and (b) a peripheral zone. The former showed evidence of decreasing enzyme activity and the latter increasing enzyme activity, which corresponded in degree with the time interval since injury, for instance of aminopeptidase at 2 hours after wounding. The results were based on experimental and human material. Post-mortem injuries showed no enzyme activity. The vital enzyme reaction was detectable for up to 5 days after death.

Although in the main experimental and human material yielded comparable results, senility, major multiple injuries, or major brain damage could impair the enzyme reaction. Raekallio has therefore warned that an estimate of the age of a wound should not be made on one histological or histochemical finding.

Jaques *et al.* (1969) and Nevelos and Gee (1970) studied the ground-substance of wounds. Malik (1971) has investigated histological and histochemical changes in experimental burns, and Brizio-Molteni *et al.* (1974) have used light- and electron-microscopy to study deep burns in human tissues. The effect of age of the individual on the rate of healing reactions has been studied by Raekallio and Makinen (1974), and Mann and Bedner (1977). The later stages of healing of experimental wounds in rats, over a period of 84 days, has been described by Williams (1970).

Most of the published work relates to wounds of the skin. Kerkola (1972) however, has applied similar techniques to the investigation of experimental liver wounds.

Fractures

In the case of any fracture it is only possible to estimate the age approximately, since a number of factors are concerned, such as the age and state of nutrition of the injured person, the site of the fracture, etc. In the skull, during the first week, the margins of the fracture are lightly adherent, being bound only by serous exudate. Within 2 to 4 weeks calcified callus forms, and the margins of the fracture become eroded; this change is first seen on the inner table of the skull. In due course the fragments are firmly united by bone. If, however, there has been appreciable separation of the fragments, the gap may persist or be filled only by fibrous tissue; the margins of the fragments are then rounded and smooth. This takes several weeks and is not likely to occur before the end of about 3 months. It is not unusual for some excess of new bone to remain, perhaps indefinitely, on the inner table, in the neighbourhood of a fracture, and this local roughening may be the means of identifying an old, but otherwise obscure, fracture. Roughening of the inner table of the left middle fossa of the skull, and old-standing damage of the cortex of the right frontal lobe was found at a necropsy in 1948; the subject had been knocked down by a pedal cyclist in 1937 and had then sustained a fracture of his skull (F.M. 619).

Repaired fractures of known age are rarely seen in the post-mortem room. It seems worthwhile, therefore, to describe an example:

A man, aged 58, fell on the back of his head on 19 May 1948. He was in hospital for 11 days and then went home, but he was unable to resume work and suffered from headache—"he always seemed to hold his head at the back in the middle". His sight was impaired and he could no longer read his newspaper. His body was recovered from a canal on 29 July 1948. Death was due to drowning, but he had sub-acute softening of the cortex of the right occipital lobe. A fissured fracture, $1\frac{1}{2}$ in. long, had occurred immediately to the left of the middle line, in the occipital bone. Bony union was complete, but the site of the fracture was marked by a shallow furrow on the surface of each table of the skull. This repair had not taken more than $11^1/_2$ weeks (.M. 460).

In the long bones, Moritz (1954) indicates that the initial haematoma formed at the site of fracture is usually clotted within 12–24 hours. The organisation of the haematoma commences in about 48 hours and is complete in 7–10 days. Osteoid formation at the periphery of the haematoma is apparent in 72 hours, and the osteoid commences to calcify at about 7 days, being complete in about 6 weeks. There have been several publications indicating the possible application of histochemical methods to the investigation of the age of fractures (Raekallio and Makinen, 1969; Raekallio *et al.* 1970).

An extensive review of the rate and nature of healing in different organs was published by McMinn (1969); see also Hunt, (1980) Irwin (1981) and Sevitt (1981).

Disseminated Intravascular Coagulation

Recently many investigations have been made into the physiological and metabolic effects of injury on the body (Sevitt, 1974). Most of these, while of clinical importance, are not of much value in autopsy diagnosis. A relevant effect, however, is the condition known as "disseminated intravascular coagulation" or D.I.C. Injury is one of its predisposing factors. It has been defined as an acceleration of the coagulation process in the dynamic circulation with consumption of coagulation factors and platelets, microvascular obstruction by fibrin deposition and secondary activation of fibrinolysis (For details of this the reader should consult Stalker (1978); Simpson and Stalker (1973) McKay (1965) Hamilton *et al.* (1978)) and Timperley (1978).

Its relevance to forensic pathology is that it is of frequent occurrence in the victims of injury who survive for hours or days but who then die and the cause is not immediately explicable, except in the sense of the general term "shock". It is valuable in these circumstances to look for microthrombi in the vessels of the lung, kidney or brain, using such stains as MSB (Lendrum, 1962). On occasion fibrin may not be detectable but the condition may be suspected in the presence of massive haemorrhage following the injury, untreatable even by blood replacement.

A man had sustained a stab wound of the abdomen which penetrated pelvic blood vessels. Attempts to combat blood loss by transfusion of a vast amount of blood, 40 units, failed (F.M. 27950A).

Another consequence of injury, mainly fracture of long bones, is fat or bone marrow embolism. A vast literature on this subject has accumulated, and in particular in relation to the source of the fat droplets. Are they derived from fat depots or from chylomicrons? (Further information is to be had in Mason's article, 1978.)

The detection of fat emboli is a useful indication of the ante-mortem origin of any injuries present. The fat can be detected by any of the conventional stains. It should be sought in the lungs and brain. Massive cerebral fat embolism is a fatal condition and may account for death occurring 1 or 2 days after injury.

Fat embolism may also be found in the severely burned. It is suggested that burning of a body after death may release fat into the circulation sufficient to simulate ante-mortem fat embolism (Sevitt, 1962).

References

ARCHBOLD, J. F. (1959) Pleading, Evidence and Practice in Criminal Cases, 34th, ed., T. R. F. Butler and M. Garsia. London: Sweet and Maxwell.

BEDDOE, H. (1958) *Police*, **3**, no. 2, 24–28.

BRIZIO-MOLTENI, L., NICKERSON, P. A., DJIEKAN, F., and CLOUTIER, L. C. (1974) *Arch. Pathol*, **98** (5), 308–311.

CAMERON, J. M., GRANT, J. H., and RUDDICK, R. (1973) J. *Forensic Photogr.* **2**, 9.

CATHCART, C. W. (1909–10). *Trans. Med.-chi. Soc. Edinburgh*, **29**, 1901.

COLLINS, D. H. (1948) *J. Path. Bact.*, **60**, 205–10.

DALGAARD, J. B. (1957) *J. Forens. Med.*, **4**, 110.

DUNKERLEY, G. E. (1956) *Lancet*, **ii**, 819.

EVANS, E. G. (1958) Re R. v. Cook (1958): Personal communication and photograph.

FATTEH, A. (1966) *J. Forens. Sci.*, **11**, 17.

FATTEH, A. (1971) *Forensic Science*, **16**, 393–396.

FAZEKAS, I. G. and KIS, E. V. (1971) *Z. Rechtsmedizin*, **68**, 86.

GONZALES, T. A., VANCE, M., HELPERN, M. and UMBERGER, G. J. (1954) Legal Medicine and Toxicology, 2nd ed., pp. 337 and 372–99. New York: Appleton Century.

GORDON, I., TURNER, R. and PRICE, T. W. (1953) Medical Jurisprudence, 3rd ed. Edinburgh and London: Livingstone.

GORMSEN, H. (1961) Kerr Memorial Lecture, *Brit. Ass. Forens. Med.*

GREEN, M. A. (1978) *J. Forensic Sci. Soc.*, **18**, 161–163.

HAMILTON, P. J. STALKER, A. L., and DOUGLAS, A. S. (1978). *J. Clin. path.*, 31–609–619.

HELPERN, M. (1946) *Ann. Intern. Med.*, **24**, 673–4.

HEMPLING, S. M. (1981) *Med. Sci. Law.* **21**, 215–222.

HIRVONEN, J. (1968) *J. Forens. Med.* **15**, 161.

HUNT, D. K. (1980) Wound Healing and Wound Infection. New York, Appleton, Crofts-Century.

IRWIN, T. T. (1981) Wound Healing, Principles and Practice London: New York, Chapman & Hall.

JAMES, W. R. L. (1961) Personal communication and photograph of specimen.

JAQUES, J. and CAMERON, H. C. S. (1969) *J. Pathol.*, **90**, 337–340.

KERKOLA, (1972) *Acta Path. Microbiol Scand.* (suppl.) **228**, 1–56.

KERR, D. A. J. (1957) Forensic Medicine, 6th ed., p. 77. London: Adam and Charles Black.

KNIGHT, B. H. (1966) *Medicine, Science and Law*, **6**, 150.

KNIGHT, B. (1975) *Forensic Sci.*, **6**, 249–255.

KNIGHT, B. (1979) *Brit. Med. J.*, **i**, 350–51.

KUKULL, W. A. and PETERSON, D. R. (1977) *Am. J. Epidermiol*, **106** (6) 485–6.

LAIHO, K. and UOTILA, V. (1966) *Nature*, 31 Dec.

LENDRUM, A. C. (1962) *J. Clin. Path.*, **15**, 401.

LINDSAY, W. K., and BIRCH, J. R. (1964) *Canad. J. Surg.*, **7**, 297.

LITTLEJOHN, HARVEY (1925) Forensic Medicine, pp. 193 and 222–3. London: Churchill.

MCKAY, D. C. (1965) Disseminated Intravascular Coagulation. New York: Hoeber.

MCMINN, R. M. H. (1969) *Tissue Repair*. New York: Academic Press.

MALEK, M. O. (1970) *J. Forens. Sci.*, **15**, 489.

MALIK, M. O. A. (1971) *Br. J. Exper. Pathol.*, **52**, 345–352.

MANN, M. and BEDNAR, B. (1977) **23**, 277–89.

MARTIN, E. (1950) Precis de Médicine Légale, 3rd ed. Paris: Doin.

MASON, J. K. (1978) *The Pathology of Violent Injury*. London, Arnold.

MOLE, R. H. (1948) *J. Path. Bact.*, **60**, 413.

MORITZ, A. R. (1954) Pathology of Trauma, 2nd ed., p. 25. London: Henry Kimpton.

NEVELOS, A. B. and GEE, D. J. (1977) *Med. Sci. Law*, **10**, 175.

OBIGLIO, J. R. (1939) *Revista de la A. M. A.*, **53**, 1005–7.

OJALA, K., LEMPNER, M. and HIRVONEN, J. (1969) *J. Forens. Med.*, **16**, 29.

POLSON, C. J. (1955) Essentials of Forensic Medicine, 1st ed., p. 113. London: E. U. P.

POLSON, C. J. (1960) 2nd Int. Meeting on Forensic Path. and Med., New York. Program and Abstracts, p. 11.

POLSON, C. J. (1963) *J. Ind. Acad. Forens. Sci.* **2**, 5–12.

PROVENT, P. and SIMONIN, C. (1940) *Ann. Med. leg.*, **20**, 231–71.

R. V. COOK (1958) Flintshire Assizes, per Dr. Gerald Evans, also *Med. Sci. Law* (1961), **1**, 33.

R. V. CORNOCK (1947) Bristol Assizes, Manchester Guardian; also Taylor (1956) vol. i, p. 242.

R. V. DONOGHUE (1954); also Taylor (1965), **i**, 218, 497.

R. V. HEATH (1946) Trial of Neville George Cleavly Heath, Notable British Trials Series, vol. 75; ed. MacDonald Critchley, 1951. London, Edinburgh and Glasgow: Hodge.

R. V. M'LOUGHLIN (1838) 8 C. and P. 635, cited Archbold (1959), p. 1002.
R. V. SMITH (1937) 8 C. and P. 173, cited Archbold, p. 1002.
R. V. THORNE (1929) Trial of Norman Thorne, ed. Helena Normanton. London; Bles.
R. V. WARMAN (1846) 1 Den. 183; 2 C. and K. 195; cited Archbold, p. 1002.
R. V. WOOD (1830) 1 Mood, 278, cited Archbold, p. 1002.
RABINOWITSCH, A. (1959) *J. Forens. Med.*, **6**, 160–5.
RAEKALLIO, J. (1960) *Nature*, **188**, 234.
RAEKALLIO, J. (1961) *Ann. Med. Exp. Fenn.*, **39**, Suppl. **6**, 1.
RAEKALLIO, (1966) *J. Forens. Med.*, **13**, 85.
RAEKALLIO, J. (1970) *Progr. Histochem. Cytochem.*, **1**, 51.
RAEKALLIO, J. (1972) *Forensic Science*, **1**, 3–16.
RAEKALLIO, J. (1973) *Z. Rechts Med.* **73**, 83–102.
RAEKALLIO, J., KOVACS, M. and MAKINEN, P. L. (1970) *Acta Path, microbiol. scand.* A 78, 658.
RAEKALLIO, J. and MAKINEN, P. L. (1969a) *Zacchia*, **44**, 587.
RAEKALLIO, J. and MAKINEN, P. L. (1969b) *Acta path. microbiol. scand*, **75**, 415–22.
RAEKALLIO, J. and MÄKINEN, P. L. (1970) *Zacchia*, **45**, 463.
RAEKALLIO, J. and MAKINEN, P. L. (1974) *Z. Rechtsmed.* **75**: 105–11.
Restriction of Offensive Weapons Act (1959) 7 & 8 Eliz. 2, c. 37.
Restriction of Offensive Weapons Act (1961) 9 & 10 Eliz. 2, c. 22.
ROBERTSON, I. and MANSFIELD, R. A. (1957) *J. Forens. Med.*, **4**, 2–10.
SCOTT, G. D. (1928) *J. Amer. Med. Ass.*, **90**, 689–90.
SEVITT, S. (1962) *Fat Embolism.* London: Butterworths.
SEVITT, S. (1970) *J. Clin. Path.*, **23**, Suppl. (*R. Coll. Path.*), **4**, 86.
SEVITT, S. (1974) *Reactions to Injury & Burns.* London, Heinemann.
SEVITT, S. (1981) *Bone Repair & Healing in Man.* Edinburgh, Churchill Livingstone.
SHAPIRO, H. A., and ROBERTSON, I. (1962) *J. Forens. Med.*, **9**, 5.
SIMONIN, C. (1955) *Médecine Légale Judiciare*, 3rd ed., p. 67. Paris: Maloine.
SIMONSEN, J. (1967) *J. Forens. Med.*, **14**, 147.
SIMPSON, J. G. and STALKER, A. L. (1973) in *Clinics in Haematology, Vol. 2.* Edit A. S. Douglas, Eastbourne. W. B. Saunders.
SIMPSON, K. (1954) *Police J.*, **27**, 110–17.
SIMPSON, K. (1962) Personal communication.
SIMPSON, K. (1969) *Forensic Medicine*, 6th ed., pp. 49–52. London: Edward Arnold.
SIVALOGANATHAN, S., (1982) *Med. Sci. Law.*, **22**, 119–125.
SMITH, Sir SYDNEY and FIDDES, F. S. (1955) *Forensic Medicine*, 10th ed., p. 110. London: Churchill.
SPILSBURY, Sir BERNARD (1939) *Med.-leg. Rev.*, **7**, 215–23.
SPITZ, W. (1965) *J. Forens. Med.*, **12**, 105.
STALKER, A. L. (1978) in *The Pathology of Violent Injury.* Edit Mason. J. K. London, Arnold.
TAYLOR, A. S. (1965) *Principles and Practice of Medical Jurisprudence*, ed. K. Simpson 12th ed., vol. **i**, p. 42. London: Churchill.
TEARE, R. D. (1961). *Med. Sci. Law*, **1**, 429–36.
TIMPERLEY, W. R. (1978) *Med. Sci. Law*, **18**, 108–116.
WEBSTER, J. M. (1960) Personal communication, confirming report in *Birmingham Mail*, 4 June 1948.
WILLIAMS, G. (1970) *J. Pathol.*, **102**, 61–68.

CHAPTER 4

Injuries of Specific Regions

Head Injuries

It has been truly said that no injury of the head is too trivial to be ignored or so serious as to be despaired of. They are common injuries and alone account for about one-fourth of all deaths due to violence; they were responsible for 60 per cent of fatal road accidents (Rowbotham *et al.*, 1954).

The present account is concerned with the more obvious results of head injuries. This is only part of the story because it is now clear that serious damage may be present but its detection requires skilled microscopical examination by a neuropathologist. The forensic pathologist, even if he has the requisite skill, experience and facilities, has far too many other calls upon his time to enable him to undertake these time-consuming investigations. Notable contributions to this section of neuropathology have been made, for example, by Tomlinson (1970), Strich (1970), Oppenheimer (1968) and Courville (1950). Their publications must be studied in the original texts; we do not presume to be able to give any satisfactory summary of their important findings.

INJURIES OF THE SCALP

The anatomy of the vascular supply of the scalp predisposes to the spread of infection from it into the skull; there is a free communication between the vessels of the scalp and those of the meninges. It is more usual, however, and more probable, that spread of infection will take place when the scalp wound is accompanied by a fracture of the skull. It is not necessary that the fracture shall be large or obvious; it is sufficient if only of pin-head size, as is illustrated by the following case, which, moreover, also demonstrates the possible gravity of an apparently trivial scalp wound.

A boy aged 5 years fell on the gravel path at his home. He sustained a small laceration of his forehead but soon recovered from the immediate effects of the accident. During the following month he was apparently quite well. He then became ill and, within 4 days, he had the symptoms and signs of meningitis. At the postmortem examination, 10 days later, his scalp wound presented as a circular, scabbed laceration, $1/_8$ in. in diameter, situated in the centre of his forehead, just below the hair line; it had penetrated to the skull. There was also a localised, depressed fracture of the frontal bone, directly below the scalp wound. This fracture was funnel-like, being approximately $1/_8$ in. in diameter in the outer table but only of pin-head size in the inner table, which was perforated. Suppurative meningitis was accompanied by an extra-dural abscess, and an abscess in the left frontal lobe of the brain. The organism responsible was *haemolytic streptococcus* (P.M. 5393).

Wounds of the scalp may give rise to difficulty in interpretation because, being closely applied to the skull, the scalp may be split in linear fashion by blunt force. In consequence, the resulting wound may appear to be an incision. Close examination, especially under a hand lens, will detect irregularity, bruising and abrasion of the margins of the wound and will thus demonstrate its true nature, i.e. a laceration. The wound should also be examined for the presence of foreign material, e.g. soil or glass, since this may distinguish between wounds due to a fall and those due to the blow of a fist or other weapon.

Bruising of the scalp, which may be better detected by touch than sight, is at once a warning that grave internal damage, not apparent at the time of the examination, may be present, yet it may not produce symptoms and signs until some hours have elapsed.

Occasionally the scalp injuries may have a shape which suggests the nature of the agent which caused them, e.g. the butt of an axe (Fig. 21; F.M. 2958).

Three unusual lacerations, at the back of the head, in the same horizontal plane, were distributed as follows: (a) a star-shaped laceration at $^3/_4$ in. to the left of the occiput overlying a fissured fracture of the skull; (b) a

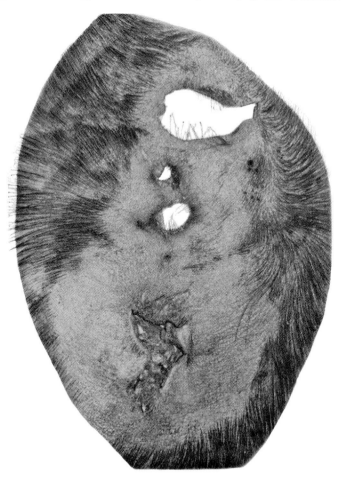

FIG. 48. Disease and trauma of scalp: healing gummata (three) above a stellate laceration due to a fall.

vertical split $1^3/_4$ in. long at $1^1/_2$ in. to the right of the middle line, and (c) a second split in the scalp 1 in. long at 3 in. to the right of the middle line. There was a recent bruise of the nose. The deceased had been drinking with companions and, en route home or to another public house, he had an argument with one of the men who hit him on the nose and he fell to the ground. This accounted for the stellate laceration and fracture. The other two injuries proved to have been accidental. The injured man had been picked up and carried for a distance. He was then sat on a wall and fell, sustaining a laceration on the right of his head. The other laceration on the right occurred when his bearers accidentally dropped him on the ground. Their first explanation of the circumstances was that he had fallen to the ground and struck his head on the bumper of a car and then the curb (F.M. 6636A).

Another unusual case was that of a syphilitic woman, aged 66, who fell downstairs. There were four lesions of the scalp, each of which, at first glance, might have been thought the result of violence. That over the occiput was a stellate, recent laceration $1^3/_4 \times 1$ in.; the other three, lying at intervals in the line between the occiput and the vertex, were approximately circular ulcers $1^1/_4$ in. in diameter. Their margins were as if punched out of the scalp and their floors had a dirty grey-green colour. These were gummatous ulcers. She had syphilitic caries of the skull and gummatous change in the dura mater (P.M. 2707, Fig. 48).

THE MECHANISM OF HEAD INJURIES

Fractures and other injuries of the head may be caused directly or indirectly.

Direct injuries may be the result of (a) compression as by midwifery forceps or crushing of the head by the wheel of a vehicle.

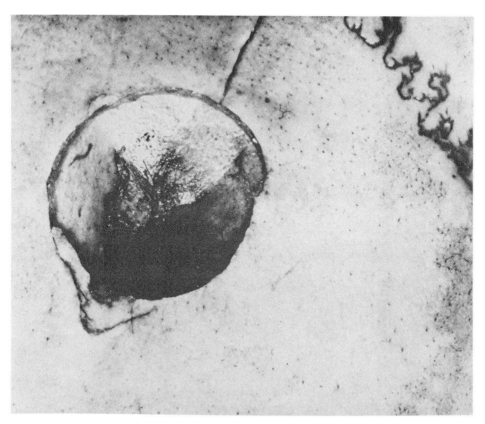

FIG. 49. Localised depressed fracture produced by a blow with a corner of a brick.

A large group of direct injuries includes those which occur when (b) the head is struck by an object in motion. These may be small missiles of high velocity which penetrate the skull, e.g. bullets, or large objects of slow velocity, e.g. bricks (Fig. 49), masonry, machinery, propeller blades. Occasionally the agent is an edged weapon, applied with moderate force and of low velocity, e.g. a dagger. Courville (1950) includes (c) repeated jars of the head by repeated sharp blows, leading to the condition of "Punch Drunk".

Another common group of direct injuries occur when (d) the head is in motion and it strikes an object, as in falls and traffic injuries.

Indirect injury of the skull follows a fall on the feet or buttocks.

The Agent

The kind of fracture which follows a blow is in part determined by the agent responsible. Weapons having a small striking face produce localised, depressed fractures but their appearances depend, in turn, upon the degree of violence used. A hammer or poker can punch a hole clean through both tables of the skull and cause comminution of the depressed portion, or there may be only partial displacement, without comminution, at the point of impact. The weight of the weapon and the distance between the parties, when it is thrown, or held in the assailant's hand, also play a part in modifying the effects of the blow and the appearances of the fracture. The effects of the blow are also modified by the thickness of the part of the skull which is struck.

Fissured and comminuted fractures rather than localised, depressed fractures are the rule following a fall or violent contact with a motor vehicle. A girl aged 13 years died of head injuries which included a localised, depressed fracture, with comminution, in an area approximately 1 in. in diameter. Hairs, which resembled those of the victim, were found on one of the nuts of the wheel of a motor vehicle. Experiments showed that the nut produced an impression in "Plasticine" which resembled the shape of the victim's scalp wound. The nut of the wheel fitted the fracture in the skull. Glaister and Rentoul (1966). A similar fracture can follow contact with a door handle (L.U. Museum, No. 125).

The Intensity of the Force

As would be anticipated, the greater the force, the greater is the damage likely to be; this is important in relation to intent. A determined attack, usually by multiple blows, will be characterised by extensive damage. It must not be assumed, however, that a single violent blow excludes the possibility of a determined attack, but it renders it less likely.

Weapons having a small striking face, e.g. hammers or pokers, do not usually damage an area of the skull greater than that of the striking face, nor cause complete detachment of the bone in that area. This, of course, is subject to qualification according to the part of the skull involved; the degree of violence necessary to produce such a fracture in the temple is less than that required to have a like effect elsewhere.

The small, fast-moving agent, e.g. a cricket ball, is more likely to cause bruising of the brain at the site of impact than contact with a broad agent, e.g. against a wall (Strich, 1970).

Heavy agents, having a large striking face, will produce extensive damage in any event, and the degree of violence need be but slight. Head injuries produced by contact with a moving motor vehicle, by the kick of a horse or a fall from a height are usually extensive fissured fractures or, according to the circumstances, there is comminution, with depression of a large area of the skull, accompanied by secondary lines of fissured fracture, radiating from the point of impact.

The question of the position of fractures resulting from impacts at different points on the skull has been studied, using stress-coat techniques of applying a film of lacquer-like substance to the skull, before striking it (Gurdjian, 1975) (Gurdjian & Webster, 1958).

The Point of Impact

The interpretation of the circumstances in which the fracture was sustained may be facilitated when the point of impact is apparent. It may be consistent with a fall from a height or contact with a part of a motor vehicle; it may indicate the probable positions of an assailant and his victim at the time of an attack. It may help to distinguish between an attack and an accidental fall, for example, whilst under the influence of drink.

Basal fractures, which can result from mild violence, are often from transmitted force, as by a fall from a height on to the feet or buttocks. Involvement of the base, however, not rarely follows as an extension of a fracture which begins at the vault or side of the head.

Fractures of the vault, back or side of the head may present with a stellate comminution at the point of impact.

The Mobility of the Skull at the Time of the Blow

The effects of a blow to the head are modified according to the mobility of the head at the moment of impact. If the head is free and unsupported, the principal effects are likely to be due to the shearing or swirling movement imparted to the brain, causing bruising and sometimes laceration of the cortex, rather than a fracture. A fall on to the back of the head or a blow from a cosh are common examples of this kind. A fracture is then likely to be a fissured one, not infrequently accompanied by a stellate comminution at the point of impact.

If the head is fixed and supported, as happens when the wheel of a vehicle passes over the head of the victim as he lies on the ground, the resulting damage is due to crushing. These fractures may be fissured, the principal line tending to encircle the skull, not infrequently passing through the base, in the region of the sella turcica. It is probable, also, that there will be comminution and gross depression of the skull where the wheel was in contact with it. The commencement of the line of fracture may be at any point between the point of contact with the wheel and the point of support. There may be almost complete separation of the nasofacial mass from the rest of the skull.

Fractures of the Skull

It has long been recognised that the importance of fractures of the skull is in reality that of the accompanying injury to the brain. A fracture, however, is a positive condition which can be demonstrated to members of a jury, and no doubt, to the layman, it may seem the more important condition.

Fractures of the skull may be fissured, depressed or comminuted fractures; mention is also made of pond or indented fractures, gutter and ring fractures. Any of them may also be compound, i.e. associated with injury to the scalp or nasal sinuses.

THE FEATURES OF FRACTURES OF THE SKULL

Fissured Fractures

These are linear fractures which usually involve both tables of the skull, but without displacement of the fragments. Rarely, they involve the inner table alone. They are notoriously difficult to detect when small, owing to negligible displacement of the fragments, and there is no certainty that they will be demonstrated by X-rays. In practice it is prudent to assume they are present, when the X-ray examination proves negative, if the circumstances and the condition of the patient suggest that a fracture may have occurred. No doubt this is a valid clinical reason for omitting X-ray examination, but, if there is a possibility of legal proceedings arising out of the injury, this examination should be made, lest it be suggested that its omission was negligent.

In some cases, as already indicated, a blow may produce a stellate or mosaic-like comminution at the point of impact and fissured fracture lines may extend from this area. The principal line of fracture is then in the direction of the force. A fissured fracture can result from a fall through a distance equivalent to the height of the victim, as after a slip on a polished floor or when knocked to the ground by the blow of a fist; a driver fractured his skull when he collapsed and fell from the platform of his tram. It is unlikely, however, that accidents of this kind will produce localised, depressed fractures, unless the head strikes some projection having a small surface and, even then, the victim must be of heavy build or the rate of fall is accelerated, e.g. by running or by a blow. Contact with a broad resisting surface, e.g. the ground, or blows with an agent having a relatively broad striking surface are likely to cause fissured fractures. A broad agent, e.g. the back of a shovel, may produce grave lacerations of the scalp and yet fail to fracture the skull or cause serious intra-cranial damage (*R.* v. *Lloyd*, 1955; F.M. 4067A, Fig. 24).

Depressed, Localised Fractures

These are also called "fractures à la signature", a descriptive term which aptly emphasises their medico-legal importance. They are often the veritable signature of the weapon or agent which caused the fracture. They therefore require careful, detailed examination. When there is comminution an attempt should be made either at operation or post-mortem examination, to preserve the fragments, which can be reconstructed for demonstration purposes. This is not always appreciated and the pieces may be thrown away.

These fractures may give reliable information concerning the probable kind of weapon, and when the skull is only dented the probable manner in which it was applied to the skull and the position of the assailant at the time may also be suggested. When there are multiple fractures, it is usual for at least one to be by the full face of the weapon, and in this manner its precise diameters may be determined.

The pattern of the fractures varies. A violent blow with the full face of a weapon can

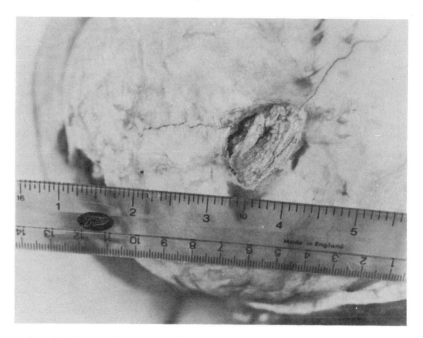

FIG. 50. Depressed fracture of skull caused by a blow with a hammer (F.M. 20891).

completely detach a portion of bone, of approximately the same diameter as its striking face, and drive it inwards. Less violence, or a glancing or tangential blow, may produce a localised fracture with only partial depression of the bone. When the striking face is circular, e.g. that of a hammer, the fracture is then circular or an arc of a circle, having the same diameter or radius as the hammer face. Depression is maximal at the point where the part of the weapon first strikes the skull. The fractured portion slopes down to this point, which is bordered by a cliff-like wall formed by compression of the tables of the skull at the margin of the fracture (Fig. 51). This appearance is sometimes described as "terracing". If a suspected weapon fits the fracture, it is possible to show not only that it was of the kind used in the attack but also to reconstruct the probable circumstances at the moment the blow was delivered. Due allowance should be made for the possibility that the assailant may have been left-handed.

Even when there is incomplete detachment of the bone, the fracture usually involves the inner table to a greater extent than the outer table. Moreover, the fracture line in the inner table is usually irregular and there may be comminution of the inner table alone.

Hammers or pokers are commonly responsible for these fractures which, however, also result from blows with an axe (Fig. 51) or a chopper. Spiked weapons, e.g. picks, sticks stones, or darts, may cause localised depressed fractures. Gardner and Simpson (1944) and Simpson (1969) in *R. v. Sangret*, Kingston Assizes, 1943, the Godalming wigwam murder, were able to demonstrate that a stick found near the body had the same width as a gross depressed fracture, of quadrilateral shape, at the back of the victim's skull. Hair resembling that of the victim was also found on the stick.

A blow from a golf ball even at long range can produce a depressed fracture. A girl aged

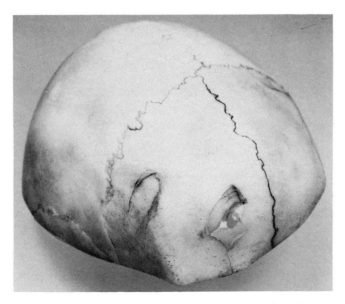

Fig. 51. Localised depressed fractures produced by the butt of an
axe: homicidal.

10 was playing near a burn which flows beside a golf course. She was not in the line of play
but a striker sliced his ball and struck her on the head, at a range of about 40 yards. She
sustained a fracture of the skull (*Glasgow Herald*, 7 June 1950). A colleague was concussed
when struck on the occiput by a golf ball; the range was several yards.

Axe and chopper blows yield distinctive depressed fractures. When the butt strikes the
skull, full face, the resulting fracture is rectangular (Fig. 51) in shape or, if only the corner
of the butt lands, the fracture is then triangular, the sides tending to be equilateral. Blows
with the cutting edge also produce linear cuts or triangular fractures but these are
isosceles; the point of maximum impact is at the narrow base; the sides of the blade
produce the long sides of the triangle (Figs. 52, 53, 54). Rarely, a depressed fracture, due
to some other cause, may superficially resemble an axe-edge injury but, when examined
more closely, the margins of the fracture may be shown to be parallel. In one of his cases,
Sir Sydney Smith was thus able to exonerate a man who was believed to have murdered his
wife with an axe. The margins of the fracture were parallel and its width coincided
precisely with that of the rim of a large metal dish on which the woman had accidentally
fallen (Smith and Fiddes, 1955).

It is becoming more common in this country to find injuries inflicted by weapons used
by ethnic minority groups. Thus in one of our cases (F.M. 28,300A) wounds had been
inflicted by a long heavy knife, or parang. This weapon, resembling a sword, produced
deep, shelving cuts several inches in length in the bone of the skull.

Depressed fractures caused by a stone may be irregular or roughly triangular; Harvey
Littlejohn (1925) depicts an excellent example and the specimen is preserved in the
Edinburgh Museum.

Fracture of the Skull by an angler's weight: A line carrying a six-ounce weight was cast

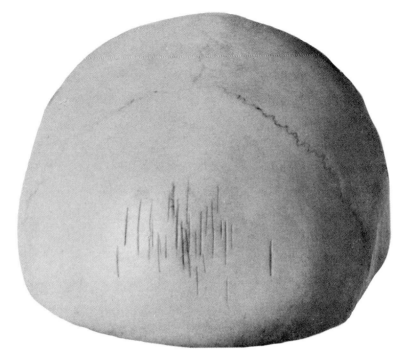

FIG. 52. Parallel chipping of outer table of skull: (simulation) suicide by hatchet (cf. Harvey Littlejohn's *Forensic Medicine*).

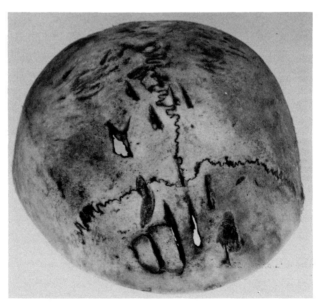

FIG. 53. Multiple localised depressed fractures of the skull: note parallel arrangement. Hatchet blows: attempted suicide.

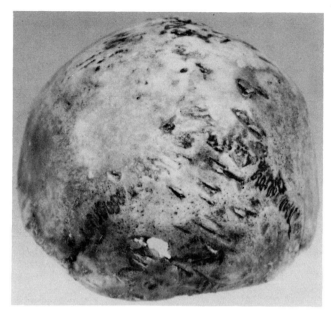

Fig. 54. Localised depressed fractures of skull. Note parallel
arrangement. Hatchet blows: attempted suicide.

and the weight struck the head of a boy aged 14. He had been rendered unconscious immediately and died later of skull fracture and brain injuries (*Yorkshire Post*, 22 Jan. 1982).

SELF INFLICTED AXE BLOWS

When a man and his friend were playing cards, the host excused himself and left the room. Shortly afterwards the guest heard repeated knocking in the cellar below. Time passed and the friend called upon his host to return. "You have chopped enough wood." The host returned with an axe in his right hand and with his head and face covered with blood. The friend immediately escaped and went for the police. He returned with an officer and they deemed it prudent to look through a window before entering the house. They saw the host laid on the floor: he was dead when they entered.

The fatal injury proved to have been a stab wound of the heart but this had been preceded by a flurry of axe blows to his head, inflicted with the cutting edge. Self-infliction was shown by the arrangement of the linear cut in parallel, gathered into areas within reach of a right-handed man. There were four fractures at the vertex, seven on the forehead and at least ten in the right occipital region. Several of the fractures involved both tables of the skull and there had also been displacement of bone. Although these injuries were severe and had been inflicted with considerable force, they were not immediately lethal nor even incapacitating. He had had time and had retained the ability to accomplish suicide by stabbing. (The notes of this case and the calvarium were presented to the Department by Dr. Eastwood. Fig. 54).

Penetrating Injuries of the Skull

These are the kind of localised, depressed fractures which are produced by pointed and, usually, sharp agents. The weapon passes through both tables of the skull, leaving a more or less clean-cut opening, the shape and size of which corresponds with the cross-section of the weapon. Likely agents include daggers or knives in civilian life, or bayonets or knives, e.g. a commando knife in war conditions. They are relatively rare injuries, of which the following is a good example.

A Pole murdered a woman by stabbing her with a sheath knife, the blade of which was strong and sharp; it was up to 1 in. in breadth. The external wound in the scalp was just at the top of her left ear; the knife entered through a clean-cut opening in the skull and severed the mid brain, in a horizontal plane, having first passed through the left tempero-sphenoidal lobe. She survived the blow for sufficient time for appreciable sub-arachnoid haemorrhage to occur at the base of the brain. The opening in the skull was a clean-cut isosceles triangle, the dimensions of which were precisely those of a cross-section of the knife at 3 in. above its tip, i.e. at the probable distance through which the blade had penetrated the skull (Fig. 38). There was slight fissuring of the outer table from the angles of the fracture and slight irregularity of its margins at the inner table. It was possible, in advance, to suggest the probable dimensions and shape of the blade, by reference to the opening in the skull, and the depth of penetration, as indicated by the extent of the injury of the brain (F.M. 3279).

In a London case the murderer had attacked his victim with a broad bladed screwdriver. The fractures were rectangular and had the dimensions of a cross-section of the weapon. A series of photographs, given to me by Dr. Holden, then director of the Home Office Forensic Science Laboratories, Scotland Yard, demonstrate the appearances of the fractures and the correspondence between them and the weapon, which fitted precisely.

In one of the victims of the series of murders known as the "Yorkshire Ripper" cases, the victim had been stabbed through the upper eyelid and the roof of the orbit by a weapon which left a clear rectangular shaped hole in the thin bone of the orbital roof. At first sight this appeared to be caused by a conventional screwdriver or chisel. However, attempts to reproduce the injury with a similar weapon against bone of corresponding thickness always resulted in the bone being shattered. It was found that the only way that a neat rectangular hole could be produced was if a particular kind of chisel, a wood carver's chisel, which had a cutting edge directed obliquely like a guillotine blade, was used. In this case, when the suspect was arrested, the weapon which he was found to have used was a normal screwdriver, but with the shaft bent so that the angle of the cutting edge was directed obliquely, as in the case of the wood carver's chisel (F.M. 27,580).

A man was stabbed in the forehead with such force that the entire length of a $4^1/_2$ in. blade penetrated the head. Externally, the wound, $1 \times {}^1/_8$ in., was situated above the inner end of the right eyebrow. The blade had traversed the frontal bone to pass deep into the brain. He was rational when admitted to hospital. The blade was extracted with difficulty but recovery was complete at the end of 40 days (Adam, 1925).

An interesting series of penetrating fractures of the base of the skull was reported by Lawford Knaggs (1907). He included: a penetrating wound of the orbit, following a fall on to a lead pencil; penetration of cheek and skull following a fall on to an iron rod, and transfixion of the cheek of a butcher by a meat hook.

A victim was stabbed, during a brawl, by the ferrule of an umbrella. This penetrated the orbit and the sphenoid bone to traverse the mid brain, almost completely separating the upper and lower parts of the brain from one another (27,780B).

These victims were unfortunate since penetrating injuries are not usually fatal. In my case, however, relatively large vessels were severed and there was extensive injury to the mid brain. Others may die when the intracranial contents are infected by the weapon. On the other hand, even if the blade breaks and a portion is left in the skull it may remain there for some time without causing trouble. Epilepsy is a probable complication, due to the formation of scar tissue (Courville, 1950).

Two more examples, in each of which the knife blade had broken and a portion remained in the skull, are described by Helpern (1946); both of these victims died of intra-cranial haemorrhage. He mentions that there may be delay for a variable period before bleeding causes unconsciousness and death; the serious nature of the injury may escape notice during this interval. Helpern also depicts a small, fatal stab wound made by an ice pick which had penetrated deep into the brain; the external wound was within the hair line and thus concealed.

It appears that in one native area the punishment for theft is to have a nail driven into the head from vault to base. The offender described by Jackson (1961) had walked 150 miles to a hospital with the nail in his head.

A company director drilled eight holes in his head, each penetrating the brain, with a portable power drill. The injuries were described as conscious, precise and accurate drilling. He was aged 57, on the eve of retirement. He was unconscious when found and died the following day. (Shrewsbury Inquest; Major Crawford-Clarke, H. M. Coroner; 25 Mar. 1971.)

Obscure Penetrating Wounds

We have drawn attention to the difficulty of detecting injury of the scalp in regions of thick hair (see p. 153). This difficulty is greatly increased when the agent is small in cross-section. Stabbing with a knitting needle, a thin-bladded knife or a hat pin of the kind in common use in the 1900s, can escape detection even by thorough and expert examination of the living patient; the pathologist also must be alert and thorough, lest he fails to detect it at autopsy, although the damage done should indicate the probable cause. These cases, fortunately, are uncommon. Hendry and Stalker reported a good example in 1967; the agent was an unusual one, namely, part of an aluminium "tail" comb.

The victim, a young man, aged 18, was involved in a fight when under the influence of drink. When found he appeared to be suffering from facial injuries. His face was bruised and abraded and he had a laceration of his upper lip. There was some blood in the hair at the back of his head but no wound was found. During the ensuing 31 hours he developed neurological signs and symptoms which were correctly diagnosed as evidence of medullary compression. A few hours before his death moisture on his pillow was recognised as cerebrospinal fluid. The post-mortem examination disclosed a puncture wound at the back of the neck, just to the left of the midline and in line with the mastoid processes. The relevant area of the scalp was excised and, in the "fixed" specimen, the wound presented as a slit, only 3 mm long, bordered by an oval band of abrasion. The track of the agent measured .3 in. from the exterior to its end in the medulla; the point had almost reached the floor of the fourth ventricle. Part of the medulla was destroyed and there was haemorrhage on its right side.

The handle of the weapon was never found but it appeared it had been resharpened. The portion of a broken comb found at the scene and an intact comb, one of aluminium alloy, are depicted in the report. The maximum dimensions of the comb's cross-section were 8×4 mm and the handle of the comb was 3.7 in. (9.3 cm) long.

Comminuted Fractures

Comminution of the skull is often a complication of fissured or localised, depressed fractures. Its occurrence, unless the skull of the victim is unduly thin, is indicative of the application of considerable force when produced by weapons having a relatively small striking face; alternatively, the blow was made by a heavy weapon with a large striking face. An attack with a heavy iron bar or poker, an axe, thick stick or bludgeon usually produces a comminuted fracture. It can follow a kick from a horse or be produced by a bullet. The majority, however, are the consequence of the all too prevalent motor vehicle accidents. Less often, comminuted fractures are due to a fall from a height or occur when a passenger or engine driver leans out of a railway train and strikes his head against the masonry of a bridge or some other structure beside the track.

Comminution may occur without displacement of the fragments and the appearances of the fracture then resemble the pattern of a spider's web, or mosaic. Fissured fractures are likely to radiate for varying distances from the area of comminution. On other occasions, when the blow has been by greater force, the broken pieces of bone are displaced; some are driven into the brain and others may be lost.

To a certain extent the amount of damage to the skull relates to its thickness. The bone in the region of the temple is always thinner than elsewhere in the skull. On rare occasions the entire skull, and in particular, the temporal region may be extremely thin; sufficiently thin for it to be possible to read newsprint held against the inner surface of the skull through the thickness of the skull itself. In our experience, (F.M. 14,503c), a blow of moderate force on the side of the head with a wooden mallet produced an extensive and deeply depressed fracture from which the victim died instantly. Demonstration of the extreme thinness of the skull in court reduced a charge from that of murder to one of manslaughter.

Comminution of the skull by a bullet is illustrated by suicide of a man who shot himself with a 0.22 automatic pistol. The bullet entered his right temple and traversed the brain and came to rest between the dura mater and the left parietal bone. The impact produced a spider-web comminution of that bone, over an area $1^1/_2$ in. to 2 in. in diameter; the central fragments were slightly displaced outwards, by less than 1 mm, and the bullet remained inside the skull (F.M. 1424; Fig. 55. See also case no. 27. p. 259–60)

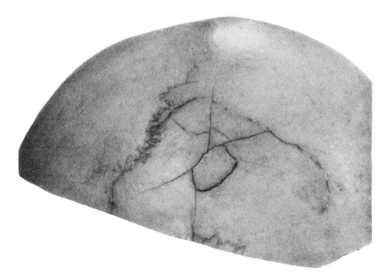

FIG. 55. "Spider web" or "mosaic" fracture of skull: suicide by 0.22 automatic pistol. Bullet inside skull at centre of the web.

Pond or Indented Fractures

Indented fractures occur only in skulls which are unduly elastic, i.e. in the skull of infants. The result of compression of their skulls can be reproduced by forcible compression of a ping-pong ball. Fissured fractures are likely to occur around the periphery of the dent.

Gutter Fractures

The glancing blow of a rifled firearm missile may plough a furrow in the outer table of the skull. Externally, these fractures present as gutters but they are usually accompanied by more extensive damage, e.g. an irregular depressed fracture, of the inner table of the skull.

Ring or Foramen Fracture (Plate 3)

Fracture of the skull occasionally results in a separation of the base; these are uncommon fractures, estimated at only 0.4 per cent of skull fractures.

The line of fracture, as depicted by Mortiz (1954) in a diagram and by Reimann (1961) in excellent photographs, runs at about 1 in. to $1^1/_2$ in. outside the foramen magnum at the back and sides of the skull; in front the fracture line is likely to traverse the middle ears and roof of the nose. This was seen where a woman aged 48 had sustained a head injury as the result of a road accident. It appeared she had been thrown forwards against the dashboard of a motor car in which she was a passenger. Her external injuries were confined to the front of the head. Abrasions were present on both sides of her forehead and on her right cheek. Bleeding had occurred from both ears and the nose. She had a ring fracture of the base of the skull. The line of fracture was at a distance of $1^1/_2$ in. outside the foramen magnum at the back and sides of the skull; it passed forwards to traverse both middle ears and the roof of the nose. In this case it would appear that the fracture was due either to a levering of the skull from its base or a shearing effect by a blow to the right side of the forehead and face (F.M. 6219; Plate 3).

The mechanism of these fractures has been described by Moritz (1954) and Reimann (1961). There are several possibilities and the precise mechanism in a given case will depend on the circumstances: (a) the base of the skull may thrust upwards and inwards by a force transmitted by the spinal column, following a fall from a height on to the feet or buttocks; (b) the vault may be driven against the base by a fall or blow; (c) a fall on to the back of the head or a blow to the occiput, or, as in F.M. 6219, a blow to the forehead, can lever the vault from the base, and (d) force, due to a fall or a blow, may twist the skull and shear the vault from the base, another possible explanation of the fracture in F.M. 6219. Moritz (1954), when mentioning this possibility, considered that such a force is more likely to cause a fracture-dislocation of the spine.

On another occasion ring fracture of the skull was one of the many injuries of the victim of an aircraft accident. The spinal column together with a portion of the base of the skull had been forced into the intracranial cavity (F.M. 5787A).

The Repair of Fractures of the Skull

It is possible only approximately to estimate the age of a fracture of the skull.

During the first week the margins of the fracture are lightly adherent, being bound only by serous exudate. Within 2 to 4 weeks calcified callus forms and the margins of the fracture become eroded; this change is first seen on the inner table of the skull. In due course the fragments are firmly united by bone. If, however, there has been appreciable separation of the fragments, the gap may persist or be filled only by fibrous tissue; the margins of the fragments are then rounded and smooth. This takes several weeks and is not likely to occur before the end of about 3 months. It is not unusual for some excess of new bone to remain, perhaps indefinitely, on the inner table in the neighbourhood of a fracture and this local roughening may be the means of identifying an old but otherwise obscure fracture. Roughening of the inner table of the left middle fossa of the skull and old-standing damage of the cortex of the right frontal lobe was found at a necropsy in 1948; the subject had been knocked down by a pedal cyclist in 1937 and had then sustained a fracture of his skull (F.M. 619). Sevitt, (1968) in his study of the repair of fractures, said that the fibrous union of fractures is the general rule, but bony union is occasionally found. In experimental work new bone trabeculer were seen at about 12 days, although these usually failed to bridge the gap. Some fractures fail to bridge at all, even months after the injury. Eventually, the fracture edges become closed by plates of new bone in continuity with the inner and outer tables.

Repaired fractures of known age are rarely seen in the post-mortem room. It seems worthwhile, therefore, to describe an example:

> A man aged 58 fell on the back of his head on 19 May 1948. He was in hospital for 11 days and then went home, but he was unable to resume work and suffered from headache. "He always seemed to hold his head at the back in the middle." His sight was impaired and he could no longer read his newspaper. His body was recovered from a canal on 29 July 1948. Death was due to drowning but he had subacute softening of the cortex of the right occipital lobe. A fissured fracture, $1\frac{1}{2}$ in. long had occurred immediately to the left of the middle line, in the occipital bone. Bony union was complete but the site of the fracture was marked by a shallow furrow on the surface of each table of the skull. This repair had taken not more than $11\frac{1}{2}$ weeks (F.M. 460).

The Circumstances of Fracture of the Skull

The majority of fractures of the skull occur as a result of an accident, which may be due to a fall or injury by a motor vehicle. A smaller number follow an attack in circumstances of murder or manslaughter, when the weapon may be a fist or some article likely to be handy, e.g. a poker, hammer, chopper, stick or bottle. The collateral circumstances are especially important when there has been only one blow, since the results may be much the same whether it be due to accident or design. Multiple fractures, however, when localised and depressed, at once raise the possibility of a determined attack.

Suicide by head injury is a rare event, since the process is painful and it is not easy to accomplish. It may be attempted by butting the head against a wall, in which event the victim is likely to be a mental patient. It has been attempted by blows with a hatchet. This is likely to produce nothing more than laceration of the scalp, with superficial damage to the outer table of the skull, as in Harvey Littlejohn's example (1925), and that of Bakke (1937). Suicide by hatchet blows, producing a large oval depressed fracture in the left half of the frontal bone, is recorded and illustrated by Hofmann-Haberda (1927, Fig. 157). The suicide described by Werkgartner (1935) was found with a hatchet in his left hand and injuries consistent with blows from a hatchet were present in his frontal and temporal bones; there were no defence wounds on his hands. Another and better example was that of a man aged 72, believed to be sane, which was described by Portigliatti-Barbos (1952), who reviewed the scanty literature. Yet another case was described by Rentoul (1954), when he invited his audience to decide whether the circumstances were those of suicide or murder. The deceased was found dead in a kitchen where blood had been shed in profusion. The victim lay on the floor and a large hammer was near his left hand. Death was due to haemorrhage from injury to the skull; an oval, comminuted fracture, in an area about 2 in. by $1^1/_4$ in. involved the vertex and twenty-eight small fragments of bone were collected from it; there were multiple lacerations of the scalp in an area approximately the same as that of the fracture. On balance, the evidence was in favour of suicide and it would appear the victim was mentally unstable; he had threatened to hit himself on the head with a hammer. We examined a man, who struck his head forcibly with a hammer before cutting his throat (see p. 138 Ch. 3).

There are two examples of self-inflicted axe blows to the skull in the museum of the Department of Forensic Medicine in Copenhagen. In the one case suicide was effected by hatchet or axe blows in the right parietal region. The target area was 5 cm in diameter, lying mid-way between the coronal and lambdoid sutures. An oval, irregular comminuted fracture, 2.5×2.0 cm in its diameter, lay in the centre of the target area and beyond there were separate cuts, either linear or triangular, in the outer table. In the second case of the skull the man had succeeded in making only superficial cuts, some 15 in all and up to 6 cm long, parallel to the middle line, in a target area, 5 cm in diameter, over the middle of the coronal suture. The appearances of the specimen coincided with that of Harvey Littlejohn (1925; see also Fig. 53).

The case of attempted suicide by head injury recorded by Eastwood (1957) is an outstanding example and the calvarium is now in the museum of our Department. This man inflicted 35 separate penetrating injuries to his skull with a hatchet, widely distributed so as to suggest at first sight that it must have been a homicidal attack. Closer examination showed, however, that these injuries were gathered into three separate target areas, frontal, high frontal or vertical, and right occipital. In each target area the fractures lay more or less parallel. Some of them had damaged the inner as well as the outer table, notably in the frontal region. The skull was of average thickness and density. Notwithstanding the gravity of these injuries he did not lose consciousness but chased his friend out of the house. When the friend returned with the police it was found that he had now stabbed himself in the abdomen and throat. He was still conscious and said he had drunk from a bottle of bleach. He survived several hours and died of peritonitis due to a perforating wound of the stomach (Figs. 53 and 54).

These cases are important because they show that there can be considerable mobility after severe head injuries. If, as I believe, Rentoul's case was one of suicide, the victim must have been capable of considerable movement after having sustained grave injury to his head; the distribution of heavy bloodstaining was widespread in the room. They are important also because they demonstrate the length to which a determined suicide can go to achieve his end. The distinction between suicide and murder is not easy and the first impressions are not unreasonably, as in Rentoul's case, those of murder. The suicidal injuries, however, may be recognised by certain criteria. They must lie in an accessible area. It is easy, for example, to strike the frontal bone with a hatchet or hammer and, if swung upwards when striking, the blows can fall upon the vertex. If a heavy weapon is held in both hands and propelled upwards from between the knees, it will land with distinct force, sufficient to fracture the skull, although, normally, several blows are required. The scalp injuries will be grouped in accessible localised target areas and will have an identical direction; a dozen or up to forty lacerations of the scalp may be present.

There will be no defence wounds on the hands nor any evidence of a struggle at the scene. There are a few reports of suicide by driving a nail or a similar object into the skull.

A woman aged 70 hammered a spike, 4 in. long into her head. It was inclined slightly to the left of the sagittal suture, at 30° to the coronal plane, near the posterior fontanelle. The spike had penetrated the upper motor gyrus, then severed the corpus collosum, and entered the left ventricle. There were also tentative punctures. She remained for some time fully conscious and coherent and had no sensory or motor disturbance. There was no mental derangement. Her condition, however, steadily deteriorated and she died at the end of 3 days. She had written a note in which she declared her intention to commit suicide (Branch, 1945). Another example, described by Thomas (1944), is that of a man aged 31 who attempted suicide by driving a 6 in. nail into his skull. He held the nail against his right temple and caused it to penetrate the bone by banging his head against a wall. He then pushed the nail into his brain by hand. It was said to have penetrated for a distance of 4 in. at right angles to the bone. The report analyses the resulting neurological disturbances. He made a complete recovery.

Head Injury as a Cause of Suicide

A bookmaker aged 53 was knocked down by a bus in September 1953; he sustained a fracture of the vault of his skull. He was able to return to work in February 1954 but his personality had changed; he became progressively difficult and abusive. His business declined and there was an overdraft at the bank. On 22 January 1955 he borrowed money from a friend and the following night he committed suicide by barbiturate poisoning. His widow sued the London Transport Executive alleging negligence and claiming damages for the death of her husband as a result of the accident. The question of whether head injuries could cause suicidal tendencies was a medical matter. There had been a conflict of opinion and the learned judge accepted the view that such injuries were reasonably capable of creating a suicidal tendency. (It was agreed that a personality change could result from a head injury). In this case, assuming that the injury was one of the possible causes of suicide, other possibilities were considered and rejected. The sequence of events which culminated in suicide could be traced back to the head injury which had created a suicidal tendency. The suicide was held to have been caused by the accident. Verdict for the plaintiff. There had been contributory negligence, the bus driver being held only one-third to blame. (*Cavanagh* v. *London Transport Executive*. Devlin, J.; 22 Oct. 1956. Reported by E. M. Wellwood *Lancet*, 1956, ii, 988.)

Intra-Cranial Haemorrhage

Although a fracture of the skull, to the layman, may well be the more spectacular change, it has long been recognised that damage to the contents of the skull, the brain in particular, following a head injury has far greater importance and danger.

Bleeding due to injury sometimes occurs in the absence of a fracture and perhaps, on occasion, in the absence of injury to the brain. There are circumstances in which the bleeding dominates the clinical picture, whereas, at other times, its effects are incidental, those of brain injury predominating. It is convenient to group intra-cranial bleeding according to its situation, a method which is to some extent justified by differences in its effects upon the patient. The site may be between the inner table of the skull and the meninges; between the dura and the arachnoid or in the subarachnoid space; injury also produces bleeding into the substance of the brain. Haemorrhage may be coincident in two or all of these situations.

EXTRA-DURAL HAEMORRHAGE

Bleeding which occurs between the inner table of the skull and the meninges is termed an extra-dural haemorrhage. It is uncommon, and, according to Rowbotham (1949), the cases represent "about 3 per cent of cases in any large series of acute cerebral trauma" and according to Tomlinson (1964) it occurs in between 1 and 3 per cent recorded cases of head injury. Their incidence amongst head injuries seen in the post-mortem room is somewhat lower since many are cured by surgical intervention.

These haemorrhages are usually the result of rupture of the middle meningeal artery or one of its branches; this occurred in 83 per cent of 125 cases (McKissock *et al.*, 1960). The main vessel is involved in at least half of the cases, whereas the frontal branch was ruptured in only two of Rowbotham's series of thirty-three cases. Complication by sub-arachnoid haemorrhage sometimes occurs and Rowbotham believes this to be one explanation of the occasional operative failure. Providing the patient is seen in good time, operative success is to be expected, since twenty-six of his thirty-three survived.

An extra-dural haemorrhage is centred near the arterial breach and, since the majority are in the temporal region following injury to the main vessel, exploration normally begins there.

The middle meningeal artery and its branches lie in grooves in the inner table of the skull. Those occupied by the anterior branches are commonly visible in X-rays and may be confused with fracture lines (Rowbotham, 1949). This arrangement is calculated to lead to rupture of the vessels whenever a fracture of the skull involves their vicinity. It is maintained by some that rupture is on all occasions a result of fracture of the skull, although the fracture may at times be small and escape detection even in radiographs.

Extra-dural haemorrhage is nearly always unilateral but rare examples of bilateral haemorrhage are known. In one case a fissured fracture of the frontal bone had extended across it so as to rupture the anterior branch of each middle meningeal artery. There were three bilateral haemorrhages in the 175 cases reviewed by McKissock *et al.* (1960).

An example of rupture of one anterior branch followed fracture of the skull in the left fronto-parietal region; it was a localised, depressed fracture, approximately 1 in. in diameter, astride the coronal suture. The wife of the victim had thrown a poker, weighing 2 lb, at his head (F.M. 3225A).

A boy was assaulted and struck on the head at a fair. Some hours later he collapsed. He was unconscious when admitted to hospital. Exploration of the skull failed to detect intra-cranial haemorrhage. X-ray examination negative. At autopsy a short fracture, fissured, was found on the right temporal bone. The posterior branch of the middle meningeal artery was ruptured. Death due to extra-dural haemorrhage.

The clinical sequence of events is traditionally characteristic, namely, that there is an initial phase in which symptoms and signs, common to any severe bump on the head, are dominant. They pass and for a period, which from case to case is of variable duration, there is a lucid interval during which the patient is apparently well, or suffers only from the local effects, notably of injury to his scalp. He may regain full consciousness and resume his employment when he may be conscious of his acts or he may perform them automatically. The symptoms and signs of cerebral compression supervene and continue to increase in severity until relieved by operation, or death occurs. Although this is indication of extra-dural haemorrhage there are often occasions when there is no lucid interval; loss of consciousness due to concussion may be maintained by cerebral compression.

A series of 125 cases of extra-dural haematoma included only thirty-five, or 27 per cent, which yielded the traditional history. As many, actually thirty-five patients, recovered from unconsciousness and remained alert, or relatively so, until treated and another thirty patients, the group which offers the worst prognosis, remained unconscious throughout. It was suggested that diagnosis of the condition is hindered by undue emphasis on the traditional history. Prompt diagnosis and urgent treatment are imperative if the continuing high mortality, which is about 50 per cent, is to approximate to the estimated level of 10 per cent, where there are adequate facilities (McKissock *et al.*, 1960). This confirmed the findings of Hancock *et al.* (1959), who found that most cases of extra-dural haemorrhage are not associated with a lucid interval. In their view arteriography is a valuable diagnostic aid.

The duration of the lucid interval is variable, it may be absent or it may last minutes or even days. In a series of thirty-three cases the range was from 2 hours to 7 days but, usually, the first sign was present at the end of about 4 hours (Rowbotham, 1949). Several factors operate to modify its duration. In some patients there may be an initial fall of blood pressure whereby bleeding from the ruptured vessel is lessened. On other occasions it may be that the injured vessel goes into spasm. If the dura is unduly adherent to the skull it will also take longer for blood to accumulate in sufficient amount to compress the brain.

Extra-dural haemorrhage, a post-mortem change, is sometimes seen in those whose heads have been exposed to intense heat as in burning building (see p. 325).

SUB-DURAL HAEMORRHAGE

A sub-dural haemorrhage is one which occurs between the dura mater and the pia-arachnoid, i.e. in the sub-dural space. Acute, sub-acute and chronic varieties are recognised and it must suffice here to consider only the acute and chronic forms, because a clear distinction exists between their clinical features and their medico-legal importance; the sub-acute haemorrhage resembles the acute form and, for present purposes, they are regarded as similar.

Sub-dural bleeding, unlike the extra-dural kind, is essentially venous or capillary and not arterial bleeding. The onset of its manifestations is therefore slower and, even when untreated by surgical operation, there can be natural arrest and repair. Increased intra-cranial pressure due to the bleeding, can, in time, attain a level which collapses the ruptured vessels and stops further bleeding. Absorption of the blood and repair by the process of organisation may lead to natural cure or it may convert an acute haemorrhage into a chronic sub-dural haematoma.

Acute (and Sub-acute) Sub-dural Haemorrhage

The majority, if not all, of these haemorrhages are the result of a head injury of which evidence is clear and recent; there is rarely, if ever, room for doubt that they are traumatic.

This view was confirmed by Rahme and Green (1961), who found that in 80 cases, injury was responsible for the sub-dural haematoma in the majority. They also found that this condition occurred more often in younger patients than is usually believed.

Not infrequently it is associated with injury to the brain, but it is by no means necessary that there is a coincident fracture of the skull or even a wound of the scalp; there may be no more than a bruising of the scalp.

Such a haemorrhage is a well-recognised fatal event in cases of non-accidental injury in children. Gutchkelch has shown that they can be caused by violent shaking of a child, without any impact having occurred to the head at all. (Gutchkelch, 1971)

They are commonly bilateral and the blood, having trickled downwards, tends to accumulate in the base of the skull, especially in the middle fossa, beside the temporal lobe. Its distribution will be determined by the position of the head, blood collecting by gravitation in the then dependent part of the skull. In the acute form the blood has not had time to disintegrate and therefore is red or dark red, part fluid and part clotted. It can be washed out of the skull since it is not adherent to the dura mater.

If a sufficient interval, one of days, elapses between injury and death, a fibrous membrane spreads over the inner surface of the clot, enclosing it. This layer is usually detectable at about 10 days, when it is firm enough to be picked up by the forceps (Crompton, 1982).

The site of the rupture of the vessel or vessels is difficult to locate. Bleeding may come from a tear in the wall of a dural sinus but usually bleeding comes from one or more of the veins which drain into the sinuses and cross the sub-dural space. On most occasions bleeding is slight but fatal compression of the brain by a large sub-dural haemorrhage can occur within a few hours (Rowbotham, 1949), death is rarely, if ever, sudden, i.e. in less than an hour.

Since the haemorrhage is of venous or capillary origin the latent period may be longer than that which may elapse after an extra-dural haemorrhage. Bleeding may cease, but a subsequent leakage may result in symptoms and signs of compression after an interval which may then be a matter of weeks. During the interim the victim may have sustained another head injury of accidental origin and apportioning the blame, when the first was inflicted by an assailant, may be sufficiently uncertain to preclude the institution of criminal proceedings. It could be maintained, even in the absence of any known subsequent head injury, that the whole of the change might have been due to natural disease or accidental causes. The difficulty created by delay between an assault and death from sub-dural haemorrhage is illustrated by the following case. A man aged 61 was attacked and hit over the head. He lost consciousness at the time, but after a few days he made what appeared to be a complete recovery. Three months later he collapsed in his shop and, when seen in hospital, he had symptoms and signs of cerebral compression. He died a few hours later and the post-mortem examination demonstrated a right sub-dural haematoma, i.e. on the side of his head struck by the assailant. Although there was no known head injury since that attack and it was probable that the attack had in fact caused his death, this was presumed accidental.

Subdural haematomas have occurred as a complication of superior saggital sinus thrombosis (two cases) (Robertson and Grove, 1958). They have occurred as a result of, or a concomitant of, anticoagulant therapy (two cases) (Strang and Tovi, 1962). A general review of the subject of subdural haematoma was published by Baker (1938). Persons suffering from haemophilia are prone to haematomata due to relatively minor violence.

Chronic Sub-dural Haematoma; Pachymeningitis interna haemorrhagica

Haemorrhage of long standing into the sub-dural space has appearances, and occurs in circumstances, which are peculiar to it. Although no doubt most, if not all, are traumatic and may well be at the end-stage of acute haemorrhages, their relationship to injury cannot be asserted with the same assurance as for extra-dural and acute sub-dural haemorrhages.

Chronic haematomas are sometimes found by chance at the post-mortem examination of alcoholic subjects and mental patients and in circumstances where there is no record of any head injury. Seemingly, therefore, they may be due to some pathological process and not trauma. On the other hand, the fact that alcoholics stumble and can sustain mild head injuries, of which they have no subsequent recollection, leaves the probability of trauma open as the cause of these haemorrhages. It is no less probable that a similar explanation holds in the case of restless mental patients. Trotter (1914) stressed the factor of injury and found that these haematomas could follow mild head injuries.

Sub-dural Haematoma following Fall from a Couch

The patient aged 76 had been put on an examination couch and had been seen by the consultant. He had left her alone in the cubicle, but quickly retraced his steps when he heard a bump. The patient had fallen off the couch and bumped her head. She died about 8 weeks later of secondary carcinoma of the pleura, following carcinoma of the breast. There was no trace of any injury to her scalp, nor of the skull, which was of normal thickness and consistence. A sub-dural haematoma, 11 × 5.5 × 1.5 cm was present in the right parietal region. It was well circumscribed and elastic to the touch. It contained dark red and brownish blood (Fig. 56). There was flattening of the brain cortex in contact with the haematoma. Although the accident was in no way the cause of her death, it could not be excluded as having played a minor part in accelerating her death. Any symptoms or signs it caused were overshadowed by those of the primary cause of death (F.M. 4303A).

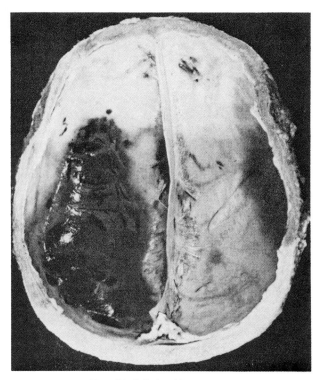

FIG. 56. Sub-dural haematoma.

The presence of blood in the sub-dural space provokes reparative changes. The dura mater provides vascular fibrous tissue which may succeed in enclosing the blood in a fibrous envelope. This may in time become sufficiently firm to permit surgical removal of the "cyst"-like structure. On the other hand, young capillaries in this tissue may rupture, even after slight injury to the head, and fresh bleeding will then occur. Whether it is by this or osmotic changes in it, swelling of a haematoma is not infrequent and may be sufficient to produce cerebral compression, even of fatal degree. Rarely, natural repair is by fibrosis of the clot and it may become calcified.

The principal medico-legal importance of this variety of intracranial haemorrhage lies in the need for caution before ascribing it to any given head injury.

Traumatic Sub-arachnoid Haemorrhage

Sub-arachnoid haemorrhage, the result of trauma causing rupture of a vertebral artery, was reported by Contostavlos (1971), Cameron and Mant (1972), and Simonsen (1976). The injury was associated with fracture of the first or second cervical vertebra and especially fracture of the transverse process of the first cervical vertebra. A blow to the neck during a fight was the usual cause of the injury.

During the decade 1972–1981 the Department of Forensic Medicine, University of Leeds, examined the subjects of 12 cases of traumatic, or apparently traumatic, sub-arachnoid haemorrhage. Techniques suggested by Contostavlos and by Cameron and Mant were employed. Eleven of the subjects were males whose ages ranged between 16 and 65 years. With one exception, all of them were involved in a fight and five of the instances occurred in, or in the vicinity of, a public house. (Gee, 1982).

Two main groups were found. Six of the subjects had sustained an injury to the neck. Of these, three also had fracture of the cervical spine but this was absent in the other three. This group is represented by the male aged 65 who was involved in a fight in the car park of a public house. A few blows were exchanged and he then suddenly collapsed and died within 2 minutes. The only external mark of injury was a small bruise of the neck below the left ear. He had a massive basal sub-arachnoid haemorrhage. X-ray examination disclosed a fracture of the transverse process of the first cervical vertebra. An injection of barium into the corresponding vertebral artery showed a leak of barium at the site of the fracture. Subsequent dissection confirmed a rupture of the artery at that site. It is noteworthy that a visit to the scene of the fight resulted in observations which suggested that he could have sustained his injury by falling against the base of a car radio aerial (F.M. 20,524A).

The second group of six included one example of the well-recognised cause of basal sub-arachnoid haemorrhage, namely, rupture of an aneurysm of a branch of the Circle of Willis, in this case a massive aneurysm of the middle cerebral artery. There were two cases where extensive search for the cause of the haemorrhage failed to find it.

In three subjects the cause of sub-arachnoid haemorrhage was rupture of a vertebral artery at a point between its emergence inside the skull and its conjunction with its fellow to form the basilar artery. This occurrence is illustrated by the case of the only female in our series, a woman, aged 38, who was involved in a quarrel with her husband. He struck her once and she collapsed immediately and was found dead soon afterwards. The blow had struck her forehead; there was no external injury to her neck. She had a massive basal sub-arachnoid haemorrhage but there was no aneurysm, no apparent injury to the spine nor left side of her neck. Search of the remaining portions of the vertebral arteries found a longitudinal tear in the wall of the left vertebral artery shortly above the point at which it had been divided in order to remove the brain from the skull (F.M. 23,537). An exactly similar rupture was found in each of the other two cases. When a basal sub-arachnoid haemorrhage is present it is therefore advisable to examine the internal part of the vertebral artery *in situ* before severence to permit removal of the brain. Rupture in these circumstances may be due to a sudden torsion or jerk of the neck when avoiding a blow; there need not be actual contact causing injury. Crompton has studied the pathology of intra-cranial aneurysms. (Crompton, 1973). (Kranland 1981).

TRAUMATIC CEREBRAL HAEMORRHAGE AND BRUISING

Contre-Coup Haemorrhage: Bruising of the Brain

Originally these superficial haemorrhages were thought to be produced by a forward, backward or lateral thrust of the brain against the skull, because some occur in situations directly opposite to the point of impact of the agent. It is true that a blow to the occiput will bruise the frontal lobes and a blow to the side of the head will bruise the brain on the opposite side; these bruises, however, rarely occur at the occipital poles following a blow in the frontal region.

They are not produced by a shuttle-like movement of the brain, but, as Holbourn (1943, 1945) has adduced from experiment, they follow sudden rotation of the head which caused swirling movement of the brain inside the skull. Bruising then results from contact with irregularities in the floor of the skull or by impact against dural partitions. These haemorrhages, therefore, should, and in fact do, occur in relation to the sides or front of the brain in preference to the occipital poles, because the floor of the skull is irregular in its front half whereas the posterior half is almost smooth and the tentorium is the only significant projection.

Bruising of the brain may also occur directly beneath the point of impact, with or without coincident fracture of the skull, because there is local deformation at the moment of impact. When fracture occurs, especially a localised, depressed fracture, fragments of bone may be driven into the brain to cause bruising and laceration. Petechial haemorrhages, which may simulate bruising, can arise in boxing contests, and are the probable basis of the condition termed "punch drunk". Similar haemorrhages, but situated in the white matter rather than in the cortex, may be seen in fat embolism and after death from delayed coal gas poisoning.

The modern study of non-penetrating injuries of the head by Strich (1970) confirms much of the foregoing but calls for its amplification. Some of us have failed to appreciate that "although some lesions due to head injury can be seen with the naked-eye, many important ones can be seen only with the microscope".

Apart from sub-arachnoid haemorrhage, contusions continue to be probably the most common macroscopical findings. They present as streaks or groups of punctate haemorrhages, accompanied by variable amounts of necrosis, and wedge-shaped areas of necrosis without haemorrhage also occur (Strich, 1970).

Although bruising of the brain may occur under the site of impact, especially by a small fast-moving object, most are found elsewhere, namely, on the under-surfaces of the frontal and temporal lobes and the sides and tips of the latter. These "contre coup" bruises occur in the same regions of the brain no matter where the blow falls. They are often more extensive on the opposite side. They are rarely seen on the occipital lobes, the convexities of the hemispheres or the cerebellum. (These findings are in accord with our experience.) The distribution of the haemorrhages is more in accord with the rotational theory, based on the elegant experiments of Holbourn (1943, 1945) than the negative pressure theory, proposed by others.

These bruises heal in a few weeks, the necrotic material is removed and the defect is lined by scar tissue which may have a pale or golden yellow colour.

Tomlinson (1970) has suggested histological criteria for dating contusions. Ischaemic changes occur in neurons as from an hour after injury. Capillary proliferation is not apparent before 5 days but is vigorous at 10–12 days. Macrophages containing fat are only present in small numbers during the first 2 weeks. Astrocytic proliferation occurs at a few weeks. The ischaemic lesion is sharply demarcated at about 2 months. Haemosiderin appears within 10 days following subarachnoid haemorrhage.

Massive Traumatic Haemorrhage

These haemorrhages are unusual but when they occur they can, as depicted by Courville (1950), damage an appreciable tract of white matter. Distinction from spontaneous haemorrhage is imperative. The latter may cause a person to fall under a car in circumstances of pure accident, whereas death from traumatic haemorrhage, with other head injuries, may be the basis of a criminal charge. A charge of manslaughter had arisen out of a fracas in which a man aged 31 was punched and fell to the ground. Gee found a laceration of the scalp over the occiput, fracture of the base of the skull and severe injury to the brain. There was *contre-coup* bruising of the poles and under surfaces of the frontal and temporal lobes, and in the substance of the left frontal lobe there was a recent haemorrhage, occupying a ragged cavity, 2 in. in diameter. Bleeding extended through the grey matter into the subarachnoid space. Natural disease was excluded and the only explanation of this haemorrhage was a head injury (F.M. 8534).

The absence of laceration of the scalp and fracture of the skull, while not excluding a traumatic cause of the haemorrhage, favours its spontaneous origin. The site of the traumatic haemorrhage is usually away from the basal ganglia, e.g. in the frontal or temporal lobes; although this does not exclude a spontaneous haemorrhage, the site points to traumatic origin. Spontaneous haemorrhage is usually accompanied by signs of essential hypertension, e.g. hypertrophy of the heart, especially of the left ventricle and, sometimes, changes of hypertensive type in the kidneys. There are cases which must be interpreted by their own particular circumstances. Very rarely the traumatic haemorrhage may be lenticular and may be bilateral; it may then be possible to show that they are only an extension of a cortical traumatic haemorrhage.

Brain-stem Injuries

Traumatic pontine haemorrhages are to be distinguished from spontaneous haemorrhages in the manner already described in respect of massive cerebral haemorrhage. In my experience the traumatic haemorrhage may produce a clinical picture which resembles that of spontaneous haemorrhage, e.g. abrupt hyperpyrexia and "pin-point" pupils. The naked-eye appearances, however, may and usually do have distinct differences.The spontaneous haemorrhage is usually single, occupying from a third to a half of the substance of the pons. Traumatic haemorrhage, on the other hand, occurs in a number of separate foci in the pons. No doubt, if the victim survives for a sufficient time, these foci can coalesce to resemble a spontaneous haemorrhage. Both kinds can rupture into the fourth ventricle; in the traumatic haemorrhage this happens when one of the foci is situated close to it.

> In a series of nine cases of traumatic pontine haemorrhage, five followed falls and four were the result of road accidents. Age was not apparently important; the ages ranged from 37 to 72; seven were males and two were females. Some of the haemorrhages were "massive", but in five the record mentions the occurrence of several small, separate haemorrhages in the middle third of the pons.

The foregoing requires amplification in the light of the valuable article by Tomlinson (1970), which must be consulted in the original text.

It contains the important lesson that "severe lesions may be present in the brain-stem although it appears normal or nearly so to the naked-eye". Therefore the brain-stem of any victim of a head injury should invariably be retained for expert examination, even though it appears to be undamaged.

Primary haemorrhages in the brain-stem may be visible to the naked-eye but some require detection by microscopy. Tomlinson pointed out that failure to appreciate this had led to under-estimates of their incidence. Too few of these brain-stems had been subjected to microscopical examination.

These haemorrhages are usually small and Tomlinson detailed their distribution, i.e. especially in relation to the walls of the third and fourth ventricles and of the aqueduct. Haemorrhages in the rostral brain-stem are usually more numerous and severe than those into the medulla in rapidly fatal injuries.

Tomlinson did not suggest that haemorrhages into the brain-stem are responsible for death; "they merely indicate damage of a type and distribution which is incompatible with life".

Secondary brain-stem injuries are produced not only by injury but may follow any increase in supra-tentorial mass. There need not have been any primary brain-stem injury but if the patient survived the head injury for sufficient time to allow the development of a sub-dural or an extra-dural haemorrhage and this is not promptly treated by surgery, there is tentorial herniation and death from secondary brain-stem lesions (Tomlinson, 1970).

Brain-stem injuries are present in the majority of those who die after a period of prolonged unconsciousness but it must be appreciated that they may also occur in some cases of minor head injury associated with temporary unconsciousness. The distribution and type of injury are similar in both groups; the difference is one of severity (Tomlinson, 1970). An extensive survey of traumatic brain damage, including evidence of hypoxic cerebral damage was published by Adams *et al.* (1980).

Boxing Injuries

Although the range of injuries to which boxers are liable is wide, as shown by Jokl (1941), the head is, obviously, most frequently damaged. In a series of forty-three fatalities in the boxing ring, intra-cranial injury, notably sub-dural haemorrhage, figured as the outstanding cause, being present in sixteen of these victims. Fracture of the skull was unusual since, as Jokl says, it is difficult to fracture the skull with a gloved fist. A few of the victims sustained a pontine haemorrhage, known to some as the "boxer's haemorrhage"; three examples were described by Carr and Moody (1939), who also reviewed the literature. Haemorrhage into the brain-stem occurred when the boxers had had a severe beating and were "out on their feet". Since the musculature is at this time relaxed and muscle tone is decreased, the motion of the head is more pronounced. In consequence acute flexion and extension can readily occur and thus the brain-stem can be pinched over the tentorium. The circumstances are probably peculiar to boxing or fisticuffs.

The condition of "punch-drunk", (traumatic encephalopathy), known to boxers under the expressive terms of "slug happy", "slug nutty", or "goofy", to mention only a selection, has long been recognised. The first account was by Martland (1928). It affects those who have been in the ring for a number of years; the risk is provided for in America by a 1 per cent levy on all boxing gates and a home for "punch-drunk" fighters is maintained by this fund. Jokl found the term applied to many conditions. "Old boxers of low intelligence and others, showing abnormal traits, are very often, without any justification, placed in the above category."

Although the precise cause of this condition has yet to be determined, it is highly probable that repeated blows to the head produce small haemorrhages in the brain, especially in the corpus striatum and the thalamic region. These haemorrhages initiate a chain of pathological changes which lead to punch drunkenness. The chief symptom of its onset is deterioration in speed and coordination, seen more readily in the "scientific" boxer than in the crude fighter. Defects in the septum pellucidum were demonstrated by Spillane in 1962. Further details were given by Corsellis *et al.*, (1973).

The need for an inquiry was emphasised by the death of a young negro boxer after he had been injured in a fight on 24 March 1962. It was alleged he had received over twenty heavy blows when propped up, possibly unconscious, before the referee stopped the fight. He died on 3 April as a result of head injuries. Yet another boxer, in May 1962, collapsed after a knock-out and later had to have an emergency operation for brain injury. He also died. These dramatic cases are relatively few but those who suffer from chronic injury of the "punch-drunk" kind may be many.

The Boxing Bill introduced by Lady Summerskill in 1962 was refused a Second Reading (*The Times*, 11 May), but it led to the setting up of a Committee on Boxing by the Royal College of Physicians, whose report was published in November 1969. The findings of the Committee related to professional boxers licensed between 1929 and 1955.

It was found that the ill-effects of boxing were progressive. Slurred speech, slow and clumsy movement, unsteadiness of gait and tremors were the commonest features. Dementia was apparent in about half of the subjects examined and six gave a history of probable epilepsy. Defect of the septum pellucidum, first demonstrated by air encephalography by Spillane (1962) in four of five cases, was confirmed; it was present in 23 per cent, i.e. twenty-eight boxers. The R.C.P. Committee did not consider this in itself to be responsible for the clumsy picture of the "punch-drunk" but it was considered evidence of permanent damage to the brain, "almost certainly due to boxing", and it was present in a large proportion of "punch-drunk" boxers. Five boxers suffered from double vision and in four of them it caused a permanent tilting of the head to one side.

Since then control of professional boxing has been stricter and, therefore, conclusions as to risk of brain damage under present conditions could not be drawn.

The Committee concluded that the evidence suggested that severe acute injury to the brain was uncommon both in professional and amateur boxers. There was, however, a high mortality in young boxers following rare accidents which caused intra-cranial bleeding.

The Committee was satisfied that there is a danger of chronic brain damage due to boxing; few boxers in their survey were severely disabled by traumatic encephalopathy "but evidence was found of lesser degrees . . . of the same disorder in an alarmingly high proportion of older boxers who had pursued their careers for over ten years".

The Committee recommended "that all forms of competitive boxing should be supervised by organisations able to undertake responsibility for the medical welfare of the boxer and that continuing personal records of all boxers engaged in competitive boxing should be maintained". Careful professional and medical supervision had probably reduced, and would continue to reduce, the chances of traumatic encephalopathy in boxers. Even so, the hazards remain and prolonged exposure carries the risk of some degree of permanent injury to the brain. This view receives support from the finding by Oppenheimer (1968) of "clusters of microglial cells and retraction balls in the brain-stem and hemispheres of patients who were briefly unconscious and died of some other cause at a later date. It may be that there is complete clinical recovery from a single incident of this kind but it is not beyond possibility that repeated knock-out blows, or for that matter severe blows, to the head may, by producing many of these areas, produce permanent damage.

The full account of this survey by the Committee was published in 1969 as a monograph by A. H. Roberts.

Retinal Detachment in Boxers

Retinal detachment is another hazard of boxing. It is possible that one important bout was lost, several years ago, because the defeated man entered the ring when suffering from undetected retinal detachment. The myope is at special risk and, if severe, he should be prevented from boxing even when his disability is corrected by lenses.

A boxer was examined prior to a bout, when wearing contact lenses, and was passed as fit; the doctor was aware of the myopia and it was so bad that without the lenses the man would not be boxing. Following the bout he suffered a retinal detachment, which, despite operative treatment, left him with severely impaired vision. Liability was admitted; his claim for negligence on the part of the medical officer of the boxing club was eventually settled for £4600 (M.D.U., 1971).

Hypothalamic and Pituitary Injuries

The effects of injury on the hypothalamus and pituitary were studied by Triep (1970), who attempted to correlate the lesions with the clinical syndrome of post-traumatic hypothalamic deficiency. He also offered an explanation of the vulnerability of the supra-optic nucleus to injury.

One of the results of injury to the hypothalamic–pituitary axis is diabetes insipidus; it is a rare event likely to follow only severe injury but Triep pointed out that minor degrees of polyuria may be overlooked. Diabetes insipidus is unlikely to occur if the neurohypophysis is alone injured.

Other possible results of injury to the axis include anterior hypopituitarism and disturbance of body temperature (causing hypothermia), which is believed to be controlled by the hypothalamus. Triep had personally observed cases of head injury in which hypothermia and bradycardia were believed to be of hypothalamic origin. (Accounts of this complex subject should, of course, be read in the original texts.)

Unusual Complications of a Head Injury

(a) *Oxyntic cell necrosis.* A man aged 31 was struck on the head by a grab and rendered unconscious; bleeding occurred from the nose and left ear. He died, at the end of 44 hours, from a fracture of the base of the skull. The fracture line traversed the pituitary fossa and there was laceration of the brain in the region of the tuber cinereum. The lesion was accompanied by oxyntic cell necrosis. The appearances paralleled those observed experimentally by Dodds and Noble (1937). They produced severe gastric lesions in animals by the injection of posterior pituitary extracts, thereby causing a sudden cessation of gastric secretion. A stomach, preserved in the Gordon Museum, Guy's Hospital, shows notable blackening and congestion of the mucosa of the cardia and body; the pyloric region appears normal. There is a superficial resemblance to poisoning by a corrosive but the change is sharply restricted to the oxyntic cell mucosa (Simpson, 1940–1).

We had experience of a similar appearance in the stomach of a girl of 20 who died following massive head injury caused in a homicidal attack. She was maintained on a life support machine, after breathing failed, within 20 minutes of admission to hospital. Artificial support of the respiration and circulation was maintained for 2 days before she was pronounced clinically brain dead and the artificial supports were withdrawn (F.M. 23184A).

(b) *Internal hydrocephalus.* Four cases of head injury followed by chronic hydrocephalus were reported by Moritz and Wartman (1938). Each patient was believed healthy prior to the head injury. Signs and symptoms of hydrocephalus first developed in from 2 weeks to 8 years, thereafter progressing rapidly to death. A chronic leptomeningitis was demonstrated in the roof of the fourth ventricle. The presence of a haemosiderin line suggested that obstruction was the result of a sub-dural haematoma caused by a head injury.

Concussion

Concussion is described by Grinker and Bucy (1951) as "a transitory period of unconsciousness resulting from a blow on the head, unrelated to any injury to the brain which is apparent to the unaided eye". This condition lasts, as a rule, for less than 5 minutes and rarely for more than 10 minutes. In the latter event it must be assumed that injury to the brain has occurred. In any event, loss of consciousness following a head injury should never be dismissed lightly, because, even when of short duration, recovery may be only an interlude before the onset of symptoms and signs which indicate serious intra-cranial changes. These, notably extra and sub-dural haemorrhages, are not manifest until sufficient time has elapsed to allow the accumulation of blood within the skull to cause dangerous compression of the brain. Even when these serious complications do not occur it is clear that head injuries, which cause loss of consciousness, however brief, have significance. In his Abbott lecture, Sir Charles Symonds (1962) confirmed his earlier conclusions (Symonds, 1940) and marshalled the evidence which showed that concussion "depends upon diffuse injury to nerve cells and fibres sustained at the moment of the accident". Even when concussion is brief and there is complete recovery of cerebral function there is the possibility that "a small number of neurons may have perished, a number so small as to be negligible at the time, but leaving the brain more susceptible as a whole to the effects of further damage of the same kind". Concussion is not "a transient and completely reversible affair".

Small irreversible lesions, from which clinical recovery may be complete, are a possibility. Strich (1970) drew attention to "the clusters of microglial cells and retraction balls" found by Oppenheimer (1968) in the brain-stem and hemispheres of patients who were briefly unconscious after a head injury, recovered, and died of some other cause at a later date. One wonders if the boxer who experiences brief unconsciousness following a knockout blow, even at infrequent intervals during his career, can be without permanent damage by an accumulation of these irreversible but apparently harmless lesions.

Although the brain-stem is the common site, Strich believes the retrograde post-traumatic amnesia and confusion, prominent features of concussion, are due to a more widespread cerebral dysfunction.

This field of pathological investigation has not been studied. Strich suggested that search for clusters of microglial cells and retraction balls should be made when a patient dies within a few weeks of a minor head injury. These changes should also be sought for in the brains of boxers not only when their deaths are due to an accident in the ring but also when it occurs at the end of their career.

The cause of concussion is still undetermined. It must suffice here to recall the experiments of Denny-Brown and Russel (1941) which showed that the rate of change in the position of the head of the subject is an important factor. Unless the agent attains or exceeds a threshold speed of 28 feet per second, the blow is unlikely to be followed by concussion. The speed of the agent is of greater importance than its size or weight. It is thus possible for a small swift penetrating agent to cause unconsciousness whereas a larger, heavier one may not, e.g. a man remained conscious after half of the side of his head was removed by the blade of a propeller. When the momentum imparted to the head is sufficient, movement of the brain inside the skull occurs and in consequence, as shown by the experiments of Holbourn (1943, 1945), the brain may be bruised by contact with irregularities in the floor of the skull, or the dural partitions, notably the tentorium. The mid brain is not the least vulnerable part, although *contre-coup* haemorrhages in the cerebral cortex are a commoner result. Acceleration or deceleration of the brain may not be the only explanation. Scott (1940) agrees that concussion is most often seen when the head is accelerated but it occurs also when the head is fixed. In his view the degree of force applied to the head is the important factor. Walker *et al.* (1944) found concussion to be associated with intense excitation of the central nervous system and detected a "marked" electrical discharge at the moment the head of the animal under experiment sustained a blow. Direct observation and photographic record of the swirling movements of the brain following the application of blunt force to the heads of monkeys was achieved by replacing the cranial vault by a transparent, artificial calvarium (Pudenz and Shelden, 1946).

Post-contusional (Post-concussional) States

The condition of the victim when ambulant following a head injury may be that of the post-contusional state. This has appreciable medico-legal importance.

The victim may exhibit automatism. He may perform acts of which he is unconscious but which, to the onlooker, may seem entirely volitional acts. The victim may fall from a horse, but, after a brief period of unconsciousness, may remount and continue his journey; during this period he may converse in an apparently normal manner. Later, however, he may be found either unconscious or dead. This is the so-called "latent period" of intra-cranial haemorrhage. It is possible that during this period he may commit some act of violence or other criminal act. Automatism leading to criminal acts is more likely to be seen following an epileptiform convulsion.

The victim of a head injury may, during the lucid interval, relate the circumstances of his accident in a manner which seems to indicate clear and precise recollection. These statements should be accepted with caution, since it may be that, when he becomes fully conscious, he has no genuine recollection of the events. Russell (1935) drew attention to the possibility that entirely false accusations may be made during this post-contusional state.

Amnesia, when prolonged after a head injury, is believed by McConnell (1944) to be a warning that there may be intra-cranial haemorrhage. One patient, whose only symptom during 9 weeks following a head injury was amnesia, was found at operation to have a large sub-dural haemorrhage.

The term post-contusional state is more usually, and perhaps more properly, confined to chronic symptoms and signs to be found in some of those who have recovered from the acute effects of a head injury. The condition can give rise to considerable difficulty if the patient is first seen at this stage. Details will be found in the account by Symonds (1941–2); only some of its features are now mentioned. Headache and dizziness are common symptoms. It may be, however, that when there is no complaint of headache, it was present during the amnesic phase. There may be vertigo; it is not a true vertigo, but "a transient disturbance of balance and often of the visual sense, experienced on stooping, or rather on rising from the stooping posture. . . . It is a common constituent of the post-traumatic syndrome." The patients may also experience sudden, transient attacks of dizziness often described by them as a "black-out". "Consciousness is often momentarily disturbed and may be lost. The main features of the attacks are syncopal rather than epileptic. Nevertheless, in some cases after repetition there is a transition into epilepsy."

Symonds found loss of sense of smell, usually bilateral, a common event, i.e. in sixty-two of his seventy-six patients; in his view failure to examine the sense of smell is a serious omission. There may be visual and auditory defects. A hemiparesis or lesser evidence of a pyramidal damage may persist. Impairment of memory, perception, and speedy, clear thinking also occurs.

This syndrome has special importance to the clinician who is required to assess the patient's disability, present and future, when there is a claim for damages or compensation following a head injury.

Secondary Ischaemic Brain Damage after Head Injury

It has been observed that many patients, who had sustained a head injury, developed a high intra-cranial pressure before death without having any focal expanding lesion. "The effect of this is ultimately to produce reduced perfusion of blood and the brain will then suffer hypoxic damage." This led Jennett (1970) to explore the aspects of the relationship between intra-cranial pressure and cerebral blood flow. His researches led him to the belief that episodes of inadequate cerebral perfusion may occur more frequently after head injury than he had suspected. He wanted neuropathologists to try to find any evidence of reduced perfusion and hypoxia in the brains of those dead of a head injury. It could be an important factor in causing secondary brain damage.

Mobility of the Victim after a Head Injury

Some remarkable instances of mobility after a head injury are recorded. Their explanation turns very largely upon the results of the experiments of Denny-Brown and Russell (1941), already mentioned. The occurrence of post-traumatic automatism must also be taken into account.

Opinion must be guarded when it is alleged that the victim of a head injury could not have accomplished this or that act, which he appeared to have performed. Mention has already been made of the man who sustained a grave head injury from the blow of the propeller of an aeroplane but did not lose consciousness. One or two more examples may be mentioned.

A man accidentally thrust the end of his umbrella through the roof of his mouth. He walked to a hospital and several hours elapsed before he died. An examination of his body then showed that the umbrella had penetrated the mid brain, in the region of the pons.

Following blows with an axe, which caused extensive comminution of the right side of his head, a man survived 10 days and was able to give details of the attack (Sydney Smith and Fiddes, 1955).

A man received a stab wound of the head. The weapon, which had a blade $4^1/_2$ in. long, penetrated deeply through a wound over the inner end of the right eyebrow. He was rational when admitted to hospital, where the blade was removed. A complete recovery followed at the end of 40 days. Examples have also been given earlier of nails driven several inches into the skull.

Recovery from traversing wounds of the head is reported from time to time. Dawson (1954) described the complete recovery of an infant aged 15 months who fell out of bed against the projecting rod of a toy. This rod, 20 cm long and 0.4 cm in diameter, penetrated the left parietal bone and traversed the head horizontally to emerge on the opposite side. There was no loss of consciousness and the child got up and walked about with the toy attached to its head. Except for slight relative weakness of the right arm, no abnormality was found in the central nervous system. The rod was withdrawn and the slight hemiparesis cleared within 48 hours. The child left hospital at the end of 14 days.

Another remarkable example was described by Louttit (1954). A young soldier attempted suicide by shooting himself through his mouth with a revolver. "After doing this, he was distressed to find he could still get up and walk round the room." The wound of entry was small and circular, in the hard palate; the exit wound was large and irregular in the left parietal region, 2 in. from the mid-line and 2 in. behind the coronal suture. The patient made an uninterrupted recovery without any mental defect or post-traumatic epilepsy.

Relatively long survival after a grave head injury is illustrated by the case. Whilst filing a steel bar, a man was being tormented by another man who, in spite of a warning to desist, kept on throwing pieces of potato.

The victim said, "If you don't give up, I will throw this [bar] at you", and shortly afterwards he threw it at his tormentor. The aim was poor and the bar, which was 18 in. long and $^1/_2$ in. in diameter, hit a boy aged 14, who was about 12 feet away. It entered the boy's forehead and traversed his skull. The boy fell to the ground and at once he became unconscious. The bar was removed and he was taken to hospital. The accident occurred at 11.30 a.m. on 7 May and he survived until 5.0 a.m. on 10 May 1947, i.e. nearly 3 days. The post-mortem, by Professor M. J. Stewart, demonstrated that the bar had entered the frontal bone on its right side and passed through the skull to emerge through the left parietal bone. There was extensive laceration of the right frontal and the left parietal lobes of the brain. The assailant was indicted for manslaughter and found not guilty (*R*. v. *Butterworth*, Leeds City Assizes, 15 July 1947).

In another case a smooth iron rod, $3^3/_4$ in. long and $1^1/_4$ in. in diameter, $13^1/_4$ lb in weight, was driven through a man's head when an accident occurred during blasting operations. The path was through the cheek upwards, with an exit at the junction of the parietal and frontal bones. There was much haemorrhage and escape of brain matter. Shortly afterwards the patient could speak and give an account of the accident. He was able to walk. After an illness lasting some weeks he recovered and suffered only the loss of an eye (*Amer. J. Med. Sci.*, 1850, **20**, 13; cited Lawford Knaggs, 1907).

NECK STRUCTURES

The majority of injuries of the neck, seen in forensic pathology practice, are described in other sections of the book (see "Incised Wounds" or "Cut-throat"; "Stab Wounds"; "Hanging"; "Strangulation"; "Firearm Injuries"). However, apart from these circumstances, other injuries sometimes occur to the neck structures, the causation of which is usually accidental.

Fractures of *the hyoid bone or thyroid cartilage* may occur due to falls. For example, an old lady was found lying dead on the floor of her living room, behind the front door, with a stepladder lying on top of her; an opened handbag with its contents scattered on the hearth rug aroused suspicion of foul-play. She had two superficial, linear abrasions, one on the head, the other on the front of the neck; the vertical distance between the injuries corresponded with the vertical distance between the edge of the treads of the ladder (F.M. 11,149ʙ). Another example is that of an elderly man who was crippled and walked with a walking frame. Pulmonary embolism from a thrombosed vein, while in the bathroom, caused him to collapse and die. He fell with his head across the lower bar of the walking frame. He had sustained fractures of both horns of the thyroid cartilage, but bleeding had occurred at the site of only one of the fractures.

Similar fractures may also occur as part of more extensive injuries sustained in motor-vehicle accidents (Nahum, 1969). They are likely to occur when the neck is in forcible contact with the handlebar of a cycle or the dashboard of a motor vehicle. They can occur in a fall against the side of a brick wall.

Subcutaneous ruptures of the trachea have been described on a few occasions (Polson and Hornback, 1960; Coetzee *et al.*, 1965) (see p. 474).

The mechanism appears to be a sharp impact on the front of the trachea when the glottis is closed causing a momentary rapid rise of pressure within the trachea.

Another consequence of blunt impacts or injuries to the neck is damage to the blood vessels, e.g. traumatic *thrombosis of the carotid artery* following compression of the neck; the actual cause of the thrombosis may be rupture of an atheromatous plaque caused by the trauma (Yamada *et al.*, 1967).

Open injuries to *the jugular veins* may cause air embolism if the wound is at a higher level than the heart, and hence it is always dangerous to attempt to make a person with a wound of the neck sit up. The air embolism may be delayed. Johnson (1971) described delayed air embolism from a stab-wound of the neck developing several hours later, apparently due to a valvular effect of tissues around the wound.

The basilar arteries are usually well protected by the transverse processes of the cervical vertebrae. Occasionally disease of the vertebrae may interfere with the vessels, e.g. thrombosis of the vertebral arteries, associated with rheumatoid arthritis. Recently there have been several descriptions of injuries to the side of the neck, especially kicks, being associated with dissecting aneurysms or rupture of the vertebral arteries, especially in the circuitous portion of their course, where they pass through the process of the 1st cervical vertebra (Contostavlos, 1971).

The cervical spine is especially liable to injury in road traffic accidents. The types of injury most often seen in Leeds have been fracture-dislocation of the first vertebra from the under-surface of the skull or fracture of the body of one of the vertebrae, usually C 5 or C 6. Sevitt (1968) reported on twenty cases of injury to the cervical spine from road accidents. There were six high cervical lesions (i.e. affecting the base of the skull, atlas or axis) and hyperextension injuries with splits of second to fourth intervertebral discs, and nine low cervical injuries, mainly hyperextension splits of the discs between C 5–C 6 and C 6–C 7. Numerous other observers have reported a peak incidence of fractures of the cervical spine in the region of C 4–C 6 and attribute the injury to whiplash movements of the neck with violent extension and flexion (Mason, 1962). Unless the injury is very gross, amounting to virtual decapitation, it is unusual, in our experience, to find macroscopic evidence of contusions of the spinal cord, though there is usually extra- or sub-dural bleeding in the spinal canal. (N.B. Artefact "fractures", due to rough handling of the body, can occur; usually these involve the intervertebral discs between C 4–C 5 and C 5–C 6 (Camps and Hunt, 1959).

Apart from injuries to *the spinal cord* associated with blunt impact or with multiple injuries in vehicular accidents, the cord may be damaged by penetrating wounds. These can be easily overlooked. Hendry and Stalker, (1967) described a fatal, penetrating injury of the upper cervical spine and brain-stem by a tail comb. In one case seen in this Department, a woman sustained 146 incised and shallow stab wounds inflicted with a fisherman's gutting knife by her attacker, while she struggled with him. The only fatal wound was a stab wound behind the left ear. Externally the wound appeared insignificant, but the agent had penetrated between the laminae of the first and second cervical vertebrae and had almost completely severed the spinal cord (F.M. 11,357A).

A knife used in a homicidal attack transfixed the spine and severed the spinal cord. It broke off and approximately 1 in. in length of the tip of the knife remained *in situ* embedded in the spine where it was disclosed at autopsy examination (F.M. 19475A).

THORAX

Heart

It is well established that a blow to the chest can cause grave damage; for instance, contusion of the heart (Hudson, 1965). These injuries are infrequent in forensic pathological practice. A consecutive series of 100 cases of multiple injuries seen in the Department at Leeds included only eighteen with injuries to the heart; of these four were contusions and fourteen lacerations.

These injuries to the heart were associated with other gross injuries, and we have not yet examined a subject whose death occurred several days after injury, from the delayed effects of cardiac damage. Such delayed effects have been described (Price, *et al.* 1968). For example, a child was run over by an automobile, and sustained a contusion of the heart and occlusion of the right coronary artery; death occurred 14 days after injury, from rupture of the post-traumatic myocardial infarct. The clinical features of non-penetrating trauma to the heart are described elsewhere by Golding *et al.* (1966) and Lasky *et al.* (1969). Moritz (1954) has described contusions of the myocardium from a blow on the front of the chest, e.g. by a steering-wheel boss in a motor-car accident. Demuth *et al.* (1967) describe the pathological features as similar to infarcts, but with more sharply demarcated margins.

Cardiac Contusion

The subject of cardiac contusion, with particular reference to litigation alleging failure to diagnose the condition, was reviewed by Menzies (1978); it may well be the subject of cross examination in relation to cardiac lesions found by the forensic pathologist. Menzies drew attention to the problems associated with the histological distinction between myocardial contusion and myocardial infarction. Such a distinction may be important in an autopsy following a road accident.

The cause of sudden death following immediately upon a blow to the chest, which may have caused cardiac contusion, can indeed be difficult to diagnose. A young man who had been involved in a street altercation and was thought by witnesses to have received only one blow to the front of his chest, collapsed and died immediately. No naked eye signs of injury were found at autopsy but histology revealed a tiny area of myocarditis effecting one bundle branch of the heart conducting tissue. This was deemed the cause of death. Froede, Lindsey and Steinbronn (1979) when reporting a sudden death from cardiac contusion referred to experiments with animals which had shown that a blunt impact on the chest may cause complete heart block and ventricular arrest or fibrillation. Viano and Artiman (1978) discuss the effect of thoracic trauma on the myocardial conducting tissue.

An additional problem may be to determine, years after an episode of cranial injury, whether a chronic myocardial lesion may be related to that injury, or is a distinct disease entity. Rajs *et al* (1976) describe the autopsy findings in four young males with cardiac lesions, dying at intervals from 1 year to 10 years after severe cranial injury. Each case showed cardiac hypertrophy with focal myocardial fibrosis and sclerosis of minor branches of the coronary arteries. It is suggested that general hypoxia, or a release of catecholamines at the time of the original injury may have caused the heart lesions.

Lacerations of the heart, in our experience, may occur in any of the chambers, but usually the ventricles, and almost invariably on the anterior or inferior surfaces. Moritz illustrates lacerations of the anterior surfaces of both ventricles, and of the inter-ventricular septum, but he had only experience of laceration of the left ventricle. We have found injuries equally frequent in the left or right ventricles. Bloch and Meir (1977) reported a case of an isolated tear of the intraventricular septum.

The sites of damage in the auricles are most often close to the attachments of the large veins. It is theoretically possible for the heart to be lacerated by the jagged ends of broken ribs, but we only rarely see clear examples of such injuries (once in a series of 100 deaths from multiple injuries); broken ribs more often injure the lungs.

Mason (1962) rarely found laceration of the heart by broken ribs in aviation accidents notwithstanding the frequency of broken ribs in such cases.

Fatal stab wounds of the heart by external agents are relatively common.

Stab wounds of the right ventricle are more likely to prove rapidly fatal than are those of the left ventricle, presumably because the pull of muscle in the wall of the left chamber tends to close the wound track during contraction of the heart, but, in our experience, the right ventricle is more often injured possibly because it forms a greater part of the anterior surface of the heart. Such wounds are often L-shaped or even have a Z-shaped outline, presumably due to pulsation of the heart while the blade is entering and lies within the wall of the chamber.

Transfixion of the heart may occur, but is uncommon. The cause of death from the stab-wound may be transection of a coronary artery, leading to haemopericardium. The amount of blood in the pericardial sac is often less in amount than that seen in haemopericardium due to rupture of a cardiac infarct, but this may be a misleading distinction; blood will have escaped through the accompanying stab-wound in the pericardial sac (Yào et al., 1967).

A stab-wound of the heart is often only one of several, each causing haemorrhage, of differing degree, in different regions of the body; cardiac tamponade is then only one factor in the death.

Stab-wounds of the heart, though usually fatal, may be associated with unexpectedly long survival, as described by Ranasinghe (1957). A man stabbed in the heart was able to walk or run a hundred yards along a street, and into another thoroughfare, before collapsing at the kerb edge. He was dead when admitted to hospital (F.M. 15,591A).

Blunt impact on the heart may also cause damage to a coronary artery. It is generally held that coronary thrombosis occurring after an accident in which there has been a blunt impact on the chest is in most cases coincidental. According to the American Cardiological Association no causative relationship can be considered unless the symptoms occur within minutes of the impact. At autopsy it is difficult to demonstrate a connection between injury and coronary thrombosis, although the theoretical considerations make such a relationship possible, as an accident associated with shock is likely to be accompanied by a period of hypotension, during which thrombosis could begin, and moreover it is known that there is an increased tendency to thrombus formation, coupled with an increased fibrolytic activity, after trauma or surgery. Coronary thrombosis has been recorded in young persons, without previous coronary artery disease, who have sustained burns or other injuries. (For a full discussion of this aspect of coronary and other thrombosis, see the section on Coagulation, Thrombosis and Embolism, *J. Clin. Path.* (1970), 23 Suppl. Royal Coll. Path., **4**, 84–120, in the *Symposium of the Royal College of Pathologists on the Pathology of Trauma*).

Generalised injury to the body may be associated with lesions of the myocardium, even when there has been no direct impact to the chest. Head injuries resulting in death after a few days in a coma or injuries affecting respiration, with resulting hypoxia, may be associated with diffuse inflammatory changes in the heart muscle; these have been termed "traumatic myocarditis" (Pluekhahn and Cameron, 1968). Our own experience of this is as yet limited to the case of a man who sustained a fractured spine and quadraplegia and survived for several days. His injuries were caused by a man who attempted suicide by leaping from the roof of a hotel; he landed on the roof of the deceased's car, crushing it. The "suicide" sustained only minor injuries (F.M. 13,417).

Aorta

Although spontaneous rupture of an aneurysm of the aorta, due to disease, may occur at any part along its length, and is frequent in the ascending aorta, yet rupture due to trauma occurs almost constantly at one site, at the junction of the arch and descending parts of the thoracic aorta, approximately 1 in. distal to the origin of the left sub-clavian artery. It has been suggested that the reason for the predilection of injury for this site is that the vessel is tethered to the spine at this part and so is relatively immobile compared to the rest of its length; downward pull on the vessel, due to deceleration, causes rupture (Marshall, 1958; Sevitt, 1968). Often the vessel shows a complete, circumferential tear at this point, and there may be multiple incomplete tears in adjacent parts of the vessel wall.

Less commonly the vessel may rupture in the ascending part, just above the aortic valve; there is usually a horizontal tear which does not completely encircle the vessel. The mechanism in these cases is presumably direct trauma to the vessel wall or raised intravascular pressure associated with other injuries.

In our cases there were thirty-three instances of ruptured aorta in 100 deaths from multiple injuries; twenty-seven occurred at the junction of arch and descending aorta, and six involved the ascending aorta. Mason (1962) says that traumatic rupture has until recently been regarded as a relatively uncommon occurrence, but the incidence is rising with higher travel speeds. Mason's experience in aircraft accidents includes many lacerations of the aorta associated with fractures of the thoracic spine, but in our experience this is not a common feature of civilian automobile accidents; only one instance being seen in a series of 100 cases of multiple injuries.

Lungs

Accidental blows to the chest, especially in automobile accidents, commonly cause bruising of the lungs. Such bruising may be seen diffusely spread over the lung surface, but it is often most pronounced in band-like areas along the backs of the lungs, lying in the recesses of the chest on either side of the spine. In these areas the pleural surfaces of the lungs are deeply discoloured purple, and here there may be multiple, sub-pleural emphysematous blebs, some large and containing blood, but most small, glistening and air-filled.

Such areas of bruising are also often seen on the pleural surfaces of the interlobar fissures. Moritz (1954) says that the sub-pleural contusions are frequently to be found along the line of the ribs, but in our experience they are usually much more diffusely spread over the lung surface and do not have a pattern to suggest rib marking. Since in most vehicle accidents the primary impact is at the front of the chest, while the maximum distribution of bruising is at the back of the lungs, the injuries appear to be *contre-coup* in type, as suggested by Osborn (1943).

Major blows to the chest, in addition to bruising of the lung surface, produce damage of the tissue within the substance of the individual lobes. This may consist of small circumscribed areas of bleeding up to 1 cm, scattered throughout the tissue, or more uniform bleeding, spread diffusely through the lobe. If the impact is substantial there may be internal laceration of the tissue, either as multiple small areas of damage or there may be a large, irregular cavity, ramifying through the lung. Mason (1962) terms this type of lesion "traumatic cavitation". Sevitt (1968) describes central lung rupture as a "burst" injury, following violent compression of the thorax, possibly with the glottis closed. The parenchyma is then torn by air expressed forcibly from the alveoli. There may also be lacerations of the pleural surfaces and especially in the region of the hila, often with rupture of the bronchi.

Major blows to the chest often cause broken ribs and the sharp ends may be forced into the chest cavity and lacerate the underlying lung. Usually the injuries take the form of small penetrating wounds, but occasionally, in severe injuries, several ribs may penetrate the lung deeply and produce a large irregular wound which almost transects part of the lung. This kind of injury is uncommon in our experience, but Mason (1962) often found them in victims of aircraft crashes.

In addition to penetrating wounds caused by broken ends of ribs, the lungs may be penetrated by agents thrust at the chest wall, such as knives. The wounds are often small and, since the lung collapses, they may be difficult to find at autopsy. They are unlikely to prove fatal or be associated with much intrathoracic bleeding if only the peripheral part of the lung is damaged, but most often, especially in homicidal stabbings, the agent has penetrated deeply into the tissue and a major blood vessel, or even the main pulmonary artery has been pierced. For example a knife, having entered the back of the chest, transfixed the lung and entered the pulmonary artery, and the track of the blade within the artery could be traced by a long scratch on the inner surface of the posterior wall of the artery; the point had reached the pulmonary trunk.

Such injuries are not usually associated with a tension pneumothorax, probably because death occurs soon after the wounding.

Penetrating wounds by firearms may also be produced and shotgun injuries may show multiple holes on the pleural surfaces caused by individual shot; these may be associated with severe and rapidly fatal intra-pleural bleeding, although each of the shot wounds individually may be quite small. On other occasions if the contents of the shotgun cartridge pass through the body adjacent to, but not actually through the chest cavity, as when the discharge is through the neck, the lung may nevertheless show extensive bruising, due to the effects of blast waves radiating out laterally from the track of the missiles. Bruising is then confined to those parts of the lung which are close to the track, e.g. the apex; the parietal pleura in such cases will usually be found to be intact.

Similar changes have been described affecting the whole of the lungs in blast damage caused by detonation of high explosives, as in victims of air-raids in wartime, and also of persons in water, as when depth charges are detonated. Such injuries are seen in civilian practice, perhaps in mine disasters and major industrial explosions. They may be a feature of explosion of natural gas in the home. They are becoming more frequent following the increase in terrorist activities. The lesions described include widespread haemorrhage and traumatic emphysema.

In persons who survive injuries for a time, and are subjected to care in hospital, characteristic lesions may develop as a result of treatment. Thus, after severe head injuries, where the victim has been maintained for some time in a respirator, characteristic appearances of "respirator lung" develop; these are seen as areas of collapse and haemorrhage with the formation of hyaline membranes (Fattal and Wyatt, 1969). A form of haemorrhagic pneumonitis has also been described in patients with head injuries (Bronwell *et al.*, 1968).

More recently the changes produced in the lung by the condition of "shock" have been described by Corrin and Spencer (1981). The lungs are heavy, airless and bloody or watery. Histological examination demonstrates congested pulmonary capillaries and the alveoli are collapsed and oedematous. The capillaries contain an accumulation of leucocytes, clumps of platelets and often with micro-thrombi. There may also be hyaline membranes and, later, interstitial fibrosis.

OESOPHAGUS

Injuries of the oesophagus are comparatively uncommon; they rarely follow blows to the chest and penetrating injuries by knives or firearms are infrequent. The swallowing of sharp foreign bodies may lead to perforation.

An example of this was a woman aged 46 who was eating stew one evening with no ill effects, and who continued to work until the following noon. She was then suddenly attacked by severe pain in the chest and began to cough, which aggravated her pain and she was compelled to go to bed. When admitted to hospital, except for severe pain, there was no other abnormality and no physical sign was detected. Poultices were applied to her chest but they gave no relief. Seven days after the onset of her symptoms she had a moderate haematemesis and then suddenly collapsed and died within a few minutes.

Examination of the body showed that the stomach was distended by a blood clot weighing 1.5 kg, representing approximately 3 pints of blood. It had formed a cast of the distended stomach. There was a little fresh blood in the intestines. A diamond-shaped fragment of bone 2.5 × 1.5 cm in its axis with sharp points, being part of the cortex of a animal's long bone, had perforated the wall of the oesophagus at 12.5 cm below its origin. Half of the foreign body lay in the lumen of the oesophagus and was lodged in a wound 2 × 1 cm. The other half of the foreign body had passed forwards and its sharp tip had perforated the wall of the arch of the aorta where there was a small circular wound 5.3 mm in diameter. The trachea, which lay to the right, was undamaged (F.M. 5341).

This case resembled that of Spry (1868); that patient was a trooper in the Life Guards, who had a similar clinical history. A sharp spicule of bone had perforated the wall of the middle third of his oesophagus, and later, the ascending aorta. The immediate cause of death was massive haematemesis. (See also Tucker, 1932 and Simanovsky, 1890; death from perforation of the common carotid artery by a foreign body in the oesophagus.)

Others have died from infection of the mediastinum or pleura. Watson-Williams (1937) reported a case of "overlooked" foreign body in the oesophagus, complicated by retropharyngeal abscess and septicaemia. This was a boy aged 4 months who had had a brass tack 1 cm long forced into his throat. The boy was illegitimate and a congenital syphilitic. (An early report of "Battered Baby".)

A bride-to-be aged 22 swallowed a dagger-like bone splinter which several X-Rays examinations had failed to reveal. Death was due to a tear in the aorta. (Daily Telegraph: 1st Sept. 1981.)

Rupture of the oesophagus has been described as a spontaneous event but it is probable that the wall had been weakened by prior ulceration; ruptures, or perforations, occur in the lower third, in the area in which ante-mortem digestion occurs. These ruptures are usually longitudinal splits in the oesophageal wall, involving all layers. In the case reported by Harrison (1893) there was no apparent antecedent damage to the oesophagus but in the case of Adams (1878) there was scarring due to healing of peptic ulceration; similar scarring was seen in the stomach. Spontaneous rupture may also be due to sudden rise in intra-oesophageal pressure, as by vomiting, the Mallory–Weiss syndrome (Editorial, *Brit. Med. J.*, 1967).

Rupture ante-mortem has to be distinguished from post-mortem rupture, e.g. due to exposure to heat when the body has been partly consumed by fire in a burning building.

Ante-mortem digestion is an uncommon but well-recognised event. Its recognition at autopsy is easy, once it has been seen on a previous occasion. The brown, or even black, discoloration of the mucosa of the lower third of the oesophagus, sharply limited to the cardio-oesophageal junction, is most striking. There can be coincident, acute perforation, with escape of fluid and food into the pleura. It is normally a terminal event in patients debilitated by disease. It is recorded as a complication of injury or disease of the central nervous system (Wilson, 1959).

Only on rare occasions may ante-mortem digestion of the oesophagus give rise to suspicion as to the circumstances of the death. (It might be more accurate to describe the condition as "acute peptic ulceration" of the oesophagus.) This can cause fatal haemorrhage of abrupt onset.

Example

A man aged 67 was found collapsed in a public toilet. It was apparent that he had vomited a quantity of blood and he complained of epigastric pain. He was moribund when admitted to hospital and died 2 hours later. The post-mortem examination showed that there was a quantity of fresh blood within the intestines, from jejunum to colon; there was a little altered blood in the stomach and duodenum but this was without trace of any peptic ulceration. The mucosa of the lower third of the oesophagus had a deep brown colour, the lower limit of which was sharply limited to the cardio-oesophageal junction. Microscopical examination demonstrated acute peptic ulceration of the oesophagus (Polson, 1936).

Perforation of the oesophagus can also result from the passage of instruments. The passage of a stomach tube in poisoning by corrosives is an age old contra-indication (although the risk is then more to the stomach than the oesophagus). It is a hazard of the introduction of an oesophagoscope, especially in the presence of a carcinoma of the oesophagus. We have not seen an example, but we have seen perforation of the stomach by a gastroscope.

DIAPHRAGM

Rupture of the diaphragm may be the result of a blow to the chest or abdomen; it can be caused by firearm injury. The injury is not necessarily immediately fatal. On the contrary, death due to herniation of the abdominal contents into the chest may be delayed for months or even years. On many occasions the rupture is only one of many coincident injuries which cause immediate death.

Rupture of the diaphragm is relatively uncommon in road accidents but Mason (1962) observed these ruptures in 30 per cent of aircraft accidents; the ruptures were mostly on the left side, postero-lateral to the heart.

Epstein and Lempke (1965) found laceration of the diaphragm in about 4.5 per cent of deaths from multiple injuries; rupture of the left dome was 20 times more frequent than rupture of the right dome, presumably due to protection by the liver.

Example. Long delay in the ill-effects of injury to the diaphragm ("Traumatic diaphragmatic hernia")

A man aged 43 years was moribund when admitted to hospital in 1930, with symptoms of an acute abdomen, but he had vomited only once; he died a few hours later. At post-mortem examination it was at once apparent that parts of the stomach, small intestine and colon had herniated into the left side of the chest. There was a healed tear, 3 in. in diameter, in the left dome of the diaphragm. The herniation had been abrupt, without any premonitory warning of illness. It appeared that he had been injured 13 years previously when he had been shot in the right thigh on 4 November 1917, during war service. A fragment of shell was found in the lower lobe of his left lung and it had damaged the left dome of the diaphragm in the course of its journey from the right thigh to the left lung (Polson, 1930).

ABDOMEN

Liver

The liver is a bulky and friable organ and not surprisingly it is frequently injured in accidents involving blows to the lower chest and abdomen. In our experience laceration of the liver occurs in about 40 per cent of the cases of multiple injuries.

The lacerations are often shallow splits of the capsule, ramifying in a cobweb-like pattern across the surface of the organ, especially over the right lobe. Less often there may be a parallel series of lacerations, corresponding to the position of the lower ribs. Greater force may produce more extensive disruption of the organ and the lobe may be virtually pulped. Extensive infarction may be found in those who survive for some time (Foster and Chandler, 1967). Localised force applied to the midline of the body is liable to split the liver along the line of the fissure for the ligamentum teres, and the injuries may range from a shallow split, confined to the capsule at the apex of the fissure, to a deep laceration, almost separating right and left lobe of the liver, associated with gross bleeding into the peritoneal cavity. Occasionally one lobe of the liver may be detached and lie free in the peritoneal cavity. Such injuries seem to be more liable to occur in children, but this is possibly due to the fact that in road accidents young children are more liable to be run over than are adults, who are usually thrown clear and sustain injuries from impacts with the vehicle and the ground, walls, etc. Tank *et al.* (1968) consider that it is due to the less rigid thoracic cage. Kindling *et al.* (1969) describe lacerations along the line of the falciform ligament as being found characteristically in drivers and passengers in automobiles and stellate lacerations, or fractures in pedestrians. The former injuries are ascribed to upward or downward displacement of the liver while the latter are due to severe compression causing bursting of the organ (Kindling *et al.*, 1969).

The liver may be bruised, but bleeding due to injury is usually in localised areas (sub-capsular haematomas). This is of course a well-recognised complication of delivery; new born infants may have massive sub-capsular haematomas. In adults greater force than that necessary to cause sub-capsular haematomas sometimes causes extensive disruption of the tissue within the liver, usually in the centre of the right lobe, producing multiple interconnecting ramifying fissures, bordered by softened haemorrhagic liver tissue. Such internal damage may be quite extensive in amount, but with very little injury on the surface of the liver to suggest its presence (see p. 646). It may be compatible with prolonged survival, and result in the formation of bile collections within the tissues. The tissues around the central area of disruption, when the victim survives for some time, will show infarction, which may be quite extensive (Foster and Chandler, 1967).

Penetrating wounds of the liver, in civilian practice, are usually caused by knives, and most often the liver is only one of several organs injured by multiple thrusts with the agent. Bleeding from such wounds is usually limited. Complete transfixion of the organ may occur. Carey and Worman (1966) described extensive bleeding occurring along the track of penetrating wounds within the liver, with massive disruption of that lobe of the organ. Puncture of the liver by needles, when taking liver biopsies, has caused severe haemorrhage and even death, if liver disease was more extensive than was expected.

Example. A patient under treatment with Cavodil became jaundiced; liver biopsy was performed. The patient died within a few hours from massive intra-peritoneal bleeding. At autopsy there was widespread liver necrosis, apparently from the effects of the drug; the track of the liver biopsy was traced from the lateral surface, through the right lobe; the needle had transfixed a large hepatic vein situated in the floor of an unusually deep fissure on the under surface of the liver; so that the total length of the track was only approximately 2 in. (F.M. 7682A).

A survey of injuries to the liver and spleen occurring in fatal road accidents was published by Bowen (1970).

SPLEEN

The spleen is generally held to be the abdominal organ most vulnerable to blunt force, though we have found it less often injured than the liver, as did McCarroll *et al.* (1965).

In countries where disease of the spleen, notably malaria, renders it larger and more friable, the incidence of its injury may be even higher than elsewhere.

In our area in Yorkshire it was injured in about 23 per cent of cases of multiple injury. The organ may bear a single laceration of the capsule, most often on the lateral surface or running up to the hilum, or there may be multiple lacerations traversing its surface, and almost bisecting the organ. It is uncommon for the spleen to be completely detached from its hilum.

Moritz (1954) describes sub-capsular haematomas and traumatic cysts of the spleen, but such abnormalities are outside our experience.

It must be remembered that apart from severe abdominal injuries the spleen, if diseased, may rupture after minimal trauma, or apparently spontaneously in pregnancy, in infectious mononucleosis, malaria, leishmaniasis, etc. (Spingate and Adelson, 1966).

Delayed rupture of the spleen occurring days or weeks after the injury to the abdomen has been described (Wilson, 1946).

KIDNEY

In most authors' experience the kidneys are found at autopsy to be injured comparatively infrequently. In one series of 100 cases we found only nine examples. This relative immunity from injury is presumably because of their anatomical position; they are protected in their deep situation alongside the spine. They may, of course, be damaged by penetrating injuries, such as stab-wounds. Otherwise, the normal impacts which rupture the liver or spleen do not affect the kidneys, but in very heavy crushing of the abdomen, or in automobile running-over injuries, they may be lacerated.

It has been suggested (Eckert, 1959) that when a single abdominal organ is injured this indicates impact restricted to the location of that organ; for instance, rupture of a kidney, in the absence of other abdominal injury, indicates impact localised to the flank, or posterior abdominal region of that side; this finding, especially in pedestrian fatalities, may be valuable in reconstructing the victim's position at the time of impact.

Occasionally there is a single massive laceration, radiating from the hilum towards the lateral margins of the kidneys and sometimes bisecting the organ. More often damage consists of a series of parallel splits of the capsular surface, not penetrating deeply into the tissue, and apparently due to the force of compression passing across the kidney. Single impacts due to blows are more likely to damage the kidneys if directed to the loins, e.g. when a victim, lying on the ground, is kicked by an assailant.

Sometimes in fatal automobile accidents, autopsy reveals bleeding into the fat surrounding the pelvis of the kidney, although there is no sign of injury of the organ itself. Presumably this is due to rupture of small vessels which are relatively unsupported in the fatty tissue.

More severe crushing injury may cause partial or complete rupture of the renal artery. In such a case the intima or media of the vessel may rupture while the outermost layers of the adventitia remains almost intact, though surrounded by massive haemorrhage in the retroperitoneal space.

ADRENAL

The adrenal gland may be injured by the same force which damages the associated kidney, and may be lacerated or crushed. However, haemorrhage of the adrenals, or adrenal apoplexy may rarely be found associated with other injuries. Sevitt (1968) found central apoplexy of one or both adrenal glands in 20 per cent of a series of thirty patients showing severe closed injuries of the chest or abdomen. In his view crushing of the glands tears the medullary venules and this is responsible for the central haemorrhage.

Unilateral adrenal haemorrhage and necrosis has been noted after operations on the stomach (Fox, 1969).

PANCREAS

Although, like the kidneys, the deep-seated position of this organ protects it to some extent from injuries, it may be damaged both by penetrating wounds and by blunt trauma. Nevertheless, we have found it to be injured in only 1 per cent of our cases of multiple injuries.

Blunt force may cause contusion or laceration of the organ, and is usually due to a localised impact in the upper abdomen. In automobile accidents this is particularly likely to happen from impact of the victim against the edge of the steering wheel, and Wilson *et al.* (1967) describe a characteristic pattern of crushing of the head of the pancreas and the second part of the duodenum and tearing of the vessels, ducts and the mesentery attached to the liver, and transverse colon.

Similar impacts may occur in fights or brawls. A patient in a mental hospital, noted for his violent behaviour, became involved in a fracas with other patients. He was later found collapsed. Examination at that stage revealed a bruise, apparently in the shape of the heel of a shoe, in the skin of the epigastrium. Death occurred within a few hours, and at autopsy a large haematoma of the head of the pancreas compressing the bile duct was disclosed. Similar injuries are described in children (Adams *et al.*, 1966). The isolated injury apparently results from a direct blow, delivered to the upper abdomen which compresses the pancreas against the underlying rigid vertebral column, or injures it by a *contre-coup* force. An example of the cause of the injury is a fall against the handlebar of a bicycle. The seemingly trivial force of the blow which may result in pancreatic trauma in children is emphasised. A late result of haemorrhage into the gland and disruption of ducts is the formation of a pseudo-cyst.

STOMACH AND INTESTINES

The stomach is not often injured in automobile accidents. We found this five times in 100 cases of multiple injuries. Compression may result in partial rupture of the wall, with longitudinal mucosal tears on the inner surface, parallel to the lesser curvature. Similar injuries may be seen after the forcible vomiting, for instance in poisoning, and we have seen several examples associated with carbon monoxide poisoning.

More severe injury may cause laceration of the full thickness of the wall of the viscus, and rarely the stomach may be completely transected (Rooney and Pesek, 1968).

The stomach is frequently injured by stab-wounds of the abdomen.

The *duodenum* is liable to be damaged by blunt trauma of the same type which injures the pancreas, but its injury is also uncommon. We have found it to occur in automobile accidents and also in one "battered baby", where the father of a 2-year-old child lost his temper at its whining and struck it repeated blows in the abdomen. The child died a few hours after the operation to repair the ruptured bowel (F.M. 13,341A). Blunt injury may also cause bleeding into the wall of the bowel, an intra-mural haematoma, with the production of a dark red or black sausage-shaped mass, causing obstruction of the lumen (F.M. 14,910A).

According to Resnicoff and Morton (1969) the extent of the haematoma is usually from Ampulla of Vater to the jejunum, and is caused by oozing of blood from the vessels deep to the muscularis.

Morton and Jordon (1968) classify four categories of duodenal injury: (1) tearing wounds resulting from sudden deceleration and occurring when the organ changes from an intra-peritoneal to a retro-peritoneal location; (2) crushing wounds where the third or fourth portion is caught between the anterior abdominal wall and the vertebral column; (3) "blow-out" injuries in which the fluid-filled duodenum is compressed with its two ends effectively closed by the pylorus and the ligament of Treitz, and (4) penetrating injuries.

Ruptures or penetrating *wounds of the intestines* may also occur and we have found them in seven cases of a series of 100 deaths from multiple injuries. The transverse colon may be crushed against the front of the spine, or the small bowel bruised or ruptured, and the mesentery torn. According to Williams and Sergent (1963) the mechanism of rupture is a shearing force, causing compression, with tearing, between the abdominal wall and the spine. They did not find it related to intra-luminal pressure, fixed points of pressure or absence of air in the lumen, when conducting experiments on animals.

Ruptures of the bowel, with eversion of the margins, have also been described in blast injuries of the abdomen.

Intestinal ruptures followed the presentation of a jet of compressed air at several centimetres from the anus; in no case was the nozzle inserted into the anus. The circumstances were those of accident, jest or revenge. Of seventeen victims subjected to surgical treatment only seven were cured; ten of them died (Bonté, 1926).

BLADDER AND GENITALIA

Rupture of the *bladder* usually occurs in association with fracture of the pelvis. This was the case in seven of the eight cases of bruised or lacerated bladder seen by us in 100 cases of multiple injuries. In such cases death usually occurs rapidly from the associated injuries, but if life is prolonged extravasation of urine into the retroperitoneal tissues may be a serious complication.

The *genitalia*, in our experience, are very rarely injured, by blast and trauma producing multiple injuries, but lacerations of the penis or contusions of testicles may occur. Incised wounds may occur in homicidal attacks, or may be self-inflicted by the male in a bizarre effort at self-mutilation. On one occasion at the Department at Leeds a case of homicidal strangulation, and stabbing by a pitchfork, of one mental patient by another was associated with castration (see p. 133).

Injuries to the *female genitalia* are usually associated with rape or abortion, and are considered in those chapters. Self-mutilation of the female genitalia is extremely rare.

SKELETAL SYSTEM

In the practice of forensic pathology injuries to the skeletal system usually consist of fractures of the skull, caused in accidents or from homicidal violence, or of fractures of the spine and limbs, sustained in motor-vehicle accidents.

Injuries to the *spine* are especially liable to be found in the cervical spine (see p. 180). In the thoracic region they are liable to occur in the mid or lower thoracic spine. McCarroll *et al.* (1965) describe characteristic injuries in pedestrian victims of automobile accidents; namely, fracture of the thoracic vertebrae and of the posterior parts of the adjacent ribs, associated with gliding forward of the separated portion of the spine, transecting the spinal cord and aorta. They attribute this to a blow on the back with acute dorsiflexion of the spine. Similar features of hyperflexion chest injury are described by Sevitt (1968). We have seen hyperextension of the spine causing fatal injuries (see p. 180).

Other characteristic fractures are of *ribs*, either near the costo-chondral junctions or near the spine and of the sternum, near the junction of the manubrium and body. These injuries can also be produced by unskilled and even skilled external cardiac massage. In such cases if death has occurred there is usually little or no bleeding at the sites of fracture;

the anterior pericardial wall may exhibit a peculiar brownish slightly parchmented appearance.

Fractures of the *pelvis and femora* may occur in occupants of motor vehicles and in pedestrians. Fractures of one or both lower legs, involving both the tibia and fibula, at a height of about 8 10 in. above the soles of the feet, are characteristic, e.g. the "bumper-bar fractures". Eckert (1959) found such fractures in 53 per cent of his series of road traffic fatalities. Abrasions of the overlying skin may indicate the site of impact on the leg, i.e. at the front or back. Measurement of the levels of the various injuries of the limbs may be of great assistance in reconstructing the accident later. Following a "hit and run" car accident there was bruising at the back of the calf of one leg, and laceration and fracture of the thigh and abrasion on the loin of the victim, and their position corresponded closely at the heights of the bumper, upper edge of the headlamps, and wing-mirror of the suspect's car (F.M. 16,022A).

Recent reviews of injuries sustained in motor vehicles accidents include those by Mason (1981), Mant (1978), Cullen (1978) and Ashton and Mackay (1978).

Falls from Heights

Falls from heights are another source of multiple injuries. In a series of 49 victims of such falls examined in our Department, in falls from the same height as the victim's the only significant injuries were to the skull, brain and ribs. Damage to the abdominal organs, e.g., liver and spleen, were rare in falls of less than 70 ft. (21 m). Goonetileke (1980) published an extensive study of such injuries.

Injuries due to Explosions

Formerly we described these as rare but they are becoming commonplace, due to the incessant activities of terrorist groups. Although mainly restricted to "established" areas, the forensic pathologist elsewhere may be involved with the victims of an infrequent event in his area. But each incident, for example the "Dropping Well" hotel explosion in 1982, can involve a number of persons simultaneously and constitute a disaster. There are then the difficulties of the identification of the victims the reconstruction of the circumstances, and the cause of death to be resolved.

As yet, our experience of such disasters is limited but there was the occasion when a terrorist bomb exploded in the luggage compartment of a coach carrying soldiers and their families in 1974 along the M62 motor way. The bodies were taken from the scene to a large public mortuary, where each was subjected to a series of investigations. First, the body was photographed; next, the clothing and valuables were removed by the Coroner's officers. Prior to autopsy each body was submitted to X-Ray examination. The autopsy followed. By means of this orderly procedure it was possible to make an adequate examination of all of the eleven victims relatively rapidly and in the knowledge that no necessary investigation had been overlooked.

In this group of fatalities all had suffered superficial bruising and had multiple abrasions. There was singeing of the hair or superficial burns. Some had more severe injuries, e.g. lacerations or destruction of the head; these victims had been closer to the position of the bomb. Internally, all had bruising of the lungs, with bloody oedema fluid;

all had lacerations of the spleen. Liver and kidney laceration also occurred. Fractures were, in the main, restricted to the lower limbs.

Marshall, State Pathologist of Northern Ireland, has had a unique experience of injuries following bomb explosions. His reports (1976, 1978a, and 1978b) should be consulted in the original text.

Marshall described possible results: namely, complete disruption of the body: explosive injury, with mangling of part of the body, small discrete bruises, abrasions, punctures, dust tattooing; masonry injury due to collapse of buildings, damage by flying missiles, e.g. sheet metal or glass; burns; blast effects causing bleeding into the lungs and intestinal wall.

Nor is the recognition of all these awful injuries the sole problem of the pathologist. He is involved in the identification of the victims and the reconstruction of the circumstances of the explosion. Marshall also indicates the need to bear in mind the possibility of associated injuries and, in particular, the possible presence of bullet wounds.

References

ADAM, J. C. (1925) *Brit. Med. J.*, ii, 546.
ADAMS, J. T., ELEBUTE, E. A. and SCHWARTZ, S. J. (1966) *J. Trauma*, 6, 86.
ADAMS, J. HUME, GRAHAM, D. I., SCOTT, G., PARKER, L. S., and DOYLE, D. (1980) *J. Clin. Pathol.*, 33, 1132–45.
ADAMS, W. (1878) *Trans. Path. Soc., Lond.*, 29, 113.
ASHTON, S. J., and MACKAY, G. M. (1978) in *The Pathology of Violent Injury*. Ed. Mason, J. K. London. Ed. Arnold.
BAKER, A. B. (1938) *Arch. Path.*, 26, 535–59.
BAKKE, S. N. (1937) Abstr., *Med.-leg. Rev.,* 1, 317–18.
BLOCH, B., and MEIR, J. (1977) *Forensic Sci.*, 9, 81–85.
BONTÉ (1926) *Thèse de Paris*; abstr. Annls. *Méd.-lég.*, 1927, 7, 331
BOWEN, D. A. L. (1970) *J. Forens. Med.*, 17, 12.
BRANCH, A. (1945) *Canad. Med. Ass. J.*, 53, 584, also *Med.-leg. Rev.*, 1946, 14, 62. This case is re-reported anonymously in *Internat. Crim. Police Rev.*, 1951, p. 68.
BRONWELL, A. W., DALTON, M. L., NANNINI, L. and RUTLEDGE, R. (1968) *J. Trauma*, 8, 449.
CAMERON, J. M. and MANT, A. K. (1972) *Med. Sci. Law*, 12, 66.
CAMPS, F. E. and HUNT, A. C. (1959) *J. Forens. Med.*, 6, 116.
CAREY, L. C. and WORMAN, L. W. (1966) *J. Trauma*, 6, 48.
CARR, J. E. and MOODY, A. M. (1939) *Calif. West. Med.*, 51, 227–30.
CAVANAGH V. LONDON TRANSPORT EXECUTIVE (1956) *Lancet*, ii, 988. Reported by E. M. Wellwood.
COETZEE, T. and VAN NIEKERK, J. P. DE V. (1965) *J. Trauma*, 5, 458.
CONTOSTAVLOS, D. L. (1971) *J. Forens. Sci.*, 16, 40.
CORRIN, B., and SPENCER, H. (1981) in *Recent Advances in Histopathology. 11*. Ed. Anthony, P. P. and MacSween, R. N. M. Edinbrugh. Churchill-Livingstone.
CORSELLIS, J. A. N., BRUTON, C. J. and FREEMAN-BROWNE, D. (1973) *Psychol. Med.* 3, 270.
COURVILLE, C. B. (1950) *Pathology of the Central Nervous System*, 3rd ed. Mountain View, California: Pacific Press.
CROMPTON, M. R. (1973) *J. Roy. Coll. Phys.*, 7, 235–37.
CULLEN, S. A. (1978) in *The Pathology of Violent Injury*. Ed. Mason, J. K. London. Ed. Arnold.
DAWSON, B. H. (1954) *Lancet*, i, 1059–60.
DeMUTH, W. E., BAUE, A. E. and ODOM, J. A. (1967) *J. Trauma*, 7, 443.
DENNY-BROWN, D., and RUSSELL, W. R. (1941) *Brain*, 64, 93–164.
DODDS, E. C. and NOBLE, R. L. (1937) *Brit. Med. J.*, i, 629–30.
EASTWOOD, J. (1957) *Med.-leg. J.*, 25, 125–8.
ECKERT, W. G. (1959) *J. Forens. Sci.*, 4, 309.
EDITORIAL (1967) *Brit. Med. J.*, 2, 261.
EPSTEIN, L. I. and LEMPKE, R. E. (1965) *J. Trauma*, 8, 19.
FATTAL, G. A. and WYATT, J. P. (1969) *Pathology Annual*, Ed. Sommers, S. C., p. 43. London: Butterworths.
FOSTER, J. H. and CHANDLER, J. J. (1967) *J. Trauma*, 7, 3.
FOX, B. (1969) *J. Path.*, 97, 127.

FROEDE, R. C., LINDSEY, D. and STEINBRONN, K. (1979) *J. Forensic Sci.*, **24**, 752–6.
GARDNER, E. and SIMPSON, K. (1944) *Police J.*, **17**, 212–20.
GEE, D. J. (1982) Report of the 12th Congress of the International Academy of Forensic and Social Medicine Vienna. May 17–22; pp. 495–498.
GLAISTER, J. and RENTOUL, E. (1966). *Medical Jurisprudence and Toxicology*, 11th ed., pp. 299–30. Edinburgh: Livingstone.
GOLDING, D., BEHRER, M. R., ANTONIOU, C. A. and HARTMAN, A. F. (1966) *J. Pediat.* **68**, 677.
GOONETELEKE, U. K. D. A. (1980) *Med. Sci. Law*, **20**, 262–275.
GRINKER, R. R. and BUCY, P. C. (1951) *Neurology*, 4th ed. Illinois: Thomas.
GURDJIAN, E. S. (1975) *Impact Head Injury*. Springfield. Charles J. Thomas.
GURDJIAN, E. S. and WEBSTER, J. E. (1958) *Head Injuries*. London. Churchill.
HANCOCK, D. O., ALEXANDER, G. L., PHILLIPS, D. G., HULME, A. and THOMSON, J. L. G. (1959) *Lancet*, **ii**, 969–70.
HARRISON, C. E. (1893) *Lancet*, April 8; abstr. *J. Laryng. Rhin. Otol.*, **7**, 586.
HELPERN, M. (1946) *Ann. Int. Med.*, **24**, 666–700.
HENDRY, W. T. and STALKER, A. L. (1967) *Med. Sci. Law*, **7**, 213.
HOFFMAN, E. VON (1927) *Lehrbuch d. gerichtl. Med.*, 11th ed. A Haberda, Berlin: Urban and Schwarzenberg.
HOLBOURN, A. H. S. (1943) *Lancet*, **i**, 438–41.
HOLBOURN, A. H. S. (1945) *Brit. Med. Bull.*, **3**, 47.
HUDSON, R. E. B. (1965) *Cardiovascular Pathology*. London: Edward Arnold.
J. Clin. Path. (1970) **23**; *Suppl.* (*R. C. Path.*), **4**, 84–120. Symposium of the Royal College of Pathologists on the Pathology of Trauma.
JACKSON, H. (1961) *Med. Sci. Law*, **1**, 410.
JENNETT, W. B. (1970) *J. Clin. Path.*, **23**; *Suppl.* (*R. C. Path.*) **4**, 172.
JOHNSON, H. (1971) In paper read to the British Association in Forensic Medicine.
JOKL, E. (1941) *The Medical Aspect of Boxing*, Pretoria: Schaik.
KINDLING, P. H., WILSON, R. F. and WALT, A. J. (1969) *J. Trauma*, **9**, 17.
KNAGGS, R. L. (1907) *Lancet*, **i**, 1477–81.
KRAULAND, W. (1981) *Zeit. Rechtsmed.*, **87**, 1–18.
LASKY, I. I., NAHUM, A. M. and SIEGEL, A. W. (1969) *J. Forens. Sci.*, **14**, 13.
LENDRUM, A. C., FRASER, D. S., SLIDDERS, W. and HENDERSON, R. (1962) *J. Clin. Path.*, **15**, 401.
LITTLEJOHN, HARVEY (1925) *Forensic Medicine*, figs. 156, 157 and p. 238. London: Churchill.
LOUTTIT, R. T. S. (1954) *Lancet*, **i**, 1348.
McCARROLL, J. R., BRAUNSTEIN, P. W., WEINBERG, C. B., SEREMETIS, M. G. and COOPER, W. (1965) *J. Trauma*, **5**, 421.
McCONNELL, A. A. (1944) *Lancet*, **i**, 273–4.
McKISSOCK, W., TAYLOR, J. C., BLOOM, W. H. and TILL, K. (1960) *Lancet*, **ii**, 167–75.
MANT, A. K. (1972) *J. Forensic Sci. Soc.*, **12**, 567.
MANT, A. K. (1978) in *The Pathology of Violent Injury*. Ed. Mason, J. K. London. Ed. Arnold.
MARSHALL, T. K. (1958) *J. Clin. Path.*, **11**, 36.
MARSHALL, T. K. (1976) *Med. Sci. Law*, **16**, 235–239.
MARSHALL, T. K. (1978a) Leg. Med. Annual, p 37; Ed. Wecht, C. K. New York. Appleton-Century-Crofts.
MARSHALL, T. K. (1978b) in *The Pathology of Violent Injury*. Ed. Mason, J. K. London. Ed. Arnold.
MARTLAND, H. S. (1928) *J. Amer. Med. Ass.*, **91**, 1103.
MASON, J. K. (1962). *Aviation Accident Pathology*. London: Butterworths.
MASON, J. K. (1981) in *Recent Advances in Histopathology*. Ed. Anthony, P. P. and MacSWEEN, R. N. M. Edinburgh. Churchill-Livingstone.
MEDICAL DEFENCE UNION (1971) *Annual Report*. London: M.D.U.
MENZIES, R. C. (1978) *Med. Sci. Law*, **18**, 3–12.
MORITZ, A. R. (1954) *Pathology of Trauma*, 2nd ed., pp. 346–7. London: Henry Kimpton.
MORITZ, A. R. and WARTMAN, W. B. (1938) *Amer. J. Med. Sci.*, **195**, 65–70.
MORTON, J. R. and JORDAN, G. L. (1968) *J. Trauma*, **8**, 127.
NAHUM, A. M. (1969) *J. Trauma*, **9**, 112.
OPPENHEIMER, D. R. (1968) *J. Neurol. Neurosurg., Psychiat.*, **31**, 299.
OSBORN, G. R. (1943) *Lancet*, **ii**, 277.
PLUEKHAHN, V. D. and CAMERON, J. M. (1968) *Med. Sci. Law.* **8**, 177.
POLSON, C. J. (1930) *Brit. J. Surg.*, **18**, 170.
POLSON, C. J. (1936) *J. Path. Bact.*, **42**, 317.
POLSON, C. J. and HORNBACK, H. (1960) *Med.-leg. J.* (*Camb.*) **28**, 88.
PORTIGLIATTI-BARBOS, M (1952) *Minerva Medicolegale*, **72**, 79–81.
PRICE, A. C., VAN PRAAGH, R., SEARS, W. P. and NADAS, A. S. (1968) *J. Pediat.*, **72**, 656.
PUDENZ, R. H. and SHELDEN, C. H. (1946) *J. Neurosurg.*, **3**, 487–505.

R. v. LEY and SMITH (1947) *Notable British Trials*, ed. F. Tennyson Jesse. Edinburgh: Hodge.

R. v. SANGRET (1943) *Godalming "Wigwam" Murder*; see Simpson (1966).

RAHME, E. S. and GREEN, D. (1961) *J. Amer. Med. Ass.*, **176**, 424.

RAJS, J. and JAKOBSSON, S. (1976) *Forensic Sci.*, **8**, 13–31.

RANASINGHE, J. (1957) *J. Forens. Med.*, **4**, 128.

REIMANN, W. (1961) *Dtsch. Z. ges. gerichtl. Med.*, **51**, 601–8.

RENTOUL, E. (1954) Paper before Brit. Assoc. For. Med., Glasgow.

RESNICOFF, S. A. and MORTON, J. H. (1969) *J. Trauma*, **9**, 561.

ROBERTS, A. H. (1969) *Brain Damage in Boxers: A Study of the Prevalence of Traumatic Encephalopathy among ex-Professional Boxers*. London: Pitman Medical Scientific.

ROBERTSON, I. and GROVE, S. S. (1958) *J. Forensic Med.*, **5**, 78–83.

ROONEY, J. A. and PESEK, I. G. (1968) *J. Trauma*, **8**, 487.

ROWBOTHAM, T. F. (1949) *Acute Injuries of the Head*, 4th ed. Edinburgh: Livingstone (1964).

ROWBOTHAM, T. E., MACIVER, I. N., DICKSON, J. and BOUSFIELD, M. E. (1954) *Brit. Med. J.*, i, 726–30.

ROYAL COLLEGE OF PHYSICIANS, LONDON (1969) *Report on the Medical Aspects of Boxing*. London: R.C.P.

RUSSELL, W. R. (1935) *Lancet*, ii, 762–3.

SCHMIDT, G. (1979) *Forensic Sci. Internat.*, **13**, 103–110.

SCOTT, W. (1940) *Arch. Neurol. Psychiat.*, **43**, 270.

SEVITT, S. (1968) *Med. Sci. Law*, **8**, 271.

SIMANOVSKY, N. P. (1890) *Vratch.*, **38**, 868; abstr. *J. Laryng. Rhin.* (1890), **4**, 513.

SIMONSEN, J. (1976) *Med. Sci. Law*, **16**, 13–16.

SIMPSON, K. (1940–1) *Guy's Hosp. Rep.*, **90** (20; 4th series), 21–22.

SIMPSON, K. (1944) *Guy's Hosp. Rep.*, **93**, 67–73.

SIMPSON, K. (1969) *Forensic Medicine*, 6th ed., pp. 30–31. London: Edward Arnold.

SMITH, SIR SYDNEY and FIDDES, F. S. (1955) *Forensic Medicine*, 10th ed., p. 138, fig. 64, and p. 146. London: Churchill.

SPILLANE, J. D. (1962) *Brit. Med. J.*, **2**, 1205.

SPINGATE, L. S. and ADELSON, L. (1966) *Med. Sci. Law*, **6**, 215.

SPRY, F. (1868) *Trans. Path. Soc. Lond.*, **19**, 219.

STRANG, R. R. and TOVI, D. (1962) *Brit. Med. J.*, i, 845.

STRICH, S. J. (1970) *J. Clin. Path.*, **23**; *Suppl. (R. C. Path.)*, **4**, 166.

SYMONDS, C. (1940) *Injuries of the Skull, Brain and Spinal Cord*, ed. S. Brock, Baltimore.

SYMONDS, C. (1941–42) *Proc. Roy. Soc. Med.*, **35**, 601–7.

SYMONDS, C. SIR CHARLES (1962) *Lancet*, i, 1–5.

TANK, E. S., ERAKLIS, A. J. and GROSS, R. E. (1968) *J. Trauma*, **8**, 439.

THOMAS, J. C. S. (1944) *J. Ment. Sci.*, **90**, 588–91.

TOMLINSON, B. E. (1964) in Acute Injuries of the Head, ed. Rowbotham, Edinburgh: Livingstone.

TOMLINSON, B. E. (1970) *J. Clin. Path.*, **23**; *Suppl.*, *(R. C. Path.)*, **4**, 154.

TRIEP, C. S. (1970) *J. Clin. Path.*, **23**; *Suppl. (R. C. Path.)*, **4**, 178.

TROTTER, W. (1914) *Brit. J. Surg.*, **2**, 271–91.

TUCKER (1932) *Amm. Otol.-Rhin. Laryng.* **41**, 1228.

VIANO, D. C. and ARTIMAN, C. G. (1978) *J. Trauma*, **18**, 452–59.

WALKER, G. E., KOLLROSS, J. J. and CASE, T. J. (1944) *J. Neurosurg.*, **1**, 103–16.

WATSON-WILLIAMS, E. (1937). *J. Laryng. Otol.*, **52**, 179.

WERKGARTNER, A. (1935) *Arch. Kriminol.*, **97**, 1; abstr. *Med.-leg. Rev.* (1936) **4**, 242.

WILLIAMS, R. D. and SERGENT, F. T. (1963) *J. Trauma*, **3**, 288.

WILSON, G. E. (1946) *The Pathology of Traumatic Injury*. Edinburgh: Livingstone.

WILSON, G. E. (1959) *J. Forens. Sci.*, **4**, 431.

WILSON, R. F., TAGETT, J. P., PUCELIK, J. P. and WALT, A. J. (1967) *J. Trauma*, **7**, 643.

YAMADA, S., KINDT, G. W. and YOUMANS, J. R. (1967) *J. Trauma*, **7**, 333.

YAO, S. T., CAREY, J. S., SHOEMAKER, W. C., WEINBERG, M. and FREEARK, R. J. (1967) *J. Trauma*, **7**, 783.

(I am indebted to the late Dr. Edgar Rentoul for a photostat of the paper by Portigliatti-Barbos.)

CHAPTER 5

Firearms and Injuries Caused by Firearms

The Elements of Ballistics

An elementary knowledge of ballistics and firearms is essential to the proper understanding and interpretation of firearm injuries and, therefore, a brief account is given of the salient features of firearms and their ammunition. (Authoritative works on this subject include: Smith and Glaister (1939), Chapters 1 to 4; Piédelièvre and Desoille (1939); Burrard's *Identification of Firearms* (1956) and his comprehensive *Modern Shot Gun*, in 3 vols. (1960); also Price (1960) and Drake (1962a, b).)

Firearms are of one of two principal kinds, namely those which have a smooth bore and those which are rifled. Although these are the usual weapons which cause serious injuries, it must not be overlooked that an airgun or airpistol, often regarded as a safe weapon to give a boy, is capable of producing grave injury.

Even a toy pistol, which fires a paper cap containing a small charge of explosive, can cause injury to an eye, if pieces of the cap are blown into it at close range.

AIRGUNS

These smooth-bored weapons, available as pistols or rifles, discharge single leaden pellets of about 0.2 in. in diameter, or darts, which are propelled by compressed atmospheric air.

They were for long regarded as innocent weapons; the majority were "merely toys" (Anon., *Encyc. Brit.*, 1929) but ophthalmologists have long known that a pellet can destroy an eye. It is now realised that a pellet can kill although as yet fatalities are rare.

The Air Guns and Shot Guns, Etc., Act 1962, was repealed but its provisions, re-enacted in the Firearms Act, 1968, section 22, ss. (4) and (5), make it an offence for a person under the age of 14 to have with him an air weapon or ammunition for an air weapon. It is also an offence for a person under the age of 17 to have an air weapon with him in a public place, except when it is so covered that it cannot be fired. It could be that even wider restrictions are needed since these weapons are used in the furtherance of robbery. Indeed, they were used in 650 of 1670 firearm offences. It is small comfort to know that only 55 per cent of the airgun robberies succeed (Weatherhead and Robinson, 1970).

The lethal power of an air rifle is indicated by the case of Lester James (1962). This little girl was shot in the forehead at a range of about 2 ft, with a 0.177 B.S.A. air rifle. The pellet entered the skull and traversed the brain and was recovered at autopsy jn the right occipital lobe; the track of the missile resembled that of a 0.22 bullet. Cf. the case reported by Wolff and Laufer (1966).

A boy shot in the chest by a pellet fired by a high-powered air rifle was more fortunate but had to undergo major surgery. The missile traversed his right ventricle and the interventricular septum; after entry into the left ventricle it became an embolus. The pellet was recovered from the right brachial artery and cardiac tamponade was treated by pericardotomy; the boy recovered (Neerken and Clement, 1964). Another boy received fatal injury when a pellet entered his skull after traversing his eye.

We are indebted to Dr. G. R. F. Harriman for the details of the following case and permission to publish them.

Example: *Fatal Air Gun Injury*

Site: head. *Range*: near. Accident.

This boy, aged 8 years, was accidentally shot in the left temple at 3.30 p.m. on 12 December 1965. He cried a little and called his mother. Soon his lower jaw was fixed, and at 4 p.m. when seen in hospital he was unconscious but could be awakened quite easily. He had a convulsion and his pupils became dilated and fixed. Breathing ceased, but his life was sustained by artificial respiration. He was transferred to the Leeds General Infirmary and at 6 p.m. his skull was explored. There was no bleeding, neither extra-dural nor intra-dural, in the left temporal region. No clot was found on cannulation. The brain was distinctly swollen. He died next day at 5.40 p.m.

The entrance wound in the skull had been modified by surgical intervention; a left temporal craniectomy, 4 cm diameter, had been performed. There was no bleeding on the left side, but on the right side the vertex was covered by a thin film of glistening blood, of about 40 ml. There was an oval tear in the dura at the junction of the squamous temporal bone and the great wing of the sphenoid. No clot in the venous sinuses.

The cerebral convolutions were flattened and there was a distinct cerebellar pressure zone. No tentorial notching. The entrance hole of a pellet was present in the left middle temporal convolution. Sub-arachnoid blood clot was present in both Sylvian fissures and at the exit of the fourth ventricle.

The brain: an airgun pellet was found in the right pre-central cortex, 2 cm above the Sylvian fissure. The track, lined by blood-stained tissue, ran horizontally from the left middle temporal convolution through the hypothalamus immediately above the chiasma. Both optic tracts were damaged. There was bleeding into the ventricles. The pellet had emerged through the cortex of the right temporal lobe and had rebounded upwards and slightly inwards to the place where it was found.

No secondary brain-stem haemorrhage. No exit wound.

(Autopsy by Dr. D. F. G. Harriman. Ref. No. N.P.A. 185/65.)

SMOOTH BORE FIREARMS

The shotgun of the sportsman is the common example of a firearm with a smooth bore; it has an overall length of about 40 to 48 in. It is usually double-barrelled, when the interior of the right barrel is a true cylinder, but that of the left is narrowed or "choked" towards the muzzle.

Choke is introduced to keep the charge of shot in a compact group over a longer distance after discharge from the barrel and thus to increase the lethal range. Three grades of choke are used; narrowing by 3 to 5 thousandths of an inch is an "improved cylinder", narrowing by 15 to 20 thousandths represents "half choke" and "full choke" is a narrowing by from 35 to 40 thousandths of an inch.

The lethal range for game is normally in an area of 30 in. in diameter at from 30 to 40 yards according to the degree of choke.

The weapon is fitted with a *safety catch* which should be applied at all times when the weapon is not in actual use. This device locks the triggers and prevents accidental discharge.

A further safety precaution is to "break" or open the gun in order to see whether it is loaded before handling a strange weapon, or prior to cleaning one or making any other examination. On no account should the triggers be released unless the weapon is known to be empty or when it is in use during a shoot. It should be carried in such a manner that any accidental discharge cannot harm anyone, e.g. with the muzzle pointing to the ground or the sky. Mr. Pickwick, it will be recalled, was particular about this.

Bore. Shotguns are described by their bore or diameter of the barrel. The usual model for an adult is called a 12-bore gun. The size of the bore is determined by the size of the lead ball which will precisely fit the barrel, and by the number of such balls as can be made from one pound of lead. Thus the 12-bore gun is one whose diameter is that of a ball of lead of such a size that 12 may be made from a pound of lead. In more modern terms, the bore has a diameter of approximately 0.7 in. or 18 mm. Another common sporting gun, the 0.410 in. shotgun, has a single barrel, about 40 in. long overall, of which the bore has a diameter of 0.410 in. or 11 mm.

Ammunition

The cartridge used in a shotgun is a cylinder of cardboard, mounted in a brass head into which a small detonator cap of copper, holding fulminate of mercury, is set. The lower part of the cylinder contains an explosive powder the composition of which differs with the make. The propellant may be smokeless or black. This is covered by a wad of felt, on either side of which is a disc of cardboard. The felt expands when the cartridge is fired and, by fitting closely in the barrel, it conserves the power of the exploding powder behind it. The felt may be waxed or greased to lubricate its passage through the gun. If the cartridge is a homemade one, its wad may be made of paper. On one occasion, the criminal was identified by his use of part of a page of a book for a wad; the rest of the page was found in a book at his house. The missiles, which are small pellets or shot of lead, or lead alloy, lie in the outer half of the cartridge and are held in place by a disc of cardboard or the case is closed by a crimped turnover. The shot are manufactured by moulding or dropping from a shot tower and are graduated in sizes of from one to ten for use according to the target. The usual kind, used to kill game, is the No. 5 for pheasants and No. 6 for partridges.

Balling or Welding of Shot

Balling of shotgun pellets results in the conversion of shot into a compact mass, which can travel for several feet in this form when the accompanying shot have spread fanwise. The result is a complex injury; in part the picture is that of a shotgun injury at distant range but one which includes a circular or oval wound, resembling that of a rifled weapon. It could lead to the fruitless search for two weapons, of different kind, when in fact a shotgun alone had been used.

It is possible for balling to be caused by faulty manufacture or deterioration of old ammunition, but this is rare. It can result from hand-loading of cartridges, if too much powder be used, if wads of incorrect kind are inserted or sealing pressure on the wads is too high. The most likely cause is deliberate interference with the cartridge with the intention to increase its lethal power. It appears that in certain areas it is the practice to remove the over-shot card and introduce a little molten paraffin wax. Alternatively, some of the pellets are replaced by a large ball bearing, which is held in place with wax.

This interference increases the lethal range to 20 yards or over (Mant, 1968).

A girl aged 14 was killed when shot in the back by a 0.410 shotgun, loaded with No. 5 shot, at a range of 50 ft. At this range the normal result would be superficial, multiple puncturing of the skin and subcutaneous tissues. Seventy of the 95–100 pellets had produced superficial punctures in an area of 20 × 15 in. Twenty of the shot, however, had balled and, entering as if a single missile, produced an entrance wound, almost circular, half an inch in diameter, just to the left of the second dorsal vertebra. The track was upwards and the shot severed the spinal cord at the level of the third dorsal vertebra. The exit wound, irregular and $^3/_4$ in. wide, was situated 2 in. above the left collar bone. The left common carotid artery was lacerated. It was at first thought that she had been shot with two kinds of firearm, namely a shotgun and a rifle (Mant, 1968).

Rifled Shotgun Slugs

The substitution of pellets by a single rifled missile of lead adds considerable power to the shotgun. It then has a shock effect equivalent to that of a rifle and is used in hunting deer and other game in the United States.

At near range the entrance wound is a clean-cut circle or oval, of about $^1/_2$ in. in diameter, bordered by fouling and stippling. The missile may disintegrate or it is flattened into a disc with a "daisy-head" surface.

Petty and Hauser (1968) describe the ammunition and the appearances in the bodies of two victims, who were shot with a 0.410 shotgun (Stevens Model 39A) loaded with Remington Express rifled slugs. The young girl, who called for help, had three wounds in her chest and her male companion had shot himself in the chest. Fragments of a slug and wads were found in his abdomen.

Rifled slug shooting was also described by Glanton and Morgan (1968).

RIFLED FIREARMS

Rifled firearms fall into two categories, those of low, e.g. 600 ft per second, or those of high velocity, e.g. 1200–3000 ft per second.

The revolver is the common example of a low-velocity weapon and the self-loading or "automatic" pistol or the service rifle are examples of high-velocity weapons. They are described by the maker's name and by the internal diameter of the barrel, i.e. their calibre. The range of calibre is from 0.2 in. to 0.455 or, rarely, 0.76 in. Each weapon bears a distinguishing number, peculiar to it.

Rifling refers to the manner in which the barrel is cut to produce spirally directed grooves and ridges or lands. Rifling is designed to impart stability to the bullet during its flight, by way of a gyroscopic effect. The several makers have different designs, so that there may be from four to seven lands and the spiral may twist to the right or to the left, according to the make; in the service rifle there are five lands which twist to the left.

The revolver, although longer than the automatic pistol, is only up to about 9 in. long, whereas some of the automatic pistols are sufficiently small to be concealed in the hand.

The revolver is recognised by the mechanism by which the ammunition is conveyed to the breech. The cartridges are fitted into holes in a metal drum and the mechanism operates so that each time the trigger is released the drum revolves a sufficient distance to bring another live cartridge into the breech. The drum normally holds six cartridges. The empty cartridge cases remain in the drum until it is emptied by hand.

The self-loading or automatic pistol carries its ammunition in a metal box or magazine fitted below the breech. A spring mechanism propels live cartridges into the empty breech. Spent cartridges are automatically ejected as part of the process of firing the weapon and the empty cases may be jerked several feet away from it. This is a point of practical importance since they may be left at the scene, either because the murderer has not had time to collect them or because they have escaped his search. Revolver cartridges, on the other hand, are likely to be taken away in the weapon.

Ammunition

Ammunition for rifled firearms has the same general construction. There is a metal cartridge case, in the base of which a small copper detonator cap is fitted. The missile is single and is propelled by a charge of powder, detonated by fulminate of mercury.

There is a wide range in the pattern and explosive charge of these cartridges but details concern only the expert. Certain features, however, require mention.

The cartridge case of a revolver is a metal cylinder with a base which projects as a flange; that of an automatic pistol is recognised by a shallow groove a little above the base, which does not project.

The missile may be of lead or lead alloy, as in revolver ammunition or that for the small bore rifle, i.e. 0.22 rifle. Automatic pistols and service rifles, on the other hand, usually fire missiles which have a central core of lead, covered by a sheet of hard copper alloy. Lead missiles usually flatten on impact and inflict lacerations as they traverse the tissues, whereas armoured missiles penetrate and leave a relatively clean track, providing they enter at right angles to the body surface. Since there is some degree of wobble, an armoured missile which strikes the surface side-on may produce severe lacerations of tissue and fragmentation of bone.

The powder used in revolver ammunition is usually black powder, a compound containing potassium nitrate 60–75 per cent, sulphur 10–20 per cent and carbon 2–8 per cent. Its explosion produces flame and an appreciable amount of smoke; powder grains are also expelled, unburnt.

Automatic ammunition usually contains a charge of "smokeless" powder which may include nitro-cellulose and/or nitro-glycerine. Flame and smoke are reduced but the products of the explosion include unburnt flakes or granules of the powder. Some of these have a distinctive colour and shape, e.g. orange or blue-black and they may be square or circular. They can be recovered from minute cuts in the skin.

Rifle ammunition is also smokeless but the longer barrel may retain particles of unburnt powder, especially if it be clean at the time of firing.

Blank rifle ammunition is also made for instructional purposes. These cartridges, of course, do not carry a missile and, instead, the end of the cartridge case is pinched together to retain the powder. It is not innocuous ammunition because it can cause injury at up to

10 yds. The wad is propelled with sufficient force to produce bruising and laceration within that range. At closer range, severe burns or the loss of an eye may occur, and at point blank range these cartridges can cause death. In one case the discharge of powder and wadding alone caused death by driving the wadding into the heart (*R* v. *Race*, 1840). Similarly, the discharge of blank ammunition into the mouth can kill. The foregoing relates to service weapons; blank ammunition for the 0.22 rifle is probably innocuous except at point blank range near an eye or in the mouth. The possibility of *tetanus* as a complication of injuries to the hand by blank ammunition must be borne in mind; a fatal case is recorded by Gonzales *et al.* (1954).

A grain of powder can yield from 200 to 300 ml of gas of which 50 per cent is CO. If all of this enters a chest or abdomen, and death is delayed for a few minutes, enough CO can be absorbed to yield a positive result with peripheral blood (see Case F.M. 10,847b, p. 220). The blood in the vicinity of the wound was saturated to 60 per cent; 20 per cent CO was found in peripheral blood. Blood from the wounded tissues should be tested for CO as a routine practice.

Explosive Bullets: (Leading article: Bernard Knight 1982)

American forensic journals have recently drawn attention to a new trend in gunshot wounds—the reappearance of exploding ammunition.[1-5] Explosive bullets present a considerable potential danger to both surgeon and pathologist—as well as causing frightful wounds in their victims.

The media seemed not to pick up the fact that in the assassination attempt last April on Ronald Reagan the president was shot with an exploding bullet which failed to detonate. Soon after the event the director of the Federal Bureau of Investigation laboratory disclosed that of the six bullets fired during the affray five were "Devastator" missiles, containing explosive material. The one that lodged in President Reagan's lung did not explode, but some of the lead azide from the charge spilled into the surrounding tissues and was removed during the surgical operation. Having learned that explosive ammunition was being used the surgeons, who later removed another bullet from the neck of a police officer hit during the incident, took special precautions to avoid detonating this second missile. Either bullet could have exploded during emergency surgery or might have been detonated if ultrasound or microwave techniques had been used for diagnosis.

Exploder ammunition is being used increasingly in the United States and is being manufactured both legitimately and covertly. The missiles used in the presidential shooting, Devastator bullets, are standard 0.22 long rifle ammunition modified by drilling out the bullet tips and inserting a tiny canister containing a lead azide charge.

These "advances" in the design of ammunition are claimed to allow law-enforcement personnel to reduce the risks both to themselves and to bystanders.[1] The aim is to transfer the kinetic energy of the bullet to the tissues of the target more quickly, so giving the missile greater stopping power and also reducing the risk to other persons from the exit of the bullet or a ricochet. This may be achieved by filling a hollow bullet with tiny lead shot beneath a plastic stopper; or using an exploding bullet, such as the Devastator. These modifications rapidly expand the size of the missile on detonation, so decelerating it faster and greatly increasing the energy transfer. The bullet may mushroom or fragment and destruction of tissue is likely to be increased.

The exploding bullet comes in various forms, but the common type has a tiny cylinder inserted into the tip of the bullet, commonly covered with a spot of yellow or red paint. The cylinder contains either black powder or a detonant such as lead azide. The cavity may contain a single lead shot and possibly a percussion cap and a tiny primer anvil. All these elements may be found on diagnostic radiography, at surgical exposure, or at necropsy. A suspicion that exploding ammunition may have been used should be aroused by finding a wound that is larger than usual, but Tate *et al* dispute any effect on the wound track.[2] Far greater fragmentation of the missile, as seen on radiography or visually, is also strongly suggestive—especially if a relatively low velocity weapon has been used. These effects occur only if the missile does explode, and in view of the apparently substantial failure rate the surgeon and pathologist need to be cautious. Their fingers and eyes are vulnerable to detonations of explosive missiles, during both handling the tissues and examining the missiles outside the body. In suspected cases they should wear goggles and use long-handled instruments to manipulate the missile during surgical operation or necropsy. Once removed, the bullet should be handled with long rubber-covered forceps and kept in a padded container to protect it from excess impact, vibration, and heat. Microwave equipment must not be used since it may trigger detonation.

Exploding ammunition has a long pedigree. These missiles were developed in the early 19th century for the penetration of barriers and the ignition of powder magazines, the invention being credited to a Captain Norton in 1822. In 1862 the British Army manufactured the Metford shell-bullet, which used mercury fulminate as the detonant. In 1897 the British arsenal at Dumdum in India began manufacturing mechanically expanding bullets for use against tribesmen on the north-west frontier. The Hague Convention of 1899 forbade the use of all such missiles and they fell into disuse, but the Soviet Union is now manufacturing most of its automatic ammunition with a large airspace in the tip to aid fragmentation. All-in-all, doctors concerned with firearm wounds will need to be aware of this new development.

[1] Menzies R. C., Anderson L. E. The Glaser Safety Slug and the Velex/Velet Exploding Bullet. *J. Forensic Sci* 1980; **25**: 44–52.
[2] Tate L. G., DiMaio V. J. M., Davis J. H. Rebirth of exploding ammunition—a report of six human fatalities. *J. Forensic Sci* 1981; **26**: 636–4.
[3] Eckert W. G. Exploding bullets, a hazard to the victim, physician, and investigator. *American Journal of Forensic Medicine and Pathology* 1981; **2**: 103–4.
[4] Amatuzio J. C., Coe J. I. Homicide by exploder ammunition. *American Journal of Forensic Medicine and Pathology* 1981; **2**: 111–3.
[5] Clark M. A., Smith T. D., Fisher R. S. Russian roulette with an exploding bullet. *American Journal of Forensic Medicine and Pathology* 1981; **2**: 167–9.

Unusual Firearms

INJURY BY "HUMANE KILLERS"

There are a few records of suicide by shooting with a "humane killer", normally used either in abattoirs for the slaughter of animals or by veterinary surgeons in the field, e.g. when it is necessary to shoot an injured horse. Fritz (1942), Simon (1958), Rossano *et al.* (1963) and Wolff and Laufer (1965) have recorded cases, and two more were seen by Hunt and Kon (1962), who have drawn attention to the pattern of these injuries. This is of practical importance because, when present, the pattern is distinctive and a crucial piece of evidence in distinguishing suicide from apparent murder.

There have been three of these suicides in Leeds. The first victim, a man aged 53, a slaughterer, survived for 6 hours after firing the weapon against his right temple (Leeds City Coroner, No. 539/31). The other two cases are recorded below.

Hunt and Kon (1962) give details and depict the several kinds of humane killer in use. They are one of two types: some fire a captive bolt and others, slaughtering guns, fire a free bullet, 0.310 in., of lead. Only one of these instruments resembles an orthodox pistol, the Webley 0.32 in. humane killer, and it is used by veterinary surgeons in the field. The captive bolt instruments are of two kinds, one pistol-like, and the other a metal tube with a bell-like muzzle. The captive bolt penetrates the head for a distance of 4 to 5 cm; the free bullet weapons have sufficient power to cause the bullet to pass through the head, as in one of Hunt and Kon's cases. In the latter event, failure to recognise the pattern of injury at the entrance wound may raise the possibility of murder.

All of these weapons recoil appreciably and, in consequence, there is likely to be a patterned abrasion around the entrance hole, reproducing the pattern of the muzzle of the instrument. In the case of the Webley 0.32 in., this is also accompanied by extensive powder blackening and there may be burning of the margin of the entrance wound.

The nature of the captive bolt, and the "bell-killer" weapons, is such that the production of a head injury in man is likely only in circumstances of suicide. It is remotely possible that the Webley 0.32 in. pistol could be used by a homicide. Even with this weapon it is probable that "contact" range is necessary to kill; the others are lethal only at contact range and, if that is true, then there will probably be an imprint of the muzzle around the entrance wound. The victims, so far, have been persons who have had access to these weapons in the course of their occupation. The weapons are all subject to the firearms regulations, i.e. a firearms certificate is required for each.

The "captive bolt" weapon creates difficulty in recognition of its injuries because there is no singeing, fouling by Amorce nor tattooing; there is no missile. The appearances resemble penetration by a pointed agent, e.g. a pick-axe.

Fatal·Injury by Captive Bolt "Humane Killer"

A man aged 46 shot himself in the forehead with a humane killer at 10 a.m. on 22 October 1958. When seen by his doctor at 10.30 a.m. he was conscious, but when he reached the Neuro-Surgical Unit at 2.30 p.m. he was unconscious and was having fits every 2 minutes; these were controlled with pentothal.

The corneal reflexes were absent; light reflex sluggish; slight response to painful stimuli. Deep reflexes and plantar responses were absent. His fits involved the left more than the right side. A frontal fracture was present and some superficial fragments of bone were removed. There was then some improvement in his condition On 24 October his temperature rose and his pulse and respiration rates increased. He died at 5.45 p.m. on 25 October, i.e. survival by approximately $3\frac{1}{2}$ days.

Post-mortem: the entrance wound had been sutured; bruising had occurred in the vicinity and there was slight bruising of the inner canthi. The undersurface of the frontal scalp was bruised and showed a clean-cut hole, 1 cm in diameter, near the centre of the forehead. A circular fracture 1.1 cm in diameter, appearing to have been punched in the frontal bone, was situated immediately to the right of the middle line and 1 cm above the orbital ridge (Fig. 57). The inner table of the skull had suffered more extensive damage; an irregular, jagged portion had been displaced and broken into small pieces; some of the pieces were embedded in the dura mater. A fissured fracture line extended from the circular fracture into the posterior wall of the right frontal sinus, which contained fresh blood clot. There was an irregular tear in the dura mater immediately to the right of the anterior edge of the sagittal sinus, but the sinus was intact. A small sub-dural haemorrhage had produced

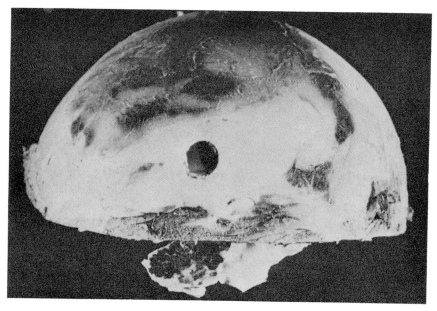

FIG. 57. Injury by "humane killer": captive bolt. Wound at centre of forehead: Suicide.
(By courtesy of Dr. Dennis Harriman.)

a shallow depression in the brain. A small area of bruising was found at the tip of the right frontal lobe, and there was a short, circular track, filled with blood clot, in the right frontal pole. There was notching of both unci, rather more of the right than the left. There was general flattening of the cerebral convolutions and an obvious cerebellar pressure cone. Terminal bronchopneumonia was also present (Leeds City Coroner, 1007/58; L.G.I. 782/58; N.P.A. 165/58; by courtesy of Dr. Dennis Harriman).

Fatal Injury by a "Free Bullet" Humane Killer.

Site: head. *Range:* contact. Self-inflicted. *Weapon:* 0.32 single-shot humane killer.

The deceased, a man aged 48, was found dead in his car. The entrance of a firearm injury was situated in the region of the right temple, 2 in. (5 cm) in front of his right ear. The wound was 0.3 in. (8 mm) in diameter and was surrounded by an area approximately 1½ in. (3.81 cm) in diameter, blackened by smoke and unburnt powder, distributed in a "butterfly" pattern. (This was later explained by the design of the gun, which had holes in the casing). Blood from the margin of the entrance wound contained 50 per cent carbon monoxide but there was no lead or nitrate present. There was an exit wound, stellate with everted margins, ½ in. in diameter, situated 2 in. above the left ear. Comminuted bone and brain tissue were seen in the floor of the wound but there was no blackening by smoke or unburnt powder.

The entrance fracture in the skull was a circular hole 0.32 in. in diameter; the exit fracture, also circular had outward bevelling. The bullet had passed through the brain to cause a track of damage, 2 in. in width, through the right frontal lobe and the left parietal lobe; the thalamus was also severely damaged.

The weapon found in the car was a 0.32 (7.65 mm) single-shot, free-bullet, humane cattle killer. A deformed bullet was found in the car and it was of soft lead and of the kind in an automatic cartridge used in these guns. The bullet had caused a dent in the roof of the car and had damaged the upholstery.

Reconstruction of the incident showed that the shot had been fired as he sat in the driving seat. It was self-inflicted; he had held the gun, at or close to his right temple. He had probably been looking directly ahead. There was no alcohol nor barbiturate in his blood. (F.M. 12,369A).

THE STUD GUN

The stud gun is an industrial tool operated on firearm principles and is used to drive studs into wood, concrete and metal. It is not classed as a firearm and no licence is required to obtain and use it.

Injuries with these tools are rare and, as yet, all have been accidental. Since the injuries have certain peculiarities Spitz and Wilhelm (1970) reported a fatality. The man sustained a head injury at a range of 3 in. He had a split, 3 in. long, with slightly everted margins, due to blow back in the skin of his forehead. It resembled the appearances of those of a contact injury by rifled firearm over hard bone. The stud traversed the head and there was an exit wound at the back of his head.

They were not aware of any intentional misuse of the tool. Its features are unsatisfactory for homicidal use but it could be used by the suicide, after the manner of a humane animal killer, and, if charged with a 0.22 bullet, it could be lethal. It appears the tool has been misused in this manner to open coin boxes in telephone booths.

GYROJET WEAPON

This lethal weapon, invented by Mainhardt and Biehl in 1960, introduces new problems in interpretation of firearm injuries.

The gun fires a miniature rocket which has a heat-resistant metal case and base plate; there are canted vents in the base plate to impart spin, to promote stability and to improve accuracy. The rocket is driven by solid fuel which, when burnt, produces considerable heat and a large volume of smokeless gas. The rocket will burn for upwards of four-tenths of a second, during which time it will have travelled for upwards of 500 yards. At less than this range the products of combustion, mainly nitrates and carbon monoxide, and unburnt fuel can contaminate a wound. Scorching of the tissues is also likely since the burning fuel attains a temperature of 500 F (250 C) or more.

In consequence, wounds by gyrojet rockets at a range of up to 500 yards may have the appearances of wounds by conventional weapons at close range, i.e. at inches.

Ballistic experts may also have difficulty in identifying the weapon because it has a smooth bore and the missile does not bear any of the characteristic marks normally imparted by rifled weapons. The sole mark is that made on the percussion sensitive primer at the base of the missile. Although available to the public in the United States in 1967, these weapons and ammunition are not yet available in this country. It is obvious that they require control by adequate restriction, even more rigid than that already applied to rifled firearms. They should be "prohibited weapons".

Identification of Firearms

This is an interesting branch of forensic science and one of considerable practical importance. The ballistic expert, given an empty cartridge case from the scene of a crime, or a missile from the body of a victim, can often prove the identity of the weapon used. Occasionally the weapon itself is left at the scene.

Identification of firearms rests upon the fact that they leave their signature upon the cartridges they fire. These marks are present on the cartridge case and, with rifled weapons, also on the missile. The signature of the shotgun is the least clear, whereas an automatic pistol, as will be seen, nearly always produces several distinctive and unequivocal marks.

The Weapon

(a) *Its number.* Each rifled firearm bears a number which is peculiar to it. A wrongdoer may erase the number and perhaps add a new one, a practice similar to that of motor car thieves who tamper with the engine numbers. Any weapon which does not bear a number is at once suspect and suitable treatment with acid of the area in which these numbers are usually stamped can reveal the number, apart from any other added over it.

(b) *Fingerprints.* Fingerprints on the weapon may be of paramount importance as a means of distinction between suicide and murder and in the identification of a murderer. It is imperative therefore that a weapon found at a scene is not handled carelessly. The unskilled or thoughtless can easily blur or erase the impressions and thus destroy valuable evidence. Even police officers do not always remember this and on one occasion the only clear impression was that of a detective officer engaged on the case (*R. v. Barney*, 1932).

(c) *Fouling of the barrel.* Chemical analysis of washings from the barrel may show that the weapon was recently fired.

(d) *Trigger pressure.* The pressure required to operate the trigger may be relevant when the question of accidental discharge arises (see p. 229). This pressure, often determined by a spring balance, should be determined by means of a dead weight. For the shotgun the trigger pressure is about 4 lb ($3^1/_2$–$4^1/_2$ lb); for a self-loading pistol, 3 to 4– lb; revolver, 3 to 5 lb and for a service rifle, 6 to 7 lb (Burrard, 1956).

The Missile

Surgical Removal and Preservation of the Missile

Surgical removal of a missile must be undertaken in a manner calculated to avoid interference with any marks on it. It should not be grasped with metal instruments in any way likely to obliterate or add marks; it should be protected by gauze during its extraction, whenever practicable. The surgeon, also, should personally supervise the safe deposit of the missile in a properly labelled and secured container. He should retain the specimen under his immediate control until it can be handed to a police officer. Its safe custody and freedom from interference is thus ensured. Similarly, any other parts of a cartridge, whether cards, felts or wads, in a wound must be carefully extracted and preserved.

Shotgun missiles. The pellets from a shotgun can be measured, weighed and subjected to chemical analysis, although the results have a relatively limited value.

Rifled weapon missiles. These are capable of similar examination. Valuable information is obtained by comparison of the missile from the scene of crime or the body of the victim with one fired from the suspected weapon. This is practicable with the comparison microscope. Each missile is mounted in a like position on a table under a microscope, a pair of which are so arranged that selected parts of each missile are simultaneously under examination, under like conditions of magnification and lighting. The instrument is also designed to permit rotation of the missiles to bring other areas into view. The object is to demonstrate similar marks in similar positions on each of the missiles. Photographic records are also made. The investigation is limited to the extent that it is of value only when precise agreement is demonstrated between the marks on the chance and test missiles.

When a number of missiles are fired from the same weapon, some may be unmarked and there may be an appreciable variation in the marking of others. It is not possible, therefore, to exclude a given weapon by the test, although, if the marks are consistently at variance with those on the chance missile, it is unlikely that it was fired by the weapon under test.

The missile will be marked, in the first place, by the rifling of the weapon, which cuts its pattern in the metal as the bullet traverses the barrel. The number of the grooves are shown and it is possible to determine their depth, width, pitch and direction. Secondary marks, produced by local defects in the barrel, although no more than scratches on the missile, may be important; they can, however, be produced by rust or fouling.

The diameter of the missile is important since it narrows the range of weapons for examination; the calibre is from 0.22 to 0.48 in. Some of the missiles are made to a standard weight and, when flattened or distorted to prevent other examination, the weight may suggest the kind of weapon used. A missile which weighs 125 grains probably fitted a weapon of 0.36 bore, whereas one of 265 grains was fired from one of 0.455 bore. This is only a general observation. When Sharpe and Lannen killed their victim in 1949, the cartridge was of a 0.310 (cattle killing) bullet fired from a 0.38 revolver (Case no. 39, p. 257).

The chemical composition may be of some assistance since an alloy of lead and arsenic or of lead and antimony is used only in certain makes of cartridge.

It is suggested, particularly by French authors, that examination of the nose of the missile may reveal a pattern when there has been contact with cloth. Silk, linen or cotton cloths produce a characteristic marking on lead missiles. Details, with illustrations, are given by Piédelièvre and Desoille (1939) in their monograph on firearm injuries.

The Cartridge Case

The weapon may make several marks on the cartridge case and these permit identification of the weapon. The more complex its mechanism, the more marks are likely to appear on the cartridge case; automatic ammunition is thus of special importance. The cartridge case is usually of greater value than the missile in these investigations. Any cartridge case at the scene, therefore, must be carefully preserved and a thorough search must be made for spent ammunition.

The empty cartridge case of an *automatic* or *self-loading pistol* may bear one or more of four distinctive marks, at different points on its surface. The firing pin dents the detonator cap in a fashion peculiar to the weapon; the marks may be central or eccentric in position. The extractor bar or hook may make a characteristic depression on the rim and its position and depth must be noted. Marks are also made by the breech block when the cartridge recoils against it. Scratches on the sides may be made by the walls of the magazine as the cartridge is pushed up into the firing chamber.

The comparison microscope will show how far the chance and test cartridge cases agree in their markings.

Revolvers and shotguns also mark their cartridge cases but in less complicated fashion. The shotgun, for example, may only dent the detonator cap by a blow with the firing pin.

Weapons which still contain ammunition, whether live or spent, should not be "broken" and opened except by the expert. In the case of revolvers it may be most important to note the sequence in which the cartridges are placed in the drum. If the gun is "broken" and the drum emptied carelessly this cannot then be determined.

Test firing. When the weapon believed to have been used is available, it is loaded with appropriate ammunition. The weapon is mounted in an apparatus which collects the missiles when fired into a box packed with wool or rag, backed by sand. This minimises distortion of the missile and simplifies its collection. Six rounds are usually fired and the weapon is cleaned. The test is then repeated as may be necessary. The missiles and cartridge cases are collected and examined as already described. The patterns at predetermined ranges are described and depicted by Drake (1962a, b).

HANDLING OF WEAPONS

It seems necessary for all who are concerned with firearm injuries to be reminded from time to time of certain simple rules:

Do not handle weapons at the scene until they have been subjected to examination by fingerprint and ballistic experts.

When a weapon is handled, the first step, on all occasions, is to "break" it in order to see if it is loaded. Failure to do this can have grave consequences.

Never point the weapon at anyone. Failure to observe this rule, no doubt, is likely only by children. A boy aged 16 was shot by his friend, who picked up a shotgun in the house, pointed it at the boy and pretended to shoot him; he pressed the trigger; the gun was loaded. The boy's lower jaw was shot away and he died a few days later from gas gangrene (Leeds City Coroner: 855/31).

Never leave loaded, nor for that matter unloaded, weapons in places where they are accessible to unauthorised persons. The gun of a farmer or a sportsman is not rarely left, loaded, in the kitchen or outhouse. Shotguns should be unloaded immediately after use and kept in a safe place, preferably under lock and key.

Firearm Injuries

Introduction

The majority of firearm injuries, by reason of their characteristic features, are readily recognised even by the inexperienced. It is a rare event for injury by a pointed stick, pick or red hot poker to produce injuries which resemble bullet wounds. It is unusual for a firearm, unless a "humane killer" with a fixed bolt, to produce injuries which resemble those produced by an ice pick or similar agent.

Although a circular hole or a stellate wound is the characteristic appearance of firearm injuries, the literature contains reports of some strange effects of firearm injury. Smith and Glaister (1939) depict a linear wound traversing the outer ear diagonally. Although produced by a bullet, it resembled an incised wound. It was a glancing wound. Close examination revealed grooving and loss of tissue with bruising of the margins. They also depict a chest wound which simulated a stab wound but radiological examination demonstrated a bullet in the chest.

The investigation, however, only begins with the recognition that the injury was caused by a firearm. It is necessary to ascertain the circumstances in which the injury was sustained, i.e. whether by accident or design and, if by design, whether self-inflicted or otherwise.

This investigation involves, in particular, the determination of the range of fire, and the direction of aim. These are matters which can only be ascertained satisfactorily by the combined efforts of medical and scientific experts. The inexperienced can readily reach erroneous conclusions which, even if they do not lead to a miscarriage of justice, may result in unwarranted suspicion of innocent persons. For example, failure to recognise a "contact" injury of an elbow and concentration on concomitant chest injuries led to the belief that the victim had been shot at a range well beyond that of self-infliction. This erroneous conclusion was reinforced by amateur tests with the gun at predetermined ranges. The true story of the deceased boy's companion was discredited and the possibility of homicide was canvassed. (Case No. 22, p. 238, fig. 22).

Some of the factors which have to be taken into account when reconstructing these incidents and interpreting them are now summarised. It is not intended to be a complete survey, because however long one continues in practice, additional possibilities are encountered.

Interference with the scene and, in particular, with the weapon, when present, is well recognised as something to avoid until the team of experts have completed their investigations. Members of the public may not always realise this but interference is not restricted to them.

When a woman is found dead of a firearm injury it is reasonable to consider homicide in the first instance. Occasionally, however, the injury may have been self-inflicted. On one occasion it is highly probable that the weapon was firmly gripped, by instantaneous rigor, in her right hand. This single feature, the "hallmark" of self-infliction, is a strong contra-indication of homicide. By the time the team arrived, the revolver had been forced from her hand, "broken", and its cartridge removed by a relatively senior person, whose training should have prevented him from interfering with it. Fortunately, in that case, suspicion of the dead woman's husband was promptly cleared (Case No. 30, pages 249/50).

Interference with the weapon may preclude satisfactory fingerprint examination. In the case of Mrs. Barney (1932) it was important to determine whether she had handled the gun. The only clear impressions on it were those of a detective officer engaged on the case.

Of course, if the victim be still alive, some interference, the least possible, is unavoidable in order to remove him to hospital.

The kind of weapon responsible is not always obvious. It may be of an unusual and unfamiliar kind, e.g. a humane killer or some special device fashioned by the suicide (Collins, 1948). The initial interpretation of a man's death by firearm injury was that of homicide because no weapon appeared to be at the scene. A metal object near the body was cast aside as one of the fire irons. Later this was recognised as a "humane killer" which fired a free bullet, and the injuries had been inflicted by the deceased at "contact" range (Hunt and Kon, 1962).

In ascertaining the probable range of fire due account must be taken of the modifying effects of reducing the length of the gun barrel, i.e. when a "sawn-off" shotgun is used. Again, modification of range occurs when the shot first travels through the panel of a door before striking the victim (Case No. 15, p. 227).

Deflection of the missile or missiles, causing contact by ricochet, or with bone in the victim's body, has to be taken into account in ascertaining the direction of aim.

The kind of ammunition has importance. There are times when bullets of smaller calibre than the gun have been used. Again, there may have been a defect in, or interference with, a shotgun cartridge. In certain areas it appears to be the practice to remove the over-shot card and to pour in a little molten wax. (Alternatively, some of the shots are replaced by a ball bearing.) This results in "balling" of the shot and, at "distant" range, the injuries may appear to have been inflicted by two weapons of an entirely different kind, i.e. a shotgun and a rifled weapon (Mant, 1968). New difficulties are created by the introduction of shotgun slugs, i.e. rifled bullets for use in shotguns (Petty and Hauser, 1968).

Defect in the ammunition or the weapon may result in a misfire, which causes the bullet to remain in the gun barrel. The next discharge then forces the reluctant bullet out of the gun and the two bullets travel in tandem. When they strike the victim, they enter by the same hole. It is then important to explain the presence of two bullets in the body. A man suspected of murder, truthfully insisted he had fired but once and that it was an accidental discharge (Michaux and Thiodet, 1960; see p. 268).

The invention of gyrojet ammunition will create problems in interpretation because, at a range of several yards, it produces injuries which simulate those produced by normal ammunition at "contact" or "near" range (see p. 243).

Damage by blast has to be distinguished from injury by missiles. Blast can cause fatal injury when none of the shot enters the body (see p. 240).

Entrance wounds are not always apparent. They may be obscured by dark hair or, by swollen eyelids (Gonzales *et al.*, 1954). In some of these cases, where an exit wound is present, it may be deemed a laceration by a blunt instrument or the result of a fall.

Rarely, there may be two "contact" injuries, self-inflicted; they may be in the left temple (Tesař, 1958).

The site, if unusual, does not exclude self-infliction. The foregoing suicide was left-handed. A left- or right-handed person can shoot themselves in the left temple (Case No. 31, p. 250). It is also possible for a suicide to shoot himself in the back of the head or anus (Simonin, 1955).

There are occasions when difficulty is experienced in finding the missile which lies inside the victim's body. This may be due to disintegration of the bullet after impact with hard bone or embolism of the bullet. A victim can survive long enough for the bullet to reach a brachial or femoral artery. On these occasions facilities for X-ray examination are invaluable. (Whenever practicable, for reasons of safety as well as skill, the apparatus should be operated only by a trained radiographer).

Firearm Wounds in the Living

It is imperative that casualty surgeons and neurosurgeons are knowledgeable about firearm injuries and make detailed records of the appearances of the injuries prior to surgical toilet and operation. The pathologist and others then receive valuable assistance in the interpretation of the circumstances. Failure to make proper records results in confusion of the kind which occurred in the Merrett case (1927). It was then important to distinguish between a self-inflicted and a distant firearm wound. In consequence of unsatisfactory medical and scientific evidence Merrett escaped conviction (not proven) of the murder of his mother. He shot himself in 1954 when strongly suspected of the murder of his wife and his mother-in-law (Teare, 1955).

It is also imperative that the surgeon (or pathologist) who removes the missile, exercises care to avoid interference with markings it may bear. Comparison studies with bullets fired from the suspected gun may be seriously impaired by blurring of the marks or the addition of marks by surgical instruments.

"Peppering" with a shotgun should not be regarded as a minor matter. It may be that the majority of the pellets produce only superficial injuries, but some may penetrate the body cavities and cause internal bleeding by damage to blood vessels or organs, e.g. a single pellet, fired at a range of about 30 ft, punctured the left external carotid artery and caused fatal haemorrhage (Case No. 21, p. 237). It is a wise course to keep patients under observation for about 24 hours when they have been shot at distant range and have sustained chest or abdominal punctures, even though the appearances of the injuries and condition of the patient do not suggest major injury.

Samples of blood and urine should be submitted for the determination of their alcohol content, because many, e.g. 78 per cent (Canfield, 1969), are under the influence of alcohol (see p. 217).

If, on admission to hospital, there is a simple dressing on the face or head, it should be removed in order to determine the reason for its application. Failure to do this led to failure to detect a small firearm entrance wound. The fact that the victim had been shot, and was not suffering from hypertension and cerebral haemorrhage, was not realised until a routine X-ray of the skull disclosed a bullet in his left cerebral hemisphere (Heulley *et al.*, 1965).

Prompt diagnosis and surgical intervention can save a patient. Haller (1962) reported the case of a man whose common carotid arteries were transected by a 0.22 bullet. The swelling in each carotid sheath was promptly diagnosed and immediate operation followed. The damaged portion of each artery was excised and an end-to-end anastomosis restored cerebral circulation.

Shotgun Injuries

The features peculiar to shotgun injuries are primarily determined by the fact that the charge is composed of several small missiles. At close range these travel in a compact mass and make a single wound as if by a solid missile of large size. As the range increases the individual pellets continue at their own speed and direction, which results in a fanwise distribution, the surface area covered by the shot increasing with the distance travelled. Meantime, the penetrating power of each pellet decreases until, at about 10 yards, penetration is normally limited to the clothing and skin of the victim.

Test patterns at different ranges, from contact to 15 ft, are reproduced by Drake (1962a, b).

Accurate interpretation of firearm injuries demands inspection of the clothing as well as a post-mortem examination; the clothing should not be removed until the pathologist and, whenever practicable, the forensic scientist are present. It is, of course, for the latter to make a detailed examination of the clothing, but the pathologist should have opportunity to see it and learn the findings of the scientist.

The importance of the examination of the clothing is illustrated by Case No. 18, p. 233. The entrance wound on the body had the appearance of a contact injury but examination of the clothing showed the presence of smoke and unburnt powder around the hole in it which indicated that the gun had been fired at a distance of several inches and less than a yard. The boy had been shot accidentally in his back at a range of about 2 ft.

An examination of the clothing may also give information concerning the direction of aim and the relative positions of the victim and his assailant. Gonzales *et al.* (1954) drew attention to the presence of a single hole in the clothing but a "through and through" wound in the body of the victim. There are occasions when the bullet traverses the body but comes to rest between the body and the clothing. Incidentally, this calls for care in removing the clothing lest the bullet be lost. They illustrated this with the case of a man who, according to the assailant, had been shot in front of the body. Surgical treatment had obliterated the entrance wound in the abdomen and the exit wound, at the back of the body, was identified erroneously as the entrance wound. When the clothing was examined there was a hole at the front but none at the back. Although the accused's statement was not challenged, the circumstances of one of our cases were similar: the bullet was recovered when the clothing was removed, prior to autopsy.

Shotgun Entrance Wounds

Their appearances are appreciably modified by the range of fire, i.e. contact, "near" (within a yard), and distant. Contact injuries also differ in their appearances according to site, i.e. whether over resistant bone, e.g. in the head, or the relatively non-resistant chest or abdominal wall.

Although contact injuries to the head normally result in gross disruption, certain differences may occur following contact with the temple, forehead, palate or back of the head.

(a) CONTACT WOUNDS

(i) *Temple or Cheek* The usual site is the right temple, but the left-handed choose the left temple and, in certain circumstances, a victim arranges matters to enable him to fire the gun at the left temple with his right hand.

The combined effects of the entry of the shot and the products of detonation, i.e. injury by shot and blast, produce gross disruption of the tissues. The scalp and skull may be burst open and parts of the scalp, skull and brain blown from the body for a distance of several feet.

Disruption and detachment of the scalp may obscure the site of contact. Extensive splits in the scalp and comminution of the skull may then lead the inexperienced to ascribe the damage to an agent other than a firearm, e.g. an axe, which in the absence of the agent suggests homicide. Expert examination on one occasion, however, established that it was a shotgun injury at contact range in the right temple (Case No. 1, p. 214; Plate 1).

Search should be made for evidence of bruising or blackening in the remains of the scalp in the known sites of suicidal injury. The occurrence of recoil injury, e.g. by the unfired barrel of a double-barrelled gun, in the form of superficial laceration or bruising in these sites, is also a possibility (F.M. 11,703 and 13,177A).

In general the results do not differ materially with the 12-bore and 0.410 shotguns because, at contact range, each causes grave damage. Disruption with either weapon may be contained within the scalp, or even within the skull. Thus, on some occasions, blast raises the scalp from the skull and the majority of the shot may be recovered from the widened space between the scalp and the skull, at the back or side of the head; the wad and cards may accompany the shot or be found inside the skull. On other occasions when the top of the head is blown away, all the contents of the cartridge may leave the body.

Comminution of the vault of the skull is usually accompanied by extensive fissured fractures, or "crazy-paving" fracture, of the base of the skull and the roofs of the orbits and middle ears. The delicate bones, e.g. ethmoid and sphenoid are often shattered; the nasal bones may be broken. An eye may be blown out of its socket.

Damage to the brain normally involves the hemispheres, but when direction of aim is to a lower level they may suffer less than the mid brain, hind brain and cerebellum. Secondary missiles, e.g. portions of broken bone, can also cause serious injury to the brain.

(ii) *Forehead* Contact between the muzzle and the forehead is not infrequently tangential, i.e. at an angle of less than 90°, and, in consequence, the major damage is restricted to the frontal region. An entrance wound at eyebrow level may then be accompanied by an exit wound a little higher in the forehead, extending to the hair line, the two injuries being separated by a narrow band of intact skin (Case No. 2, p. 214). A variation is provided by the coalescence of entrance and exit wounds in the form of a wedge-shaped gash, with its base uppermost near the vertex, on the front of the head (Case No. 3, p. 215).

(iii) *Mouth* An entrance wound in the mouth or nose may or may not be accompanied by an exit wound. Resistance by the hard palate reduces the power of the shot so that even if a substantial piece of skull, e.g. in the occipital bone, be detached, the shot may lie within the head; most of them may be in the space widened by blast between the skull and scalp, at the back or side of the head. In these circumstances it is possible that death due to firearm injury may be initially overlooked. This is more likely when a rifled weapon was used. Laceration or bruising of the lips, a usual feature, might be deemed the result of a blow on the forehead, as in one case the direction of aim was upwards and forwards, producing an exit wound in the forehead (F.M. 12,038A).

There should be little difficulty at autopsy in recognising the entrance wound, certainly not when the "Y"-shaped skin incision and dissection of the neck structures gives a clear view of the roof of the mouth.

The wound presents as a circular hole in the roof of the mouth, of from 0.45 in. to 1.0 in., according to the weapon used. The mucosa is likely to be stripped from the hard palate and the margins of the hole in the bone are blackened by smoke and powder. Abrasion or bruising of one or both lips, with or without laceration, is usual, and this is due to recoil of the gun sight. Splitting of the angle of the mouth may be due to blast.

The hand which held the gun in position may bear spatters of blood on the base of the thumb and the index finger. A swab for nitrates may be positive, unless free bleeding has washed them from the wound.

As might be expected, the nose, nasal sinuses and basal vessels are shattered. The external carotid arteries and basal vessels are ruptured, and there is major damage to the nervous system; its distribution depends on the direction of aim; it may be in the frontal lobes or the mid brain and occipital lobes, or mid brain, medulla, cerebellum and spinal cord. The base of the skull is likely to be extensively damaged and again, according to direction of aim, the occipital bone or a parietal bone may be fractured and a substantial portion of the bone detached. The scalp, however, may remain intact but be detached from the skull by blast; the space may contain not only blood but shot.

The direction is usually upwards and backwards but the damage done depends on the angle of the gun.

(iv) *Back of Head* Although an entrance wound in the nape of the neck or over the occiput is presumptive evidence of homicide, which, incidentally, may be accidental, it is then likely to be a "near" and not a contact injury. If a "contact" injury, the possibility of self-infliction must be considered. For obvious reasons it is a rare choice, but there has been one instance in Leeds (Leeds City Coroner, 309/42).

The upper two vertebrae and base of the skull sustain the major damage. It is possible for the cord and brain to escape and death is then probably due to destruction of major blood vessels on one side of the neck. This can happen when the direction of aim is to the right or left of the middle line.

Examples of Contact Shotgun Injuries

Case No. 1 (Plate 1)

   Site: temple, right, *Range:* contact. Self-inflicted. *Weapon:* 12-bore shotgun.

   This man, aged 39, was found dead in the potting shed of his nursery garden; he had fallen backwards and was propped up against an agricultural implement.
   It was obvious that he had gross injuries. The top of his head had been burst open and the scalp torn into flaps, the margins of which suggested to the lay observers that the injuries might have been inflicted with an axe. A 12-bore shotgun lay on the floor of the shed but because it was at a distance, actually 4 ft from the body, it was not considered as the agent.
   It was later shown that at the base of a skin flap on the right side, in the region of the temple, there was a band $1/8$ in. wide of blackening by soot and unburnt powder. This indicated a firearm injury and at close, probably contact, range.
   A pool of blood had collected beneath his head. There were traces of blood at the front of the lower parts of his trousers and on his boots, and traces of blood on his hands. He was erect when he shot himself and he then collapsed into the position in which his body was found.
   The skull was comminuted and portions of its vault and the brain had been scattered, some inside the shed and others outside it up to a distance of 30 ft. A wad and card were found in a corner of the shed to the left of the body. The cerebral hemispheres were absent but the mid brain, hind brain and cerebellum remained, apparently undamaged (F.M. 10,610B).

Case No. 2 (Plate 11)

   Site: forehead. *Range:* contact. Self-inflicted. *Weapon:* 0.410 shotgun. *Ammunition:* No. 6 shot.
   Special feature: a tangential wound.

   This man, aged 50, when found dead in his scullery, was in a crouching posture with a 0.410 single-barrelled shotgun beside him.
   An entrance wound was situated in the middle line of the forehead just above the level of the eye-brows; the

lower border of the wound was at the root of the nose. This was an oval wound of which the vertical and horizontal diameters were respectively $1^9/_{16}$ in. and 1 in. The opening was bordered by a band of abraded, blackened skin, $^3/_4$ in. broad. The forehead sloped backwards and was depressed owing to comminution of the underlying bone.

There was a second irregular laceration, 3 in. long, somewhat mushroom-shaped, situated directly above the entrance wound, and separated from it by a band of intact skin, $^1/_4$ in. broad. The stem of the laceration, angled to the left, below, was $^1/_4$ in. broad but the upper part of the "mushroom" was up to 2 in. broad, where it abutted the hair line. The margins of this laceration were everted; they were not abraded, nor soiled by soot. It was the exit wound.

A series of linear splits, each approximately $^1/_4-^1/_2$ in. long, were present in the outer layers of the skin, approximately $^1/_8$ in. outside the margins of the exit wound.

Bleeding had occurred into the eyelids and from the right ear.

The internal damage included: comminution of the anterior half of the vault of the skull with fissured fractures radiating into the orbital roofs and each middle ear; the nasal bones were fractured. The formal lobes of the brain were lacerated, but the mid brain, hind brain and cerebellum were intact. Pellets and a wad were found between the scalp and the vertex of the skull, directly behind the comminuted bone.

His blood contained 97 mg/100 ml alcohol; no barbiturate present.

This case is of interest because of the close approximation of the entrance and exit wounds. Although a contact injury, the gun must have been held at less than a right angle to the forehead, an angle of about 45°, instead of the more usual 90°. Even so, fatal damage was done (F.M. 8270B).

Case No. 3 (Fig. 58)

Site: (a) chin; (b) forehead. *Range:* contact. Self-inflicted. *Weapon:* 12-bore shotgun. *Ammunition:* No. 6 shot.

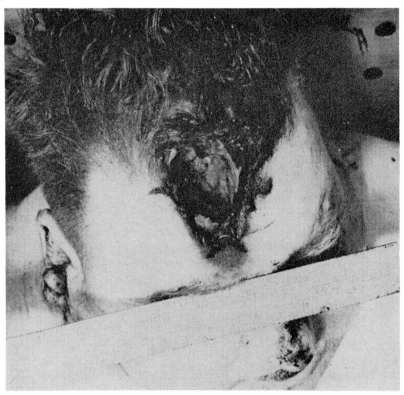

FIG. 58. Shotgun, contact, wound: tangential; wedge-shaped split of front of head.
(Case No. 3.)

Following the murder of his wife by shooting her (see Case No. 20, p. 235) he went to his bedroom and shot himself with the gun. His first attempt was made with the muzzle of the gun near his chin and he failed to cause major damage. He then shot himself in the forehead, at contact range.

The first injury. With the gun against his chin, directed to the right, he had produced a triangular laceration of the superficial tissues, opened the right external jugular vein and broken his lower jaw. It was a "through and through" injury at close range; there was blackening of the skin by soot and unburnt powder in a fan-shaped band of skin in the right side of his neck, 6 in. long and 3 in. broad, extending from the point of the chin to the right ear. There was bruising of his right shoulder and a few pellets were found beneath the skin in this region.

The second injury. This was a contact wound in the middle line of the forehead, $1^1/_2$ in. above the bridge of the nose. It presented as a wedge-shaped wound 4 in. long and 2 in. broad at its base near the vertex. The margins were ragged and bruised; four small splits extended out from them. The skin beyond the margins of the wound was soiled by smoke and unburnt powder. There were no satellite punctures. The shot had shattered the frontal bone, fragments of which had been driven into the brain.

The distance between his forehead and index finger (arm extended) was 39 in. and that between his chin and index finger was 33 in. The length of the barrel of the gun was 28 in.; trigger pressures $3^3/_4$ lb right and 6 lb left (F.M. 13,232A, Fig. 58).

Case No. 4 (Fig. 59)

Site: face. *Range:* contact. Self-inflicted. *Weapon:* 12-bore double-barrelled shotgun. *Ammunition:* No. 5 shot Eley.

This man, aged 60, was half reclining against the fireplace in his living room. Gross injury of the face was apparent. A 12-bore was beside him with the muzzle on the floor and the butt resting against the fireplace at 2 ft above the floor. His right eye and tissue from his right cheek, the cerebral hemispheres and left eye had been blown out of his head and lay at 5 ft from the body. Blood splashes were on the ceiling. An empty 12-bore cartridge lay on the body.

The entrance wound was in the right cheek near the outer corner of the right eye. It was ragged and $^1/_2$ in. across. A circular "cut", 0.8 in. in diameter was adjacent (a recoil injury by the empty right barrel of the gun,

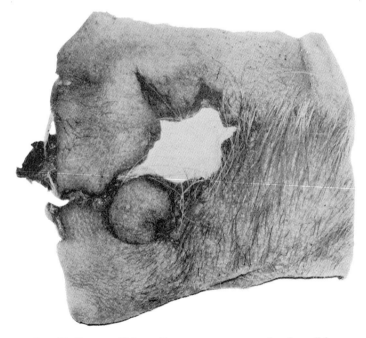

FIG. 59. Shotgun: 12-bore. Contact entrance wound and recoil imprint. (Case No. 4.)

Fig. 59). The margins of the entrance wound were blackened by powder. The damage principally confined to the face and anterior compartment of the skull; the middle and posterior compartments were, by comparison, almost intact.

There was a mark on the left support of the fireplace at 2 ft above the ground; it was identified as the recoil mark of the butt of the gun, with the heel uppermost.

Reconstruction of the scene led to the conclusion that he had knelt or squatted in front of the muzzle of the gun. He had held it, trigger guard uppermost, with the butt wedged against the fireplace. He had held the muzzle against his cheek with his left hand and fired the trigger with his right.

It was a new gun and both barrels had recently been fired. The right barrel was now empty but the left contained a discharged cartridge. The overall length of the gun was 45 in.; muzzle to trigger 31 in. Deceased's arm length, armpit to thumb 25 in. Despite this discrepancy it was found by test that he could have fired the gun when fixed in the manner described. (F.M. 11,703B).

Case No. 5

Site: palate. *Range:* contact. Self-inflicted. *Weapon:* 0.410 shotgun. *Ammunition:* No. 5 shot.

This man, aged 47, had bled from both nostrils and bleeding had occurred into each orbit. There were blood splashes on the chin and left cheek. The vault of the skull had been opened and the sagittal suture sprung apart to a width of $^1/_2$ in. The upper lip was split just to the right of the middle line, the damage being due to contact with the foresight of the gun.

Internal examination showed that the anterior two-thirds of the tongue were scorched and there was a circular hole 0.45 in. in the palate. The mucosa had been stripped from the palate. The bony margins of the hole in the palate were blackened by soot and powder. The roof of each orbit was shattered. Both internal carotid arteries were destroyed. There was extensive fracturing of the vault of the skull involving both parietal bones and there was a transverse fracture 3 in. long in the occipital bone. A semicircular fracture (having the diameter of a 0.410 wad) of the inner table of this bone, just to the left of the middle line, was also present. A wad was nearby.

Most of the shot had left the skull but several pellets were found in blood which had collected between the skull and scalp in the occipital region. The meninges had been stripped from the skull and contained at least forty punctures by pellets. There was extensive brain damage partly by shot and partly by fragments of bone. The hind brain was separated from the pons which had been destroyed. The cerebellum was damaged by splinters of bone. The basilar arteries were destroyed.

The gun, from muzzle to trigger, was 31 in. long, i.e. 2 in. less than the distance between his thumb and mouth. No implement was needed to reach the trigger when the muzzle was in the mouth. The trigger pressure was $5^1/_4$ lb, i.e. normal. Although the breech mechanism was faulty, the gun could be fired. He had held the gun in position with his left hand and fired it with his right. Thus the shot passed slightly to the left. There were droplets of blood on the back of the left thumb and index finger.

He had a right renal calculus and this kidney was atrophic; the left kidney was hypertrophied $\times 1^1/_2$ (F.M. 12,163E).

Case No. 6

Site: palate. *Range:* contact. Suicide. *Weapon:* 0.410 Belgian shotgun. *Ammunition:* No. 5 shot.

This man, aged 43, had bled from his ears and nostrils and there was bruising, $^1/_2 \times ^1/_{16}$ in., of his lower lip. (The bruising was due to injury by the foresight of the gun.) Bloodstaining was present on the back of the left thumb and index finger.

Dissection demonstrated a circular entrance wound on the roof of his mouth. There was a hole $^1/_2$ in. in diameter in the hard palate and the roof of the mouth was blackened by soot.

The vault of the skull was shattered; there was "crazy-paving" fracture of the base of the skull. Fracture of the skull presented as a hole in the left parieto-occipital region and a wad and cards were found in this region.

There was gross laceration of the brain; the thalamus, most of the occipital lobes and the mid brain were destroyed.

After he had shot himself the hot barrel of the gun fell against his chest. This was indicated by a band of burning $^1/_2$ in. wide and 5 in. long extending upwards from his left nipple. A swab of the skin of the chest was positive for nitrates as was also one from the margin of the wound in the palate.

Measurements showed that his potential reach was larger than the distance from the trigger to the roof of his mouth.

The range, if not direct contact, was estimated at less than $^1/_2$ in.

His blood alcohol content was 135 mg/100 ml and his urinary alcohol was 175 mg/100 ml; the equivalent of ingestion of 4 pints of beer by a man weighing 12 stones (F.M. 12,425A).

Case No. 6A

Site: face and neck. *Range:* "near" and "contact". Homicide.

This man, aged 31, was the night watchman at a warehouse, who was shot by an armed intruder. When making his escape, the latter shot and killed a police inspector who was investigating the crime (see F.M. 14,646; Case No. 21).

The dead man was found lying on his back in a small office. His head was under the central part of a desk; his feet extended to the centre of the room.

Two firearm injuries were apparent, one in his face and the other at the left side of his neck. There was spattering of blood beneath the desk and to the right of the head.

The facial injury: this was an irregular wound 2 in. in diameter, with slightly ragged edges and with narrow side splits of up to $^1/_4$ in. long at the right border. It was situated between the upper lip and nose. There was no scorching; no soiling by soot nor involuntary tattooing. The range, therefore, was beyond the range of self infliction but, in the absence of satellite punctures, it was only about 1 yard.

The neck injury; this was a circular hole, $1^1/_4$ in. in diameter, situated $1^3/_4$ in. below the right angle of the lower jaw, its lower border was on the level of the thyroid cartilage. There was an abrasion collar of up to $^1/_8$ in. broad around the wound. Except for slight blackening of the adjacent skin by fibres of cloth which adhered to the skin, soiling by smoke was absent; there was no involuntary tattooing.

The track of the shot was upwards and backwards towards the middle line where it merged with that of the facial injury.

The body of the hyoid bone was flattened and the horns were separated from the bone. The thyroid cartilage was intact. Shot had torn open the right carotid artery and jugular vein. The merged tracks passed on through the skull and the shot had produced an oblong hole 1 × $^1/_2$ in. on the floor of the left posterior compartment of the skull. Fissured fracture extended from this area to the right side of the frontal bone. In addition to subdural haemorrhage there was extensive laceration of the brain-stem and cerebellum. Portions of cloth were embedded in the brain.

Several pellets were found in the muscles at the back of the neck. A wad and cards were beside the cervical spine and another wad and card were within the skull.

There was no exit wound to either of these shots.

The neck injury had the appearance of a contact wound.

During this incident the deceased was first shot in the face when erect, at close range, about a yard, and then, after his collapse he was shot in the neck at contact range. Spattering of the desk and floor were indicative of injury while he lay with his head under the desk.

Although an incidental finding, it may be noted that he had excessive iron storage in his liver, early haemochromatosis (F.M. 14,647).

(v) *Abdomen or Chest* Contact injuries are characterised by the production of a circular or oval wound of the skin, about an inch in diameter, as if a piece had been punched out of it. The margin, which is slightly ragged, is bordered by a narrow rim of powder-blackened tissue about $^1/_{12}$ in. broad (Case No. 7, Fig. 61, abdominal wound). The band of blackening may be broader around part of the periphery and its distribution bears a relationship to the relative position of the muzzle and the body wall. When a man shot himself in the chest, with partial contact by the muzzle, the wound was oval, $1^1/_8 × ^3/_4$ in., with a band of blackening up to $^1/_2$ in. broad beside the lower half of the circumference of the wound (F.M. 3744B, Fig. 60). Although the skin wounds in these cases are relatively clean-cut, there is severe disruption of the underlying structures. Internally, these wounds present as ragged craters of about 2 in. in diameter, lined by torn muscle and, in the chest, portions of ribs; blackening by unburnt powder may also be seen. Carbon monoxide may be present in blood in the wounded tissues, and, rarely, in the peripheral blood (Case No. 8, p. 220).

Case No. 7 (Fig. 61)

Site: abdomen. *Range:* contact. Self-inflicted. *Weapon:* 12-bore shotgun.

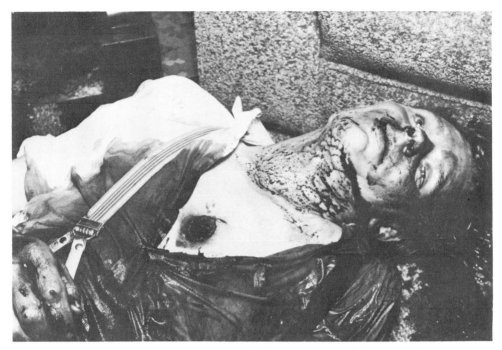

F̲ɪɢ. 60. Shotgun, 12-bore: contact wound of chest. Note opened clothing. (F.M. 3744ʙ)

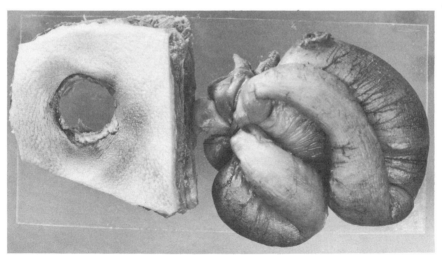

Fɪɢ. 61. Contact wound: 12-bore shotgun. Site upper abdomen; herniation of a coil of gut.
(Case No. 7.)

This body was sent to the mortuary as that of a man found collapsed in his garden. The attendants preparing it for examination, reported an injury to his abdomen. Two coils of small intestine, 11 cm and 19 cm long respectively, had herniated through an aperture in the right upper quadrant of the abdomen. It was a circular hole, 1 in. in diameter, bordered by a narrow rim of blackened tissue. Internal damage was considerable; the right lobe of the liver and the right kidney were gravely lacerated and there was comminution of the lumbar spine. Pellets, cards and a wad were within the abdomen. There was no exit wound. The deceased was a gamekeeper whose physical and mental health had deteriorated. He had been found by his wife, who took the gun into the house and put it in a cupboard. She had found it reared against a bench near the body and she thought he had been cleaning it. No cleaning apparatus was there but a metal rod, 18 in. long, was on the ground at the scene and it appeared he had used this to release the trigger. Blood at the scene was negligible (F.M. 4776, Fig. 61).

Case No. 8

Site: abdomen. *Range:* contact. Self-inflicted. *Weapon:* 12-bore shotgun, double barrelled. *Ammunition:* No. 5 or No. 6 shot.

Special interest. A female who committed suicide with a firearm. Carbon monoxide not only in the vicinity of the wound but also in the peripheral blood. (Survival for sufficient time for absorption of carbon monoxide from the abdominal cavity into the circulation.)

This woman, aged 47, the wife of a farmer, was found dead in the coal shed at the farm. When first seen by her husband she lay face down on the floor; he turned the body over in order to see if she was still alive.

The body was turned back by the police and it then lay over a 12-bore shotgun, parts of which protruded, showing that the breech was partly opened, the barrels and stock being at an angle. Blood at the scene was confined to a pool beneath the body. Her collapse had been immediate and mobility thereafter ceased. She was dressed in a nightdress, vest and knickers; her feet were bare. Scorching of the nightdress in an oval area $1 \times {}^{7}/_{8}$ in. was observed in relation to a circular hole; three similar holes were in the vest; it had been folded when on the body.

External examination of the body. A circular entrance wound, ${}^{5}/_{8}$ in. in diameter, was centred in the middle line of the upper abdomen, $2{}^{1}/_{2}$ in. below the xiphisternum. The margins of the wound were serrated by pellets and were blackened by melted nylon. It was a contact injury by shotgun, its diameter being less than that of the gun barrel due to stretching of the skin over the muzzle at the moment of firing; subsequently the skin had contracted.

A crescentic, bruised abrasion was present at ${}^{3}/_{4}$ in. to the left and ${}^{3}/_{4}$ in. above the centre of the entrance wound. This was a recoil injury by the left barrel of the gun.

Blood from the vicinity of the wound was saturated to 60 per cent carbon monoxide, and blood from the abdominal cavity was saturated to 30 per cent carbon monoxide. The surprise result was that of 20 per cent saturation of blood taken from a vein in the left arm.

Internal examination. Grave damage was done by the shot to the pylorus, small intestine, especially the jejunum, the pancreas, upper half of the left kidney and the left psoas muscle which was detached from the lumbar vertebrae (L1–L4). The transverse processes of these vertebrae were shattered and the shot had cut a groove in the left side of the vertebral bodies. The track ended in the muscles immediately to the left of the spine. There was no exit wound.

Death of a woman by firearm injury raises a presumption of accident or homicide, because females rarely choose firearms to accomplish suicide. The findings at the scene and by post-mortem examination in this case established the fact of self-infliction of the fatal injury. Thus, the injury had the characteristics of a contact shotgun injury and this received confirmation by the presence of a recoil mark in the abdominal wall and CO in blood from the margin of the wound. The recoil mark must have been made by the left barrel since this contained the live cartridge. She had shot herself with the right barrel which contained a discharged cartridge. The gun, moreover, must have been held with the trigger away from her body, in order for her to reach the triggers. Had she been shot by another person, holding the gun in the normal manner, the recoil of a left barrel would have been on the other side of the entrance wound. For fairly obvious reasons, contact injury by firearm is difficult to inflict unless the victim be incapacitated by sleep, disease, drink or injury. She was physically fit and not incapacitated by drink or injury.

It was shown that she had leant over the muzzle of the gun, held against her upper abdomen. The length of her arm from armpit to thumb was 24 in. The gun from muzzle to heel of butt was 3 ft 9 in. (She could have reached the triggers when leaning over the gun.) The wound centre was 3 ft 7 in. from the soles of her feet; its track was such that she was not erect when shot.)

The steel plate on the heel of the butt of the gun was scratched and bore concrete dust. A deep impression with curved scratches was found in the concrete floor of the shed at a point where the butt would have been, i.e. just in front of her feet as she leant over the gun.

The direction of the shot was backwards, slightly to the left and downwards. This, presuming she was right handed, indicated that she had leant over the gun with her body twisted somewhat to the right.

A minor problem was created by the fact that the gun under her body was "broken". The breech locking lever was in the open position; it had not been returned to the fully locked position after firing. It had no safety catch.

Both hammers fell when the breech was closed but not locked. It was found difficult to close the gun because of a fault in its mechanism. When she collapsed the weight of her body upon the muzzle of the gun had forced it into the "broken" position; the locking lever had not returned to the fully locked position (F.M. 10,847B).

Case No. 9.

Site: chest. *Range:* contact. Self-inflicted. *Weapon:* 12-bore shotgun, single barrelled. *Ammunition:* No. 5, shot.

A man, aged 45, found dead in scrub on the bank of the river, was fully clothed, with raincoat. The jacket and raincoat were open and the upper three buttons of the shirt were undone, but there was a ragged tear in the shirt over the heart region; a 1 in. hole was present in the vest. There was a circular hole in the left chest situated 2 in. to the left of the middle line, $2^1/_4$ in. below the nipple and $2^1/_4$ in. internal to it, over the left 5th rib. There was slight laceration of the margin and contusion in a crescentic band up to $^1/_8$ in. broad on the left half of the circumference. No singeing, blackening by smoke, or tattooing could be seen in the skin or on the clothing.

There was much destruction of tissues internally, with comminution of the 5th and 6th ribs; blood in the area was bright red, saturated to 60 per cent by CO. The lower half of the heart was lacerated and there was laceration of the inner aspect of the lower lobe of the left lung. The left half of the diaphragm was torn and some pellets had passed through the stomach. There was laceration of the spleen and of the left lobe of the liver. A card and a wad were present in the chest under the damaged heart; a second card with the bulk of the pellets lay in a ragged crater at the back of the chest near the 9th and 10th ribs on the left side; the ribs were comminuted. The direction of aim was slightly down and out, as if the deceased had leaned over the barrel in order to fire the weapon. A person whose arm was 24 in. from armpit to index finger could have fired this trigger without the aid of a stick, notwithstanding that the distance between the trigger and the end of the barrel was 29 in. (F.M. 7861A).

Case No. 10 *(Figs. 62, 63)*

Site: chest. *Range:* contact. Self-inflicted. *Weapon:* 12-bore.

Special feature. Owing to ricochet from within the chest, pellets emerged to produce an external appearance

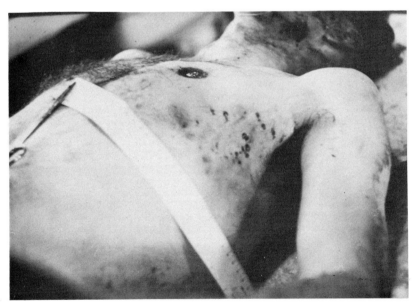

FIG. 62. Contact shotgun injury simulating distant shot. Pellets emerging from chest to the left and below entrance wound. (Case No. 10.)

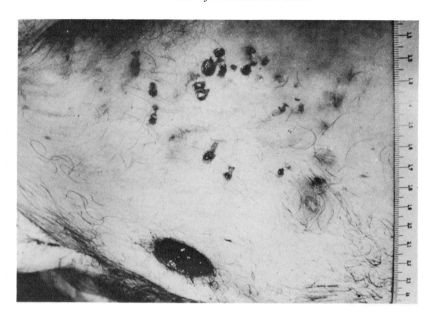

FIG. 63. Shotgun, 12-bore contact wound. Simulation of distant shot because of exit
of pellets below and to left of entrance wound. (Case No. 10.)

which simulated a range beyond that of self-infliction. Also he collapsed at a short distance from the place at
which he shot himself. Hence the gun was not beside him.

The man, aged 47, was found dead in a passage-way of some outbuildings. He was fully clothed and lay on
his left side. A pool of blood had collected beneath his chest. When the body was turned over, it was seen that
there was a circular tear, $7/_8$ in. in diameter, behind the left lapel of his jacket and similar tears were in his
waistcoat, shirt and vest. He had not opened his clothing. There were no additional small holes in any of these
garments. They were not scorched or soiled by smoke or unburnt powder. There was heavy blood saturation
of the clothing of the left side and blood had collected between it and his body; some pellets were found in the
blood.

External examination of the body showed that there was a circular punched-out firearm wound, $7/_8$ in. in
diameter, bordered by a narrow zone of blackened skin, $1/_{32}$ in. broad, on the inner (right) half of the
circumference of the wound. Its centre lay 2 in. to the left of the middle line and 3 in. below the inner end of the
left collar bone; it was about midway between the collar bone and the nipple. Gross damage to the chest cage
in the vicinity was apparent as an abnormal depression of the middle third of the chest. The appearances were
those of a contact injury, directed backwards and somewhat downwards.

The unusual feature was the presence of twenty satellite punctures and six circular bruises of pellet size;
pellets were palpated beneath the latter.

The satellite injuries were situated within an area of 3 in. in diameter, below and to the left of the contact
wound at the level of the nipple. None of these pellets had damaged the clothing.

Internal examination disclosed gross disruption of the left chest. Anteriorly, the middle third of the chest
cage was shattered. Two areas of damage were distinguished; one in front was a ragged crater, 4 × 3 in., in
which ribs 2–8 were found to have been comminuted. The other, also a crater, $1^3/_4$ × 1 in., was at the back of
the chest and it contained fragments of the 7th and 8th ribs. Pellets were present in the floor of this crater
behind the pleura.

The pleural sac contained 2 pints of blood. The left lung was collapsed and its lower lobe extensively
lacerated. A wad, cards and pellets were present in it. The heart and great vessels were intact, and there was no
injury to the spine.

It was concluded that he had leant over the gun and fired it into his chest. A piece of wood was near the gun
and he may have used this to release the trigger. Ricochet of pellets from the ribs had forced them outwards.
Some had penetrated the chest wall and lodged between his body and his clothing. Others had reached the
subcutaneous tissues but had not penetrated the skin.

Since no major vessel was damaged he could have survived for a short time, long enough for him to have walked a few paces. (It is appreciated that some of the blood in his left pleura had collected there by gravitation after death.) (F.M. 10,109A.)

NEAR WOUNDS: *at Ranges of up to 1 Yard*

If within about 6 in., the tissues, or clothing, may be singed by flame as well as blackened by smoke and unburnt powder; the zone of blackening is appreciably broader than that of a contact injury, e.g. up to $^1/_4$ in. broad. Carbon monoxide may be present in blood from the damaged tissues. The entrance wound is again likely to be circular or oval. In the skull there is less disruption than that at contact range; bursting open of the skull and scattering of its contents is not normally seen at this range. A girl, shot at a few inches with a 12-bore gun at the base of her skull, had no exit wound: the shot, wad and cards were within the skull (F.M. 3744A, Fig. 64). The scene of this murder and suicide is shown in Fig. 65; this also shows interference with the scene: gun placed on settee by third party.

Blackening of the tissues or clothing by smoke is unlikely at a range of over 12 in. and tattooing by unburnt powder is unlikely at a range of over 2 ft., nor do cards normally travel beyond a few feet; the overshot card travels for about 6 ft. The wad, however, may travel for several feet.

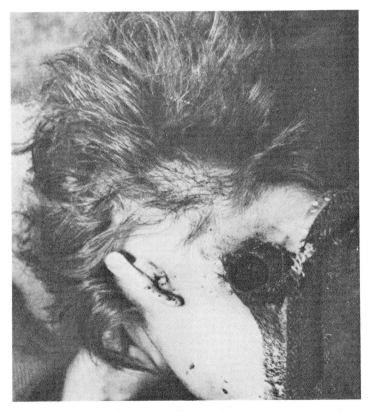

FIG. 64. Shotgun, 12-bore: "near" injury (about 4 in.) of left side of neck: homicide. (F.M. 3744A, p. 223.)

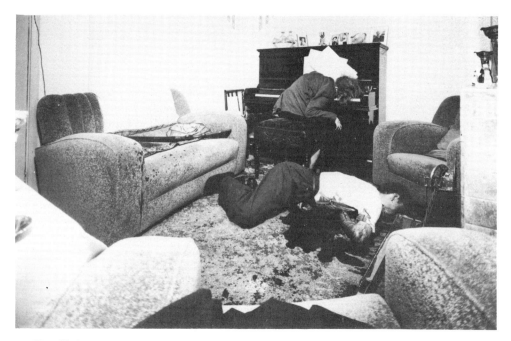

FIG. 65. Scene of murder—suicide by shotgun (picked up and placed on settee by first person at the scene). (F.M. 3744A, B.) (See figs. 60, 64).

Up to about 1 yard the shot travel in a compact mass, having the effect on impact of a solid mass of metal. The resulting entrance wound, up to about 1 yd., is a punched out, circular or oval wound of up to about $1^1/_2$ in. in diameter. At 18 in. or less the hole is about 1 in. or less in diameter. There are no outlying secondary entrance wounds produced by separate pellets. It is possible, as in the case below (F.M. 5541A, Figs. 62, 63), that after entry separate pellets at the end of their course come to lie beneath the skin or actually emerge. At this range, when the shot enters the body at an angle of less than 90°, the shape of the hole may be modified, as in Case No. 17, Fig. 73, so that the lower part of the circumference of the wound, instead of being curved may be straight—a "D"-shaped wound. This is deemed an intermediate change between the circle normally seen and the triangular lacerations which may occur at greater range, say 3 yards or so. The shot, by striking tangentially, tend to tear away a triangular flap of skin instead of punching a hole (see Case No. 23, Figs. 84, 85).

Case No. 11

Site: head. *Range:* near. Homicide. *Weapon:* 0.410 shotgun.

This man, aged 24, was in a double bed when he was shot at close range from behind his head.

He had fallen to the right so that his head rested on the floor beside the bed but his hips and legs remained covered by bedclothing. The body was partly supported by the arms.

A large pool of blood, about 2 ft in diameter, had collected on the floor beneath and in front of his face. An open clasp knife lay on the floor with its point at the edge of the pool of blood. A 0.410 shotgun, with its muzzle towards the bed head, was on the bed to the left of the body. A spent 0.410 cartridge was found in the fireplace.

The entrance wound, oval and $^7/_{16} \times ^1/_2$ in. in its diameters, was situated in the left side of the neck, $^1/_4$ in. behind the ear. Blackening by soot and unburnt powder was present in an area $1^7/_8$ in. around the entrance hole. There was a circular abrasion, $^2/_5$ in. in diameter, immediately below the wound; it had been produced by the impact of a card from the cartridge. The range of fire was estimated at 6 in.; this was confirmed by subsequent tests.

The track of the pellets was forwards and to the right at an angle of 45° to the middle line. The left sterno-mastoid muscle, common carotid artery and external jugular vein were lacerated. Both zygomatic arches were fractured and the pellets had fractured the right maxilla and had lacerated the right internal carotid artery and internal jugular vein. A wad and pellets were in the right maxillary antrum and more pellets were lying against the right ramus of the mandible which was fractured close to the right tempero-mandibular joint. A small amount of blood had been inhaled and was in the middle and lower lobes of the right lung.

The range of fire and direction of aim, and the length of the barrel of the gun precluded self infliction as the explanation. He was shot from behind and to the left while he sat up in bed. There had been no struggle or fight. The clasp knife had not been in his hand at the time and had not fallen from his hand to the floor. Its relationship to the pool of blood was consistent with its having been on the floor prior to the shooting.

He was under the influence of drink at the time; his blood alcohol level was 249 mg/100 ml and the urinary level was 196 mg/100 ml; this was estimated to represent an intake of 12 pints of beer.

The gun was his own property which he kept suspended on a hook above the bed head. He was engaged in an argument with his brother, who took down the gun and shot the deceased from behind the bed (F.M. 12,163A).

Case No. 12

Site: face. *Range:* 6 ft. Homicide. *Weapon:* 12-bore shotgun.

This Pakistani male, aged 31, had firearm injury on the right cheek, just in front of the ear. It was D-shaped with the convexity downwards. The edges were ragged and the maximum diameter was $1^3/_4$ in. It was accompanied by some twenty satellite punctures just outside its margin. The spread of shot was in an area of $2^1/_4$ in. There was no exit wound.

The shot had passed backwards and slightly upwards. The structures damaged included the upper and lower jaws, both of which were fractured, the right internal carotid artery and internal jugular vein, which were divided, the spines of the 1st and 2nd cervical vertebrae. The spinal cord was severed at this level. Shot had entered the base of the skull and had lacerated the left lobe of the cerebellum, the pons and the left occipital lobe. A wad and cards were found in the skull near the edge of the foramen magnum. About two-thirds of the shot had entered the skull and caused a crazy-paving fracture of the base, and had separated the posterior and anterior halves. The vertebral and basilar arteries were lacerated. The sphenoid sinus was shattered and portions of bone from its walls were found in the nose.

The range, estimated at 5–6 ft, was shown to have been 6 ft on test. The weapon was 12-bore shotgun which could have been fired either from the shoulder or the hip.

The man was fully dressed. Blood had run down the front of his sweater to the left of the midline. Spots of blood were on the outside of his trouser leg; he was erect when shot. (F.M. 12,329c.)

Case No. 13

Site: head. *Range:* near ($^1/_2$ in.). Self-inflicted. *Weapon:* 0.410 shotgun. *Ammunition:* No. 5 shot.
Special interest. Found dead at a distance of over 6 ft from the gun. A "near" wound; range $^1/_2$ in.

This man, aged 27 when found dead, was in a half sitting posture, propped against a bicycle in a potting shed. A 0.410 single-barrelled shotgun was leant against a wall in the angle between the shed and an adjacent greenhouse; the gun was over 6 ft away from the body. There was no evidence of a struggle.

A shotgun wound, $^1/_2$ in. in diameter, was situated just above his right ear. Powder "burning" of the skin around the wound was apparent in an area $1^1/_2$ in. in diameter. Bleeding had occurred from both ears and nostrils. Powder "burns" were at the back of his left thumb and index finger.

The track of the shot passed from right to left with a downward inclination of about 5°. The base of the skull was shattered and gas was present between the dura mater and the skull. The internal carotid arteries, the Circle of Willis and the dural sinuses were destroyed. There was laceration of the under surface of the brain and the hind brain was detached from the pons. (Fragments of bone had done as much damage as the pellets.) A wad, cards and pellets were amidst the shattered bone at the left side of the skull. There was no exit wound. No natural disease.

The gun was 27 in. from muzzle to trigger. It had no safety catch, but had a rebound safety notch. It could not be discharged by accidental dropping on the ground. The shot were the English No. 5. The wad and card

were from a 0.410 cartridge. Nitrates were present in the powder "burn" at the back of the left hand.
By test, the range was estimated at half an inch, i.e. almost "contact".

Reconstruction of the event: it appeared that he was erect when shot. He had stood half facing the potting shed door with the gun resting on the right-hand door post, between the shed and the green-house. He had held the gun with his left hand and fired with his right. The muzzle was half an inch from his head. When he was shot he was thrown off balance and his body slid along a chest of drawers inside the potting shed and it moved about 6 ft before he collapsed against the bicycle. There was no evidence to show that anyone else was responsible. It was not an accident (F.M. 12,41A7).

Case No. 14 (Figs. 66, 67)

Site: left temple. *Range:* "near" (about 1 in.). Self-inflicted. *Weapon:* 12-bore shotgun. *Ammunition:* No. 5 shot.
Special interest. Release of trigger with the aid of a fisherman's "lazy stick". Site of entrance wound: left temple.

This man's body was found on the ground behind his motor car. He was aged 35 years.

Grave damage to his head was obvious and there was evidence of a shotgun entrance wound in the left temple, $1^1/_2$ in. in front of the left ear. Scorching of the hair, soiling by smoke and involuntary tattooing by unburnt powder indicated a shot at near range, an inch or thereabouts, rather than a contact injury. An entrance hole was not apparent; it had merged with the extensive star-shaped laceration of the scalp and forehead, in the area which extended from eyebrow level to the back of the head. The skull had been burst open and much of the vault and brain had been blown away. The base of the skull was comminuted by fracture, of the "crazy-paving" type. There were fractures also of the facial bones and hard palate.

Most of the pellets had left the body, but thirteen were collected from the skull just in front of the right ear between the meninges which were punctured by shot. Pellets and brain tissue were found in the back of the car.

The direction of aim was from left to right at close range. There was powder marking on the left thumb and index finger. Swabs from them and the forehead yielded a positive nitrate test. He was sober and was not under the influence of drugs.

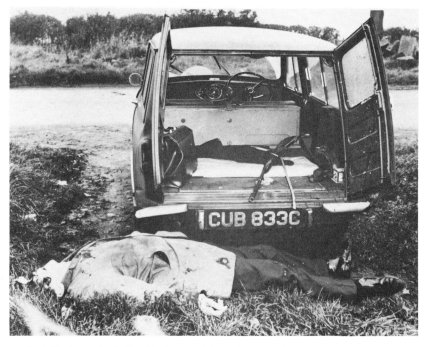

FIG. 66. Scene of suicide with shotgun: firing achieved with aid of "lazy stick". (Case No. 14.)

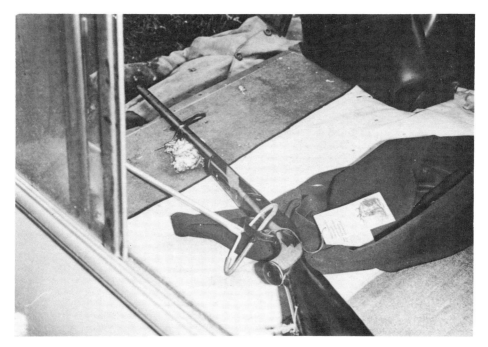

FIG. 67. Shotgun suicide: trigger released with a fisherman's (angler's) "lazy stick". (Case No. 14.)

This shooting was clearly planned. That morning he had purchased the 12-bore shotgun and the fisherman's lazy stick (the seller's label was still attached). He had taken his Mini traveller van to a quiet place and arranged matters in order to shoot himself at the back of the van. He had hooked the lazy stick inside the trigger guard of the gun and had used it to release the trigger. The stick was 32 in. long and the distance between the muzzle and the trigger was 31 in. Using the stick, a right-handed person could shoot himself in the left temple. The butt of gun was laid inside the van and he had released the trigger while standing at the back of the van and with his head bent forward to the level of, or just below, the roof. He had faced the offside of the vehicle and stood a few inches away from the open doors of the van.

The gun was in good order; the safety catch was in the off position; it was not an automatic catch (F.M. 12,635A).

Case No. 15 (Figs. 68, 69)

Site: chest and left hand. *Range:* near. Homicide. *Weapon:* 12-bore, two barrelled—trigger pressures; 5 lb and $4^1/_2$ lb. *Ammunition:* No. 5 shot.

Special interest. Victim was shot at close range through a bedroom door. It could have been an accident, precipitated by slamming the door against the muzzle of the gun.

The deceased, a man aged 32, was the former employee of a farm and had had an affair with the wife of the farmer. He had returned and been ordered out. The husband left and the deceased remained. The woman's son returned and, finding that his mother and the man were upstairs in a bedroom, he took his father's shotgun from a cupboard and went upstairs. He ordered the man out and threatened to shoot him if he did not leave. The boy stood on the landing outside the bedroom with the gun to his shoulder. The gun was discharged and the shot went through the door and struck the man in the left side of his chest. A circular dent was found beside the hole in the door and it could have been produced by forcible contact with the muzzle of the gun. The deceased may have slammed the door, causing it to hit the gun and the discharge was then involuntary. It could have been a recoil mark after intentional discharge, but the former view was accepted.

There was a circular hole in the right upper panel of the door, approximately an inch in diameter and approximately 48 in. above the floor. The woodwork around the hole on the inner side was splintered. The direction of aim was in a horizontal line, directed from left to right, i.e. towards a bed inside the room, to the

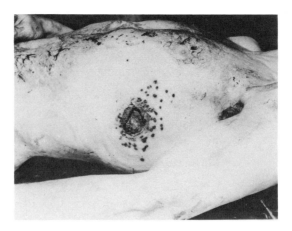

FIG. 68. Shotgun, 12-bore injury. Range: at about 2 yards. Pattern of injury to chest modified by (a) shot passing through panel of door and (b) left hand at side of chest—hence no pellet marks below main hole (see Fig. 69: the hand). (Case No. 15.)

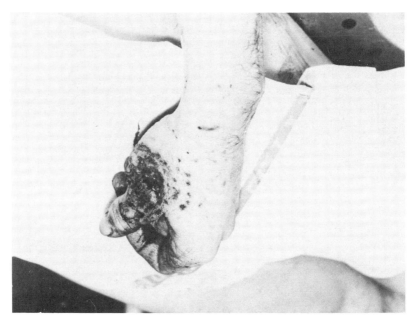

FIG. 69. Shotgun injury: Range at about 2 yards. Hand injured when held beside chest. Main and fatal injury to chest (see Fig. 68). (Case No. 15.)

right of the door. The victim was standing within a few feet of the door. This reconstruction was based on the appearances of the injuries and the distribution of blood in the bedroom.

The deceased had shotgun injuries on the left side of his chest, centred at 46 in. above the heel of his boot. They were in the form of a large entrance hole, $1 \times 1^3/_4$ in., with a serrated margin, situated 6 in. below and 3 in. behind the left nipple. It was accompanied by fifty-one satellite punctures almost all of which were in the skin above a horizontal line through the major wound; the skin below that level was intact. Had they been spread all round the major wound, the area would have been about 5 in. in diameter (Fig. 68).

The abnormal distribution of the pellet wounds was at once explained by an examination of his left hand Fig. 69. The metacarpo-phalangeal joint of the thumb was disrupted and several satellite punctures were above it in the skin between the thumb and index finger. His hand must have been raised beside his chest and received part of the charge of shot, and in turn, that part of his chest wall had been protected.

A spread of shot over 5 in. normally represents a range of about 12 ft, but the present range must have been less than 11 ft because that was the distance between the door and the outer wall of the room. Blood stains on the carpet indicated that he must have been near to the door, not more than 5 ft from it. Tests were not made, so that the effect of passage through the panel of the door on the spread of shot was not ascertained.

Internal examination demonstrated a ragged crater, 2 in. in diameter, within the chest. The left pleura contained a pint of blood together with a wad, cards and pellets. There were several punctures of the left lung. Several ribs, notably 7–10, were fractured.

The track was slightly downwards. There was a tear $2\frac{1}{2}$ in. long in the left dome of the diaphragm, and the stomach, punctured by shot, had herniated into the pleural sac. Pellet injuries were present in the splenic flexure of the colon and the spleen. Three pellets had traversed the aorta to produce pairs of punctures beside the origins of the 5th and 7th intercostal arteries. One pellet had opened a vein at the back of the left ventricle. The pericardium contained 4 ounces of blood.

There was a small cut in his left upper eyelid and an abrasion of his face, produced by splinters of wood, not pellets. This indicated he must have been near the door since the splintered wood was near to it (F.M. 9662A).

Case No. 16

Site: Head. *Range:* near. Accident. *Weapon:* shotgun

In this case the victim, a farmer, was found lying on his back, on snow and ice, near a gate into one of his fields. His shotgun was to the left of his body. His cap and glasses were still on his head (Fig. 71). An entrance wound, almost circular, $\frac{3}{8}$ in. in diameter, was at the right side of his head $2\frac{1}{2}$ in. behind and 2 in. above the outer opening of the right ear. The wound was within the hair but there was no singeing; some fouling by smoke and tattooing were apparent. Blood in the adjacent tissues was bright red and contained CO, saturation being estimated at 10 per cent. The entrance wound in the skull was somewhat pear-shaped, $\frac{7}{8} \times \frac{3}{4}$ in. in its axes; its margin was blackened by powder. Bevelling was indicative of an ingoing force. The posterior half of the skull was extensively comminuted but there was no exit wound. The pellets had passed in a more or less solid mass to plough a ragged track through the right parietal and left occipital lobes of the brain. A card was also within the skull. The site of the injury was unusual for suicide and tests with the gun, fired at portions of calvaria bearing hairy scalp, showed that the probable range was one of about three inches; it was not a contact injury. It was believed that he had slipped on the snow—the soles of his wellingtons were smooth with wear— and had been accidentally shot. The only feature inconsistent with this interpretation was the fact that the trigger of this weapon required a pull of $4\frac{1}{2}$ lb and, therefore, it was unlikely to have been discharged accidentally (Dr. F. G. Tryhorn) (F.M. 4042A, Figs. 70, 71).

Case No. 17

Site: Chest. *Range:* near. Accident. *Weapon:* sporting gun.

This man was found lying on his back close to a barbed wire fence. His 12-bore sporting gun lay at his right side (Fig. 72). He was fully clothed and wore wellington boots, the soles of which were smooth. An oval, ragged hole 2×1 in. was present in his tweed jacket, on the inner side of the left revere; fouling by powder was apparent round the hole. The entrance wound was almost circular, $1\frac{1}{8}$ in. in diameter, but the lower part of its periphery was straightened and at each end of this segment there was a small side laceration, one $\frac{3}{8}$ in. and the other $\frac{1}{8}$ in. long, at right angles to the main wound (Fig. 73). There was slight shelving of the circumference of the wound on the right side. A few small, circular, recent bruises beyond the wound marked the position of pellets in the subcutaneous tissues; one pellet was visible at the body surface. The pellets had entered the left chest at a point over the fourth rib at $\frac{3}{4}$ in. to the left of the sternum and had passed downwards and outwards. Outlying pellets, probably deflected by the ribs, had passed through the chest and were embedded in the chest wall (Fig. 73). The base of the left lung and the apex of the heart were lacerated, and the half of the diaphragm had been torn open; the stomach and part of the transverse colon had prolapsed into the thorax. The fundus of the stomach was lacerated for a distance of 4 in. along the greater curvature. There were linear tears of the left lobe of the liver. Three small, separate bruises on the front of the left kidney had been caused by pellets. The upper half of the spleen was lacerated. An oval laceration, $1\frac{1}{2} \times \frac{1}{3}$ in., was found in the pleura over the 9th

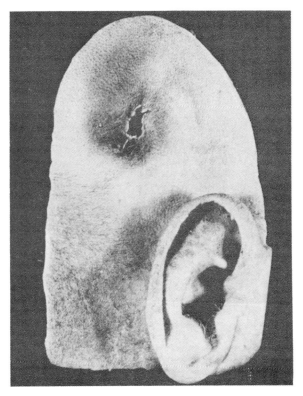

FIG. 70. Shotgun (0.410) "near" injury: above and
behind right ear. (?accidental: ??suicidal.) (Case No. 16.)

and 10th ribs at the left side of the chest. Pellets were alone recovered from the body but a wad was found
between his shirt and vest.

The appearances were consistent with a cross-shot from right to left, passing down and out, at near range.

His left woollen stocking was torn and there were linear scratches on the skin of his left leg. Fibres of wool
identical with those of his stocking were found in the barbed wire in front of the body (Fig. 74). It appeared he
had lost his footing when he had attempted to cross the fence and the gun was accidentally discharged (F.M.
5541 A).

Case No. 18

Site: back. *Range*: under 1 yard Accident. *Weapon*: shotgun. 12-bore.

A boy aged 15 handed his shotgun to a friend before he climbed a fence. It appeared that when trying to
make it safe the friend discharged the gun and the deceased was shot in the back. His clothing had a circular
hole $^7/_8$ in. in diameter punched out of the material. There was no singeing, fouling or tattooing of the
garments. A circular entrance wound, 1 in. in diameter, was centred at $2^1/_2$ in. to the right of the mid-line over
the lower ribs. The shot had entered as if a solid mass of metal; no outlying pellet injuries. The pellets lay in a
compact mass inside the body near the lower dorsal spine which was shattered; two cards and a wad were also
inside the abdomen. No exit wound. The right kidney and right lobe of the liver were lacerated and there was
bruising of the bases of the lungs. The direction of aim was horizontal. The circumstantial evidence confirmed
that this had been an accident at a range of just under 1 yard (F.M. 6873A, Fig. 75).

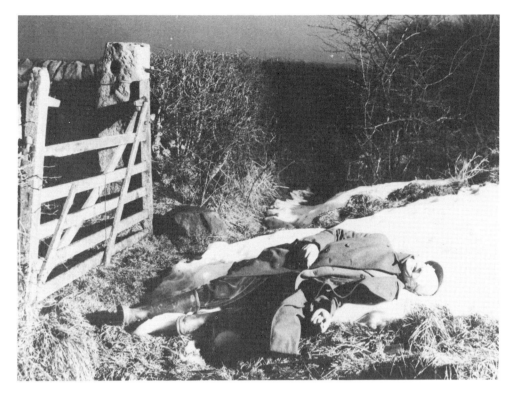

F𝚤ɢ. 71. Scene of injury to head by 0.410 shotgun: ?accident ??suicide. (Case No. 16.)

Case No. 19

Site: (a) abdomen (distant); (b) chest (near). Homicide, *Weapon*: 12-bore shotgun. *Ammunition*: No. 4 shot.

This man, aged 20, was shot twice, first at a distance, in the lower abdomen and, secondly, in the right side of the chest at near range.

The abdominal injury. Punctures by individual pellets, about 160 in all, were distributed in an area 6 × 7 in., between the pubes and umbilicus in the middle third of the front of the abdomen. Internal examination showed that there were innumerable punctures of the intestines estimated at forty in the large bowel and over 500 in the small intestine, together with twenty more in the bladder and twenty in the liver. The abdominal aorta was punctured at $^1/_2$ in. above its bifurcation and one pellet had traversed the right common iliac artery to produce two punctures in its wall. The peritoneum contained $1^1/_2$ pints of blood from which fifty pellets were recovered. There was no exit wound.

The range of fire, as judged by test with the weapon, was approximately 12 ft.

The chest injury. An oval entrance wound, 2 × 1 in., unaccompanied by satellite injuries, was situated in the upper half of the front of the right side of the chest. The wound had an irregular margin, slightly flattened below, with downward bevelling. Fragments of cloth were in the wound.

The right pleura contained 2 pints of blood in which a wad and cards were found. Shot had traversed the upper and lower lobes of the lung, of which about two-thirds were destroyed, partly by pellets and partly by portions of fractured ribs. There were a few pellets in the remains of the lower lobe. The pleura was punctured in several places close to the spine.

The pericardium contained 2 ounces of blood and four pellets. There were twenty punctures in the pericardium and in the upper part of the heart, notably in the atria. The right ventricle was intact, but two pellets were present in the left ventricle.

The range of fire was less than 3 ft and the direction of aim was downwards and backwards towards the middle line. None of the shot had caused the abdominal injuries. There was no exit wound.

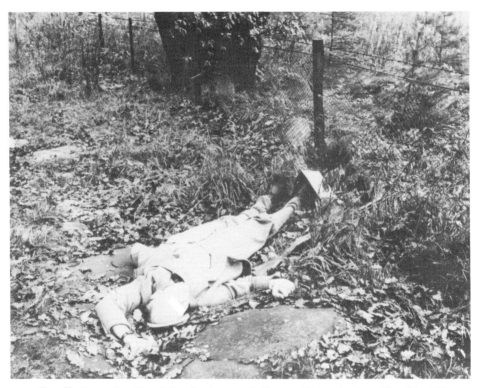

FIG. 72. Scene of accidental shooting in a wood. Shotgun 12-bore, in chest. (Case No. 17.)

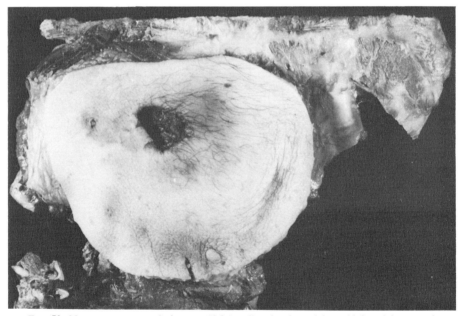

FIG. 73. Near entrance wound: shotgun, 12-bore; direction from right and left and downwards.
(Case No. 17.)

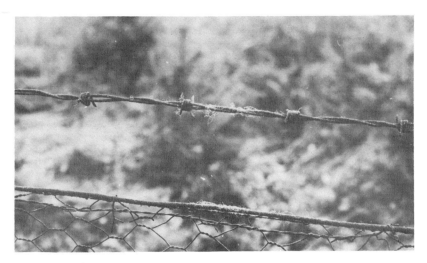

FIG. 74. Fibres of wool from deceased's stocking on barbed wire fence; indication of a
slip when attempting to climb over the fence: accidental shooting. (Case No. 17.)

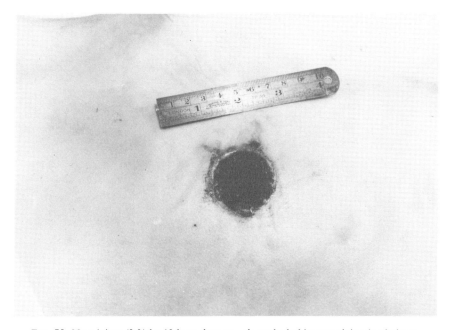

FIG. 75. Near injury (2 ft) by 12-bore shotgun—through clothing over loin; simulating a
contact injury: see the clothing as well as the body. (Case No. 18.)

The weapon was an old 12-bore shotgun in good condition; shot No. 4 Eley.

He had first been shot at a range of about 12 ft. After his collapse he was shot a second time at close range,
under 3 ft, while laid on the ground. He had a split lip and some teeth had been recently dislodged. These
injuries could have been produced by a blow with the butt of the gun or a kick (F.M. 12,907A).

Ranges of over 1 yard

The resulting injuries are normally produced by the shot alone and, as the range increases, the shot diverge more and more widely. Assuming the barrel to be a cylinder, without "choke", the diameter of the area in which the pellets lie, measured in inches, minus one, represents the approximate range in yards. Due allowance must be made for idiosyncrasy of the weapon and kind of ammunition. A fully choked barrel, keeping the shot compact over a greater distance, reduces the area by about one-quarter; over a range of, say, 19 yards the spread with a choked barrel is only about 15 in., whereas it would be about 20 in. from an unchoked one. It must be emphasised that these calculations are always only approximate and whenever practicable an estimate of the range must be based on tests with the suspected weapon.

At a range of up to about 4 yards the bulk of the shot is still in a compact mass, capable of tearing a large hole in the body. If the shot strikes it at an angle of less than 90°, e.g. from above downwards, the wound is in effect the result of tearing away a triangular flap of tissue. It will be accompanied by several secondary entrance wounds, some of which may be circular punctures and others superficial grooves, the latter made by shot striking the skin tangentially (Figs 84, 85; F.M. 4764A). When the shot enters the body at right angles, on the other hand, the shot is likely to punch a large circular hole and this will be surrounded by discrete, secondary entrance wounds (Fig. 76). The principal entrance wound was 2 ins. in diameter and the diameter of the spread was $4^1/_4$ in., the range being estimated at $3^1/_2$ yards.

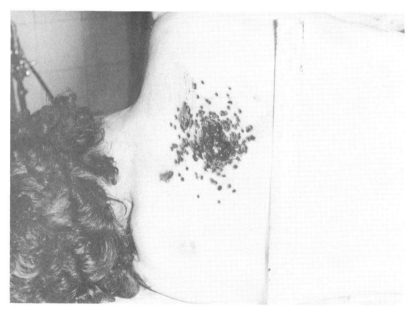

Fig. 76. Shotgun (12-bore) homicidal wound at range of about 12 ft. (At level of 4th dorsal vertebra.) (Case No. 20.)

Case No. 20

Site: Back. *Range*: 12 ft. Homicide. *Weapon*: 12-bore shotgun. *Ammunition*: No. 6 shot.

This woman, aged 65, was shot in the back by her husband (see Case No. 3, Fig. 58).

They had quarrelled and she was about to leave the house. The key to the front door was still in her left hand when her body was found on the floor between the front door and the stairs. From the appearance of the injury the range of fire was estimated at about 12 ft; this was later confirmed by tests with the gun. The husband had been standing at the top of the stairs when he shot her. He then went into the bedroom and shot himself.

Collapse was immediate and she was rendered immobile by spinal injury. Blood at the scene was restricted to a pool on the floor under her head and right arm.

The entrance wound at the back of her body, $1\,^1/_2 \times 1\,^1/_4$ in. was accompanied by a number of satellite punctures in an area 4×3 in., the centre of which was at the level of the 4th dorsal vertebra. The wad had produced a semi-lunar, bruised abrasion, just above the entrance hole.

Internal examination showed that the transverse process of the 4th dorsal vertebra had been detached and blown forwards so as to lacerate the main pulmonary artery in an area 2×1 in. The middle lobe of the right lung was lacerated by shot and portions of bone, in a track 2 in. wide. Pellets were present in the upper and lower lobes of the lung. The 5th and 6th dorsal vertebrae were also damaged.

The spinal cord was lacerated at the level of the 6th dorsal vertebra. A wad and woollen fibres were recovered from the para-spinal tissues in this region.

Four fresh bruises on the left upper arm were of the kind produced by a firm grip of the arm (F.M. 13,232B).

At a range of 10 yards or over the spread of shot is such that there is no principal entrance wound and each shot produces its own small wound. The majority are superficial injuries, the pellets for the most part penetrating no deeper than muscle. It can be, however, that one or more pellets penetrate deeply to cause fatal injury. In Dr. Gerald Evans' case (Fig. 78) death was due to injury of the liver. Should the pellets strike the neck, one or more may perforate the carotid artery and so cause fatal haemorrhage. This

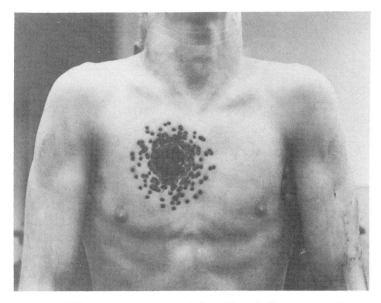

FIG. 77. Shotgun injury at range of about 12–14 ft. (By courtesy of Dr. Lester James.)

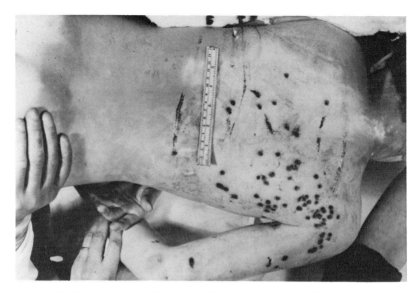

FIG. 78. Shotgun injury—12-bore—at distant range: approx. 10 yards. A few shots penetrated abdomen and injured liver. Death from internal haemorrhage. (By courtesy of the late Dr. Gerald Evans.)

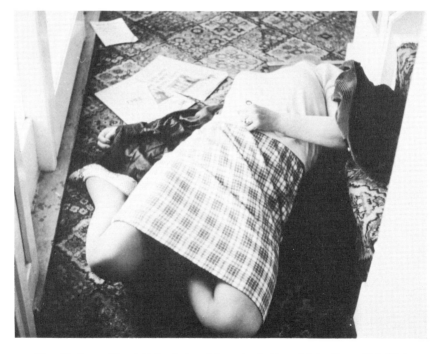

FIG. 79. Scene of homicide by shotgun injury: stood at top of stairs. Range 12 ft. (Note key held in left hand.) (Case No. 20.)

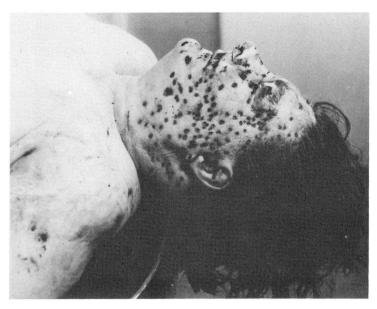

FIG. 80. Shotgun injury, 12-bore. Range of about 15 yards. Fatal haemorrhage due to severance of the left external carotid artery by one of the pellets.

occurred when a woman was shot in the head and neck at a range of about 15 yards (F.M. 9378A, Fig. 80).

When the shot have travelled for just over a yard the peripheral pellets begin to separate from the mass of shot and lie a millimetre or so apart from it. The resulting injury, although a circular or oval wound, depending on the angulation of the muzzle to the body surface, is not a clean cut injury. Naked-eye may fail to make the distinction but, under low magnification, it is possible to detect notches in the margin of the wound, produced by individual pellets, of up to about half their diameter. It is only when the range increases that these pellets produce separate satellite punctures.

Case No. 21

Site: chest. *Range*: distant. Homicide. *Weapon*: sawn-off shotgun.

The deceased, aged 30, was a police inspector who was shot by a man making his escape from a warehouse after having murdered the night watchman (see Case No. 21, Fig. 81.). The precise range was not stated but it was one of several feet.

The officer was fully clothed when he received a charge of shot in the left side of his chest. The spread of shot was such that there were over 230 separate punctures and no central hole. Each puncture was one of up to $^1/_8$ in. in diameter in an area 13 in. vertically and 8 in. horizontally, in the side of the chest between the armpit and hip. The centre of the area was 52 in. above the sole of the foot. Some of the pellets had been arrested beneath the skin, but a considerable number had penetrated the wall of the chest and abdomen. Punctures were also found at the back of the left arm; there was also some longitudinal grooving of the skin due to tangential contact by some of the pellets. An abrasion of the left cheek and laceration of the eyebrow were probably sustained when he collapsed.

The chest was penetrated on the left side in the area between the 4th-11th intercostal spaces. The track of the pellets was in a broad band across the middle third of the chest from left to right. The left pleura contained $1^1/_2$ pints of blood. Thirty-five punctures were seen in the left lung and shot had traversed the lung to lodge near

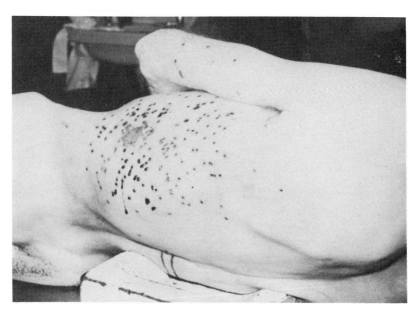

FIG. 81. Shotgun (12-bore) injury: range about 10 yards. Pellets lacerated the left
lung and three perforated the aorta. (Case No. 21.)

the spine. These pellets were found in the lower lobe of the left lung. There were eight punctures in the left side of the heart and two of the pellets had crossed through the interventricular septum to reach the outer wall of the right ventricle. The pericardium contained $^3/_4$ pint of blood.

There were at least twenty-five punctures in the left dome of the diaphragm. Fifteen pellets were found in the spleen, one in the pancreas and two in the left lobe of the liver. The aorta had been traversed by pellets; three pairs of punctures were found in its wall at a point $1^1/_2$ in. above the origin of the coeliac axis (F.M. 14,646).

Case No. 22 (*Fig. 82, 83*)

Site: arm and chest. *Range*: contact, apparently distant. Accidental. *Weapon*: 0.410 shotgun.

Special interest. The appearances, to a lay observer, were those of injury at a range beyond self-infliction because a contact injury in the right arm had escaped notice.

This boy, aged 13, was accompanied by a younger boy, in a field near his home. He was carrying a loaded 0.410 shotgun and when they were about 4 yards from a stone wall he slipped and fell on the wet, uneven and slippery ground. The gun was discharged and he was shot. He got up and turned back to run home; he had only gone about 35 yards when he collapsed, and shortly afterwards, died. This account was given by the younger boy, but it was at first doubted because, when his body was examined by the police, the only injury observed was that in the deceased's chest. Preliminary, amateur tests had been made with the gun and the range was estimated at 12 ft.

There was a small collection of blood at the place where he died. A tiny spot of blood was found on a blade of grass a few feet nearer to the wall, but there was no trail of blood; until he collapsed, all bleeding had been internal.

The body had been stripped before the investigating team arrived at the mortuary. Examination of the clothing showed the presence of two holes in the right sleeve of the boy's sweater, one at the elbow and the other near the right armpit.

The correct interpretation was ascertained when the right arm was abducted and examined. There was a contact entrance wound, presenting as a round hole $^1/_2$ in. in diameter, bordered by a zone of blackening $^1/_{16}$ in. broad, on the inner side of the right elbow joint, over the inner condyle of the humerus. The entrance wound was 14 in. above the right thumb and 44 in. above the sole of his foot. Soiling of the skin in an area $^3/_4 \times ^1/_4$ in. was also present below the wound (Fig. 83).

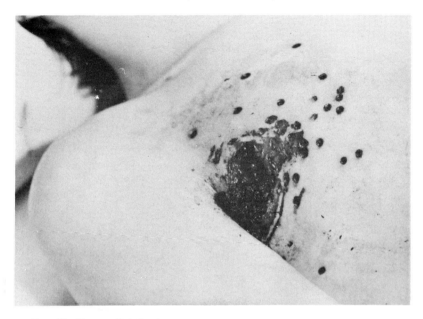

FIG. 82. Shotgun (0.410) injury: superficial resemblance of a wound inflicted at a range of about 8 ft (see Case No. 22, Fig. 83).

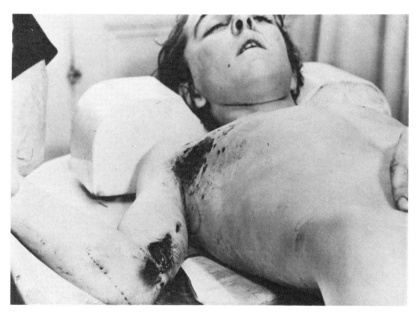

FIG. 83. Shotgun (0.410) injury. Contact wound on inner side of right elbow joint. Tangential laceration immediately above and shot passed to enter the chest, in front of the armpit. (Case No. 22.)

Pellet injuries were present in the skin of the arm. At $^1/_4$ in. above the entrance wound, pellets had produced an oval, superficial wound, 2×1 in., prolonged by furrowing of the skin by tangential contact for a further distance of $1 \times {}^1/_2$ in. A solitary pellet was found beneath the skin at 3 in. below the armpit.

The principal damage had been caused by the relatively compact mass of shot entering the chest beside the armpit. They had inflicted an oval, secondary entrance wound in the form of a hole $^1/_2$ in. in diamter, set in an area of abrasion 2×1 in. Satellite punctures by individual pellets were around the entrance hole in an area of between $3^1/_2$ in. and $4^1/_2$ in. (Fig. 82).

The shot had penetrated the pectoralis muscles, and fibres of cloth, a wad, cards and pellets were recovered from the track. No major vessel had been damaged but there were a number of punctures of the upper lobe of the right lung. The lower lobe was intact. The right pleura contained about a pint of blood. There was no damage to the heart or left lung. No natural disease to account for his death or his fall.

The internal diameter of the gun was $^1/_2$ in. and the distance from muzzle to trigger 28 in.; the distance from trigger to heel of the butt was $14^1/_2$ in.; overall length 43 in. The boy's arm, from the point of the shoulder to the thumb measured 24 in. He had released the trigger accidentally when he slipped (F.M. 15,505A).

Case No. 23. 12-bore Injury: 3 to 4 yards: Homicidal

This man was shot by his father from an upper window; the distance between the muzzle and the head of the victim, when erect, was not more than 12 ft and not less than 9 ft.

The shot had separated before they struck the victim but the majority entered in a compact mass to tear a triangular flap out of his left cheek (Figs. 84, 85). Numerous small outlying injuries by individual pellets were also present in the form of gutters or small circular pits in the skin (Fig. 85). One of the cards had struck his nose to produce a crescentic abrasion on the left nostril. The track of the pellets was down and to the right, involving the neck structures and the upper lobe of the right lung (Fig. 86). A solitary pellet had been deflected upwards and was found at the under surface of the right frontal lobe. (*R.* v. *Wharton*, 1956, F.M. 4764A.)

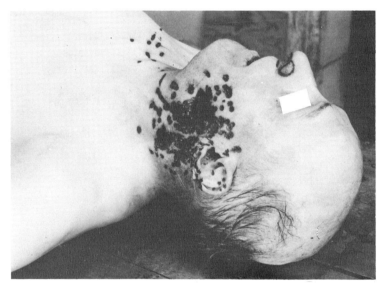

FIG. 84. Shotgun, 12-bore injury. Range approx. 12 ft; direction: from the left to right and downwards. (Case No. 23.)

INJURY BY THE BLAST OF A SHOTGUN

A man was killed by a shotgun when it was discharged at close range, notwithstanding that no pellet entered his body. A considerable area of the soft tissues of the left side of his chest had been lacerated and underlying ribs had been fractured. He had also sustained laceration of his left lung and haemothorax. There was a

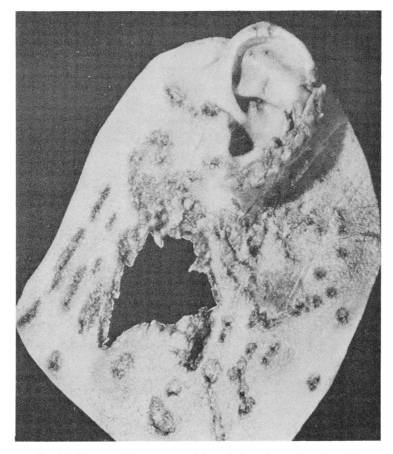

FIG. 85. Shotgun, 12-bore: range 12 ft, "D"-shaped tear. (Case No. 23.)

smaller area of laceration of the skin of the inner side of the left arm (Fig. 87). It was clear that the shot, wad and cards had passed between his chest and arm and his fatal injury was primarily due to blast (P.M. by Dr. Lester James 1959; C. P. in attendance).

EXIT WOUNDS

At contact or near range the exit wound is characterised by greater disruption of tissues than is seen in the entrance wound. There is no singeing, blackening nor tattooing of the margins. The appearances are essentially those of a gross eversion and disruption of the parts. The top or the side of the head and the intra-cranial contents may have been blown away. Shot, felt and cards will probably travel through the head and be lost, although cards and wads may be found at the scene and pellets may lodge in any adjacent woodwork. At 10 yards or over it is unlikely that the shot will penetrate beyond the subcutaneous tissues or muscles; even so, a few pellets can enter and kill.

With some contact or near injuries, the cards, wad and shot may remain in the body and there is no exit wound.

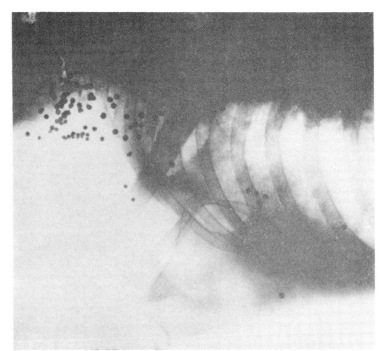

FIG. 86. Shotgun injury: X-ray of chest and neck; showing distribution of pellets inside the body (see Fig. 84). (Case No. 23.)

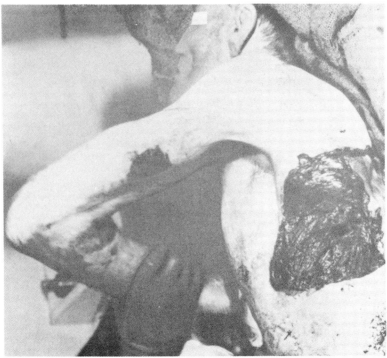

FIG. 87. Shotgun injury, 12-bore. Shot, cards and wad passed between arm and chest. Fatal injury by blast. (By courtesy of Dr. Lester James.)

TANGENTIAL, NON-FATAL INJURIES

There are occasions when the shot strike the body tangentially and fail to cause fatal injury, although there may be appreciable superficial damage. This happened in three cases of attempted suicide; two of the subjects achieved suicide by a second shot, but one of them survived. Thus, in Case No. 3, p. 215, the man's first shot was aimed from left to right, from beneath the chin towards the right side of his neck. This destroyed the superficial tissues and opened a vein. He then fired a second shot at his forehead and destroyed his skull and brain. In similar fashion, a second subject fired his first shot into the lower part of his chest, a "through and through" wound, which damaged only his large intestine. His second and fatal shot was into his forehead. The third subject, a woman, shot herself in the left side of the upper abdomen. It was a "through and through" injury but no major structure had been damaged and she recovered.

A man who shot his wife and two children then committed suicide by shooting himself. His first attempt was a tangential shot in the upper abdomen; this caused only a deep gutter in the abdominal wall. His second shot, an inch away from the first, produced a "through and through" injury but he did not succeed until he fired a third time, at contact range at his forehead (F.M. 15,916D).

Rifled Firearm Wounds

ENTRANCE WOUNDS

Contact Wounds

(i) *Over dense bone.* These wounds are characterised by their irregular, stellate shape and everted margins, which are bruised. It is also to be noted that changes in the adjacent skin due to burning, fouling by smoke and involuntary tattooing are slight or absent, notwithstanding it is a contact wound. The paradox is only apparent. When the gun is pressed firmly against dense bone, the explosion splits the skin and on expansion the gases, recoiling from hard bone, penetrate the subcutaneous tissues and evert the skin. Also, almost the whole of the products of the explosion enter the wound and blackening is then confined to the subcutaneous tissues and bone. The soft tissues are grimed and torn to a degree never seen except in contact wounds. It is sometimes possible to demonstrate carbon monoxide, even to a saturation by 60 per cent, in blood from the damaged tissues (e.g. Case No. 35, F.M. 5518; contact injury with 0.455 revolver).

Such injuries are not the invariable result of contact explosions, but when they occur they are strongly indicative of self-infliction. (The possibility that the homicide can press the weapon closely against the skull of a incapacitated victim remains.) These injuries are normally seen over the forehead (F.M. 7502A; Fig. 88) or the mastoid region (F.M. 6951B); in these sites the bone is of sufficient density to resist the explosive forces so as to lead to stellate skin wounds. They may occur in the temple, as depicted by Gonzales *et al.* (1954).

(ii) *Over thin bone.* In these situations the wound is normally a circular hole bordered by a band of bruising and abrasion, the abrasion or contusion *collar*; the overall diameter of the hole plus the collar represents the approximate diameter of the bullet.

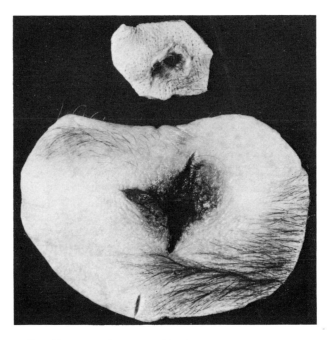

FIG. 88. Automatic pistol (P. 38) injuries: (a) upper wound: a characteristic stellate laceration of skin over dense bone—just above right eye-brow; (b) lower wound: the exit wound, in left temple. (Case No. 24.)

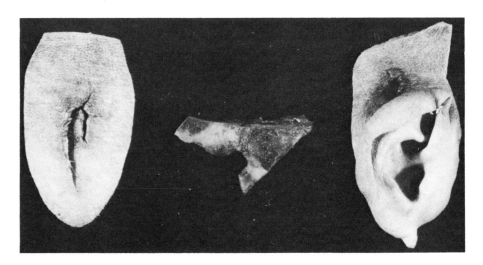

FIG. 89. Automatic pistol (0.32) entrance wound in right temple. A "near" injury—fouling of wound by smoke, and involuntary tattooing around the abrasion collar and entrance hole (see Fig. 90 for exit wound.) (Case No. 26.)

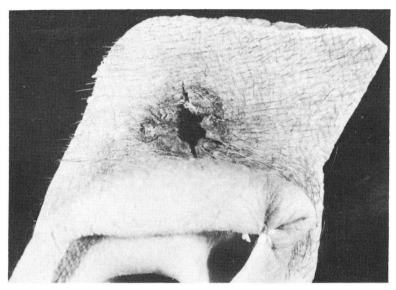

FIG. 90. Automatic pistol (0.32) exit wound (see Fig. 89 for entrance wound). (Case No. 26.)

The hair in the vicinity may be singed this is not invariable in contact injuries, notably when 0.22 ammunition is responsible; the distance which flame travels is probably only about 2 in. and less than 6 in. Some fouling by smoke and tattooing of the skin by unburnt powder may also be seen in an area about 1 in. around the entrance wound (Case No. 26A, Fig. 91). The bullet drills a circular hole in the bone and there may be fissured fractures

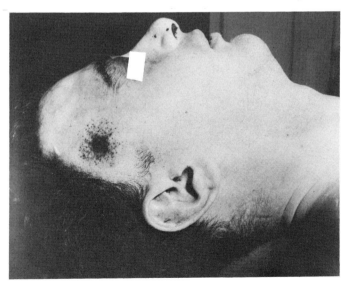

FIG. 91. Automatic pistol (0.32) entrance wound in right temple. A "near" injury—fouling of wound by smoke, and involuntary tattooing around the abrasion collar and entrance hole (see Fig. 92 for exit wound). (Case No. 26.)

running from the circumference into the adjacent bone. If the bone is unduly thin, there is local comminution and the circular hole thereby obscured; if of moderate thickness, then bevelling is apparent, i.e. the inner table bears a larger hole than the outer, as shown by the bevelled edge of the hole.

The external appearances are more or less similar, irrespective of the site, if thin bone, chest wall or abdominal wall, except that contact injury of the abdomen with rifled arms is distinctly unusual; the site of election in suicide is the right temple, as to about 80 per cent.

When the weapon is not at right angles to the surface, products of the explosion escape so as to injure the skin, within a limited zone at the circumference of the entrance wound.

Close contact against bone, in particular dense bone, may be followed by recoil injury; an imprint of the end of the gun may then accompany the entrance wound. Even when only partial, this patterned abrasion or bruised abrasion is of obvious importance as proof of a contact injury. It may be beside or overlap the entrance wound.

At times the entrance wound may be obscure; this is likely in the rare event of entry at the inner canthus of an eye. The swollen lids of the victim close over the entrance wound whilst the exit wound, at the back of the head, may then be thought to be the result of a blow from a blunt instrument.

Entrance wounds in the roof the mouth may be small and obscure (Piédelièvre and Desoille, 1939). They may be overlooked and the cause of death not ascertained.

Case No. 24. P. 38 (9 mm) Automatic Pistol Shot to the Head; Contact Injury. Split Wound of Forehead: Suicidal

A man aged 34 who was found fully clothed in his motor car. The entrance wound was a stellate split of the skin, a triangle with one or two small side splits, of up to $1^3/_8$ in. in its axes, situated over the lower part of the front of the right temple, just above the outer third of the supra-orbital margin (Fig. 88).

There was no blackening or tattooing of the skin but there was blackening of the soft subcutaneous tissues; blood in the area had a bright pink colour, due to the presence of carbon monoxide. The underlying bone was comminuted but it was apparent that there had been a circular hole driven through the bone, approximately $3/_8$ in. in diameter. The centre of the hole was situated $1/_4$ in. above the right supra-orbital margin and 1 in. to the right of the outer end of the right eye, 3 in. above the outer opening of the right ear.

The exit wound was present on the left side of the head at about the middle of the left temple in the form of a laceration $3/_4$ in. long gaping by $1/_4$ in., the long axis lying vertically (Fig. 88). There was no blackening of this wound nor any pink discoloration of the blood in the neighbourhood. There was a small herniation of brain. The wound was situated just outside the hairline, 2 in. above the outer end of the left eye.

The bullet appeared to have traversed the head from right to left in a slightly downward direction. There was some blood, in the form of small splashes, on the index finger and thumb of the right hand. There was comminution of the right anterior quadrant of the skull with fissured fractures causing separation of a large piece of bone, the right half of the frontal bone and the right parietal bone. The supra-orbital margins were also involved. The saggital suture had been sprung open. There was comminution of the floor of the anterior fossa, especially of the roof of the nose and each orbit. There had been bleeding from the right ear. The bullet had passed through the anterior part of the right frontal lobe to cause laceration of the brain and had then run under the left frontal lobe to cause a little laceration of the cortex. The exit hole was circular.

Bleeding into the skull was slight but a fair amount of blood was found in the motor vehicle; some of this blood had no doubt drained out of the skull, after death. There was a fair quantity of blood in the trachea and main bronchi but he did not appear to have inhaled blood into the lungs. Flame-shaped (shock) haemorrhages were present beneath the inner lining of the left ventricle (F.M. 7502A).

Case No. 25. Contact Wound: Suicidal: Revolver. Stellate Wound

A man aged 55 was found fully clothed on his bed; a revolver was clasped in his right hand (instant rigor). A stellate wound was present in the right side of the forehead. Powder marking of the edges and subcutaneous tissues present; entrance hole in skull $1/_4$ in. in diameter. No exit wound; bullet found in the cerebellum. (Leeds City Coroner: No. 294/41.)

Case No. 26. Contact: 0.32 (German 7.65 mm) Automatic: Suicidal

When found gravely ill on a couch he appeared to have a laceration $^3/_4$ in. long near the left temple. He had black hair which had obscured the entrance wound in his right temple. After shaving the area a circular wound with an abrasion collar $^1/_8$ in. in diameter was seen in an area of involuntary tattooing 1 in. in diameter (Fig. 91). The track of the bullet lay horizontally through each frontal lobe. The bone below the entrance wound was distinctly thin. Singeing of the hair was not detected but flame from these cartridges is probably negligible. He survived the injury by about 10 hours (F.M. 5275A, Figs. 91, 92).

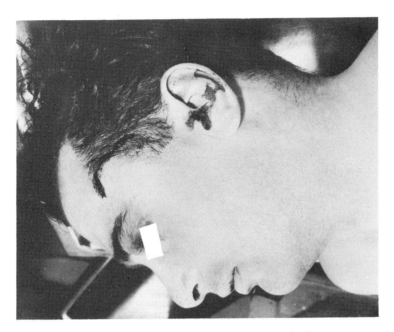

FIG. 92. Automatic pistol (0.32) exit wound (see Fig. 91 for entrance wound). (Case No. 26.)

Case No. 27. Contact Injury: Automatic 0.25: Suicidal

The victim, a man aged 49, was found lying dead on his back in a park shelter. There was an entrance wound in the right temple and an automatic pistol was on the ground near his right hand (Fig. 93). He had been in financial difficulties and was in trouble with the police. A letter to the coroner indicated his intention to commit suicide.

The entrance wound, bordered by an abrasion collar, was 5 mm in diameter. The hair and skin around the wound were scorched and blackened; the margins of the wound were inverted. No exit wound. A discharged automatic pistol cartridge case was found in the shelter and a nickel-covered lead bullet, 0.25 in. calibre, was recovered from the skull. The skull showed a spider-web comminution, without displacement of the fragments, in the left parietal region. The wound was within the hairline and was not observed by the person who found the body (F. M. 1424).

Case No. 28. Contact Wound: 0.22 Winchester Rifle: Suicidal

This man leant on the rifle and shot himself in the middle line of the forehead 2 cm above the root of the nose, 5 mm above the supra-orbital margins. Circular entrance hole with abrasion collar $^1/_3$ in., traces of blackening by powder around and beneath the hole. No singeing. Bruising of eyelids but not the eyes. Bleeding from nose and ears. No exit wound. Hole in outer table 0.7 mm and in inner table 10 mm. Comminution of roof of nose and both orbits; fissured fracture line to right middle ear. The bullet passed

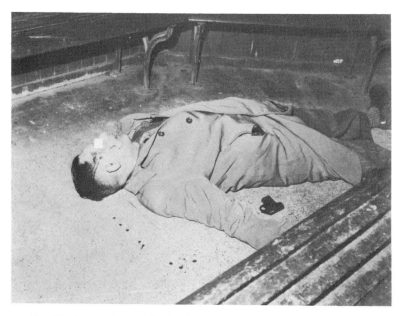

Fig. 93. Automatic pistol (0.25) suicide. Scene of death—a shelter in a park.
(Note entrance wound in right temple. Scanty bleeding at the scene.) (Case No.
27.)

between the hemispheres and was arrested just within the cortex of the left occipital lobe; it had rotated through 180°; a lead 0.22 bullet with flattened nose (F.M. 6742A).

Case No. 29. *Contact Wound: 0.22 Winchester Rifle: Suicidal*

An entrance wound, having a dark red abrasion collar, of $^1/_4$ in. in diameter, was present in the left temple. No singeing, fouling or tattooing. Surgical toilet in hospital had removed any fouling by smoke. No exit wound. The bullet was not found, but fragments of lead were present in the brain and X-ray examination confirmed the presence of opaque fragments, presumably of the bullet. A circular hole in the skull with fracture lines extending into the frontal bone. Superficial laceration of the left frontal pole.

Found seriously injured, unconscious and bleeding, in his car, slumped between the steering wheel and the offside door. A 0.22 Winchester rifle rested with its butt on the passenger seat; the muzzle was below the body. The safety catch was off; the gun had recently been fired and a spent cartridge case was found on the road at the rear of the car. His shattered spectacles lay on the floor of the car. The police believed he had shot himself in the road and found a trail of blood from the site of spent cartridge to the car. He had regained the car but had collapsed before he could turn it round in order to get help; the car went forwards into a field. He had threatened to shoot himself (F.M. 5685E).

Case No. 30

Site: head. *Range:* contact. Self-inflicted. *Weapon*: Colt 0.380 police special revolver, but altered to smaller size by amateur (Figs. 94, 95).

After forcing an entry the police found the body of a woman laid on one bed of a pair of twin beds. She held a revolver in her right hand. Her dark black hair was saturated with blood. No wound was visible at this stage. Search discovered a bullet embedded in the wall to the left of the body at 6 ft above the floor. Another bullet was embedded in the wall of an adjacent bathroom, at about 2 ft. above the floor. This bullet had come from the bedroom and had passed through the wall between it and the bathroom.

The barrel of the revolver, a Colt 0.380 police special, contained six cartridges; two live; two recently fired, and two fired some time earlier. It was the property of her husband who had a small collection of firearms in the house. He was absent.

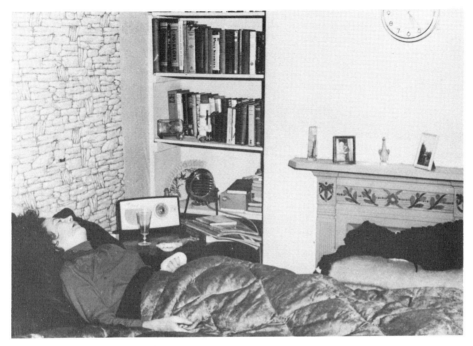

FIG. 94. Scene of suicide with revolver: female victim. Mark on wall to her left marks site of one of the two bullets fired. (Case No. 30.)

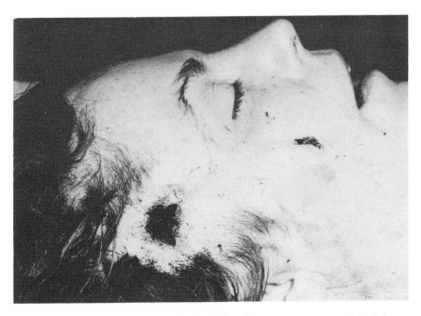

FIG. 95. Suicide with revolver: female victim. Contact entrance wound in right temple. (Case No. 30.)

The initial view of the circumstances was, understandably, one of strong suspicion. The victim was a woman who had been shot, apparently in the back of her head (the entrance wound was obscured by her dark hair). The recent firing of two shots was also suspicious as well as the discovery of a small armoury at the house and for which the necessary firearms certificates were apparently lacking.

Additional information gathered by the investigating team soon led to an entirely different view. The husband was able to satisfy the police that he had been away from home, several miles away, at the time of the shooting. The person who removed the revolver from the dead woman's hand, prior to the arrival of the team, described the grip as firm and force had been required to remove the gun. It was, in all probability, an instance of cadaveric spasm, a hallmark of self-infliction. (Incidentally the same person went further in his interference with the scene. He broke the gun open and extracted the ammunition. It was then impossible to ascertain precisely the order in which the four spent cartridges had been fired.)

Palpation of the head detected a wound in the right temple and a second rather larger one in the left parietal region. It was shown later that these were in fact the entrance and exit wounds of a bullet, and, as was probable, if she had shot herself when sat up in the bed, the bullet would have lodged where it was found in the bedroom wall.

There was now substantial evidence of suicide.

At the post-mortem examination the head hair was cut away to expose a circular entrance wound $^1/_2$ in. in diameter, with four splits each $^1/_4$ in. long at right angles to its margin. The margin was slightly everted. There was slight bruising of the lower part of the wound. The hair adjacent to it was scorched and there was slight tattooing by powder at the upper margin of the wound. There was a circular hole, 0.30×0.35 in. with its margins blackened by soot and powder, in the outer table of the underlying bone; there was bevelling inwards in the inner table (Fig. 95).

The wound was situated 2 in. behind the right eye and $1^1/_2$ in. above the pinna of the right ear. It had the characteristics of a contact wound by a bullet of about 0.380 in., slight eversion of the margin being due to rebound of pressure against resisting bone. The site was that chosen by about 80 per cent of those who use firearms for suicide.

The exit wound, $^1/_2$ in. to the right of the middle line and 4 in. above the pinna of the left ear, was star-shaped; each of its six arms were up to $1^1/_4$ in. long. It was devoid of scorching, soiling by smoke or tattooing by powder.

The underlying hole in the skull was 1 in. in diameter, with bevelling outwards. Conical plates of bone had been lifted from the outer table of the skull. Fissured fractures extended into the skull from the margins of the exit hole. This abutted the fronto-parietal suture, just to the left of its mid-point. The sagittal sinus was lacerated and the bullet had traversed the right parietal lobe of the brain.

The track of the bullet was upwards and to the left at an angle of about 45° to the horizontal.

Blood at the scene was restricted to the back of the head; it had run downwards and backwards on to the pillow. A few spots of blood were found on her right sleeve, shoulder, and front of her body over the right breast. She was fully clothed.

She was under the influence of alcohol. Her blood alcohol level was 210 mg/100 ml; urinary alcohol level 277 mg/100 ml; this was deemed the equivalent of the ingestion of half a bottle of spirits by a woman who weighed $9^1/_2$ stones. There was no natural disease.

Suicide was motivated by financial and marital problems.

There remains the minor problem of the other shot, directed from the bed into the adjacent bath-room. The possibility that she fired a second time after shooting herself, even involuntarily, as she fell back on to the bed was rejected. She might have had a trial shot before putting the revolver to her head. In all probability, having regard to her intoxication, she fired the gun accidentally before she shot herself.

The findings, as a whole, left no doubt that this death was due to a planned self-inflicted injury (F.M. 13,222A).

Case No. 31

Site: back of head. *Range:* contact. Self-inflicted. *Weapon*: Luger self-loading pistol 9 mm.

A married man, aged 33, fully clothed, was found dead in his bedroom. He had been depressed because of failure in a professional examination.

The entrance wound, at the back of his head, was midway between and in line with each outer ear. The centre of the wound was 5 ft 1 in. above the soles of his feet. It was a circular wound, $^1/_2$ in. in diameter, devoid of scorching, soiling by smoke and tattooing by unburnt powder. The muscles around the track of the bullet, however, were blackened.

The track, a well-defined cylindrical one, was demonstrated by probe to pass forwards in a horizontal line, slightly inclined to the left. The bullet had shattered the posterior arch of the atlas and had severed the spinal cord at its junction with the hind brain. It had then entered the skull near the foramen magnum and travelled forwards through the basi-sphenoid, and the left maxillary antrum, to emerge at the left side of his nose. There was comminution of the sphenoid and nasal bones and fracture of both orbits.

The exit wound, between the nose and the inner canthus of the left eye, was oval, $^3/_4 \times ^1/_4$ in. with everted margins. No scorching or blackening of the tissues present. A subsidiary wound, also $^3/_4 \times ^1/_4$ in., immediately to the left of the exit wound, had been produced by expulsion of fragments of the nasal bones, or cartilage.

The length of his arm, from shoulder to closed fist, was 24 in. Tests with the weapon showed that, when held butt uppermost, it was possible to place the muzzle at the nape of the neck and release the trigger.

A bullet (9 mm) was found on the floor of the bedroom.

There was no evidence to show that the shot had been fired by another person. It had been possible for self-infliction. It was a "planned" shot and not an accidental one. It could be that he had used the mirror in the wardrobe to check his aim (F.M. 13,658A).

Case No. 32. Contact Wound: 0.22 Winchester Rifle: Suicidal

There was an entrance wound, 5 mm in diameter, almost at the middle of the forehead. The margin of the entrance wound was blackened by abrasion and powder. Tiny linear slits ran out from the periphery of the hole. There was a band of reddish discoloration at the upper margin of this entrance wound which could have been bruising by the muzzle of the weapon. There was a circular hole in the frontal bone just to the left of the middle line, 1 cm in diameter, and it opened immediately into a large frontal sinus. A somewhat larger and more ragged hole was present in the posterior wall of that sinus immediately to the left of the crista galli. From this hole there were some fissured fracture lines extending outwards, e.g. one passing upwards and outwards into the left half of the frontal bone. There was a fracture of the cribriform plate and of the orbital plates; the fracture line went on to the roof of the right antrum, which contained blood. There was laceration of the frontal lobe and the track was traced through the brain from the left superior frontal to the posterior parietal region, also on the left side. Radiological examination had shown that a bullet had lodged in the latter place whence a somewhat flattened 0.22 lead bullet was recovered. (F.M. 7402A, Dr. Dennis Harriman; C.P. present.)

Cases No. 33 and 34

Site: forehead. *Range:* contact. Homicidal. *Weapon:* 0.22 rifle. *Circumstances:* murder and suicide.

A young woman was found dead and a young man was found unconscious in the living room of a house.

The girl, aged 19, lay on her back in front of a small bookcase. A rifle was on the floor a little distance from her outstretched right arm and a spent cartridge case was near her body. Her feet and the butt of the rifle were close to the hearth of a fireplace.

The man lay on the floor at the opposite side of the room close to an armchair; his head rested on the skirting board.

Although the girl's legs were apart there had been no interference with her clothing. A pool of blood at the left side of her head had collected from a wound in her forehead.

This was a circular entrance wound of a bullet; the hole was $^3/_{16}$ in. in diameter and there was an abrasion collar of blackened skin, the overall diameter of the wound being $^1/_2$ in.; there were tiny radiating splits in the skin around the periphery of the bullet hole (the muzzle of the gun was $^1/_2$ in. in diameter). The centre of the wound was $1^1/_2$ in. above and $^3/_4$ in. to the right of the bridge of the nose. Bleeding had occurred into the eyelids and from the left ear. There was no exit wound.

Except for the pool of the blood near her head, the only other blood present near her body was in two spots on the wall behind her, to the right of the bookcase at about 2 ft 6 ins from the floor.

A small hole was noticed in the wall at 4 ft above the floor above the bookcase; a misshapen 0.22 bullet was recovered from this hole.

Internal examination demonstrated a circular hole $^3/_4$ in. in diameter, directed upwards, in her frontal bone. Fissured fractures involved both orbits, the ethmoid bone and the base of the left anterior and middle compartments of the skull.

The track of the missile, an inch wide, presented as a deep groove in the under-surface of the left cerebral hemisphere. It ended at the occipital pole where there were two misshapen fragments of metal, the remains of a 0.22 bullet. Both frontal lobes were bruised and lacerated, as was the upper surface of the left cerebellar hemisphere. There was no exit wound.

The direction of aim was backwards, slightly to the left, in a horizontal line.

The limited distribution of blood indicated immediate collapse, after having been shot, into the posture in which her body was found.

The entrance wound had the appearance of a contact injury, i.e. the muzzle had been in contact with the skull at the moment of discharge. This is normally the "hallmark" of self-infliction. Had she sat on the arm of a chair nearby and leant over the gun with its butt on the floor she could have released the trigger since the measured length of her arm was sufficient. Collapse could have then brought her to the ground in the manner she was found. This interpretation, however, required support of the evidence that she was familiar with the use of firearms. (The firer had known how to operate the bolt and reload the gun). This is lacked. None of the fingerprints on the rifle were hers. It was necessary also to explain the injury in the young man and the occurrence of a third shot which struck the wall above the girl's body. It was concluded that she had been shot by the young man (see below), but it was not clear how he had been able to shoot her at contact range. It could have been that during their quarrel, he was angry with her because she had been out with another boy, his first shot missed and hit the wall above the bookcase. She may then have fainted and he was then able to shoot her in the forehead as she lay on the ground. There was no evidence that he had hit her so as to render her unconscious. There was no natural disease to cause her sudden collapse.

The man, aged 24, lay unconscious beside an armchair at the other side of the room; his head rested against the skirting board down which blood had run to form a pool under his head. He was removed to hospital and died a few hours after arrival. He too had the entrance wound of a bullet in his forehead. It was a contact wound but its appearances had of necessity been altered by surgical toilet and suture. There was a circular hole, $3/_{16}$ in. in diameter, in his frontal bone, situated in the middle line, 1 in. above the bridge of his nose.

Internal examination showed that the frontal sinuses, the ethmoid bone and the orbital roofs were disrupted. The track of the missile, backwards and slightly upwards, passed along the inner border of the left cerebral hemisphere to the outer part of the left occipital lobe; a 0.22 lay close to the occipital pole. There was no exit wound. No natural disease found.

He had shot himself when erect near the armchair; blood and fragments of brain on the chair were from his body. (No fragments of brain had left the girl's body). He had then fallen backwards and come to rest with his head against the skirting board. He was then immobilised.

He never regained consciousness and, therefore, the explanation of this case involves speculation. Despite the fact that the girl's injury was a contact one, the balance of probabilities suggests that he, the owner of the gun and familiar with its use, and the aggrieved party, had threatened the girl with the gun. His first shot was a "miss" but he fired again and killed her. He then shot himself. The alcohol content of the blood and urine of the victims was not ascertained. In view of the marksmanship, two bullets in a planned position, it seemed unlikely that the man was then under the influence of drink (F.M. 10,044A and 10,044B).

Contact wounds over the *heart*, i.e. over structures which offer relatively mild resistance, are normally circular. There is an abrasion collar and, when contact is made with bare skin, fouling by smoke and involuntary tattooing. Singeing of hair may or may not occur. Contact wounds of the temple or any part of the skull where the bone is thin, are likely to be similar; the stellate wound is most often seen in or near the forehead.

If the weapon be fired at contact range and the body is fully clothed, and more especially if an overcoat is worn at the time, the body injury may simulate one caused by a near discharge. It is obviously imperative on these occasions also to examine the clothing, where singeing, fouling by smoke and involuntary tattooing may be found.

Case No. 35. Contact: 0.455 Revolver: Suicidal (Fig. 96)

This male aged 62 shot himself with his service revolver when ill in bed. The entrance wound $1/_4$ in. in diameter was bordered by a dark brown discoloration of the skin of up to $1/_2$ in. in breadth. CO at 60 per cent saturation was demonstrated in blood in the subcutaneous tissues. The wound was over the 5th interspace, close to the sternum; the 6th rib was fractured. The exit wound, $3/_4$ in. in diameter, was at the back, $1^1/_2$ in. to the left of the mid-line and in the 7th interspace.

The base of the right ventricle had been lacerated and the bullet had traversed the lower lobe of the left lung. A 0.455 lead bullet, dented and marked by rifling, lay between his body and his pyjama jacket (F.M. 5558).

Case No. 36. Contact: P. 38: Suicidal

Found lying on his back, with his arms and ankles crossed, on moorland about 10 yards from his locked, parked, car. The key of the car was in his pocket. He was fully clad and his cap was on his head. A P. 38 pistol

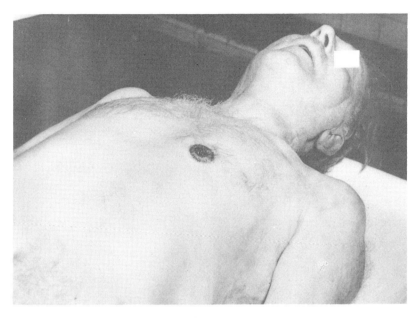

FIG. 96. Revolver: 0.45 contact entrance wound of chest. (Case No. 35.)

lay near his feet. The front of the raincoat and jacket, although blood-stained, was not damaged. There was, however, a hole in the shirt and vest at the front of the body and a hole in these and the jacket and raincoat at the back of the body. Presumably he had opened his coat and jacket before firing but had been able to fasten them afterwards, or, of course, someone who found the body had done this. The police said the coat and jacket were fastened when the body was found.

The entrance wound, 12 mm in diameter, had a purple-red abrasion collar, and was situated over the 5th interspace. There was slight fouling by smoke and tattooing by powder. The left ventricle and the inner side of the lower lobe of the left lung were lacerated. The exit wound was 4 cm, to the left of the spine near the 12th rib. Direction of aim was almost horizontal, with a slight downward direction (F.M. 5876A).

"Near" Wounds: Within about 1 Yard

These wounds are characterised by an entrance wound accompanied by damage to the skin by the products of detonation and ignition (Burrard (1956) regards "explosion" as erroneous, although commonly used). There may be singeing or scorching of the tissues and this is likely to occur only when it is indeed a near injury, i.e. well *within* 6 in. and, normally, within 3 in. It depends on the weapon and kind of ammunition. Scorching range, maximal with a service rifle, is up to 6 in., but with a revolver it is from 2 in. to 3 in. and may be less with firearms of smaller bore, e.g. 0.22 bore. We have found no scorching in some cases where a weapon of this bore had been fired at near range. Scorching range is also reduced if the skin surface is wet.

Fouling by smoke is also a feature of near wounds and the extreme limit of the range of this fouling is well within a normal arm's length, probably only about 1 ft. As Burrard points out, absence of fouling by smoke, therefore, does not exclude self-infliction.

Tattooing by unburnt powder grains is yet another feature of near wounds (Fig. 91). Its range is greater than that of fouling, but its extreme limit is normally beyond arm's length

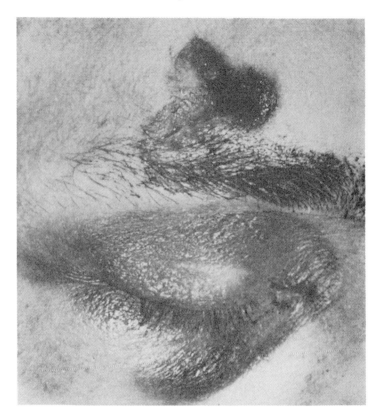

FIG. 97. Luger automatic 9-mm pistol. Entrance wound above right eye.
Range approx. 2 ft. Homicide. (Case No. 41.)

and, therefore, its absence points to injury by another. It is not conclusive evidence, since the length of the barrel of the weapon, the pressure and type of powder used must be taken into account (Burrard, 1956).

The presence of *carbon monoxide* in the blood of the injured tissues, in the track of the bullet, is also a feature of a near wound; the range is then one of only a few inches.

The entrance wound is the result of a punching inwards of the tissues by the bullet. In consequence it is circular and its margins are inverted. The skin is soiled and bruised by the missile and, therefore, the skin adjacent to the hole may show two zones. The inner one, soiled by grease and other foreign material on the nose of the bullet, is known as the "grease collar". The outer zone, easier to recognise, is dark red or red, i.e. bruised, and is slightly abraded; this is known as the "contusion" or "abrasion collar". Each of these zones is only a fraction of an inch, about $1/32$ to $1/8$ in., wide. In estimating the calibre of the bullet from the size of the wound, the measurement should be the diameter of the wound, taken to include the hole and the contusion collar.

When the wound is oval, the weapon was probably directed obliquely. In that event the bruising should be especially noted because its width is broader in the direction of the line of fire.

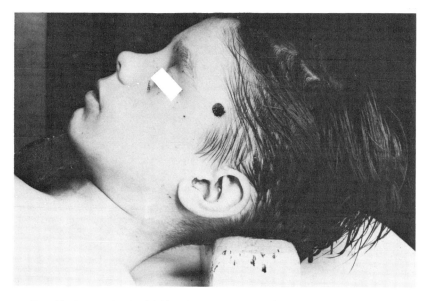

FIG. 98. Automatic pistol 0.32. Distant range (several feet). Accidental shooting. (Case No. 42.)

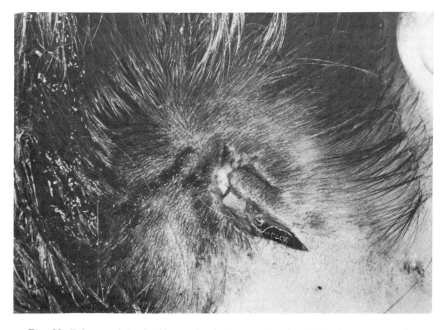

FIG. 99. Exit wound. Back of head. Simulating laceration by a fall or blow. Automatic pistol 0.32. (Case No. 42.)

A contact wound, especially when caused by 0.22 ammunition, may be a circular hole with fouling and powder marking of the adjacent skin, as opposed to a stellate wound and relatively unmarked skin. The distinction between a "contact" and "near" injury is then difficult, but it remains clear that the injury was within the range of self-infliction, assuming the weapon had been held in the hand.

If the bullet strikes, side on, the wound may have a key-hole shape (see Case No. 41, Fig. 97).

Case No. 37

Three wounds. *Range*: close range. Homicide. *Weapon*: 0.455 Smith & Wesson revolver.

This was a woman aged 35 who was found fully clothed, laid on her back between an armchair and a settee. There had been no interference with her clothing and her spectacles were in position. Bloodstaining of her clothing was seen and blood was on the floor near her body. When her clothing was removed a bullet of 0.455 calibre was found between her outer garment and her body. On external examination of the body, three firearm injuries were recognised.

Wound No. 1. This was an entrance wound in the form of a circular hole $^1/_4$ in. in diameter bordered by an abrasion collar, the injury having an overall diameter of an inch. It was situated at the front of the neck, $^1/_2$ in. to the right of the middle line at the level of the upper border of the thyroid cartilage. The skin adjacent to the wound, in an area of 4 in. in diameter, was tattooed by unburnt powder.

The bullet had passed backwards in a horizontal line and its track was traced through the thyroid cartilage, oesophagus, upper part of the body of the 2nd dorsal vertebra and spinal cord, which was severed at this level. The exit wound was beside the 3rd dorsal vertebra, an inch to the right of the middle line. It was a ragged laceration, $^1/_2 \times ^1/_4$ in., with everted margins; it was not abraded nor blackened by soot or powder.

Wound No. 2. This entrance wound was oval, $^3/_8 \times ^1/_4$ in., with slight bruising of its margin, situated $3^1/_2$ in. to the left of the middle line at the level of the collar bone. The track of the bullet was to the right at 15° below the horizontal. The bullet had penetrated the lower end of the sterno-mastoid muscle and has passed behind the oesophagus, over the upper border of the first rib on the right side. The transverse process of the 7th cervical vertebra was comminuted and the bullet travelled through the muscles at the back of the right shoulder.

The exit wound, $^3/_4 \times ^3/_8$ in. with irregular margins, was situated 5 in. to the right of the middle line at about the level of the 7th cervical vertebra.

Wound No. 3. This entrance wound, $^1/_4$ in. in diameter, with an abrasion collar $^1/_4$ in. wide, was situated 3 in. to the left of the middle line and 4 in. above the umbilicus. The track passed backwards and to the left and in its course the bullet had passed through the cartilage of the 7th rib, the stomach, upper pole of the left kidney and between the transverse processes of D12 and L1 vertebrae. Bleeding was negligible in the track of this bullet.

The exit wound, $^3/_8$ in. in diameter, and circular, was situated $^1/_2$ in. to the left of the middle line.

In reconstructing the event it was deduced that she was erect when shot the first time because one bullet was found embedded in the wall well above floor level. The first shot must have been that in the neck, since severance of the cord occurred and this would have caused immediate paralysis and collapse. Although this was a near injury at a range of under a yard, the subsequent shots were at even closer range. These were fired at her when she lay on the floor. The shot just above the collar bone preceded the abdominal one, since bleeding in relation to the latter wound was negligible; she was then dead (F.M. 10,355).

Case No. 38. 0.38 Revolver. Near wound. Self-inflicted

A youth aged 19 was found dead lying on the floor of a cabinet shop where he was employed. An American 0.38 Webley revolver was found clamped in a vice by its butt, with the trigger upwards. It was about 3 ft above the floor. A discharged cartridge case was in line with the barrel. The victim had shot himself through the right lower eyelid and the bullet had passed through the orbit to the right occipital region where it was found between the brain and the skull; the skull was fractured but there was no exit wound. Powder soiling and tattooing of the eyelids indicated a near discharge. It appeared that he had knelt in front of the gun with his eye close to the muzzle. The suggestion that the gun had been discharged accidentally while he peered into the barrel to detect some fault in it was not accepted. His object had been to avoid military service. Verdict: Suicide (Leeds City Coroner, No. 982/41).

Case No. 39. 0.38 Revolver. Homicidal. Range over 6 inches but under 1 yard (probably 18 inches)

The victim, aged 52, was a jeweller who was shot when two youths entered his shop intending robbery. The bullet entered his left chest in the 7th interspace, $3^3/_4$ in. to the left of the middle line. Its course was traced downwards into the abdomen. It had passed between the stomach and spleen apparently without injury to either, but a perforation of the stomach was later found at post-mortem. There were two perforations in the colon at the splenic flexure. The bullet had almost divided the small intestine at the duodeno-jejunal flexure and had passed through the lower pole of the left kidney. There was no exit wound. The initial search for the bullet in the abdomen was fruitless. X-ray examination was then made and a bullet was shown to have lodged in the sacral region. A somewhat distorted bullet of lead, rather less than 0.38 in., was recovered from a recess in the left side of the sacrum.

The victim had been shot with a bullet of less than the normal calibre for the weapon. He had also been struck with the butt of the weapon on the forehead and nose. Death was due to peritonitis at about 30 hours after the shooting (*R.* v. *Sharpe and Lannen*, 1950, F. M. 1124.)

Case No. 40

Site: head. *Range:* "close". Self-inflicted. *Weapon:* B.S.A. 0.22 rifle.

The body of this man, aged 23, was seen on a landing close to a ladder to the loft of a semi-detached house. He lay on his back, legs outstretched, with his arms folded over his body. There was a pillow under his head and a second pillow with a towel and sponge were near the body. A rifle was on the floor close to his feet. A small pool of blood had collected beneath the body. Blood spots and smears were on the wall of the landing and on adjacent bedroom doors. Small blood smears were on the ladder to the loft, e.g. on the fifth rung, on top of the ladder and on the border of the opening into the loft. Shotguns, ammunition and powder were in the loft. There were blood stains in the loft.

The only external injury was a small firearm wound in the left temple. This presented as a hole $^1/_8$ in. in diameter, with blackened contusion collar $1/_{16}$ in. broad; there was no singeing of the hair. The wound was centred at $1^1/_2$ in. above the left external auditory meatus. Bleeding had occurred from the nostrils, ears and mouth and into the eyelids. There was no carbon monoxide in the blood from the wound.

There was no exit wound. The bullet had traversed the right temporal bone, where there was an irregular hole with outward displacement of the fragments. A distorted 0.22 bullet was recovered from the right temporalis muscle at 2 in. above the right external auditory meatus.

The entrance hole in the left temporal region was $^1/_4$ in. in diameter, with blackened margins.

Secondary fissured fracture involved the vault of the skull, the roof of each orbit and each middle ear.

The bullet had made a track 1 in. wide and 6 in. long in the under-surface of the left temporal lobe, across the mid brain and then the right temporal lobe, i.e. it was directed from left to right and upwards to the exit on the right side of the skull. Flame-shaped haemorrhages were inside the left ventricle.

The range was estimated as "close contact" and he was injured whilst standing or crouching in the loft near the opening to the ladder. He had fallen forward through the opening on to the landing. The gun fell with him. Death was delayed, but mobility once he reached the landing was nil.

His arm length was 25 in.; the distance from temple to left index finger 34 in. Length of rifle from muzzle to trigger guard $29^1/_2$ in.; length of barrel 25 in.; muzzle to butt, $42^1/_2$ in. (F.M. 15,249A).

Distant Wounds

Any rifled firearm injury inflicted at a range beyond that at which the products of the detonation can mark the skin and where the bullet alone leaves its mark, is a "distant" wound. These, therefore, are inflicted at a range of 2 or 3 ft or over and that range is normally, if not invariably, beyond the range of self-infliction, when the weapon is held in the hand; it is probable that even a person with unduly long arms cannot shoot himself with a revolver or automatic pistol of normal size at a range of 2 ft or beyond. (The distance was 21 in. with a Colt automatic held by a man whose arm span was 7 ft.)

The entrance wound whether at, say, 3 ft or 30 ft is similar, i.e. a circular hole with an abrasion collar without any powder marking of the skin. *In that event, precise estimates of the range cannot be given; it is possible only to say that the weapon was fired beyond the range of self-infliction.*

The suicide can arrange matters so that the weapon is fired at a distance, e.g. the weapon is clamped in a vice (e.g., Case No. 38) and the trigger operated by a string, but this arrangement is then apparent. It is an unlikely mode, since it lacks certainty of effect.

Case No. 41. 9-mm Automatic Luger Pistol. Distant Range—at 1 yard or over

Entrance wound, of keyhole shape, $^1/_4$ in. above centre of right supra-orbital margin. No singeing, fouling or tattooing of skin or subcutaneous tissues. Circular hole in skull $^1/_4$ in. in diameter with considerable comminution of the left side of the skull. Exit wound, a stellate laceration, on a level with and $1^1/_4$ in. to right of occiput. Horizontal track of bullet through the left hemisphere (*R.* v. *Hirst*, 1947. F.M. 5177A; Fig. 97).

Case No. 42. 0.32 Automatic. Distant Range—at 1 yard or over

Shot by accident at over 1 yard by another boy who, unaware that the pistol was loaded, pointed it at the deceased. The entrance wound was situated in the left temple; a circular hole $^3/_8$ in. in diameter overall, with a dark red abrasion collar of up to $^1/_8$ in. broad. No singeing, fouling or tattooing of the skin or underlying tissues. The exit wound, a 'Y'-shaped laceration with everted edges, was on a level with and 2 in. to the left of the occiput. Track of bullet was traced through the left cerebral hemisphere (F.M. 4214, Figs. 98, 99).

Case No. 43. 0.22 Rifle. Distant Range

This boy aged 13 years was accidentally shot by another boy who had taken a 0.22 rifle from an armoury. The probable range was one of several yards; they were on opposite banks of a river. The entrance wound, $^1/_4$ in. in diameter overall, was a circular hole bordered by a narrow, red abrasion collar. There was no fouling of the skin by smoke and no involuntary tattooing. It was situated at the front of the chest, $^3/_8$ in. above and $^3/_8$ in. internal to the left nipple, lying directly below the lower border of the 3rd rib, $1^3/_4$ in. to the left of the middle line. The track of a bullet was traced through the upper lobe of the left lung, the aorta, trachea and upper lobe of the right lung. The bullet left the chest through the third intercostal space at 3 in. to the right of the spine and was found, with its long axis horizontal, nose directed towards the spine, in the right infra-spinatus muscle, at the outer border of the right scapula. There was no exit wound. Death was due to bilateral pneumothorax; there was about a pint of blood in the pleural sacs, and there had been some external haemorrhage.

The boy had been clothed at the time and a circular tear was present in each of the garments at the front in a position which corresponded with the chest wound. No singeing, blackening or tattooing by powder.

The direction of aim was in a diagonal line through the chest, from left to right, and from front to back. The victim and firer had been face to face and the victim erect at the time. He had been able to walk a short distance before he collapsed. His death was the result of a foolish prank (F.M. 3599A).

EXIT WOUNDS

The emerging missile pushes the tissues before it and splits the soft parts to produce an exit wound which is an irregular laceration, usually appreciably larger than the entrance wound and without any signs of blackening, singeing or tattooing by the products of the detonation (Fig. 99). The exit wound in the skull will show greater damage to the outer than to the inner table, with outward bevelling of the track through the bone.

Variation in the rule that the exit wound is the larger may occur at contact range, when the entrance wound may be the larger or both wounds may then be of like size if produced by a high velocity bullet; a rifle, fired at over 200 yards, can produce entrance and exit wounds which are almost alike. The distinction may be made, if one wound has an inverted and the other an everted margin.

Contact between the missile and bone can introduce factors which obscure interpretation. A piece of bone separated by the bullet may become a secondary missile. Pieces of clothing, buttons, etc., driven in by the missile, may also complicate the appearances by becoming secondary missiles.

DIRECTION OF AIM

The entrance wound is at all times of greater importance than the exit wound, in particular for the purpose of determining the direction of aim.

This problem might seem a simple one which calls only for accurate recognition of the line which joins the entrance and exit wounds and then prolonging it to the range suggested by the appearances of the entrance wound. This should fix the position of the weapon, when fired. Unfortunately this simple method is beset by one or more of several difficulties which complicate interpretation. The missile, for example, may have struck some object and been deflected by it before it strikes the victim, i.e. by ricochet; the missile may have been deflected by bone or other body tissues before it left the body of the victim; it may have been a tangential shot. In consequence, the path between the weapon and the exit wound, or between the entrance and exit wounds is not in fact always straight but may be a zig-zag or curved line. (Piédelièvre and Desoille (1939) deal with this problem in some detail; their work should be consulted.) An examination of the clothing is important.

THE "ODD AND EVEN" RULE

Whenever the firearm wounds are an odd number, it must be presumed that a missile is still inside the body of the deceased. There are exceptions when, for example, the missile splits into two portions inside the body and produces two exit wounds (Ellis, 1959). An odd number of wounds also occurs when the missile breaks off a piece of bone which then becomes a secondary missile, producing its own exit wound. Yet another exception is provided by the entry and exit of one missile and a glancing blow, merely grooving or grazing the part by another. It is well also to remember that some exit wounds are obscure. Piédelièvre and Desoille (1939) described one in the ear, hidden by the helix.

When it is likely that a missile remains in the body and facilities exist, an X-ray examination is of considerable value. On one occasion a missile lay inside the abdomen but its site was obscure to ordinary examination. The radiogram, however, promptly located it in a crevice beside the sacrum, whence the bullet was extracted (Case No. 39, p. 257). On another occasion, when no bullet could be found, X-ray examination of the skull demonstrated fragments of opaque material, which showed that the bullet had disintegrated. Later, small fragments of lead were recovered from the interior of the skull (F.M. 5685E).

When the missile lies inside the skull due care must be taken to collect it, lest it fall out and be lost when the skull-cap is removed. A dish should be held in position to receive it, otherwise it may fall into the drain, sometimes situated directly below the position of the head.

The search for a missile, in the presence of an odd number of external wounds, must be exhaustive. Radiological examination in an invaluable aid.

If lodged in bone, the portion of bone should be removed together with the bullet, no attempt being made at the post-mortem examination to dislodge it. It is important not to blur marks made by the weapon by rough handling with forceps or other instruments.

The Sites of Firearm Injuries

(a) ACCIDENTAL INJURIES

These may involve any part of the body, from head to foot, in the front, at the back or at the sides. In short, they are devoid of plan or pattern.

(b) SUICIDAL INJURIES

As one would expect, the suicide, intending death, will aim at an area which he believes especially important to life and its destruction will result in death and probably sudden death. Be that as it may, the majority aim either at the head or the praecordium, with the intention of injuring the brain or heart. An abdominal wound is distinctly uncommon since the layman appears to be aware that the result is less certain. It is also less easy to achieve. The majority of those who aim at the head, aim at the temple and, since the majority are righthanded, the right temple is the commonest site; it is the choice of at least 60 per cent, if not 80 per cent, of firearm suicides. The left-handed fire at the left temple but it is also possible for the right-handed person to shoot himself in the left temple, with a shotgun, if not a hand gun (see Case No. 14, p. 226).

The forehead is not infrequently the site of suicidal firearm injury. In that event there is usually evidence that the victim took care to select the centre or near centre of the forehead at about midway between the eyebrows and the hair line.

When a rifled weapon is used the contact injury may have a stellate pattern, with slightly everted edges. The identification of the entrance wound as a contact injury is important when the site in the forehead is significantly distant from the centre, i.e. even by an inch.

An unusual but recognised variant of suicidal head injury is that in which the victim interposes his hand between the muzzle and his head. The contact entrance wound is then usually in the palm. This procedure suggests that the hand is used to grip the muzzle to keep it in position. (We are indebted to Professor Keith Mant for information and photographs of his case.)

Some suicides choose a site behind and sometimes above the ear but within at least 2 in. of the pinna; some shoot into the external auditory meatus. An extrance wound in the region of an ear calls for special care in its interpretation, especially when it is a "near" and not a "contact" injury. If left-handedness be excluded, we agree with Keith Simpson that the near discharge of a pistol behind the LEFT ear justifies "the strongest presumption of foul play". We go further and say that a near injury in the region of the left or right ear must always be considered, in the first instance, as probably homicidal. It may later be established, as in our two cases below, that they were suicides.

Suicide: Entrance Wound Behind the Right Ear

The victim was a man aged 37, who had served as an officer in the British Army and was in unlawful possession of a 0.45 automatic Colt pistol, U.S. Army pattern. His marriage had been unhappy and he had had psychiatric treatment for anxiety neurosis. He had threatened suicide. One night he went out and, when he did not return, a search was made for him. He was found dead, lying in a yard with the weapon beside his body. He was fully clothed. His clothing was wet and he lay on his back with the legs extended. His left arm was flexed and the right was extended. A circular entrance wound, $^7/_8$ in. in diameter, was situated behind the *right* ear. Its centre was 1 in. behind and $1^1/_2$ in. above the right external auditory meatus. Singeing was not apparent, but there was soiling of the skin by smoke, in an area $^1/_2$ in. in diameter, and there was some involuntary tattooing. There was a dark grey abrasion collar, $^1/_{16}$ in. broad, with tiny side lacerations extending out from the entrance hole. A small abrasion, $^1/_8$ in. in diameter, lay directly behind the entrance wound. There was comminution of the underlying skull, with a central hole $^7/_{10}$ in. in diameter. The bony margins were blackened by powder. This was an in-going injury, as shown by shelving of the skull, which in this region was $^1/_8$ in. thick. Blood in the tissues around the wound contained CO, estimated at 15 per cent saturation. The exit wound was in the left parietal region, $2^1/_2$ in. to the left of the middle line and 5 in. above the left external auditory meatus. There was comminution of the vault of the skull and the suture lines had been opened by the force of the explosion (F.M. 6951B).

Another male, 19 years old, also shot himself behind the *right* ear. An entrance wound $^3/_8$ in. in diameter with a red abrasion collar was situated $1^3/_8$ in. above and $^1/_2$ in. behind the pinna. There was blackening by smoke and tattooing in an area $1^1/_4$ in. in diameter around the wound. The exit wound was in the left frontal region, 3 in. above the inner end of the left supra-orbital margin; its margins were lacerated and everted. A suicide note had been left (Leeds City Coroner, No. 446/40).

Suicide/Homicide, "Near" Wound Behind Right Ear

The site of the wound may be an important issue in a trial, as in that of J. D. Merrett in 1927. He was accused of the murder of his mother by shooting her with an automatic pistol; his defence was that she had shot herself. The wound was situated at the back of the right ear, immediately behind the external auditory meatus; the bullet had passed forwards to the base of the skull and lodged near the sella turcica, without causing injury to the brain; she died, about a fortnight later, from meningitis. The site of the wound is unusual for suicide but Sir Bernard Spilsbury, who gave evidence for the defence, believed that this site and the direction of aim were not inconsistent with suicide. He instanced a similar case of his own in which the victim was found with the weapon firmly grasped in his hand; death had been instantaneous and there was no doubt that the circumstances were then those of suicide. In the Merrett case, a verdict of "Not Proven" was due, in the main, to the fact that the medical witnesses were unable to agree on the range of fire (Roughead, 1929).

Other sites occasionally chosen by the suicide include the nose, beneath the chin, side of the head and eye; there are also instances of the back of the head, and the rarest site is the top of the head.

All require interpretation with care and in the light of all the available evidence. The circumstances of an entrance wound well above and behind the right ear were, on the balance of probabilities, those of an accident (Case No. 16, p. 229). There were two instances of a suicidal entrance wound at the back of the head in our series (Leeds City Coroner 309/42 and Case No. 31, p. 250).

Keith Simpson (1965) had seen three cases of suicide by a shot in the eye. In our case the man had fixed a revolver in a vice and knelt before the muzzle (Case No. 38, p. 256). Gonzales *et al.* (1954) mention the possibility that swelling of the lids following the injury may obscure the entrance wound. They depict an example; the shattered right lens of his spectacles drew attention to the eye injury.

The chest is not rarely the site of suicidal firearm injuries, but the incidence is only about half of that of head cases. The majority shoot themselves over the praecordium and succeed in causing damage to the heart and/or the major vessels. Some open their clothing in order to bring the muzzle into direct contact with the skin.

Our experience confirms the infrequent choice of an abdominal site by the suicide and, when chosen it is nearly always in the upper abdomen.

Canfield (1969) analysed forty-six cases of firearm suicide and only two chose the abdomen. The injuries in this region are, as we have found, usually penetrating but not perforating, "through and through" injuries.

Olivier *et al.* (1966a, b) reported two unusual suicides, one with a rifle and the other with a fowling piece.

(c) HOMICIDAL FIREARM INJURIES

These tend to have a pattern which differs from that of suicide. For obvious reasons when the intent is to kill, aim is directed at the head or heart but not rarely the back is the target; the abdomen is more often the site in homicide than in suicide. In their series of 274 cases of homicide by firearms, Gonzales *et al.* (1954) reported that 25 per cent had been shot in the abdomen, 23 per cent in the chest and only 10 per cent in the head; 7 per cent were shot in the spine. The majority were shot with a single shot. There were only four victims of multiple shots.

Firearm Injury of the Pregnant Uterus

Firearm injury of the pregnant uterus is a rare event and, fortunately, not normally fatal. Beattie and Daly (1960) recorded the case of a pregnant woman who, in her 7th month, was shot with a 0.22 bullet in the abdomen. She was delivered a week later of a macerated infant. They reviewed the literature and collected thirty-eight other cases. In their view, if the victim be at the 7th month or later, and the child is still alive, it should be removed by caesarean section and the wound repaired. (The literature on firearm injuries of the uterus was reviewed by Kobak and Hurwitz (1954) when they reported two cases and by Wright *et al.* (1954)). Three more cases were reported by Bochner (1961) and one by Kracke (1963). The latter was an example of congenital paraplegia following bullet injury to the spine while *in utero*; delivery by Caesarean section at the 28th month.

Firearm Injury of the Heart

Firearm injury of the heart is not necessarily fatal, especially in view of the modern advances in thoracic surgery. It would appear that masterly inactivity might be a safe course on some occasions. Shoemaker and Eckels (1930) reported the case of a woman aged 23 who sustained two bullet wounds in her chest. One bullet was removed from beneath the skin near the spine. The other was shown by radiology to have lodged in the heart muscle. No attempt was made to remove it and at 2 months the patient appeared to be perfectly well. Their view was that the majority require no surgery. Interference with function, however, is not the only factor to be considered. There is the possibility that retention of a lead bullet could cause lead poisoning. This occurred in a man who had carried a bullet in his right femur for 6 or 7 years (Machle, 1940).

The Circumstances of Firearm Injuries

Although it is the duty of a coroner or a jury to determine the final interpretation of the circumstances of a firearm injury, the pathologist assists them in arriving at their verdict. He is also required to assist the police in forming an initial interpretation, so that the appropriate lines of inquiry are promptly instituted.

There are occasions when there is little doubt about the nature of the circumstances, but careful and detailed investigation at the scene, as well as in the post-mortem room and laboratory, is always necessary. Some of the features which give a lead to the probable interpretation are next considered.

Firearm Suicide

The victim is rarely a female.

A few of the suicides leave a note or letter in which their intention is clear; some had threatened suicide. The forgery of a suicide note is a remote possibility.

There may be evidence of preparation at the scene. An outstanding example was that of the man who fixed his revolver in a vice and knelt in front of it in order to shoot himself. The relatives failed to convince the coroner that he had been repairing the gun and had been looking into the barrel to discover a defect in it (Case No. 38, p. 256). There is also an account of the man who wedged the butt of his loaded gun in the grate, lit the fire and seated himself in front of the muzzle to await the discharge.

When a shotgun or rifle has been used, some agent, e.g. a piece of stick, a poker or a fisherman's "lazy stick", may be near the weapon.

It is not imperative to use an implement with which to fire a shotgun or rifle. It is a routine step at autopsy to measure the length of the deceased's arm. Even if it appears too short to have reached the trigger, due allowance must be made for the possibility that he had adopted a posture in which he was able to reach and release the trigger.

The weapon is almost invariably at the scene and usually near or on the body. A suicide, however, can fling the gun away from his body when he collapses, or his body may slide a few feet from the weapon (Case No. 13, p. 225). The weapon may be firmly gripped in his hand by instant rigor; a rare event but the hallmark of suicide. Absence of the weapon at the scene does not exclude suicide. A relative or friend, in an attempt to avoid a suicide verdict, may remove the gun (Fig. 65, p. 224). The gun may have slipped into water, out of sight, if suicide occurs on the bank of a pond (Simpson, 1965).

Ownership of the gun is to be ascertained. Although a person may be murdered by his own weapon, it is unusual for the suicide to use a gun other than his own or one which is accessible to him in his home or place of employment.

Fingerprints on the gun, if exclusively those of the deceased, point to suicide. It could be, as has sometimes been alleged, that the prints of another were applied in an attempt to prevent suicide by pulling the weapon from his hands.

The posture of the body and its relationship to the surroundings requires careful note and record, *by sketch* as well as photographic record.

If clothed, note is taken of the fact that it has been opened. Some, who shoot themselves in the chest or abdomen, open their clothing, ostensibly to bring the muzzle into direct contact with the skin; it would be a most unusual murderer who had opened the victim's clothing before shooting him.

The site of the entrance wound is especially important because it is almost always readily accessible and is planned. The temple, forehead or roof of the mouth are examples and, if the wound be a contact one, there is a strong presumption of suicide. Deviation, even by an inch, from the centre of the forehead, on the other hand, calls for caution in interpretation. Similarly, when the entrance wound is above and behind the ear. Homicide through the roof of the mouth is rare. There is the story of the girl who asked her boy friend to shut his eyes and open his mouth and she then shot him in the mouth. A man who murdered his family shot one of his children in the mouth.

Examination of the hands is especially important. In suicide it is likely that the hand which fired the gun, if a hand gun, or the hand which steadied the shotgun or rifle may bear traces of the products of detonation, notably powder grains. These may not be obvious when modern cartridges are used. The hand, and in particular the skin at the base of the thumb and index finger, should be swabbed and the swabs examined for nitrates, etc. The hand may bear flecks of blood. There may be a thermal burn in the palm following contact with the hot barrel of the gun.

Suicide is usually accomplished by one shot but multiple entrance wounds are known. For example, the first shot may be under the chin and directed to one side so that there is relatively minor damage, restricted to the superficial neck tissues, and the major vessels remain intact; he may shoot himself in the upper abdomen but the direction of the shot although taking a "through and through" course, may result in damage restricted to the abdominal wall and, perhaps, the colon; the man may then be able to fire a second shot. Mention has been made elsewhere (see p. 215) of multiple shots by suicides before they succeeded in their attempt.

Homicidal Firearm Injuries

The site of the entrance wound in an inaccessible part, e.g. the back of the body, or a deviation from the normal position of a suicidal injury of the head, raises a presumption of homicide. In does not follow that an entrance wound at the back of the head is always homicidal. The Leeds series includes the case of a Portuguese student who shot himself in the back of the head with a shotgun (Leeds City Coroner 309/42) and the man who shot himself with a revolver at the centre point between the ears at the back of his head.

A range of fire outside that of self-infliction is at once presumptive evidence of homicide, unless special steps had been taken by the victim to effect suicide at a distance. In the latter circumstances there will be evidence of the arrangements he had made. Contact injuries are presumptive evidence of suicide; although it is true that the majority of contact injuries are suicidal, there are occasions when they are homicidal. When homicidal, it is probable that the victim was incapacitated by disease, drink or drugs, was asleep, or, as in the case of prisoners in World War II, under restraint.

A body "riddled" with bullets excludes suicide but multiple firearm injuries, up to at least six, have been self-inflicted. It is possible for a suicide to shoot himself coincidentally with each of two weapons. The Chinese man mentioned by Gonzales *et al.* (1954) did so in the presence of witnesses. Although the record does not mention two separate wounds, a man who shot himself in Leeds held an automatic pistol in each hand (Leeds City Coroner, 608/37). The weapon may be one which discharges a succession of bullets when the trigger is released and continues to fire as long as there is pressure on it; the suicide could continue to exert pressure for a brief period before he lost consciousness and thus be shot by more than one bullet. In the case of a shotgun the first shot may not have been lethal and the suicide is able to fire the second barrel.

It is important to distinguish multiple exit wounds from those of entrance. A single missile can disintegrate and produce two or more exit wounds. Secondary missiles, e.g. portions of broken bone, clothing or buttons, may also produce exit wounds.

Curious results may be expected if the bullet splits on contact with bone. Ellis (1959) described two cases of this kind. The victims had apparently sustained two firearm injuries, yet only one bullet had been fired. The bullet, 0.22 calibre, when it struck the forehead, had split in two; one portion, later recovered from the brain, had entered through a hole in the skull between the two external wounds. The other fragment had ricocheted off the skull to leave by the second upper wound in the forehead. The lower wound presented as a "contact" injury but the upper one, an inch higher, was without the signs of a contact injury.

The weapon is usually absent but, if an automatic pistol, spent cartridge cases may be left at the scene either because the assailant did not have time to collect them or they had been lost to sight. These should be sought for since they may bear important marks by which a suspected weapon could be identified. Rarely a murderer may leave the weapon at the scene and arrange it so as to simulate suicide. The gun may be placed in the victim's hand but it is highly improbable that it will be held by a firm grip; that of instantaneous rigor is a vital phenomenon and its firmness is rarely if ever equalled by the normal stiffening of muscles after death.

Accidental Firearm Injuries

Sometimes there are witnesses. In their absence the features which suggest an accident are, first, a single shot; second, a range of fire and direction of aim which are consistent with the firer's account of the shooting. A careful examination of the scene may yield insignificant yet important evidence. When a man was found shot in a wood the first impressions were those of suicide. It was possible to prove that he had slipped and fallen when negotiating a barbed wire fence. Fibres of wool, identical with that of his stockings, were found on the barbed wire. His left stocking was torn as by wire and he had linear scratches of the left leg. On that occasion it was especially important to distinguish between suicide and accidental death since a considerable sum was forfeit in the event of a verdict of suicide (Case No. 17, p. 229).

SUMMARY

The foregoing is not intended to be a complete account of the features on which the interpretation of firearm injuries is based. Each case must be approached with an open mind and all require close attention to detail, no matter how obvious their circumstances appear to be.

The medical and scientific evidence in the case of J. D. Merrett (Roughead, 1929) should be obligatory reading for all engaged in crime detection. It is an outstanding example of how the investigation of firearm injuries should NOT be undertaken.

EMBOLISM OF MISSILES

Although a rare event, embolism of missiles is well recognised. Keeley (1951), when adding a new case, summarised the reports of twenty-two published cases. A bullet which enters the left ventricle can be carried in the blood stream and lodge in a femoral artery (Keeley, 1951; Iskeceli, 1962), axillary (Saltzstein and Freeark, 1963) or a brachial artery (Neerken and Clement, 1964). Even more remarkable, and as yet unique, was the case of bullet embolism in the right pulmonary artery, reported by the late Douglas Collins (1948). The patient shot himself in the chest and the bullet entered his right ventricle. It lodged for a time in the interventricular septum and was then carried to the right pulmonary artery. The immediate cause of death was massive infarction of the right lung. The patient survived 19 days.

The weapon was a block of aluminium to which he had added a clip to fasten it to his braces. He had drilled a hole in the block to take a Sten gun cartridge. He had detonated it by a blow with a spanner.

Shotgun pellets which enter the heart may become emboli.

Kinmonth *et al.* (1961) described the case of a boy aged 12 who was injured by a 0.410 shotgun at a range of 35 yards. Loose shot had entered the right side of the heart and some had been transferred to the lungs. A few had traversed the septum to enter the left ventricle; these could have become cerebral emboli. Fortunately operative removal of the pellets prevented this and, but for transient pain and hyperaesthesia of the right foot, due to popliteal embolism, the boy made an uneventful recovery. Shot of size 5, i.e. 3 mm in diameter, are large enough to obstruct the bifurcation of the carotid artery and cause hemiplegia as in one of the two cases reported by Barrett (1950).

MOBILITY AFTER INJURY BY FIREARM

On many, if not most, occasions firearm injury to the brain, heart or aorta causes immediate collapse and rapid, if not instantaneous, death. There are occasions, however, when collapse and death are delayed following grave injury to the head or chest. It may be possible for the victim to take but a few steps; on the other hand he may survive for several days before he dies of sepsis. Mrs. Merrett, for example, survived for about 14 days before she died of meningitis; a boy, who was shot in the face and suffered destruction of his lower jaw, survived for a few days before he died of gas gangrene (Leeds City Coroner: 855/31).

Mobility in these cases depends on the particular part of the brain or heart involved. An horizontal shot, which passes from temple to temple, may travel below the brain and, although it could then sever the optic nerves and cause blindness, the victim may not collapse; indeed, even if the shot passed through the frontal lobes he could remain mobile. Severance of the spinal cord, on the other hand, results in immediate paralysis.

Concussion following a head injury may produce a state of automatism in which the victim performs acts in an apparently normal fashion, but is himself unaware of his conduct.

Firearm injuries of the lungs may well be followed by a period of mobility when, as by shotgun, there are multiple small perforations without damage to a major blood vessel. These victims can run a distance of yards before they collapse from blood loss and shock

(Case No. 22, p. 238). Similarly, firearm injuries of the abdomen may not cause immediate immobility, unless the aorta or common iliac artery be damaged.

The degree of mobility after a severe head injury is well illustrated by the following case:

> An elderly man left his hotel one evening and did not return that night. This occasioned no comment because he was accustomed to absent himself without notice. He returned at 7.30 a.m. and when seen by the maid at the door, he had his umbrella over his arm and his hat on his head. The maid, however, noticed blood stains on his face and called her mistress. The man placed his umbrella in the hall, took off his overcoat and then, saying "I will just go upstairs", did so. He was found unconscious in the bathroom and transferred to hospital, where he died 3 hours later. He had a bullet wound of entry at a point beneath the chin 2 in. to the left of the middle line. There was no external blackening or tattooing round the wound but powder was found amongst the disrupted tissues in the floor of the mouth (see "Contact wounds", p. 212). The bullet had traversed the base of the tongue, the frontal and temporal lobes of the brain, which were extensively damaged, and had left the skull at the left side of the frontal bone; the exit wound was that of a 0.45 bullet which had turned on its side inside the skull. A 0.45 revolver, the property of the deceased, was found in some gardens, near the hotel. Investigation of the scene showed that the man must have shot himself before 6.30 a.m. and, for some time, had walked about before he returned to his hotel, when he still appeared to be reasonable and intelligible. He had left letters in which he declared his intention to commit suicide because he believed that he was the victim of cancer (Sydney Smith, 1943).

Firearm injury of the abdomen, is not necessarily immediately fatal, nor even, if grave, will severely incapacitate. This is illustrated by the following case:

> A man, aged 34, under pressure of heavy over-spending and demand for payment of debts, shot his wife and two sons in the parental bedroom. He then went into the bathroom and committed suicide.
>
> The weapon was a 12-bore shotgun. He made two attempts before the fatal shot. His first was a "near" shot on the left side of his abdomen. This produced a large, oval, gutter-like wound, $4^1/_2 \times 2^1/_2$ in., the floor of which was formed by lacerated muscle; the abdomen had not been opened.
>
> The second attempt produced a contact wound, with a recoil bruise from the second barrel of the gun, within 1 in. of his first attempt. The shot travelled in a horizontal line, backwards and to the left, and the exit wound was an irregular hole 4 in. in diameter in the left loin. It was centred 12 in. below the top of his shoulder. The skin adjacent to the hole was punctured by pellets, and a wad and pellets were recovered from the tissues around the hole. Coils of intestine had herniated through the hole, but the colon was the only major structure damaged by the shot.
>
> Despite the shock and pain which these two injuries must have produced he then proceeded to the third and fatal shot, which was a contact injury to the forehead just above the left eye.
>
> The gun was found beside his body with the trigger guard uppermost, and the butt lodged behind the pedestal of the w.c. His right arm measured 28 in. from top of shoulder to tip of middle finger, i.e. long enough for him to have fired the gun, when arranged as it was found.

MULTIPLE CONTACT ENTRANCE WOUNDS

It is a reasonable presumption that a contact firearm injury in the temple, or elsewhere in the head, for that matter, will be fatal. There are always exceptions. Tesař (1958) recorded the occurrence of two separate, unequivocal entrance wounds, each accompanied by a recoil imprint of the muzzle of the gun, in the left temple of a left-handed man, aged 35. The gun was a 6.35 Browning automatic pistol. His first shot had taken an oblique course and damage was restricted to the frontal lobes; his second shot had destroyed the basal ganglia.

An even more remarkable case was that of a man aged 74 whose suicide began with the firing of no less than four shots at his head. Possibly because of an unusual consistence of construction of his skull, and a relatively low muzzle velocity, none of the shot penetrated or fractured the skull; the flattened projectiles were found lying against the skull. He had not lost consciousness. He accomplished suicide by a fifth shot into his chest; the bullet pierced his heart and came to rest in his stomach. The gun was a 0.32 Colt Short and he had used lead alloy bullets, 80 grain instead of the proper 98 grain; this had reduced the muzzle velocity from 780 ft/sec to 346 (± 57) ft/sec (Mason *et al.*, 1966). This case is not unique. Gonzales *et al.* (1954) recalled the old man who fired five shots through the anterior part of his temple; he perforated the skull five times without touching the brain. He survived for several days and then died of sepsis.

It is possible for the suicide to fire two shots into his temple, when the first cartridge is defective. Gonzales *et al.* depict the case of suicide in which the first bullet, owing to defect in the cartridge, lodged in the temple but failed to enter the skull; the second, fatal shot entered just in front of the other one.

Alcoholic Intoxication and Firearm Injuries

It should be a routine practice to determine the alcoholic content of the blood and, if available, the urine of all victims of firearm injuries. The majority of the suicides in the series analysed by Canfield (1969), namely 18 or 78 per cent, were under the influence of alcohol. The range in our series was from 97 mg/100 ml to 210 mg/100 ml blood; the latter result was from a woman who shot herself with a revolver while on her bed (Case No. 30, p. 248). By contrast, a suicide, who planned a shotgun head injury, firing the weapon with a fisherman's "lazy stick", was cold sober (Case No. 14, p. 226).

Guerin (1960) found that 59 per cent of the 167 subjects in his series had a blood alcohol content which exceeded 100 mg/100 ml; the maximum level was 390 mg/100 ml; the level was 100 mg/100 ml or over in seventeen of fifty-seven homicides but only ninety-one suicides were intoxicated. In one of our cases of homicide it was 249 mg/100 ml in the blood and 196 mg/100 ml in the urine, a result which represented the ingestion of 12 pints of beer. Intoxication to this degree must facilitate homicide; it could provoke an argument or quarrel.

The absence of alcohol, or a low content, in the body is likely in those shot by accident and this finding would support an explanation of accidental shooting.

Tandem-Bullet Injuries

In the event of a misfire or a defect in the cartridge, a bullet may remain in the barrel of the weapon until it is moved by a second discharge. The two bullets may then travel in tandem and enter the target through a single hole. Unless this is realised, the presence of two bullets in the victim's body may throw doubt on the statement by the firer that he had fired but once. The ballistic expert can confirm that the bullets had travelled in tandem.

Gonzales *et al.* (1954) describe and depict an example. Owing to defect in the cartridge a 9-mm bullet remained in the gun. The second discharge carried both bullets in tandem. There was one entrance hole in his head but two bullets were found half an inch apart embedded in the skull on the opposite side of the head. The illustration shows how the impacted bullet could be stood on top of the second one.

Michaux and Thiodet (1960) reported the case of a woman who was shot in the right breast. At operation a bullet was removed from the base of the right side of her chest and the wound was closed. Subsequent X-ray examination disclosed the presence of a second bullet which was extracted through the same incision. Her husband maintained, and his mother confirmed, that he had fired only one shot and it had been an accident. Examination of the bullets showed that they had travelled in tandem.

A detailed report by Lowbeer (1961) concerned a woman who was shot by her husband during a quarrel; he contended he had fired in self-defence. There had been a misfire, ascribed to faulty ammunition, and the 0.32 bullet lodged in the gun until it was moved by the subsequent discharge. There was a single bullet wound in the head had a track through the brain as by a single bullet, but at its end two bullets were found lying "like peas in a pod". It was not the fatal shot. He had fired a prior shot, which fractured the base of the skull and the ethmoid sinuses and which caused considerable bleeding into the air passages; the immediate cause of death was inhalation of blood and pulmonary oedema.

The jury acquitted the accused "assuming homicide justifiable because of self-defence and temporary insanity". It appears they were influenced by evidence concerning the characters of the couple, who had been about to be divorced.

References

ANON. (1929) *Encycl. Britannica*, 14th ed., Vol. 1, p. 457.
BARRETT, N. R. (1950) *Brit. J. Surg.*, 37, 416.
BEATTIE, J. F. and DALY, R. J. (1960) *Amer. J. Obstet. Gynec.*, 80, 772–4.
BOCHNER, K. (1961) *Obstet. Gynec.*, 17, 520.
BURRARD, Sir GERALD (1956) *Identification of Fire-arms and Forensic Ballistics, 3rd* ed. London: Herbert Jenkins.
BURRARD, Sir GERALD (1960) *Modern Shotgun*, 3 vols. London: Herbert Jenkins.
CANFIELD, T. M. (1969) *J. Forens. Sci.*, 14, 445.
COLLINS, D. H. (1948) *J. Path. Bact.*, 60, 205.
DRAKE, V. (1962a) *J. Forens. Sci. Soc.*, 2, 85.
DRAKE, V. (1962b) *J. Forens. Sci. Soc.*, 3, 22.
ELLIS, H. D. (1959) *Police*, 3, 51–52.
FRITZ, E. (1942) *Arch. Kriminol*, 3, 51–52.
GLANTON, A. and MORGAN, H. C. (1968) *American Rifleman*, Aug., 35.
GONZALES, T. A., VANCE, M., HELPERN, M. and UMBERGER, C. J. (1954) *Legal Medicine and Toxicology*, 2nd ed., pp. 397442, New York: Appleton Century.
GUERIN, P. F. (1960) *J. Forens. Sci.*, 5, 294–318.
HALLER, J. A. (1962) *Amer. J. Surg.*, 103, 532.
HASTINGS, Sir Patrick (1949) *Cases in Court*, London, pp. 263–78. Melbourne and Toronto; Heinemann.
HEULLY, F., DE REN, G. and PICARD, L. (1965) *Annls Méd.-lég. Crimin. Police Scient.*, 45, 298.
HUNT, A. C. and KON, V. M. (1962) *Med. Sci. Law*, 2, 197–203.
ISKECELI, O. K. (1962) *Arch. Surg., Chicago*, 85, 184.
JAMES, W. R. L. (1962) *Med. Sci. Law*, 2, 153–4.
KEELEY, J. L. (1951) *J. Thor. Surg.*, 21, 608.
KINMONTH, J. B., BURTON, J. D., LONGMORE, D. B. and COOK, W. A. (1961) *Brit. Med. J.*, ii, 1666–8.
KOBAK, A. J. and HURWITZ, C. H. (1954) *Obstet. Gynec.*, 4, 383.
KNIGHT, B. (1982) Leading Article *Brit Med. J.* 284, 768–9.
KRACKE, A. D. (1963) *J. Pediat.*, 63, 1184.
LOWBEER, L. (1961) *J. Forens. Sci.*, 6, 88–97.
MACHLE, W. (1940) *J. Amer. Med. Ass.*, 115, ii, 1536–41.
MANT, A. K. (1968) *Med. Sci. Law*, 8, 256.
MASON, M. F., ROSE, E. and ALEXANDER, F. (1966) Abstract of Papers IVth International Meeting in Forensic Medicine, 15–18 August, Copenhagen, p. 190.
MERRETT, J. D. the trial of (1927) See Roughead (1929); Teare (1955).
MICHAUX, P. and THIODET, J. (1960) *Annls Méd.-lég. Crimin. Police Scient.*, 40, 68.
NEERKEN, A. J. and CLEMENT, F. L. (1964) *J. Amer. Med. Ass.*, 189, 579.
OLLIVIER, H., LEVY-LEROY, J. C. and VUILLET, F. (1962a) *Annls Méd.-lég. Crimin. Police Scient.*, 42, 245.
OLLIVIER, H., VUILLET, F. and BASTARET, M. (1962b) *Annls Méd.-lég. Crimin. Police Scient.*, 42, 167.
PETTY, C. S. and HAUSER, J. E. (1968) *J. Forens. Sci.*, 13, 114.
PIÉDELIÈVRE, R., and DESOILLE, H. (1939) *Blessures par coups de feu*. Paris: Baillière.

PIÉDELIÈVRE, R., DESOILLE, H. and MICHONI, R. (1956) *Med. Biol.* (11.), **6**, 225–9.
PRICE, G. (1960) *Crim. L. R.* 404; 478; 543; 611.
R. v. BARNEY (1932) Cited Hastings (1949).
R. v. RACE (1840) Cited Taylor (1965).
ROSSANO, Y., GALLET, F., VUILLET, F. and OLLIVIER, H. (1964) *Annls Méd.-lég. Crimin. Police Scient.*, **44**, 87.
ROUGHEAD, W. (1929) *Trial of John Donald Merrett.* Edinburgh and London; Hodge.
SALTZSTEIN, E. C. and FREEARK, R. J. (1963) *Ann. Surg. Chicago.* **158**, 65.
SHOEMAKER, R. and ECKELS, J. C. (1930) *New Engl. J. Med.*, **203**, 195–201.
SIMON, G. (1958) *Arch. Psychiat. Nervenkr.*, **197**, 124–47.
SIMONIN, C. (1955). *Médicine Légale Judiciare*, 3rd ed. Paris: Maloine.
SIMPSON, K. (1965) in *Taylor* (1965), pp. 303, 305.
SIMPSON, K. (1969) *Forensic Medicine*, 6th ed., p. 80, Fig. 66. London: Edward Arnold.
SMITH, SYDNEY (1943) *Police J.*, **16**, 108–10.
SMITH, SYDNEY and GLAISTER, JOHN (1939) *Recent Advances in Forensic Medicine*, 2nd ed., pp. 1–85. London: Churchill.
SPITZ, W. U. and WILHELM, R. M. (1970) *J. Forens. Med.*, **17**, 5.
TAYLOR, A. S. (1965) *Principles and Practice of Medical Jurisprudence*, 12th ed., pp. 303, 305, ed. K. Simpson. London: Churchill.
TEARE, R. D. (1955) *Med. Leg. J. (Camb.)* **23**, 57.·
TESAŘ, J. (1958) *Soudni Lek. pro Prevniky*, p. 280; English trans.: *J. Forens. Med.* (1964), **11**, 106.
WEATHERHEAD, A. D. and ROBINSON, B. M. (1970) *Firearms in Crime*, No. 4. H.O. Statistical Division Report; London, H.M.S.O.
WOLFF, F. and LAUFER, M. (1965) *Dtsch. Z. ges. gerichtl. Med.*, **56**, 87.
WOLFF, F. and LAUFER, M. (1966), *Arch. Kriminol.* **137**, 38.
WRIGHT, C. H., POSNER, A. C. and GILCHRIST, J. (1954) *Amer. J. Obstet. Gynec.* **67**, 1085.

CHAPTER 6

Electrical Injuries and Lightning Stroke

Historical Note

Lightning stroke was recorded at least as early as the first century AD. Pliny the Elder, in his "Natural History" (77 AD) recorded the stroke of a pregnant woman; her child was killed but she survived (Wagner and McCann, 1941). Benjamin Franklin (1706–1790) read a paper, entitled "The sameness of lightning with electricity", in about 1750, before the Royal Society. It was received with derisive laughter but, a few years later, his experiments were better appreciated; he was then invited to accept the fellowship and excused the customary payments and, in 1753, he was awarded the Copley gold medal. His principal experiment, of which he did not appear to realise its danger, was the demonstration that lightning flashes were electrical discharges and not, as formerly believed, gaseous explosions. He arranged the collection of electricity from the clouds by flying a kite during a storm and connecting the lower end of its string with a Leyden jar. This experiment led on to the invention of lightning rods or conductors which, today, give protection to buildings and other prominent structures.

The scientific study of electricity was greatly advanced by the invention of the Leyden jar by van Musschenhoek in 1746. It was the product of a delightfully simple experiment. A gun barrel was suspended by two silk threads. A wire, fixed to the middle of the barrel, was led through a cork into a flask filled with water. When the gun was charged with electricity the charge was stored in the flask. The experiment exceeded his expectations but nearly put an end to his further research. When he touched the barrel with one hand and put his other on the flask the discharge prostrated him for two days. (deVille, 1955). News of this experiment soon spread and in England experience of the effects of electric shocks became a popular and fashionable activity. Abbé Nollet, "electrician" to Louis xv, on hearing of the experiment, sought to repeat it, not on himself, but on others. It became a source of innocent merriment at the French court. He connected 180 soldiers of the Guard with a capacitator; at the moment of discharge the men leapt as one into the air. A better spectacle was provided by 700 monks who were connected with each other and with a capacitator. At the moment of discharge they leapt into the air "with a simultaneity of precision out-rivalling the timing of the most perfect corps de ballet" (Cohen, 1941).

In the latter half of the 19th and the early 20th century an outstanding advance in the use of electricity was in the field of electric traction. The earliest electric railway in this country was constructed in 1883 at Port Rush in N. Ireland. Thomas Parker (1843–1915), of Ironbridge, Shropshire, was a notable pioneer in this country. He was consultant engineer of the Blackpool tramway, 1884–86, and of the Liverpool Overhead Railway, (1883) the first of its kind in Europe, if not of the world. His principal work was as consultant engineer for the electrification of the Metropolitan and District Railway, the first section of the London Underground to be electrified. The line had been opened in 1863 but, until 1900–06, the trains were hauled by steam engines and the passengers had to suffer the effects of smoke and soot when they passed through the tunnels. (It was an appropriate gesture, which would have given him great pleasure, when the local authority commemorated his memory by naming the school for handicapped children in Telford, the Thomas Parker School).

Incidence of Fatalities

Despite the widespread increase in the distribution of electricity in the home, as well as in industry, whereby millions of the population have access to this dangerous but invaluable source of light and power, fatalities continue to be few, less than 200 a year in a population of over 50 millions, which consumes over 100,000 million kW hours a year. Although its potential danger is at least that of coal gas, the latter, in its hey-day, claimed an average of 2580 deaths a year, during 1948–53. Electricity also is, as yet, an uncommon choice of the suicide whereas 1961 of the deaths by inhaling coal gas during 1948–53 were suicidal.

There has been a steady fall in the number of deaths by electrocution in relation to the amount of electricity supplied; this is indicated by the statistics of fatalities per million kW hours consumed (Lee, 1965a).

The precise total of electrical accidents, however, is difficult to ascertain since non-fatal accidents in the home are not recorded and those which occur in industry may not come to notice unless the premises are subject to the Factory Act. Nor is it certain that all fatalities are included in the Registrar General's list. Lee (1965a) found that there were nine deaths during 1963 which were not in the list. Incidentally, not all of those which were included were deaths by electrocution. Lee had to exclude twelve cases, since seven of the deaths had occurred in 1962, four were deaths by burning and one died in an explosion. Despite the difficulty in obtaining precise figures, the fact remains that fatalities are relatively few. Lee estimated them at about 140 a year.

Lee (1965a) furnished statistics which indicated that since the beginning of this century there had been a steady increase of these fatalities; an average death rate of 11.25 per year in 1901–4 had risen to 128 in 1955–59 and during 1960–62 the rate was 130.3. Further increase was anticipated; contrary to expectation, there was a notable decrease during 1967–69; i.e. about 90 deaths/year. The peak year still seems to have been 1943, when, under wartime conditions, it was difficult to maintain a high degree of safety. In that year fatal electrical accidents totalled 183. Industrial accidents totalled 1255, of which 58 were fatal.

Incidence: Danger of Imported Appliances

The classification of deaths due to electrical shock was changed by the I.C.D in 1968 and placed in classification E 925, which includes not only deaths due to faulty domestic wiring and appliances but also fatal accidents in power generating units, etc. The annual totals of these deaths during 1975–79 were: 93, 115, 101, 98 and 75 (Lee and McNamee, 1982). Even if it be assumed that for each of these deaths there were at least two non-fatal accidents, the incidence of serious injury by electrical current is low.

There is no room for complacency. From time to time cheap dangerous appliances are imported. Hair driers, power driven tools and, now, the latest menace is a three-way adaptor, L Y 7387, imported from Hong Kong. It was found to be inadequately earthed. The director of the W. Yorks. County trading standards, Mr. John Bennett, is reported to have described it as the most dangerous accessory (as yet) examined in their laboratory (*Yorkshire Post*, Friday, 19 Nov., 1982). Constant vigilance in the observance of safety precautions, and their extension as may be required, is needed to maintain the present high degree of safety in industry and the home.

Domestic wiring and appliances must be kept in good order. Frayed flex should be promptly replaced or repaired and appliances should receive periodical checks, e.g. electric blankets, vacuum cleaners and kettles. Education of the public, especially children in respect of potential dangers is a worthwhile investment.

Lee drew attention to the earth-leak circuit breaker devised by Dalziel (1962), and its potential safety value, if universally installed and correctly maintained and adjusted. This fitting prevents the occurrence of ventricular fibrillation and, since this is the immediate cause of death in the majority of fatal electrical accidents, it would of itself be a major factor in the reduction in these deaths. Lee thought it probable that most of those who had died of shocks which passed from limb to limb and through the thorax, as happens in about 75 per cent, would have been saved; in his view it is also probable that electrocution in a bath is due to the thorax being in the route of the current and they too might have been saved.

Gordon (1968), in the discussion of Dalziel and Lee's (1968) paper, reported that dogs he had subjected to electrical shocks from a 115 volt supply, with a G.F.I. inserted between the animals and the supply, were immune to ventricular fibrillation when the current passed arm to leg or arm to arm. It occurred in only a few animals when there was maximum contact with the chest to chest route, which is in accidental electrocution in man.

Although pathologists, individually, see few cases in any one year, or for that matter, during their whole career, it is important that they are prompt to recognise this cause of death.

The Goulstonian Lectures of 1913, delivered by Jex-Blake, remain a principal account of electrical injuries, surpassed only by the review by Jaffé (1928). Reviews by Langworthy and Kouwenhoven (1932), Long (1935) and Alexander (1938) are also noteworthy; another review was by Polson (1959). The outstanding work, and one which includes several excellent plates in colour, is *Die Elektrischen Verletzungen* by Jellinek (1932), which is considerably better than his earlier *Der Elektrische Unfall* of 1927, although the latter is valuable. The research by Ferris *et al.* (1936) and the publications of Dalziel and his colleagues since 1941 and by Lee and his colleagues since 1961 are also major contributions to the subject. The early researches of Oliver and Bolam (1898) are at least of historical interest. Electrical injuries of the nervous system were described by Critchley (1934, 1935), Panse (1930), Hassin (1933, 1937) and Dickson (1947). The review by Goldie and Lee (1976) is a comprehensive account of current knowledge of lightning death.

Factors Which Influence the Effect of Electrical Shocks

The electrical voltage or tension, although less important than the amperage, i.e. intensity, is a convenient index of the danger of an electrical current. Low tensions, of 50 volts or under, as used therapeutically, rarely cause accidents, but fatalities due to alternating current of low tension have been recorded, e.g. Capello and Pellegrini's case (cited Jaffé, 1928), where the tension was 46 volts. Jellinek believed a tension which exceeded 25 volts can be dangerous; Jex-Blake regarded one of 65 volts dangerous if the current passed through the heart. A few fatalities with 60 and 65 volt a.c. current have been recorded, a death from contact with 24 volt d.c. is reported below.

Steps were taken by H.M. Factory Department to ensure the operation of portable electric tools by a supply of not more than 110 volts, i.e. 55 volts to earth (H.M. Chief Inspector of Factories, 1951).

Most of the fatalities follow shocks from currents at a tension of 220–250 volts, i.e. the usual household supply. Emmerson (1961, cited and confirmed by Lee, 1961) found that approximately two-thirds of all fatalities were from voltages below 250. A proportion are due to contact with high tension circuits of which the voltage is measured in thousands. It does not follow, however, that death is then inevitable. Other factors, e.g. brief duration of contact, may appreciably minimise the effects. A boy aged 15 failed in his attempt at suicide when he touched a wire carrying a supply of 8000 volts (Gey, 1926). A man survived the immediate effects of contact with 4000 volts but later died of tetanus infection of his injuries (Chiari, 1919, cited by Jaffé, 1928).

Conversely, medium voltages, i.e. under 500, predispose to prolonged contact because the victim grips and holds on to the conductor; this is actually dependent on the amperage rather than the voltage of the current. Lee found that only one of fourteen "held on" cases occurred at high voltage (6000 volts); all the others were associated with medium voltage. The liability to Joule burns is not surprisingly related to holding on to the conductor, fourteen of fifteen Joule burns occurred in "held on" accidents (Lee, 1961).

Notwithstanding the wide distribution of high-tension circuits in industry, the majority of industrial accidents were due to contact with a low or medium voltage supply. Thus, in a series of 250 accidents 206 were due to low-voltage contacts and only forty-four were with high tension (3300 volts or over) and in industry as a whole, the proportion was 427 to 75 accidents (Wood, 1965). Incidentally, he found that it was quite common to work with 240 volt supplies "live".

The agents commonly responsible for fatal accidents in industry were hand tools (8), over-head lines (9), switch gear (7) and lamps (4); these accounted for 28/41 or 68 per cent (Corney, 1961).

Amperage is important and probably the most important factor in electrocution. It is the cause of "hold-on" to conductors which, in turn, is the cause of serious local damage and fatal shock. It is determined by dividing the voltage or tension by the resistance of the conductor. This formula, $A = V \div R$, applies to direct current and alternating current when in phase.

Contact with current at only 1 mA can yield a sensation of tingling. As the amperage rises the sensation becomes increasingly unpleasant and then painful. There is inability to release the conductor at relatively low amperage. Experiments have shown that healthy young men can tolerate a current of up to 21.6 mA but, normally, "hold on" occurs at about 8.8 to 9.4 mA. Women are somewhat less tolerant. For them the maximum level is 14 mA and the average upper limit is 6 mA with a.c. current at 50 cycles (Wood, 1965; Lee, 1965a, b). Currents between 10 mA and 60 mA cause "hold on", loss of muscular control, asphyxia or ventricular fibrillation. Contact with a current of 60 mA for a second or longer is dangerous. The critical level, i.e. that calculated to prove fatal, is about 100 mA for one-fifth of a second with a.c. at 50 cycles. With d.c. the critical amperage is of the order of 200 to 250 mA. The danger increases when amperage rises above 100 mA to about 4 A. Thereafter it decreases and if the heart be fibrillating an increase of amperage above 4 A arrests fibrillation; this is the principle of treatment with a defibrillator.

It is possible that shocks at a high voltage may be in circumstances of low amperage and, therefore, much less dangerous than contact with a current of moderate voltage but of which amperage is high. An example of this occurred when a photographer received a shock from an electronic flash unit (see p. 298).

Conversely there is the apparent paradox of death from low-voltage d.c., normally considered incapable of producing serious ill-effects. In the case reported below, where 24-volt d.c. caused electrocution, contact was prolonged because the man was wedged beneath the vehicle; conditions were damp and contact was with areas of skin of relatively low resistance, i.e. shoulder and thigh. It was possible therefore for a current of over 60 mA to have passed through his body. He was well earthed at the time.

Case Report: Electrocution by Low-voltage, 24-volt d.c.

The victim was a milk roundsman aged 52, who was found dead beneath a hand-controlled milk float on 26 December 1956. The vehicle was powered by two 12-volt batteries, yielding a 24-volt d.c. supply of electricity. Snow and ice were on the ground at the time. He was wedged under the vehicle with his right shoulder blade near, if not in contact with, an uninsulated coil; his right thigh was pressed against the chassis. Two electric marks were present on his body. That over the right shoulderblade measured 3.5 × 1.0 cm; this presented as on oval, shallow crater lined by grey-white skin which was slightly translucent: it was bordered by a faint but distinct zone of hyperaemia (Fig. 100). Minute haemorrhages were present in the subcutaneous tissues related to the mark. The other mark, over the outer aspect of the right hip joint, was also an oval, shallow crater, 3 × 1.8 cm; this was lined by light brown skin, in parts translucent; this skin was somewhat parchmented (Fig. 100). Small haemorrhages and disruption of the subcutaneous tissues were apparent to the unaided eye.

Microscopical examination of the marks, more especially that on the thigh, demonstrated a honey-comb disruption of the corium.

Except for the electric marks and a few petechial haemorrhages beneath the epicardium at the back of the heart, there was no sign of injury or disease. There seems little doubt that death was due to electrocution, although tests applied to the vehicle failed to demonstrate any defect in it, beyond a slight leak from the batteries. This appeared capable of yielding an amperage of about 5 mA, i.e. well below the danger level. The fact remains that this healthy man died in circumstances which could only be explained by accidental contact with an electrically-powered vehicle and he had two unequivocal electric marks on his body. There were no other injuries to account for his death (F.M. 5097; post-mortem by Dr. H. Thompson and C.P.).

A fatal case of electrocution with low voltage and low amperage was reported by Balbo (1957).

The density of the current is believed by some to be a major factor.

The resistance of the body tissues also plays an important part. The effects of a shock will be materially modified according to the part of the body which comes into contact with the current and, again, whether the skin be dry or moist. The dry skin of the palms offers the greatest resistance and, in a labourer, it was estimated by Jellinek at from a million to two million ohms. Sweating appreciably reduces resistance; the fall was estimated by Cardieu (cited Jaffé, 1928) to be from 30,000 ohms to 2500 ohms; when the skin was moistened with water or saline there was a further fall to between 1200 to 1500 ohms. (A. S. Curry and C. J. Polson confirmed this.) Furthermore, changes in the skin produced by the current decreased resistance to only 380 ohms, but, once burnt, the resistance of the skin rises and this may cause a break in the circuit. If, however, the tissues be carbonised, conduction through them improves.

There is a considerable range in the resistance offered by the skin, this being greatest in the palms, especially of labourers, and least on the inner side of the thigh. The average skin resistance is of the order of 500 to 10,000 ohms. Vascular areas, e.g. the cheek, are better conductors; the mucosae offer a resistance of only about 1500 to 2000 ohms, but bone has a resistance of about 900,000 ohms. The blood is the best conductor in the body and Jellinek believed, and Langworthy and Kouwenhoven (1932) have shown, that most of the current passes along the blood vessels. Jellinek has pointed out, however, that the effects in man are not dependent on a simple ohmic resistance; the capacity of the body for polarization permits it to act as a condenser. Some of the effects due to lightning stroke have been explained on this basis (Pritchard, 1934).

In industry the risk is greater than in domestic circumstances because the workers may be on concrete which is rarely quite dry, or on damp ground or flooring; they may be wearing steel-shod boots or worn boots. They are often near steelwork. In the home the person is likely to be dry shod, stood on wood or a carpeted floor. Here the greatest risk is in the bathroom and, above all, in the bath. In the home glancing contact with the electric current may result only in a sensation of tingling or, at worst, an unpleasant shock and

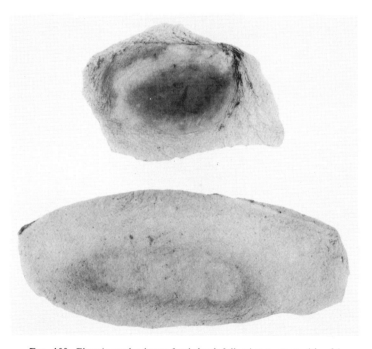

Fig. 100. Electric marks due to fatal shock following contact with a 24-volt d.c. circuit. (a) Left: mark on right should—hyperaemia border; (b) right; mark on left hip—a mild Joule burn.

temporary increase in heart and respiration rate, as happened when a finger was put on a live floor plug socket. If, however, the conductor is grasped there is the likelihood of "hold on" and fatal shock; similarly, if the subject is well earthed. This can result in a hand to hand shock from the mains and, according to Wood (1965); it is a common cause of electrocution.

INSULATION

Stout rubber gloves and rubber boots, in good condition (not infrequently the boots of the victim have worn soles), are a considerable protection but the wrist may still come into contact with the supply. All tools used should be adequately insulated, e.g. the handles are made of non-conducting material or, in the case of mechanical drills and the like, the casing is adequately earthed. It is indeed hazardous to effect repairs of domestic appliances with scissors or other household implements, while the apparatus, as is not rarely the case, is still connected with the supply. A woman was electrocuted when she attempted to repair a vacuum cleaner with scissors. She had taken the precaution to pull the plug from the wall socket but, unknown to her, her son, aged 3, had reinserted the plug. "About half the deaths of women over 60 were due to the use of metal scissors in the investigation of connectors of electric irons and kettles" (Lee, 1965).

CONTACT WITH THE ELECTRICAL SUPPLY

Electrocution is normally the result of direct contact with the 240-volt a.c. supply, and the closer the contact the greater the danger, especially when it results in "hold on". A glancing contact or a fall against the conductor, on the other hand, is followed by a break in the circuit; in the case of high-tension supplies the victim is usually repelled violently and, if on a pylon or ladder, thrown to the ground. The fatal injuries may then be due to his fall.

Broad, good contact reduces skin resistance appreciably, e.g. from 100,000 ohms to 1000 ohms (Simonin, 1955).

Indirect contact with high-tension current not only results in arcing but there may be direct flow of current in an indirect fashion. Jellinek (1927) told of the boy who was electrocuted when he urinated on to a high-tension conductor; the current ascended the stream of urine. It appears cows have sustained electric shocks in this manner.

The area of contact modifies the external appearances. A conductor which has a small surface area, e.g. the end of a rod or wire, can produce a circular hole in the tissues and simulate a bullet injury; wire wound round a wrist produces a linear groove. On the other hand, a broad conductor, closely applied, may electrocute without producing any external mark. This may explain the fact that not infrequently electrocution in a bath is without any external mark and the diagnosis of electrocution may then have to be by exclusion of all other possible causes. There is close contact with wet skin in circumstances of good earthing. The flow of current is almost unimpeded and occurs without the generation of heat.

Duration of contact, obviously, determines the amount of damage following "hold on" contacts with low or medium voltage. The longer the contact the greater the damage, increasing from an electric mark or blister to charring, the Joule burn, and destruction of the tissues, so as to expose muscle and bone.

The site of contact has an important bearing on the effects of the shock. If it be the thickened palm of a manual worker, the resistance offered may prevent electrocution whereas contact with the arm or face is always serious.

Contact is most often with a hand; Jaffé (1928, citing Schridde) said that the left hand was most often involved, in 88 per cent, and advised those near electrical gear to keep that hand in their pocket. However, the right hand is not immune and, therefore, it is better to keep both protected.

An analysis of 118 cases by Lee (1965a) showed that the usual route, i.e. in forty-five, was arm to leg; it was arm to arm in thirty-two cases and arm–leg–arm in another eighteen cases. The thorax but not the head was also involved. It should be noted that electrocution in a bath occurred in 13 or 10 per cent of this series and Lee (1965b) believed that the thorax was probably involved in these circumstances. The finding that a limb to limb route occurred in 80 per cent is in accord with general experience. Entry by the head is uncommon, both in industrial and domestic accidents; when the face is the site of entrance it is usually the result of a fall against live apparatus, e.g. an electric fire in a bathroom (F.M. 1309) or a television set (Polson, 1959) or live cable (F.M. 11,992).

According to Simonin (1955) the right hand–leg route delivers 1.5–2.5 times the amount of current to the heart than the left arm to leg route.

The kind of electrode and its position plays a part but in Jellinek's view this is a factor of secondary importance. It is not necessary for the area of contact to be large, because a fatal shock may be sustained when contact is made with only a small area on the tip of a finger. Jellinek found that the area of contact did not determine the severity of the shock; others believe it to be an important factor.

Alternating current is more dangerous than direct current. In one series of 212 fatalities, only eight were due to direct current (Boruttau, 1918, cited Jaffé, 1928). Several fatalities from alternating current of under 220 volts have been recorded but they are rare from direct current at voltages under 220; one instance of a death from direct current of 120 volts is mentioned by Langworthy and Kouwenhoven (1932). It may be that the greater danger of a.c. is only apparent; direct current supplies are unusual and, therefore, there is less opportunity of injury by d.c. The number of cycles of alternating current is material and there is danger when the rate is between 39 and 150 c/s; the critical frequency is one of 50 to 60 c/s. An increase in the rate above this range decreases the danger; when the rate was raised to 1720 c/s, it was found that the heart was about 20 times more tolerant to the current than to one at 150 c/s (Prevost and Battelli, 1899). It is a question of the number of separate shocks received in a short period of time.

Personal idiosyncrasies of human beings may be a material factor. Jellinek considered that the individual's personality and physical condition, and the existence of mental or bodily distress at the time, influence the effect of a shock.

Disease, notably cardiac disease, may predispose to death from electrical currents of low tension. Jellinek, however, found that those who suffered from heart disease appeared better able than healthy persons to withstand severe shocks. Electro-convulsive therapy, it appears, is not contra-indicated for those who have coronary disease. Severe coronary disease may have played a material part in one death (Leeds City Coroner, No. 290/52).

Anticipation of a shock is a valuable but not infallible protection. When aware of the possibility of a shock, the victim can then withstand one which might otherwise be dangerous. Reported cases show that a person taken by surprise may succumb to shocks which normally produce no ill-effects. An engine driver was accustomed to exposing himself to shocks from an electric lamp, supplied by tension of 50 volts, as a means of earning drinks. This he did with impunity until one day his arm made accidental contact with the lamp and he died of the unexpected shock (Taylor, 1948). Jellinek conducted experiments in which eighty electricians, aware that they would receive a shock, were exposed to electrical tensions of from 50 to 500 volts. The experiments with lower voltages lasted up to 10 seconds but in those with higher voltages, exposure was limited to a fraction of a second. None of the men suffered any disturbance of function; fright and paralysing effect were absent.

Sleep is said to increase resistance to an electrical current. This belief, which at best has a slender foundation, may be based on nothing more than a statement attributed to Seneca, namely, that sleep protects against lightning stroke.

Familiarity Leading to Carelessness

Under-estimation of the danger of "live" circuits and carelessness play a part in industrial accidents. Ignorance accounts for some of the domestic accidents but the low incidence of accidents in industry is largely due to the wide recognition of the dangers and the use of safety measures. Some workmen, and they include those with experience, undoubtedly fall victims because they underestimate the danger. Rather than take the trouble to switch off the current, they risk manipulation of live wires and other gear. In his report, H.M. Chief Inspector of Factories (1951) said, "The Inspector was told, with a glance sideways, that electric shock would not hurt anyone except an old woman". Many have no doubt sustained shocks without ill-effects but fail to realise that "a dry pair of shoes on a pavement are very different electrically from a wet pair in the mud". On other occasions the circumstances are inexplicable. The victims are conscientious men, of long and wide experience, who cannot but be fully aware of the dangers. The Chief Inspector could account for these accidents only by the suggestion that they arise out of "a form of mental aberration, affecting even the experienced and conscientious persons", who are thus led to take some stupid risk or to omit some obvious precaution, when dealing with a live circuit (H.M. Chief Inspector of Factories, 1946).

The Important Factors

In Jellinek's view the effects of an electrical shock are primarily the product of voltage, amperage and duration of contact. Long (1935) estimated the effect on a more elaborate basis:

The effect = (voltage × amperage × duration)-tolerance and alertness.

The Mortality and Mechanism of Death by Electrical Shock

Mortality from electrical shock is estimated at about 5–50 per cent of known accidents, the latter rate relating to contact with high-tension current. Immediate and competent resuscitation can appreciably reduce the mortality rate, for not a few of the victims are only in a state of suspended animation, or, in the view of Urquhart and Noble (1929), of inhibition of the central nervous system. If however, this is not relieved without delay, death ensues. The majority die immediately, or the interval may be no longer than permits them to cry out at the moment of contact; death is then delayed for a short period, during which time the current may continue to pass through their bodies. A few, who after shock are found at a distance from the source of electrical current, may die notwithstanding that contact has been broken. Death may be delayed on these occasions for several minutes, and during this period the victim may recover consciousness, free himself and then die.

Presumption of death before its signs are unequivocal, e.g. a rectal temperature of only 70°F (21°C) or lower is always unwise. Long (1935) mentioned a man, whose death certificate had been issued, who revived and sat up. Jellinek also mentioned a Russian, who was believed dead after contact with high-tension current; 7 hours later the man exhaled frothy mucus. Resuscitation has been successful following the persistence of suspended animation for upwards of 2 hours (Payne, 1940; H.M. Inspector of Factories, 1946). There were 323 recoveries in the series of 479 cases studied by MacLachlan (1930) and he found artificial respiration was likely to succeed if begun within 3 minutes of the accident. He described a remarkable recovery, when resuscitation was begun at once, after the victim had received a shock from a current of 22,000 volts. Relays of rescuers maintained artificial respiration from 2 p.m. onwards. The victim remained cyanosed until 8 p.m. but began to breathe voluntarily at 10 p.m. and recovered.

On occasion, delay in death may be a matter of hours or even days. These victims probably suffered from coronary disease at the time of shock. There is also a small group of those who recover from the immediate effects of the shock but die from one or more of the complications of electrical injury, namely, burns, haemorrhage, infection, gangrene or embolism.

THE MECHANISM OF ELECTROCUTION

Despite the considerable experimental studies, the precise mechanism of electrocution has yet to be ascertained. Those who have contributed to this research include: Urquhart (1927), Urquhart and Noble (1929), Ferris *et al.* (1936), Kouwenhoven *et al.* (1959), Dalziel (1943 and later), Lee (1961 and later) and Lee *et al.* (1965).

It is outside my competence to assess these researches. They appear to show that ventricular fibrillation is an important, if not the principal, factor in electrocution by low and medium tension current.

It is clear that the same mechanism does not operate in all cases. Most deaths are due to ventricular fibrillation and in others it is asphyxia. If the head be in the circuit there may be respiratory arrest, due to paralysis of the respiratory centre. High-tension current not rarely is the indirect cause of death; the immediate cause of death is then more often thermal burns, either the result of arcing (flash-over) or the ignition of clothing. Some of these victims die because of injuries sustained as the result of a fall caused by the pressure generated in arcing.

(a) *Ventricular Fibrillation* This mechanism of electrocution was first described by Prevost and Battelli in 1899. As the result of clinical and experimental studies, ventricular fribrillation is now recognised as a principal, if not the commonest immediate cause of death by electrocution. Lee (1964) also pointed out that it is not always associated with immediate loss of consciousness nor arrest of respiration. This, again, is not a new observation; a report by Oliver and Bolam in 1898 was of a man who breathed for a few minutes before he died from the shock; some can walk about before they die (Lee, 1965a).

(b) *Tetanic Asphyxia* Low or medium current passing through the chest, when sustained at an amperage of 20 mA to 30 mA, can induce tetanic contraction of the extrinsic muscles of respiration, and thus cause death by mechanical asphyxia (*l'électocuté bleu*, Simonin, 1955). These victims are likely to be cyanosed whereas those who die of ventricular fibrillation are not (*l'électrocuté blanc*, Simonin, 1955). The production of a Joule burn at the point of contact may lower resistance and thus increase the amperage above the critical level at which ventricular fibrillation occurs.

Ventricular fibrillation occurred when a current of between 70 mA and 300 mA passed for 5 seconds but it required only 0.01 second to induce it when the current was one of from 1800 A to 8000 A (Dalziel, 1943).

Ventricular fibrillation is reversible, the basic fact in its modern treatment. This is possible even after the passage of a current of 1 A, if of very short duration, although there may then be subsequent disturbance of rhythm, but if the shock lasts a second or longer, fibrillation is irreversible and fatal (Simonin, 1955).

Fibrillation is arrested by the passage of a massive electric current through the heart (Kouwenhoven *et al.*, 1960), e.g. a current of 5 A, at 440 volts for 0.25 second (Knicker-bocker and Kouwenhoven, 1961).

A single strong surge of current, with the ventricles between the electrodes, can arrest fibrillation and the heart then starts to beat normally. A current of about 3 A forces the heart into maximal contraction and thus arrests fibrillation (Noordijk *et al.*, 1961).

(c) *Respiratory Arrest* In the event that the route of the current passes through the respiratory centre, and this is likely only when the head is involved, there may be paralysis of the centre and respiratory arrest.

Continued respiratory arrest after the shock has ceased is doubted by Lee (1965b) and, in his view, an unlikely event when the route is arm to arm.

(d) *Cerebral Anoxia* Prolonged ventricular fibrillation may cause brain damage due to an inadequate blood supply, i.e. cerebral anoxia. In the event of survival, the patient may have sustained permanent cerebral damage.

(e) *Neurological Damage* Some of the deaths are due to injury to the central nervous system. It is not necessary for the current to pass through the head to cause loss of consciousness; this may happen when the two contacts are with the same hand, e.g. following contact with a light socket (Jellinek, 1927). Serious nervous damage, however, is unusual unless the current passes through the head. Under experimental conditions, as found by Urquhart (1927) and Urquhart and Noble (1929), it would appear that the effect is a profound paralysis or block of the nerve centres. Recovery occurred after an interval following break of the alternating current, providing that artificial respiration was applied and there was no charring of the nerve structures. The block caused a failure of respiration and the usual cardio-vascular and conjunctival responses were not obtained. It was also shown that temporary block occurred in the conducting pathways in the spinal cord and in nerves. This view that electrical shock causes paralysis of the central nervous system was not new, because it had been advanced by d'Arsonval in 1885–87. In some cases the structural changes are irreversible. This has been demonstrated by Hassin (1933, 1937) and Dickson (1947). The changes were likened by Hassin to those which follow concussion of the central nervous system, as after fracture of the skull or increased intra-cranial pressure. The current may cause a tearing of the nervous tissue. Hassin found that histological changes were invariably present, although death was practically instantaneous. Haemorrhages were not a principal feature. In addition to tearing of the nervous tissue he observed shrinkage around the smaller blood vessels and rupture of the layers of the larger blood vessels, notably of the elastic membrane. The latter was considered by him to be a specific change in electrocution.

Signs of Death by Electrocution

Confusion has arisen because the effects peculiar to electrical shock are still described by some as "burns". Jellinek, however, makes a clear distinction between them. It is better to adopt his view and to speak of the electric mark and to distinguish it from the effects of a flash, which produce burns of a kind wholly akin to those produced by any other naked flame; ignition of clothing is responsible for some of the burns which follow electrical shock.

Although Joule burns are the result of the same mechanism which produces the electric mark and occur after more prolonged contact, and greater heat production in the tissues, it is deemed clearer if they are described separately.

Visible damage due to electrocution ranges within wide limits from nil to gross, appalling destruction of the tissues. This depends to a large extent on the strength of the current; gross damage is normally the result of contact with high-tension current, although it can be caused by prolonged contact with low or medium current. It is convenient and of practical importance to consider the injuries in two groups; first, those due to low or medium current, i.e. of up to 400 V and, second, those caused by high-tension circuits.

I. LOW- OR MEDIUM-TENSION INJURIES

The Electric Mark

An electric mark is to be found at the point of entry of the current; unfortunately the coincidence of a thermal burn is not unusual and it then masks the mark. It may be trivial (Fig. 103) but the recognition of a mark of this kind at once furnishes an explanation of death in circumstances which might otherwise seem inexplicable. Rarely, there may be no external mark but such a report may mean inadequate search rather than complete absence of a mark, or electrocution occurred in a bath.

The *electric mark* is specific and diagnostic of contact with electricity, but it is not, of itself, proof of electrocution (Figs. 102, 104, 108). Dr. Hainsworth and I confirmed the observations of Schridde and Beckmann (1924) and Strassmann (1933) that such marks, indistinguishable from those found on the victims of electrocution, can be produced after death (Figs. 104, 108). The finding of an electric mark, however, raises a strong presumption of death by electrocution, especially, as Jaffé said, when it occurs on an uncovered part of the body.

Characteristically these marks are round or oval, shallow craters, bordered by a ridge of skin of about 1 to 3 mm high, around part or the whole of their circumference. The crater floor is lined by pale flattened skin; the ridge pattern is usually preserved, but because of flattening, the ridges are broad and scarcely above the general level. In some marks there may be a breach of the skin within or near the margin of the crater, resembling that of a broken blister (Figs. 101, 102). The skin of the mark as a whole is distinctly pale, but there

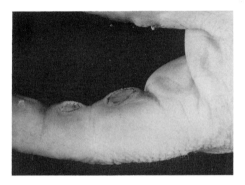

FIG. 101. Electric marks on index finger and thumb.

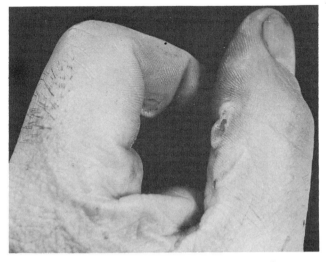

FIG. 102. Electric marks on index finger and thumb.

may be mild hyperaemia of the intact skin immediately beyond it. (In one of our experiments, in which we used a hand after its storage in a refrigerator for a week, we noted faint, apparent hyperaemia outside the electric mark.)

The shape of the mark is determined by the shape of the conductor or that part of it which is in contact with the skin. Usually the mark is circular or oval, but when the conductor is a rod-like structure, such as a flex or wire, or when it has a pattern, like that of a wire screen or fire guard, the mark is then a negative reproduction of the rod or patterned wire (F.M. 13,642A): Contact with the long axis of the wire yields a linear mark or groove, but contact with the end of the wire produces a hole, which can go deep into the tissues to involve not only skin and muscle but also bone. Jellinek (1927) recorded an example of such a mark, which resembled the entrance wound of a bullet.

Eight specimens depicting electric marks were examined in Professor Gormsen's Institute at Copenhagen. Three, in particular, bear a reproduction of the pattern of the conductors. In one the current was conveyed by coins and the entrance and exit marks were both circular; in a second case, when the terminal was a metal hinge, the mark was rectangular and in a third, a rectangular metal label fixed inside a bathing dress with a safety pin produced a rectangular mark crossed at the top by a horizontal linear mark, representing the position of the safety pin (Fig. 105). Some blurring of the outline is likely, as in the latter two specimens, because of imperfect contact, continued effects after death and, possibly, movement of the victim at the moment of electrocution. Even so, the mark gave an indication of the shape of the terminal in each of these three cases.

Jaffé (1928) has recorded an instance where an inexplicable death was subsequently recognised as a case of electrocution by the fact that the man had a patterned electric mark

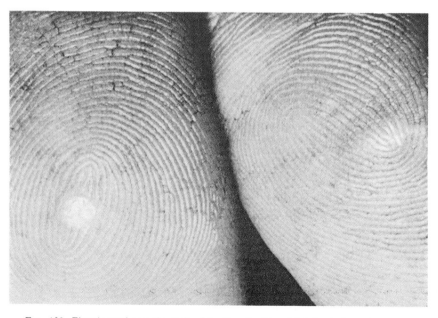

FIG. 103. Electric marks on the pads of the thumbs. Non-fatal shock through contact with condenser of an electronic flash unit.

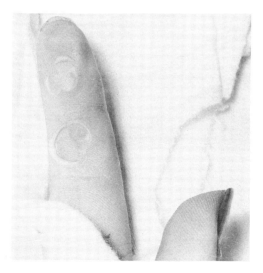

FIG. 104. Electric marks produced post-
mortem.

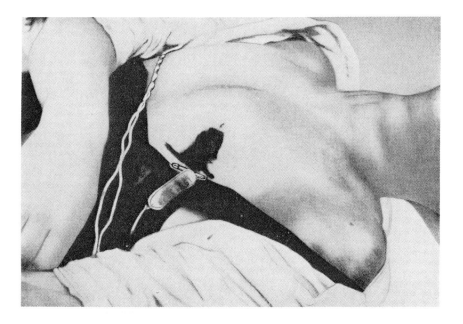

FIG. 105. Joule burn: reproducing the pattern of the conductor, a metal label attached to
a bathing costume by a safety pin. Professor Willy Munck's Case. (By courtesy of
Professor Munck and the Publishers of the *Deutsche Zeitschrift für gerichtliche Medizin*.)

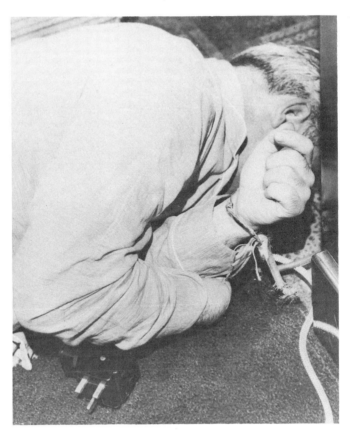

FIG. 106. Electrocution by wiring the wrists to the domestic 240-volt circuit. Suicide. (See Fig. 107 for mark on wrist.)

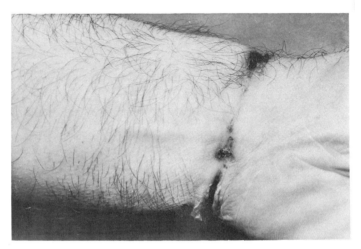

FIG. 107. Electric mark on wrist of man who committed suicide by wiring his wrists to the domestic 240-volt circuit (see Fig. 106).

on his left palm; the mark reproduced the pattern of part of a faulty inspection lamp which he was holding at the time of his death.

The Joule Burn (Endogenous Burn)

When contact is more prolonged the skin in the mark acquires a biscuit or brown tint and, with yet further contact, there may be charring. These changes are due to burning, the so-called *Joule burn*, a term which distinguishes it from the changes caused by exogenous thermal heat, following contact with high voltage, i.e. flash burn.

Electric marks and Joule burns are most often found on exposed parts of the body and, in particular, on the hands. As might be expected, since contact is usually due to grasping the electrode, the palmar aspect, i.e. the flexor aspect, is far more frequently the site than the back or extensor aspect. Lee (1961) found that, in thirteen of fifteen cases, the mark was on the flexor aspect of the hand.

It is possible for the mark to be almost anywhere on the body surface and it can be produced beneath intact clothing and then it may be undamaged by thermal heat (see F.M. 5097; electrocution by 24-volt d.c., p. 275). In that case the entrance mark was either on the shoulder or thigh. We have seen them on the inner aspect of the forearm (F.M. 5020), the side of the neck (F.M. 12,210), cheek (F.M. 1309 and 5020) and lips (F.M. 11,992); annular marks were also seen in those who had wired their wrists to the domestic circuit (F.M. 8701; 10,490; and 13,899). The marks were on the back of the body of the man who was electrocuted by a blanket (F.M. 12,698).

We have noted that marks produced on the back of the hand, where the skin is relatively

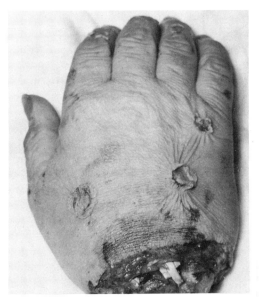

FIG. 108. Electric marks produced post-mortem. (Note furrowed elevation of the skin around the marks especially those on the right.)

loosely applied, may take the form of craters which have ridged, sloping external walls. The appearances suggest that during the production of the mark the adjacent skin was pulled towards its base (Fig. 108). A somewhat similar appearance is reproduced when the skin at the back of the hand is pinched and pulled away from the hand.

There is little doubt that these electric marks are produced, as described by Jaffé, by the conversion of electricity into heat within the tissues. They might be termed "endogenous burns" to distinguish them from "flash" or "exogenous" burns. Dr. Hainsworth and I watched electric marks develop. When the smooth, polished, face of a brass conductor, 1 cm in diameter, was applied to the skin, at a voltage of 240 a.c., tiny discrete pale blisters soon appeared around the perimeter of the conductor. In another second or so, these blisters grew bigger and coalesced to produce the usual wall to the crater. When the conductor was removed we had then produced a characteristic electric mark. If contact continued for a few more seconds, the skin in the mark turned brown and became a Joule burn. This may reproduce the pattern of the conductor (Fig. 105). Heat generated in the skin and, more especially, in the corium and subcutaneous tissues had caused the fluid to boil to produce blisters. By prolonging the process, the steam thus generated bursts through the skin.

Jaeger (1921) described the appearances of electric marks sustained when a joint was flexed at the moment of contact. In this position the path of the current may be shortened so that it passes through adjacent folds of the skin.

II. HIGH-TENSION INJURIES (EXOGENOUS BURNS)

Injury by high-tension current is either by direct contact or, as is not infrequent, an indirect result of arcing or flash-over. There is then the risk of grave thermal burns because of the considerable heat generated in the flash and of "knock down" by the sudden and appreciable increase in local atmospheric pressure.

The indirect production of high-tension injuries is likely to occur when anyone climbs an electric pylon supporting high-tension cables with a view to suicide or theft of cable. There is a grave risk of arcing if he comes close to the cables.

The distance between the person and the cable leading to arcing is related to the voltage. Thus a tension of 5000 volts will not arc until the distance is only 1 mm but when the tension is one of 100,000 volts arcing will occur at 35 mm (Mueller, cited by Simonin, 1955).

On most of these occasions survival of the victim implies that the current had passed by and not through the body. Fitzsimmons (1924) reported a survival after contact with a 20-kV circuit, when the man did not wear rubber gloves or rubber boots; at the time he was standing on a dry concrete floor. His only permanent disability was sloughing of the sole of one of his feet. It could be that contact with high voltage, even 13.2 kV, is not immediately lethal because, in such circumstances, the amperage of the supply, if it passes through the body, could exceed 4 A and, in consequence, ventricular fibrillation would not occur. Survival in these circumstances is to be attributed to high amperage, rather than one below the "critical" amperage of 0.1 A. The former is possible when skin resistance is 30,000 ohms or less, whereas the latter would imply a skin resistance of over a million ohms. In the Preston case, cited by Taylor (1956), the survivor was a boy and not a hornyhanded labourer. It is more probable that the current had passed over him, but its passage through his body was not impossible. The usual course of events in these pylon cases is a flash-over of explosive character, which knocks the victim down without any actual contact with the supply. He then suffers more from injuries due to the fall than burns and from both of these rather than electrical shock. The man who climbed a pylon with intent to commit suicide caused a short circuit and flash-over, which knocked him down and burnt his clothing. He fell to the ground below and died of multiple injuries and burns; electricity played only an indirect part (Leeds City Coroner, No. 432/37).

Although flash burns may be extensive and severe and may be exaggerated by burns from ignited clothing, gross destruction of the soft tissues and charring of bone or fusion of bone into pearl-like bodies, as depicted by Jellinek (1927), imply direct contact with the supply; similarly, sequestration of dead bone, as depicted by Jellinek (1932) and Glaister and Rentoul (1966).

Bone injuries are usually due to a fall following an electric shock; carbonisation by heat is uncommon, e.g. once in a series of 100 cases (Boemke ahd Piroth, 1959).

Flash-over burns are liable to delayed resolution, since there appears to be greater devitalisation of tissues in these circumstances; they remain unhealed for a long time, even 6 years (Moorhead, 1910). Pain is less pronounced and suppuration is unusual in flash-over burns.

Exit marks. These are variable in appearance, but they have some of the features of entrance marks. There may be more disruption of tissue and, instead of presenting as craters, they are often seen as splits in the skin at points where the skin has been raised into ridges by the passage of current; splitting of these ridges may be continuous or interrupted (Leeds City Coroner, No. 116/58 (Plate 4); also specimen in Univ. Copenhagen, F.M. Museum No. VIa. 1). The microscopical appearances are dominated by the honeycomb structure of the damaged tissues.

Metallisation

This is a specific feature of electrical injury and lightning stroke, likely to be seen in full development only in the latter circumstance. The face of a victim may, as depicted by Jellinek, become darkened, the shade being brown or even black. The colour is varied by the composition of the conductor, i.e. brown or black if of iron, or yellow-brown if of copper, although copper salts may leave a blue mark on the skin. This feature is due to the volatilisation of the metal, particles of which are driven into the skin. We have found it can occur when medium voltage (220–240) current is passed through the skin (F.M. 13,899). Small grey-green areas were present in the floor of the electric mark and the face of the brass conductor, originally smooth and polished, had become finely pitted and dull.

Metallisation in most of the marks produced by low or medium voltages may be detected only under low magnification or by histological or chemical examination.

Metallisation can occur "even when the current drawn from a 110-V d.c. power supply is no more than 20 mA (Adjutantis and Skalos, 1962). If the injury be an electric mark, a metallic deposit is probably invariable; if indefinite or invisible, the acroreaction should be tested. This is a delicate test and positive results can be obtained up to the onset of putrefaction. It is claimed to be proof of electrocution and a positive result can also indicate the composition of the conductor.

Schäffner (1965) found the metallic deposit mainly in the superficial layers of the skin but some was in the hair follicles. There was no relationship between voltage and metallisation.

Using ring-shaped copper electrodes, connected to a 220-volt supply, Bosch (1965) produced imprints of the electrodes with bark-like pieces of copper in the marks. Epithelium adhered to the electrodes.

The Acroreaction Test

A microchemical test for metals, devised by Skalos in 1944, was applied by him and Adjutantis to the identification of electric marks. The test is based, primarily, on the solubility of the metal present, e.g. iron, copper, aluminium, nickel or zinc, in either hydrochloric or nitric acid.

All of the metals mentioned, except copper, are soluble in hydrochloric acid and all, except iron, are soluble in nitric acid. The first step is to dissolve the metal in the mark with acid and then take up a portion of the solution with a tiny wedge of filter paper treated with reagent. The demonstration of iron, for example, is by the production of prussian blue with fresh potassium ferrocyanide or the production of Turnbull's blue with fresh potassium ferricyanide.

The details of the procedure are given in their article (Adjutantis and Skalos, 1962) which should be consulted by those interested.

Experiments showed that burns with hot wires, of copper, iron, nickel and aluminium, yielded only negative results with the test and served as controls for tests of electrical marks produced by electrodes made of these metals. It is a sensitive test and, it appears, valid even when putrefaction has begun.

Microscopical examination. The epidermis is apparently flattened, but this is in reality due to distortion of the cells, which are stretched as if orientated in the direction of the current (Jellinek, 1957). The cells are otherwise unchanged; there is no evidence of disintegration, but they may stain more readily with haematoxylin. Separation of the epidermis from the corium also occurs to the extent of blister formation. The outstanding feature, however, is the occurrence of spaces of varying size, some elliptical, others circular, in the corium and epidermis to impart a lace-like or honeycomb appearance. Small haemorrhages may also occur in the corium.

Elongation of the cells in the *Str. germinatorum* and *Str. basalis* was observed by Schäffner (1965), who found that similar appearances were caused by cold.

Hassin (1933, 1937) found that even when death was instantaneous microscopical changes were invariably present in the brain. In his experience haemorrhages were not the principal change. He laid stress on tearing of nervous tissue and shrinkage of it around the smaller blood vessels. He also demonstrated rupture of the elastic membrane of the larger vessels. Critchley (1934) found focal petechial haemorrhages scattered through the brain, especially in the medulla, and they were sometimes to be seen also in the spinal cord, especially in its grey matter. By experiment he found that these were commoner after contact with alternating current. Large tears were also seen in the brain when the head had been directly struck by lightning. Microscopically, the nerve cells showed chromatolysis, especially in the pyramidal cells, the cells of the medullary nuclei and in the Purkinje cells of the cerebellum. Critchley found wide dilatation of the perivascular spaces. There was sometimes swelling and softening of the nervous tissue, even to diffluence of the brain. This usually followed very severe injury. Brain injury was deemed to be determined by one or more of several factors, for example, the duration of contact, duration of survival and, more especially, on whether or not the head was in the path of the current. In his experience, the most striking change was a localized ballooning of the myelin sheaths of the peripheral nerves and he depicts an example in the ulnar nerve of a boy who sustained a shock of 12,000 volts. The arm had to be amputated on account of gangrene. This case has something in common with that recorded by Jellinek (1957). A man sustained immediate necrosis of a hand and had intense pain is his arm, pain which did not resolve to any medical treatment and, in consequence, it was decided to perform a high amputation of the limb. Later, when the amputated arm was dissected, it was found that the cause of his pain was a clean break through the ulnar nerve in the region of the elbow.

The blood vessels also suffer from the effects of electricity and, in consequence, become brittle.

Diagnosis: Post-mortem

The pathognomonic features of electrocution are the electric mark and the Joule burn, when low- or medium-voltage current is involved. Electric marks are not always obvious especially on the hands of a manual workers; when the circumstances suggest electrocution the hands should be closely scrutinised. Proof of an electric mark is obtained by histological and histochemical (the acroreaction) examination.

The pattern of a Joule burn may be the "signature" of the conductor as in the case of Munck (p. 285). The acroreaction can also assist in the identification of the conductor.

Electrocution by high tension is usually associated with gross thermal injuries, the result of direct contact, or flash-over or thermal burns, or due to the ignition of clothing. The circumstances rarely leave room for doubt as to the cause of death.

There are occasions, notably electrocution in a bath, when there are no external signs of injury. Moreover, the internal examination fails to disclose any specific changes. On these occasions details of the scene, e.g. the presence of a "live" appliance or wiring in the bath, are important, as also is the exclusion of any other possible cause of death, especially natural disease, poisoning or an overdose of a drug.

The internal examination is rarely if ever productive of characteristic findings. In the event that the immediate cause of death is mechanical asphyxia, the changes present will be those common to any cause of this state. Cyanosis of the face, petechial haemorrhages in the skin of the face and beneath the pleura and epicardium may be seen. There may be congestion of the viscera and oedema of the lungs and dilatation of the heart, and so forth, but these are not specific changes. Moreover, if, as is probable, the immediate cause of death be ventricular fibrillation (*l'électrocuté-blanc*, Simonin, 1955), "remarkably little change may be found" (Taylor, 1965). In the event that the brain was in the route of the current, certain histological or even macroscopic changes may be found. The most striking example is that reported by Dickson (1947), see p. 302.

The recognition of electrocution is important, because it draws attention to wiring or equipment which is dangerous to others. A man, aged 21, died suddenly when operating an electrical drill. Post-mortem examination and microscopical examination of the tissues yielded entirely negative results, but electrocution was the probable cause of death. The drill was examined and a short circuit was present, whereby its casing was live (Taylor, 1965). Sometimes the electrical examination may fail to yield a satisfactory solution, although there was no doubt from the pathological stand-point that the death was due to electrocution, and there were unequivocal electric marks on the body (F.M. 5097).

When present, the electric mark is of first importance, but it must be realized that such a mark, unaccompanied by hyperaemia, can be produced after death. It is also possible to produce changes in the skin which resemble an electric mark by applying a glowing wire or the flame of a micro-bunsen burner to the skin. The distinction between an electric mark and a thermal burn can be made by the acroreaction test (see p. 290).

Delayed Effect of Electrical Injuries

Gangrene and Haemorrhage

Necrosis of tissue following electrical injury may be extensive and, as seen in Jellinek's illustrations, gangrene may involve, for example, the whole of an upper limb. Moreover, the probable extent of the damage cannot be accurately assessed until some time has elapsed, because arterial damage extends beyond the field of obvious injury. Gangrene, or necrosis of a hand or hand and forearm, may be immediate. Demarcation is astonishingly sharp and a true geometrical plane separates the dead and living tissues (Jellinek, 1957).

Arterial damage is also a feature of electrical injury and it often extends beyond the area of obvious necrosis of other tissues. This is a point which has a bearing on the plan for amputation. Severe haemorrhage is one of the late complications of electrical injury and attempts to control it by ligature or forceps fail, because brittleness of the vessel results in tearing at the point of application. Satisfactory control is practicable only by compression of the part.

Neurological Changes

Loss of consciousness is often immediate, especially after contact with high current; it is estimated to happen in 63 per cent of high-tension and 31 per cent of low-tension accidents (Jaffé, 1928). Its duration may be brief and the victim not only recalls the circumstances of the shock but is able to get up and resume his work. Others may remain unconscious for long periods and some remain so until coma and death supervene. There may be retrograde amnesia.

When treatment has restored the victim to consciousness, prognosis should be guarded and several days must elapse before the full extent of any neurological changes can be assessed. They may be indefinite, for example, changes in personality, changes which resemble those of the post-concussional state, or they may be overt changes such as hemiplegia, with or without aphasia. The possibilities are discussed, e.g. by Panse (1930) and by Macdonald Critchley (1934, 1935).

Amnesia may last several days and it occurred in all fourteen cases studied by Silversides (1964). He also found that when the head was in the route of the current unconsciousness was immediate and could last for 4 days.

Narcolepsy following injury by electric current was reported by Roberts (1966). Three patients suffered from catalepsy, sleep paralysis and hypnologic hallucinations. All three responded to conventional analeptic treatment. Organic disturbances, e.g. epileptiform convulsions, headache and vertigo, may also occur but permanent organic disease is an infrequent sequel to electrocution (Roberts, 1966).

Prolonged unconsciousness will not necessarily lead to complications, Jellinek (1927) mentioned the patient who was unconscious for two hours, following a shock from a 4500-volt supply at 75 mA, sustained for several minutes. He was revived by artificial respiration and, but for thermal burns having local effect, he made a complete recovery.

Eye Injury

A guarded prognosis is also wise when the current has entered through the head because cataract is another possible result, which may not be apparent until several weeks after the accident. Changes in the lens, in the form of flaky opacities, can be produced by currents at tensions which range from 220 to 50,000 volts (Jaffé, 1928). Bilateral cataract due to electrical injury was reported by Bégué (1935). Fortunately, it would seem, lasting forms of eye injury are uncommon, if not rare (Lee, 1961). Optic atrophy and choroido-retinitis following electrical injury has also been recorded (Bainbridge, 1930).

Arc eye: this condition may be seen in those exposed at close range, within a yard, of a short-lived flash. There may be coincident singeing of the eyebrows, eyelashes or hair and first degree burns of the face. In the majority the injury is a mild one with prompt resolution within a day or so. Serious injury occasioning prolonged absence from work occurred in only one of sixteen cases of arc eye (Lee, 1961).

Prognosis

In general, the prognosis after recovery from electrical shock is good. The majority of those who survive make a complete recovery, which is often rapid but in some it may be delayed for several weeks. Complications, when they occur, are usually a result of contact with high-tension current.

Repair of Electrical Injuries

Jellinek emphasized the unique character of the healing process following electrical injury. From the outset these injuries are painless; they do not suppurate. Gross injury is unassociated with fever or general disturbance. The end result is often astonishingly good—for instance, the spontaneous resolution of cataract, the excellent healing of a perforated ear-drum and the complete regeneration of a joint capsule, despite extensive damage, and the perfect reconstruction of a disintegrated radial annular ligament. The regeneration of a full-thickness loss of skin is by delicate soft skin, which can be easily moved over the underlying tissues. A characteristic feature of this repair is the formation of an exceedingly fine and beautifully constructed network of elastic fibres which is never seen in non-electrical burns or chemical injury (Jellinek, 1957).

The changes in electrical injuries may begin with a period of quiescence and this is followed by a stage of disintegration when the dead tissue is shed and the wound becomes clean. There follows a phase of regeneration characterised by the formation of highly vascular granulations. The danger from profuse haemorrhage arises at this stage (Jellinek, 1957).

Repair of fractures caused by electricity can be by callus which is radiotranslucent. Jellinek (1957) reproduced an X-ray of a crack in the ulna at the back of a right elbow. Although united by callus, this is radio-translucent and the fragment appears as a sequestrum.

Jellinek pleaded for conservative treatment of electrical injuries. All too often, he said, in defiance of their natural history, electrical injuries are treated actively like burns, instead of conservatively.

The Circumstances of Electrocution

ACCIDENTAL ELECTROCUTION

The majority of fatalities are the result of accidental contact with low voltage, normally 210–250 volts, which is the domestic supply.

There are a number of possible hazards in the home and a frequent cause of electric shocks is *frayed or broken flex*; the particular site of damage is at the point where a flex enters the appliance since this is the point of special stress and strain. Flex or cable which runs along a floor also needs attention since it may be damaged by feet or furniture. The connections of appliances and lengths of flex or cable liable to damage should be inspected periodically and any defects promptly remedied. (A colleague's wife was electrocuted by her vacuum cleaner because the wiring at the plug was faulty).

It is also important to check the *earthing* of appliances operated by hand. At the same time it is advisable to check the *wiring of the sockets* into which these appliances are plugged. It is not rare that the wiring of the socket is such that, although the switch is in the "off" position, the socket is "live". Moreover, this is possible although the switch appears to operate the appliance satisfactorily. The appliance itself may be of *defective design*, for example a radiogram has been constructed with the outer casing in contact with the "live" chassis.

The domestic appliances which call for special attention include portable electric fires, hair dryers, kettles, irons and vacuum cleaners, radios and tape recorders. Hand inspection lamps, electric drills or soldering irons are also potential hazards. Electric blankets, now in wide use, need annual inspection to check their efficiency and, even when efficient, they require intelligent use.

If the householder wishes to limit his risk of fire and electrocution to the minimum he should not only have had the wiring of the house approved by the Electricity Board but also any correction made only by a professional of repute. New power or light points or repairs of defective flex or appliances, are not work for the do-it-yourself enthusiast. Unless he has the necessary skill and experience he is far safer employed in painting or decorating the house.

Examples of domestic accidents are well known but merit recapitulation. Our experience includes fatalities when an electric dryer was used by a woman in her bath (F.M. 903); another two persons died after contact with an electric fire in the bathroom (F.M. 1309 and F.M. 10,346, in the latter case the fire was plugged into a light socket).

Two persons committed suicide by putting a "live" fire in the bath (F.M. 375; F.M. 15,191).

Defective wiring was responsible for the death of a man aged 31, who was found dead beside his van. He was holding a plug connected by a length of wire to the domestic supply. The switch was in the "off" position but the wiring was faulty and the line conductor had not been isolated. For some years a socket in a certain garage, unknown to the owner, had been in this condition; it was detected and remedied when he had cause to use the socket for a new appliance.

Accidents due to faults in an installation are uncommon. For example, death from coal-gas poisoning was the indirect result of a fault in an electrical junction box. The conduit from it was close to a gas pipe, which formed an earth; the gas pipe melted and gas was released. Electrical wiring and gas pipes should be separated by a distance of at least 2 in.

Electric blankets are indeed a boon but unfortunately perfection of design has yet to be attained and it is not the general practice to have blankets tested each autumn before they are put into use.

The hazards created by these blankets include not only electrocution and thermal burns but also fire. When not in use blankets should be stored flat to prevent damage to the wiring by folding.

(a) *Fire: Unattended Electric Blanket*

It is indeed unwise to heat an unoccupied bed for an indefinite period, unattended, even when the blanket is thermostatically controlled. It is also a risk to use the blanket for this purpose if covered with too many blankets, etc. A doctor sustained loss by fire of an expensive bed and there was serious damage to his newly decorated bedroom when an electric blanket had been left unattended for several hours.

Lustig (1961) found that the incidence of fires caused by electric blankets was 780 in 1960. This was not ascribable to increasing use of these blankets because a four-fold increase in use was accompanied by a ten-fold increase in the number of fires during the same period. It was possible that some of the newer blankets were not as safe as the older models.

(b) *Electrocution*

It may be that some of these victims not only sustain thermal burns but also are electrocuted.

Example No. 1

A man aged 22 retired to bed when under the influence of drink. He lay on an electric blanket and during the night he urinated into the bed. When found dead he had electrical and thermal injuries in the region of his shoulder blades, buttocks and thigh. There was a band of reddening 4×5 in. in the shoulder region traversed by two horizontal strips of whitened, hardened skin, $1 \times \frac{1}{4}$ in., lying 2 in. apart; the appearances were those of electric marks. Reddening of the skin, with central charring, occurred over the buttocks, in an area 8×4 in. on the right and 6×4 in. on the left; there was another burn on the outer side of the left thigh. His blood alcohol content was 131 mg/100 ml, and the urine content was 159 mg/100 ml (F.M. 12,698).

Example No. 2: Electrocution by a Blanket

> The victim was a woman aged 50, who was found dead in a bed heated by an electric blanket. There was no natural disease to account for her death. Joule burns were found on her trunk as follows: (a) a burn, 22 in. long and 3 in. wide, extended from the left shoulder blade to the natal cleft; the central two-thirds of this burn were formed by yellow, parchmented skin, beyond which was a pale zone, $^1/_2$ in. wide, and beyond that another zone, $^1/_2$ in. wide, of hyperaemia: (b) at the right-hand side of the centre of burn there were two superficial burns, slightly blistered: one measured 2×1 in. and the other was 1 in. in diameter: (c) a burn, 5 in. in diameter, was behind the right shoulder; this too had three distinct zones, a central yellow parchmented one, a pale zone and, outside that, a zone of hyperaemia. A few petechial haemorrhages were found beneath the epicardium of the right ventricle and on the outer aspect of the first part of the aorta (F.M. 7451 B).

(c) *Thermal Burns*

It may be a counsel of perfection to insist on a rule that no electric blanket should be operated when the bed is occupied. At least the precaution should be taken to switch off and, preferably, disconnect the blanket before going to sleep. The risk of using these blankets when a patient is unconscious, or when he is a diabetic liable to fall into coma, is indeed real. Although they may not be electrocuted, they may sustain serious burns. Bull and Cason (1959) recorded the case of a diabetic who passed into coma while lying on an electric blanket.

He sustained a full thickness burn, 8×7 in. of his left thigh, and there was charring of the blanket. He had sweated profusely and his pyjamas and parts of the blanket were soaked with sweat. The blanket was on the low switch position and this, with the wiring intact, produced a just-perceptible warmth, not enough to burn the skin. Moistening of the blanket, however, caused the damp areas rapidly to become warmer and saline fluid, such as sweat, reduced the insulation of the wiring. In consequence, local overheating, sufficient to cause burns, occurred. Bull and Cason recommended that electric blankets should not be used if they are liable to be moistened by sweat or urine. The blankets, also, should be designed so that the heating elements are not arranged in a manner which allows a high potential difference between adjacent wires. Fry (1962) believes it probable that a low-voltage blanket with a transformer would reduce the danger of shock. Some blanket manufacturers incorporate a continuous sensing element; running the full length of the heating element, it is designed to cut out when any overheating occurs. The Fire Research Station cannot say how effective this is.

(d) *Hyperpyrexia*

There is risk if an infant is kept in a cot heated by an electric blanket. The risk here is not necessarily that of fire, burns or electrocution, but overheating. In one of my cases a baby was gravely ill when found by its father in a cot heated by an electric blanket; it died a few hours later. It appears that the child had been left alone in that cot for at least 3 hours. The blanket was not thermostatically controlled and tests showed that it could become heated to about 64°C. The death of that child was probably due in part, if not entirely, to heat hyperpyrexia (F.M. 6882 A).

Electrocution in the Bath

This is a common mode of electrocution in the home. Each case requires careful investigation. The first step is to determine whether the death was due to electrocution, not always as obvious as it might seem, and then to determine whether it was by accident or design. If by design, the possibility of murder must be considered, especially when the victim is a baby or child.

Example

A woman, aged 54, was found dead in her bath on 18 January 1965. (Three months later her husband, aged 58, committed suicide by electrocution, see Case No. 1, p. 304).

A portable electric fire was stood on a ledge at the sloping end of the bath, i.e. opposite the taps. Her body was forced down in the water; the face and chest rested against the sloping end of the bath; the feet touched the bath directly below the taps. There was no disorder in the room. The fire was not over-turned; it is presumed to have been switched on at the time of her death.

She had sustained grave, deep, thermal burns. Loss of skin and exposure of charred muscle had occurred over the greater part of the front of the chest and right shoulder; the right side of her face was also severely damaged. Deep heat ruptures were present. The right half of the lower jaw bone, right clavicle and upper part of the right humerus were exposed and charred. These grave injuries were unaccompanied by evidence of vital reaction.

Electric marks, in the form of "blisters" of from $1/4$ in. to 1 in. in diameter, were present on the back of each of the fingers at the level of the proximal interphalangeal joints. There was also an electric mark on the ball of the left thumb.

Sub-pericardial petechial haemorrhages were present at the back of the ventricles. There was a little froth in the trachea and bronchi. The lungs were damaged by heat. A "heat haematoma" in the form of chocolate-coloured blood clot was present in the extra-dural space of the right middle fossa of the skull. There was no injury to the scalp and no fracture of the skull. The right cerebral hemisphere was damaged by heat. She had been a healthy women and there was no natural disease to account for her death or to cause sudden collapse.

The woman had touched the fire with her hands, especially the right and received a fatal shock which caused collapse close to the fire, and she lay near to it, if not on it, for some considerable time. The major, visible injuries, namely gross charring of tissues, occurred after her death, since there was no vital reaction. The injuries on the hands were characteristic electric marks, unassociated with any charring.

The circumstances were those of an accident and an illustration of the danger of placing electrical equipment on or near a bath whereby the person in the bath can come into contact with the apparatus (F.M. 10,346).

Other examples. A man, aged 72, who put a "live" flex in his bath was electrocuted but had no external sign of injury (F.M. 15,191). Electrocution, by a faulty fire on the floor beside the bath, when the person in the bath touched it (F.M. 1309), and also Leeds City Coroner's Cases 301/35 and 142/44 in similar circumstances.

We have also seen electrocution by a hair dryer when it was used by a woman in her bath (F.M. 903).

There are now several reports of electrocution in the bath. Dérobert and Grèzes-Rueff (1958) examined a man, aged 67, who was found dead in his bath with a bedside lamp in the water and it was connected to a plug under the wash basin. Drowning and poisoning by carbon monoxide were excluded. He was suffering from mental illness; suicide.

The suicide recorded by L'Èpée *et al.* (1965), a woman aged 60, had plugged in a wire to the domestic supply and plunged the "live" end in her bath. She had an exit mark on her right buttock, a reproduction of the pattern of the plug hole of the bath; a veritable signature of it.

Other reports include those by Schwerd (1959), who described the formation of electric marks following electrocution in water, and Dürwald *et al.* (1964), who gave details, with illustrations, of a series of six cases.

A radio or tape recorder in the bathroom can also be the source of a lethal shock.

OTHER EXAMPLES OF ELECTRIC SHOCK BY LOW- AND MEDIUM-TENSION CIRCUITS

Flooding from a cistern can damage electrical wiring. A woman who had been away from her home returned to find water cascading from the ceiling and sparks coming from the water taps. They had become "live". The police were summoned and promptly cut off the water and electricity supplies at the main. Fortunately no injury was sustained by anyone on that occasion.

A boy aged 8 sustained an electric shock when he put his foot on a foot-rest in a cinema. It was shown that he had made contact with a conduit which ran beneath the foot-rest and, owing to faulty installation, the conduit was "live".

A traffic light and the adjacent pavement became "live" as the result of a short circuit. The curious behaviour of a dog which approached the lamp standard attracted the attention of a police officer. It stopped suddenly, yelped and leapt into the air. A pedestrian crossing the adjacent pavement dropped her handbang and complained of an electric shock. Snow and ice had earthed the standard to the pavement.

Electric shock from a photographic flash unit

An experienced photographer was repairing his flash unit at a time when it was connected with the 240 V mains for charging. He was pressing wire to the rectifier, on the red side of the circuit, with his right thumb. Meantime, his left thumb was in contact with the condenser at a point where there was a tear in its insulating cover. He received a shock of about $2^{1}/_{2}$ kV direct current. He felt the shock pass up his arms and across his

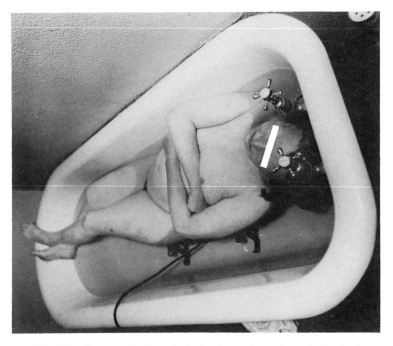

Fig. 109. Electrocution in a bath by live radiator beneath the body: probably suicidal. (see p. 305)

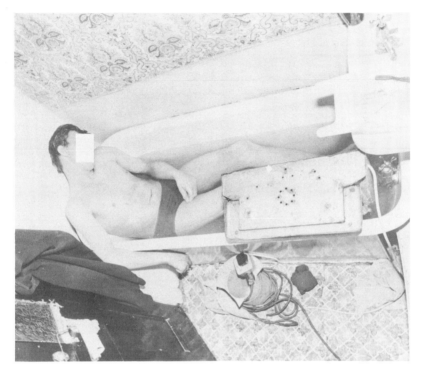

FIG. 110a. Suicidal drowning in bath by wire led into water (F.M. 20456).

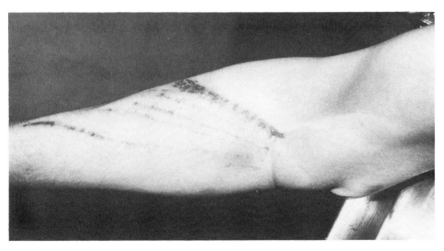

FIG. 110b. Electric marks on arm in case of Fig. 110a, caused by the inside of the arm contacting bare metal under the lip of the bath edge.

shoulders; he was immediately thrown to the ground, but did not lose consciousness. The devotion to photography in his department was such that his assistant, who rushed to him, was primarily concerned to obtain a photograph of his injuries! His recovery was prompt and the only after-effect was a sensation of tingling in the skin of his wrist beneath the wristlet of his watch. He sustained two small electric marks, one on each thumb. That on the left was approximately $1/_8$ in. diameter; the skin in it was pale and its ridge pattern was lost (Fig. 103). With his ready co-operation the initial appearance of these marks and subsequent changes in them, during the ensuing 5 weeks which elapsed before resolution was complete, were recorded by colour photography. This risk has been minimized, if not eliminated, in more recent models of these units.

During a game of bowls, one of the "woods" ran out of play. A player stopped to pick it up and, to steady himself, he grabbed an electric cable. He collapsed immediately and died. He had an electric mark on his right hand (Rossano *et al.*, 1964). (The voltage was not stated but the wiring was for electric light; presumably, therefore, low tension.)

A man was electrocuted when he was making an extension of the lighting system from an inn to a hen-house nearby. The new electric point cable was connected to the mains by a plug which was inserted into a socket in the house. When he was found dead he had the cable in his left hand and uninsulated pliers in his right hand gripped it. The control switch of the socket indoors was in the "off" position, but the cable was still live. Moreover, if he had fitted a lamp to his end of the cable it would not have lit up and he would have concluded that the cable had been disconnected (H.M. Coroner for the East Riding of Yorkshire, H. W. Rennison, Esq., 11 October 1957).

There is risk also from electrified hedgeclippers. A distinguished soldier received a severe shock and injury of his right hand when he flicked a speck of dirt from the cable-joint of one of these clippers. Portable tools and transportable equipment are common sources of electric shock in industry. The Chief Inspector of Factories repeatedly pressed for their operation by a current at 110 volts, whereby the danger would be materially reduced.

Electrocution of a boy whose face made contact with the grille of a television set was due to faulty design or assembly, so that the chassis, which is normally live, was in contact with the grille (H. M. Coroner for the County of Leicester, Mr. J. H. Deane, 7 May 1951).

A man, aged 54, had trespassed on the railway, possibly with the intention to steal copper wire. He was found dead in a yard with his head against a brick wall, along which there were wires carrying a 240-volt supply of electricity; it appeared he had slipped and fallen against the wires; the ground was damp. He had an electric mark on the back of his right hand and another on his lips. Hair at the vertex of his head was scorched, and, when the scalp was shaved, a circular area of charring, the exit mark was seen (F.M. 11,992).

A man, aged 57, was checking the wiring of a gantry crane. The wires from a fuse box on one of its pillars passed in a metal conduit to porcelain insulators, but the last 6 in. of this wiring was bare. It appeared he had lost his balance and, to steady himself, he had clutched the bare wires with his right hand and the conduit with his left hand; he sustained a shock from a 440-volt supply and was thrown to the ground from the 15-ft ladder on which he had been standing. He had also leant forward while on the ladder and thus brought the side of his neck close to the conduit. He sustained burns of both hands and the side of his neck; laceration of the back of his head was due to his fall (F.M. 12,210).

EXAMPLES OF HIGH-TENSION ACCIDENTS

Accidents due to contact with high-voltage supplies are uncommon outside the electrical industry. One industrial accident may be mentioned to show the importance of attention to detail if accidents are to be prevented. The victim was employed in cleaning equipment at a generating station. His job was to wipe some metal bars which were "live" and this was apparently quite safe. One day, when engaged on this task, there was a violent explosion due to a short circuit and he was blown out of the building. Investigation of the accident showed that he had been using a piece of brocade to wipe the bars. The cloth had touched two adjacent bars and the short circuit occurred because it contained metal as well as other non-conducting fibres. It was subsequently discovered that the supplies of rags, believed to be entirely safe, included several pieces of brocade which contained metal fibres.

Outside the electrical industry, individuals are likely to come into contact with high-voltage circuits only when they disregard warning signs or forget the presence of high-voltage cables when moving ladders and the like. Electricity Boards are at some pains to make it clear that the climbing of pylons is dangerous and provide guards to these and to power stations, which most people would find insurmountable. Cables have to be at least 17 ft above ground level. In spite of these precautions, accidents occur. A boy may climb a pylon to retrieve his toy arrow, or surmount the spiked metal fencing round a sub-station and overcome yet other obstacles in order to reach a bird's nest.

Forgetfulness of the existence of overhead cables led to the electrocution of a man who was moving a ladder when erecting lamp standards near one of them, which was 22 ft 3 in. above ground level. Contact occurred and the 11-kV supply was conducted by reinforcing metal strips at each side of the $22^1/_2$-ft ladder to the victim's hands (F.M. 116/1958 Plate 4, P.M. by Dr. H. Thompson and C.P.). On another occasion a fatal accident occurred when men were engaged in moving a yacht; its mast made contact with an overhead cable.

Indirect contact with high voltage occurred when a man was flying a kite attached to a length of steel wire instead of string. The kite descended on high-voltage cables and he received a shock from the 33-kV supply. Although he survived, unsuccessfuly to sue the Electricity Board for alleged negligence on their part, he lost not only this action but also the part of his right arm below the elbow (*Moyle* v. *Southern Electricity Board*, *The Times*, 24 Oct. 1961).

Shocks can be received in similar circumstances, even if the kite be attached to string, because if the string becomes wet with rain it will act as a conductor. Indirect contact with high voltage also occurred when a boy urinated on an electrified rail; the current passed upwards through the stream of urine.

Examples from our area include contact by accident and by misadventure.

In 1961 a man sustained appalling and extensive injuries when he climbed a ladder and grasped a high-tension cable. He and an accomplice had intended to steal some of the cable. (Dr. Thomson's case, Leeds Infirmary, August 1961.)

A scrap-metal dealer was found by his companion at the foot of a 24-ft pole which carried a 1000-volt current. He had been seated in the cradle at the top of the pole, used by service engineers. He was working in the dark, in wet conditions, and had failed to see some low-tension cable, which led a 400-volt supply from the main cable. When he leant over them, arcing occurred and he sustained injury to his right hand (thumb and index finger) and severe flash burns of each eye; there was half-thickness damage of the cornea of each eye. The route of the current appeared to have been hand–heart–foot but there was no exit mark (F.M. 11,586 E).

In a similar accident, a man aged 22 was electrocuted while attempting to steal copper cable. He was found at the foot of a high-tension pylon with a pair of wire cutters beside him. He had been seated on an iron bracket at the top of the pylon and had already cut several lengths of wire. He had worn thick PVC gloves to protect himself from the 6000-volt supply. Arcing occurred and he sustained grave burns of his body especially of the wrists, upper arms and chest. Although his clothing had been damp it was set on fire by the flash. This had probably been the cause of the thermal burns of his abdomen and thighs. Although he had fallen about 20 ft this had not caused additional injury because the ground was soft (F.M. 14,595 A).

A variation of contact between a kite and high-tension cable was provided by the case of a man flying a model aeroplane which he guided by a wire fitted with a metal handle. The control wire made contact with cable carrying 20,000 volts. He was electrocuted and had a Joule's burn on the palm and fingers of his right hand. Then was an exit wound, a crater $^3/_4$ in. in diameter, in the sole of his left foot. Although he was wearing rubber boots, the left boot was defective (Ennis, 1968).

A man was loading hay on to a stack in damp conditions; there were frequent showers. As the stack grew, the man came nearer and nearer to overhead cable, carrying 20,000 volts. His clothing was damp. Arcing occurred and he fell off the stack and broke his neck. He had not touched the cable but there was an entrance mark behind the tip of his right ear (Ennis, 1967).

Two men, unaware that the current had been automatically cut off by an accident, did not hesitate to climb a pylon in order to save a boy who was suspended from one of its girders. This boy had climbed the pylon and received a shock from the 33-kV supply. The explosion which resulted knocked him over and set his clothing on fire, but his fall was broken when one of his boots became entangled in the girders.

Underground cables are another source of accident, and those who excavate in their neighbourhood should be aware of their precise distribution. A man received a severe shock when he drove a steel spike into a 20-kV cable. He was standing in water at the time, but he escaped electrocution because he was wearing gumboots and he used a wooden mallet.

Aldrich (1943) reported an accident which befell a technical student, following contact with a high-tension circuit of 33,000 volts. The current entered his left hand when he was earthed to a steel girder under his right foot. Natural breathing was suspended for 3 hours and 10 minutes but he was kept alive by artificial respiration. His convalescence was stormy, and permanent injury to the left kidney and his left arm, which was charred and useless, resulted from burns.

IATROGENIC ELECTROCUTION

A number of mishaps, which occurred in the course of investigation or treatment of patients with electrical apparatus, are now on record. It is clear that there should be constant watch to ensure that the instruments are of safe design and in good working order. Since there is always a risk, those who use them should satisfy themselves that their use is necessary; the tests or treatments should not be "routine" procedures.

Accidents arising out of the use of electrical equipment in the course of diagnosis and treatment should not be overlooked. They are a potential source of litigation. The Medical Defence Union (1961) gave information concerning four of these electrical accidents. One occurred when diathermy to remove warts was begun before the surgical spirit used to clean the skin had dried. The spirit caught fire and the patient sustained burns. Her claim was settled for £1000. In a similar accident, spirit was set on fire by an electric cautery (£250 damages).

"The ever-present hazard in patient monitoring is electrocution resulting in ventricular fibrillation". Electrocution can occur when more than one piece of electrical equipment is connected with the patient; when the distal end of an intracardiac catheter is handled and when pericardiocentesis is carried out with ECG monitoring. Small currents of the order of 100–200 μA may then cause ventricular fibrillation. The threshold is substantially lowered by anoxia and acidosis but not, it seems, by barbiturate anaesthesia (Lee, 1970).

The following examples illustrate some of the possible hazards:

Dickson (1947) examined the brain of a woman who died of accidental electrocution when the shock was direct to the brain itself. Alternating current of 240 volts was in contact with the right temporal pole of the brain, through a trephine opening immediately in front of and slightly above the level of the right ear; this had been made in the course of an operation on the trigeminal nerve. The conductor was an electrically lit retractor, which had been inserted into the wound. An assistant nurse, standing by the apparatus and the patient, "also received a shock and, having her hand on the patient, presumably acted as a conductor of the current from patient to earth". The shock caused immediate unconsciousness and this continued until the death of the patient, 21$^1/_4$ hours later, but the shock itself was of brief duration. The precise cause of the short-circuit was not determined. The resulting changes in the brain were in the form of an extensive disruptive process, both of the grey and white matter, to produce a remarkable foamy appearance, apparent to the unaided eye. The appearances are consistent with the generation of bubbles of steam or gas, due to intense heat and electrolytic action; they are also consistent with an electrostatic disturbance.

Two accidents, one fatal, were due to faulty insulation of an electrocardiograph when used in conjunction with a mains-operated cardiac pace monitor. The electrodes in the myocardium caused ventricular fibrillation. If the heart be outside the route of the current, e.g. right thumb and right finger, the danger is minimal but if the heart be directly involved, as by the insertion of electrodes, only a small amount of current will cause fibrillation (Noordijk *et al.*, 1961). The probability, if not the truth, of the latter observation one dares to say is self-evident.

Ventricular fibrillation occurred during cardiac catheterisation and four separate electrical faults were later traced in the apparatus (Mody and Richings, 1962). Electrocution as a hazard of angiocardiography was also reported by Bousvaros *et al.* (1962).

Three deaths due to electrocution by defective medical instruments were reported by Furman *et al.* (1961); an electrical pace-maker caused one death, an oscilloscope another and the third was caused by a fluoroscope. Electrocution by a faulty cardiac monitor was reported in the *Lancet* (1960, **i**, 872).

To date, it appears that the biggest total of accidents due to any one group of iatrogenic electrocutions is that of accidents in the course of, or related to, electro-convulsive treatment.

A woman aged 43 died, while under the anaesthesia, when she received the first application of the shock apparatus; she stopped breathing and resuscitation was unsuccessful; she had acute pulmonary oedema and the immediate cause of death was left ventricular fibrillation. It was stated at the inquest that up to that date there had been only thirty-three of these accidents ("Medicine and The Law", *Lancet*, 1963, **i**, 1155).

Two deaths in the course of electro-convulsive therapy were investigated by the Leeds City Coroner:

Case No. 1

A man, aged 64, died immediately after the fourth of a series of these treatments, each of a dosage of 25 joules. During the 4-day interval between the third and last of these treatments he had complained of severe pain in his chest. Heart trouble was suspected and an ECG was taken. This showed no abnormality and the patient ceased to complain of pain. Although he was not re-examined immediately before the last shock, there was no reason to suspect that there was a contra-indication to further treatment. He was therefore prepared by the administration of hyoscine and scoline. After an interval, he received a shock of 25 joules, passed quickly into the tonic phase, and died. The late Dr. William Goldie found a haemopericardium due to rupture of the heart, which had occurred through a large infarcted area, involving the greater part of the left ventricle. The appearances of this infarct were consistent with coronary arterial obstruction of about a week's duration. The left coronary artery was almost completely closed by a clot which was in the process of organisation. In his opinion death had been accelerated by treatment (Leeds City Coroner, No. 290/52).

Case No. 2

A patient, aged 43, died during the fifth of a series of shocks which had been administered to him for the treatment of depression. No untoward effects had followed the first four shocks, but during the fifth he passed into a tonic convulsion in which he remained until he died. Although artificial respiration was begun at once and continued for three-quarters of an hour, it was unavailing. Post-mortem examination showed that there was recently clotted blood in the nasal fossae and there was a little blood, insufficient to cause severe obstruction, in the trachea. A slight laceration of the undersurface of the tongue on one side was the only detected source of bleeding. The appearances were those of a death from asphyxia, which was deemed to be due to the prolonged fit, perhaps accelerated by the inhalation of blood (F.M. 292).

Patient monitoring carries the "ever-present" hazard of electrocution, with resulting ventricular fibrillation. Lee (1970) has drawn attention to the hazards surrounding a patient with a clutch of these electrical gadgets, e.g. handling the distal end of an intra-cardiac electrode, and pericardiocentesis with ECG monitoring. Only a small current, one of 100–200 mA, can then cause ventricular fibrillation and this threshold is lowered by anoxia and acidosis.

AUTO-EROTIC ELECTROCUTION

Electrical stimulation has joined hanging and suffocation as a mode of auto-erotic practice and shares with them comparable dangers and the penalty of death, in the event of ignorance or miscalculation.

It also shares with them some of the criteria of sexual deviation by which this is distinguished from suicide. The victims are males, either nude or, if clothed, they wear female garments, or their own clothing is opened to allow access to the genitalia. The wiring is either arranged to include the genitalia or to stimulate erotic zones, or both. The possession of pornographic literature or pictures, or the arrangement of the scene to permit personal observation of the procedure, or the making of a photographic record of it, are other possible features.

Schollmeyer (1959) reported the death of a man, aged 47, who was found dead beside his bed, nude, with electrical wiring round his penis; he had been in direct contact with the domestic supply of 220 V. A linear, grooved electric mark was close to the base of the penis and extended for a distance in the skin of the groin and lower abdomen.

Schollmeyer cited the case of Kopczyk (1957), where death was due to accidental contact with electricity in the course of masturbation, and also the cases of Kosyra (1957) and Schwarz (1952). Another case was reported by Hirth (1959); that of Holzhausen and Hunger (1963) was of a man, aged 27, who, when found dead, was dressed in female undergarments and corsets. Wiring had been arranged to stimulate erotic zones and the penis; there was an extensive electric mark in the left groin and lower abdomen. (See also the atlas of Weimann and Prokop, 1963.)

SUICIDAL ELECTROCUTION

Although it requires no profound knowledge of electricity and electrical wiring to commit suicide by electrocution and the requisite materials are easy to acquire, suicide by electrocution is still uncommon. When Munck described four new cases in 1934, he summarised the reports published during 1885–1932, a total of only twenty-nine cases; one of the first cases was reported by Nippe (1921). Incidentally, when I had the privilege of meeting Professor Munck at Aarhus in 1962, he told me he had never seen another case since 1934.

A common mode, if not the most frequent choice, is wiring of the wrists in connection with the domestic supply of electricity. The following are examples in our practice:

Case No. 1

A few weeks after his wife had been accidentally electrocuted in her bath (see p. 297) a man, aged 58, was found dead in his locked bathroom. He was seated on a chair, his feet were bare and in a bowl of water on the floor. His wrists were wired to the domestic supply. He had linear Joule burns around each wrist. He had threatened suicide and had left a "suicide note". It appeared that he had felt himself responsible for the faulty condition of the heater which had caused his wife's death (F.M. 10,496).

Case No. 2

A man aged 29 had wound the red lead to his right wrist and the blue lead to his left wrist and plugged the wires into a wall socket. He was under the influence of alcohol at the time; his blood contained 158 mg/100 ml and his urine contained 189 mg/100 ml. He died from ventricular fibrillation (F.M. 13,899 Figs. 106, 107).

Case No. 3

A man aged 72 died of electrocution in his bath; he had introduced a "live" flex into the water. No trace of external injury and no internal abnormality to account for the death. Diagnosis was by a process of elimination of other possible causes (F.M. 15,191).

This case was not unlike that of Dr. J. V. Wilson in 1967. The man aged 29 had wound the wires of an electric flex to the horizontal rod which had formed the base of wooden coat hanger. The wires were at each end of the rod, about a foot apart. It appears he was found dead in his bath, holding this appliance.

Case No. 4: *Probable suicide by Electrocution, Open Verdict*

The victim was a middle-aged woman, who had been treated for thyro-toxicosis and neurasthenia. She had been left alone in the house and, when found, she was dead in the bath. Both taps were open, the bath was full and water was escaping through the overflow and over the edge of the bath. A flex ran from an electric point outside the bathroom and was connected with an electric fire, which was in the bath, beneath the woman's body. The elements of the fire were against the bottom of the bath and they were switched on. The woman lay as if asleep in the water, with her arms folded across her chest and with her legs crossed (Fig. 109). No electric mark nor any other external injury was found on her body, except four small recent bruises in the scalp over the occiput, and another at the right elbow.

It may be that, when carrying the fire into the bathroom to warm the place, she had tripped over the flex and had then fallen into the bath, carrying the fire with her. It seems more probable that she had placed the fire, back uppermost, in the bath, turned on the taps, and had then lain on top of the fire, to wait until the water rose and electrocuted her.

The probability of murder seems the least likely explanation. Her husband prepared her breakfast at 6.45 a.m. and took it to her bedroom. She then seemed in rather better spirits. He left early for his work and did not return until midday, by which time the body had been found and the house was in an uproar. He was shocked at the news. Arrangements had been made for his wife to be visited by neighbours. One, who was due at 9.30 a.m., found the house locked and could not get in. This surprised her, since the door was usually left open. When she returned later it was open and she then gave the deceased a light meal. The deceased, when told of the earlier visit, said "I heard you and came down and opened the door", but her visitor had then gone. When another neighbour called at 11.15 a.m. to prepare dinner she found both doors locked. This was unusual. She got no response when she rang the bell, so she sent for the deceased's son, who opened the door, and returned to his work. It was then 11.40 a.m. Since the husband was due to return at 12.10 p.m., attention was first given to the preparation of his dinner. A little later the woman went upstairs to see the deceased and found her in the bath. The electric fire was "twitching" in the bath. The police were summoned and turned off the supply.

The husband married again shortly after his wife's death, but in any event, his movements during the interval between the visits of the two neighbours, and during which interval she had died, were satisfactorily determined, and it is scarcely possible that the first of the neighbours put her in the bath with the fire (F.M. 375).

Case No. 5

This woman aged 29 connected her wrists with wires to the domestic supply of electricity. She was under the influence of alcohol at the time.

She was laid on her back in her living room on a carpeted floor. There was an electric plug socket and switch on the wainscot of the wall, near her feet. She was clad in a nightdress. Her right leg was extended and the left leg was doubled under her right; her arms were flexed over her chest.

There was a length of black rubber-coated flex attached to a plug to the right of her body. The free end of the flex had been opened to expose the two leads, red and blue. Their wires had been bared and wrapped round her wrists, the red lead to her right and the blue lead to her left wrist. The skin of the right wrist was scorched and blackened. She had an electric mark on the right side of her abdomen.

The immediate cause of death was ventricular fibrillation.

Her blood alcohol content was 158 mg/100 ml and her urine alcohol content was 189 mg/100 ml. This was deemed the equivalent of the consumption of two-fifths of a bottle of spirits. (F.M. 13,899).

Reported cases include the series of four by Munck (1934), of which we are privileged to reproduce one of his illustrations (see Fig. 105). Examples of suicide by throwing a weighted wire over a high-tension cable were reported by Buhtz (1930) and Breitenecker (1938). A recent example is that of Ollivier *et al.* (1961). This suicide fixed a loop of copper wire round his neck and threw the free end over a high-tension cable carrying 60,000 volts.

L'Épée *et al.* (1965) described the suicide of a man who put a live plug into his bath; the water became the electrode. On this occasion there was an exit mark in the form of a circular burn, 5–6 cm in diameter, on his right buttock. It reproduced the shape of the exit hole in the floor of the bath.

Randall (1966) reported the suicide of a boy aged 13. He held a $5^1/_2$ in. Meccano metal rod in each hand; these electrodes were connected to a wall plug and he had wired his right leg to a metal rod in the garden. The smell of burning attracted the attention of his mother who switched off the current but was too late to save him.

The case of Nippe (1942) is a variant of our Case No. 1. The current was wired to a bucket of water. Suicide was accomplished by plunging the arms into the water.

Suicide by a combination of hanging and electrocution was reported by Petit *et al.* (1962).

> A man aged 60 was found suspended by a metal cable which was high up under his neck; it was arranged neither in a running noose nor in a fixed loop. He had an abrasion of his nose and a small bruise on his forehead. There was also an injury of his left hand and wrist; this injury had been initially described as a drying wound (*plaie sèche*) but was later identified as an electric mark. It was deduced that he had attempted suicide by putting his hand on an electric motor. The shock had caused him to fall and sustain facial injury. He then had recourse to hanging. The absence of a noose was accounted for by the inability to tie the ligature because of injury to his left hand.

Four cases of suicide by electrocution are represented by specimens in Professor Gormsen's Institute. One victim used a brass disc, 3.2 cm in diameter, and a metal key, 5.2 cm long, as terminals; another wired coins to the domestic supply, 225 volts; the third used a pair of brass door hinges, 4.5 × 3.0 cm. The fourth man, when found dead in a room at the back of his shop, was clad in pyjamas and beneath them he wore a bathing dress. In this case the terminals were rectangular, numbered, metal labels, fastened with safety pins to the inside of the bathing dress. In each of these cases it appears that one terminal was applied over the heart and the other at the back of the body. (Details of these four cases were published by Willy Munck, 1934.)

HOMICIDAL ELECTROCUTION

Murder by electrocution is as yet rare. Whybrow was convicted of attempted murder by electrocution in 1951 and sentenced to 10 years imprisonment. His appeal was dismissed (*R. v. Whybrow*, [1951] 35 Cr. App. R. 141). It appears he had connected the soap-dish in his bathroom to the household supply of electricity in such a manner that, operating a switch in his bedroom, he could cause his wife to receive a shock when she touched the soap-dish. She had received shocks while taking baths and eventually called in an electrician, who discovered the trap.

A woman, intending suicide and the death of her child, took her into the bath into which she put an electric fire. She survived, but the child died. When her mother-in-law found them in the bath, she received a shock on putting her hand into the water. The mother was later charged with murder of her child.

A man is reported to have murdered his wife by electrocution (Carrieri, 1957).

A father murdered his child aged 22 months by inflicting electric shocks with the flex of the radio. He bared the ends of the wires and plugged the flex into the domestic circuit. The bared wires were then put into the cot with the intention that the child would play with them. That was one version he gave of the incident, but there were many peculiar marks on the child's body, some tiny and pin point, others elongated up to 4 cm in length. They appeared to have been produced by a pointed agent; some had a sharp ring around them and others had depressed centres; several were in pairs, about 4 mm apart. The appearances were those of repeated applications of the ends of "live" wires. It was when he learnt this, that the father abandoned his initial explanation that, while using his soldering iron, repairing a radio set, the wires made contact by accident with the child, asleep in its cot nearby. The child had a number of convulsions; and father said he saw it flopping about in its cot like a fish out of water. These no doubt occurred when he made repeated application of the wires to the child's body.

The child had come between him and its mother. He did not wish to kill the child but intended to hurt him. He was acquitted on the ground of mental irresponsibility—paranoid schizophrenia (Bornstein, 1962).

A man planned to injure his wife by connecting the exit and overflow of their bath with the domestic electrical supply. It was intended that when her heel made contact with the exit plug she would receive a shock. It appears that she did but was able to get out of the bath and go in search of a pencil with which she flicked the plug out of the exit. There was a bluish flash and the electric lights fused. Her husband said he had intended only "to take the mickey out of her" because she had taunted him about a personal matter. He was acquitted of attempted murder but found guilty of administering an electric shock with intent to annoy (*R.* v. *Donald,* C.C.C. May 1958).

MANSLAUGHTER BY ELECTROCUTION

In 1927 a man, who was ratting near some coal bunkers, was electrocuted because he came into contact with an electrified wire which had been erected to protect them. A charge of manslaughter was preferred against the colliery proprietors (Smith and Fiddes, 1955). In 1958 the owner of a workshop was similarly charged when a boy, aged 14, was electrocuted by a fence which was intended to protect the place from robbers. The owner normally switched off the 230-volt current during the day, but on this occasion he had forgotten to do so.

Low-voltage electric wiring is used to keep cattle within bounds.

The electrification of door knobs and the like, as a practical joke, may miscarry. Glaister and Rentoul (1966) record a death which occurred when a door handle had been connected to an electric light switch. The intention was to play a trick. When the victim tried to open the door, he received a shock from a 230–250 volt supply, while standing on damp soil.

LIGHTNING STROKE

The avoidance of lightning stroke during a storm is always the first consideration. It is not to be assumed, however, that those who have the misfortune to be struck must die. On the contrary, *prompt* and persistent treatment by artificial respiration proved successful on more occasions than is usually imagined. Only 250 of 601 victims of lightning stroke died; apparent death in the survivors lasted from 6 minutes to 6 hours (Sestier, 1880). Recovery may be complete or, as described later, there may be permanent effects due to injury of the central nervous system.

The examples cited below indicate some of the circumstances in which lightning stroke occurs and the precautions which should be taken to avoid injury. Further examples, of which there are nearly fifty, are cited by Tidy (1882). A valuable account of lightning stroke is given by Spencer (1932), who for a quarter of a century was a district surgeon in the Transvaal. The report of the Ascot accident in 1955 is also noteworthy (Arden *et al.,* 1956). The comprehension review by Goldie and Lee (1976) should be consulted.

Examples of Lightning Stroke

In August 1947 four walkers were overtaken by a storm and took shelter under an oak tree which was struck by lightning. One man was killed; the other three suffered shock and burns (*Manchester Guardian*, 6 Aug, 1947). This is an example of the well-recognised danger of sheltering under a tree during a storm.

There is, however, no guarantee that the shelter of a house will preclude injury, although the effects directly due to the electrical discharge may then be greatly minimised. A boy aged 15 years was killed when listening to the wireless in the kitchen of his home during a storm. His father felt the shock pass through his feet and his mother felt a shock in her arm when lightning struck the chimney of the house (*The Yorkshire Post*, 3 June, 1949). The danger inside a house is due to the effects of the blast of superheated air produced by the flash, or falling masonry, notably the chimney, e.g. a boy aged 13 was thus injured (*Manchester Guardian*, 8 Aug., 1950). Innes, cited by Spencer (1932), advised the occupants of a house should avoid the line between open windows or an open door and a window or the fireplace, since the blast will leave the house by these routes.

Tent poles are particularly likely to be struck, therefore shelter in tents is unwise.

When a farmer aged 54 took shelter under a large bombing aeroplane during a storm, a "thunderbolt" fell in the field. His body was found beneath the machine; there was a cross-piece of metal, 6 in. long each way, under his body. There was no trace of damage to the aeroplane, the aerial of which had been earthed by a wire to a metal rod in the ground. There was a small hole in the cloth cap of the victim; its margins were not burnt; a small hairless spot, resembling an abrasion of the scalp, was directly below this hole. Recent superficial burns, $1^1/_2$ in. in diameter, were present on each buttock over the ischial tuberosity. His boots were shod with iron heel- and toe-plates. His watch was still going. It appeared that at the time of the shock he was squatting on the ground. Dill (1942), who reported the case, drew attention to the danger of sheltering beneath an aeroplane; had the man been inside it, he would in all probability have seen safe.

Lightning stroke may claim victims who are in the open. In one of our cases, the victim was near a stile in the open moorland. On another occasion two men were walking on the Great North Road in search of shelter when they were struck. One of the men, who was carrying a steel billhook on his shoulder, was killed but his companion felt only a heavy pressure between his shoulders. The dead man sustained fractures of both legs and, with the exception of part of his left sleeve, his clothing was stripped from his body. The blast also made a hole 18 in. deep in the road (*The Yorkshire Post*, 4 Sept. 1948).

Two youths, aged 18 and 20, were killed by lightning when they were working on a haystack; the farmer, who was with them, suffered shock. They were using hay forks at the time; the farmer and one youth were on top of the stack and the other youth was in a cart below. It appeared that the youth on the stack was struck first and fell on to the one in the cart (*The Yorkshire Post*, 29 July 1950).

When five people ran for shelter during a storm two were killed and the others were injured (*Manchester Guardian*, 22 May 1950).

When two men were driving in a dog-cart during a storm, the vehicle was struck and both men fell out of it. Five minutes after the flash their bodies were found lying side by side on the road. The seat of the cart was beneath them and the driving apron was still around their legs. One of the men had an extensive burn over his chest and abdomen, and circular holes of from $^{1}/_{16}$ in. to $^{1}/_{4}$ in. in diameter were scattered over the burnt area. His metal collar stud had fused and the underlying skin was deeply burned. His watch was still going. The other victim had no external injury. The horse was uninjured and trotted home (Whichello, 1899).

Injuries, at first sight suggestive of murder, were sustained by an African native when struck by lightning in his small hut, made of sticks and with a low thatched roof. A coconut tree nearby had been blasted. His body lay in a posture consistent with sleep at the time of the flash. The blast had produced a laceration of the left side of his neck where all the soft tissues between the trachea and spine had been blown out; the wound admitted a closed fist. His left shoulder had also been gravely lacerated and there was a double fracture of the humerus; one at the neck and the other about 4 in. lower down; the broken bone was denuded of muscle and lay in the wound. There were superficial injuries of the face, chest and of the genitalia. Deep lacerations were present on the inner aspect of each thigh, extending from groin to knee. The skin of the right side of the abdomen was slate-grey in colour and parchmented but no burning or singeing was seen. The scalp was intact but there was an extensive fracture, with comminution, of the base of the skull; the brain, however, presented no naked-eye abnormality. The hut was shared by his brother, who only suffered shock (Skan, 1949).

Multiple casualities from the same lightning stroke occurred during a football match. During the second half of the game, a terrific storm broke and a brilliant flash of forked lightning struck the field. The referee and most of the players near him, together with several of the spectators, were struck down. The spectators, although dazed, got up but the referee and the players remained motionless on the ground. Two of the players died and the referee and the others suffered shock. When reporting this case reference was made to another during which the referee's whistle was struck as he was about to blow it for a penalty. "He stood transfixed with his arm outstretched but continued his duties after a rest" (*Daily Telegraph*, 20 April 1948).

The fashionable event, Ascot races, was marred by a severe thunderstorm, preceded by a heavy fall of rain, in 1955, when lightning claimed forty-five victims, of whom two died. The clinical features were analysed by Arden *et al.* (1956) in their report of the incident. The two fatalities were caused by head injuries. Twelve persons were rendered unconscious and others were momentarily dazed. Those thrown to the ground found that when they attempted to rise, they were unable to move their limbs. Twenty-six of thirty-seven patients seen in hospital complained of paraesthesiae in one or more limbs. The characteristic story was one of a sudden shooting pain in the arm, followed by weakness and "pins and needles", persisting for 2 to 3 hours. In a few cases paraesthesiae persisted for several weeks. Only a few rendered unconscious suffered any symptoms of a post-contusional state. Diminished hearing and emotional disturbances occurred in a few of the patients.

Fifteen sustained burns, but none required skin grafting. " Feathering" was transient, lasting at most only a few days. Some had flash burns, which presented as a brown discoloration of the superficial layers of the skin. Five had erythema and blistering, which healed in less than 10 days. Punctate, full thickness burns were the commonest finding. Linear charring of the skin, but only of partial thickness, was also seen. Although this did not require grafting, the eschars in one patient took 6 weeks to separate. Some of the burns were related to overlying metal.

Nearly all of the casualties had crowded together, in their wet clothes, near a tea stall in or near a tent with metal-topped props. The latter acted as a lightning rod. Being wet and well earthed, the victims sustained burns. Had they been dry and well insulated, they could have suffered the disruptive effects of lightning.

Spencer discussed the apparent immunity of motor vehicles from lightning stroke; he knew of no instance of a car being directly struck; this might be due to insulation by the tyres. A car may be indirectly struck, however, by a "splash" from some other object struck nearby. He instanced a motorist whose car was indirectly struck when it passed under the veranda of a house which was struck by lightning at that moment. Although the flash traversed the front of the car and the driver could watch its course, he felt no electric shock. It appears that the flash was conducted by water streaming from the car during the storm.

This immunity to lightning stroke may have an entirely different explanation. Dr. A. S. Curry, recalling Faraday's experiments which showed there was no circuit within an empty metal box, suggested to me that a motor car is such a box. Immunity within it is preserved even if a window be opened to call for help, but would be lost if a fist or even a finger be put outside. The protection would be similar, if an overhead "live" cable fell on the car.

Side Flash

The danger of sheltering under a tree during a storm is appreciable because, if the tree be struck by lightning, the current, in passing down the trunk to the earth, may be deflected to enter the head, neck or shoulder of a person standing beside the trunk. About 10 per cent of lightning casualties in the U.S.A. are persons who had sheltered under a tree during a thunder storm.

The occurrence of a side flash may be confirmed by the presence of clear marks of entry of the current into the head, neck or shoulder. Goldie and Lee (1976) detailed a most unusual and instructive case. The victim had taken up a telephone during a storm. He was stood near a refrigerator and other metal equipment from which a metal tube projected and was close to his right ear, to which he had applied the telephone receiver. He had rested his buttocks against the refrigerator. At the time he was wearing a gold necklace which undoubtedly saved his life by diverting the current from his heart. The necklace was destroyed; it had left a patterned burn on the right side of his neck and over the clavicle. The accident was attributed to faulty installation of the lightning conductor. By error, a bonding connection between the sheath of the telephone cable had been omitted. The current was deemed to have passed from the metal tube and the refrigerator through his buttocks and abdomen to the telephone. Electric marks were present below his right ear, below the melted gold necklace and on his buttocks. The ear piece of the telephone had formed part of the return pathway and had deflected the current from his respiratory centre.

Flash Over

When two or more persons are close together during a thunder storm, all or several of them may be killed or severely injured although only one of them suffered a direct strike.

Examples include players in a game of football. Two men, marking each other, were awaiting a throw-in when lightning struck one of them. Both were violently thrown apart and died. Lichtenberg figures were on the sides of their bodies turned towards each other before they were thrown apart. No burn marks were present neither on their bodies nor on their clothing. It could have been that delay in immediate skilled treatment led to death from respiratory arrest or, possibly, ventricular fibrillation (Lynch and Shorthouse, 1949).

Twenty three climbers caught in a thunderstorm when climbing on a steep mountain ridge in Japan. Only one of the boys was struck, but all of one group of 20–25 boys were killed. There was clear signs of entry by flash over and side flash damage. This and step voltage were deemed the cause of the death. (Goldie and Lee, 1976).

When four boys were affected by lightning while playing football, one was struck fatally and the others, at from 30–100 feet away from him, suffered non-fatal effects. The one struck survived 7 days but never regained consciousness. Cerebral function ceased by the sixth day and at post-mortem examination there was oedema of the brain and extensive softening of grey and white matter.

A second boy, aged 11 who had been at about 30–50 feet from the deceased, was knocked unconscious and had arrested breathing. Cardio-respiratory resuscitation, administered by a nurse enabled him to resume spontaneous respiration within 5 minutes. Ten minutes after the accident he was found to be disorientated and amnesic to the event. Later he complained of presternal pain and pain in his arms. The particular feature of this case was the development, at 3 weeks after the accident of severe agitation and emotional liability, with frequent expression of fear of dying. This feature required psychotherapy for several months and the pain in his chest and arms continued at intervals for about 6 months.

A third boy, aged 11 who had been about 100 feet from the deceased, was unconscious for about 1 to 2 minutes but maintained spontaneous breathing throughout. A week after the accident he was found to be amnesic for a significant portion of the game prior to the accident. He continued to have frequent episodes of depression, emotional liability and impaired concentration on schoolwork. Spontaneous resolution at 3 months after the accident.

The fourth boy, also aged 11, who had been within 30–50 feet of the deceased, regained consciousness spontaneously within a few minutes. He suffered from mental disability for about 6 weeks but the trouble then resolved spontaneously. He had had difficulty in abstract thinking and his calculation ability had been impaired (Kotagal *et al.* 1982).

LIGHTNING STROKE (AND ELECTRICAL SHOCK DURING PREGNANCY)

The occasions on which pregnant women have suffered lightning stroke or, for that matter, any electrical shock, are rare. Rees (1965) recorded an incident in which a married couple, and the man's father, were struck by lightning on a Welsh mountain near their farm. At the moment of being struck the woman was sheltering under a sheet of zinc, which rested on the nape of her neck. She felt as if she had been struck in the back of her neck and this sensation persisted for several hours. Her clothing was not burnt. She had a "fern-leaf" burn at the back of her neck and right shoulder; there were exit burns on her buttocks. She was able to walk back to the farm, but was admitted to hospital, where she stayed 2 days. A few days later she complained of nausea and was then found to be pregnant. In due course she was delivered of a female infant whose birth weight was 5 lb 10 oz.

Rees was able to trace only five instances of electrical shock or lightning stroke during pregnancy reported since 1930. The women were all at or beyond the sixth month of pregnancy; they all survived but all of them lost their infants. In Baldi's case (1957, cited Rees) there was spontaneous delivery of a macerated foetus at 5 days after receiving a shock from 220 volts; she had passed the eighth month. Samsvenarjo's report (1959, cited Rees) was of a woman who had passed the sixth month of pregnancy when struck by lightning. She lost consciousness and sustained severe burns directly below the umbilicus. Her uterus ruptured and she was delivered of a dead infant by Caesarean section.

The Diagnosis of Death by Lightning Stroke

The history of the recent occurrence of a storm is of first importance. This may be confirmed by evidence of blasting of trees, buildings or other objects. The clothing may be completely torn off the body but there may be only a small entrance hole or no mark at all. The bursting open of the clothing is characteristic and the tears may be scorched and smell of singeing. Boots, shoes and belts also can be burst open and the tear is usually at the back (Spencer, 1932).

Injuries of a disruptive kind, particularly well illustrated by Skan's case cited above, may be extensive or there may be no external mark on the body. In most cases it is usual to find areas of burning, if not of laceration. The burns may be restricted to the area of a collar stud or other metal object, e.g. metal support of a corset, or steel hairpins. Fracture of the skull by direct impact, without any burns, is not uncommon (Humphreys, 1940); the fracture can be produced by the disruptive effects of lightning rather than a fall to the ground; this was the interpretation preferred by Arden *et al.* (1956) in respect of their fatal case.

Spencer (1932) grouped the external marks or burns into three classes. These may be *surface burns*, which are tissue burns and are usually related to metallic objects worn or carried by the victim. *Linear burns*, of from 1 to 12 in. long and $^1/_8$ to 1 in. wide, may be found where an area of skin offers less resistance, notably in the moist creases and folds of the skin. His third group is that of *arborescent* or *filigree* "*burns*" or feathering (Fig. 111, 112). The latter indicate a severe stroke and, in Spencer's experience, were "invariably seen upon the electrocuted". Arborescent marking is characteristic when present, but it fades rapidly if the victim survives (see the Ascot experience, Arden *et al.*, 1956). An excellent example is given in a woodcut which illustrates the report of two men, injured by lightning (Cook and Boulting, 1888). They are not thermal burns. Goldie and Lee (1976) prefer to call them Lichtenberg figures.

Metal objects, e.g. a steel penknife or parts of a watch may become magnetised. This is to be sought for especially when bodily injuries are negligible or absent. In view of the gravity of the injuries on other occasions care must be exercised lest an erroneous diagnosis of criminal violence is made. The presence of magnetised objects on or near the body may assist in making the distinction.

In Spencer's experience the head is invariably struck and this may cause obvious bruising, usually at the back of the head. The injury is distinguished from the effects of a

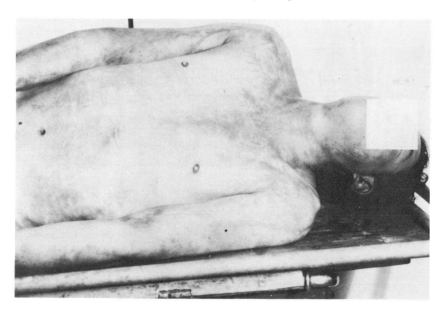

Fig. 111. Lightning stroke: arborescent marks. (By courtesy of Dr. Leopold.)

blow by a weapon because abrasions and lacerations are absent. If a hat was worn it is likely to have a hole in it at a point corresponding with the bruise of the scalp.

Recoveries from Lightning Stroke

Those who recover may do so without any residual ill-effects. Some, however, may complain of neurological abnormalities, which can vary appreciably in character and severity. There may be no more than areas of anaesthesia or, as in Eulenberg's (1875) case (cited Tidy, 1882), these may be hemiplegia; it was 7 months before this victim recovered. In Lane's case (1872, cited Tidy, 1882) the right tympanic membrane was lacerated. The disturbance of the brain cortex by the shock may leave permanent damage resulting in mental deterioration.

Spencer (1932) described the history of a man who, even 8 years after lightning stroke, was still deaf. His personality had changed; formerly a cheerful man, he became consistently morose and pessimistic. Like others who have been able to give an account of the stroke, all he knew at the time was that "a smashing sledge-hammer blow" on the back of his head had "knocked him out". It is wise to defer a final prognosis until sufficient time has elapsed to permit a satisfactory assessment of the probable permanent damage to the nervous system. Due allowance must also be made for intercurrent or incidental, unrelated mental illness (Langworthy and Kouwenhoven, 1932).

The occurrence of psychological disturbance, requiring psychiatric treatment, as a sequel of non-fatal injury by "flash over" was reported by Kotagal *et al.* (1982) (see page 311).

The neurological effects of lightning and or electricity were described by Macdonald

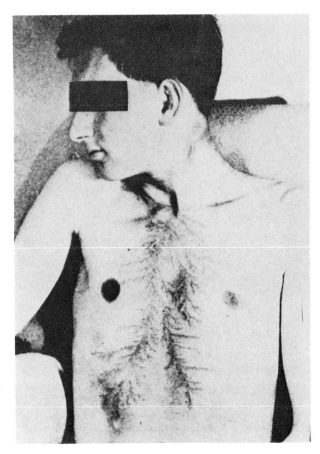

Fɪɢ. 112. Lightning stroke: arborescent marking. (Reproduced by courtesy of the Editor of the *British Medical Journal* (1963, i. 1329) and by Professor Chassar Moir and Professor Fraenkel.)

Critchley (1934, 1935). In his view the poor conductivity of nervous tissue probably accounts for the comparative infrequency of neurological signs after electrical and lightning accidents. Their occurrence also depends on the course taken by the current. If it passes from arm to arm, the central nervous system may escape completely, on the other hand it is almost certain to be involved if the head is a point of contact. (The papers by Panse, 1930; Hassin, 1933 and 1937; and by Dickson, 1947, should also be consulted.)

Resuscitation

Respiratory arrest should be treated by the best current method, which is mouth-to-mouth assisted respiration. It should be continued for at least 10 minutes, if spontaneous breathing has not already been resumed. If still needed, the treatment should be continued until the patient is admitted to an intensive care unit, assuming the patient be still alive. In short, dont be too quick to assume that death has occurred nor too diligent in attempting to restore the dead.

Cardiac arrest is to be treated, in the first instance, by external cardiac massage. Care must be taken to avoid undue force. It is not unknown for several ribs, and even a breast bone, to be broken by an enthusiastic operator of powerful physique.

Prognosis

Even when the best facilities are promptly available, complete recovery is likely in only about 49 per cent; where these facilities are not available the recovery rate is only about 17 per cent (Goldie and Lee, 1982).

Protection from Lightning Stroke

Indoors. If a large building, or one which is appreciably higher than its neighbours, fitting it with a lightning conductor is a wise precaution. It is important, also, that the fitting be done by a competent person.

During a storm the inmates should avoid the vicinity of fireplaces and especially positions which place them in direct line between a fire place and an open window, since that is the likely line of the current if a chimney be struck and the current passes down the interior of the chimney to the fireplace. Shelter in a garage may be safe and the best place is then within a motor car. As stated earlier, the interior of a closed motor car is well insulated.

Out-of-doors. The increasing number of fatalities from lightning stroke amongst hikers, climbers and others, involved in a storm, when in the open, (the football field should not be forgotten as another area of special risk), calls for renewed attention to the precautions which reduce the hazard. Standing on the top of a vehicle or building must not occur. The vertical posture should be avoided and squatting be assumed. Umbrellas should not be used, no matter how tempting the apparent protection of a "golf" umbrella may be. These and tools fitted with a metal implement are distinctly dangerous, potential, lightning conductors.

Swimming is dangerous during a storm. A boat fitted with a metal mast or keel is also dangerous. If in a tent, keep clear of the tentpole and wet canvas.

A group of persons caught in a storm should keep well apart, if possible by at least 100 feet (30 m) to avoid the effects of "flash over" if one or more be struck. Never shelter under large trees, since there is grave risk of "fatal flash over" if a tree be struck.

References

ADJUTANTIS, G. and SKALOS, G. (1962) *J. Forens. Med.*, **9**, 101.
ALDRICH, R. H. (1943) *Ann. Surg.*, **117**, 576–84.
ALEXANDER, L. (1938) *J. Industr. Hyg.*, **20**, 191–243.
ANNOTATION (1888) *Brit. Med. J.*, **ii**, 242 (see Sestier).
ARDEN, G. P., HARRISON, S. H., LISTER, J. and MAUDSLEY, R. H. (1956) *Brit. Med. J.*, **i**, 1450–3.
BAINBRIDGE, W. (1930) *Brit. Med. J.*, **ii**, 955–6.
BALBO, W. (1957) *Zacchia* , **20**, 449.
BÉGUÉ, MONS. (1935) *Bull. Soc. Ophthal.*, Paris, March, 167–70.
BOEMKE, F. and PIROTH, M. (1959) *Frankfurt*, Z. Path., 70, 1–35; obstr. *Med.-leg. J.* (Chamb.), 1960, **28**, 162–3.
BORNSTEIN, F. P. (1962) *J. Forens. Sci.*, **7**, 516.

Bosch, K. (1965) *Dtsch. Z. ges. gerichtl. Med.*, **56**, 318.
Bousvaros, G. A., Don, C. and Hopps, J. A. (1962) *Canad. Med. Ass. J.*, **87**, 286.
Breitenecker, L. (1938) Internat. Kongr. ger. soz. Med., Bonn.
Buhtz, G. (1930) *Dtsch. Z. ges. gerichtl. Med.*, **14**, 443–8.
Bull, T. P. and Cason, J. S. (1959) *Brit. Med. J.*, **ii**, 189.
Carrieri, F. (1957) *G. Méd.-lég. infortunistica e tossicologia*, **3**, 103. (Reference not available in U.K.)
Chardack, W. M., Gage, A. A. and Greatbatch, W. (1960) *Surgery (St. Louis, Mo.)*, **48**, 643; cited Knickerbocker and Kouwenhoven (1961).
Cohen, L. B. (1941) *Benjamin Franklin's Experiments*. Havard University Press.
Cook, A. H. and Boulting, W. (1888) *Brit. Med. J.*, **ii**, 234–5.
Corney, L. A. (1961) Area Boards' Medical Advisers Conference, Nov. 16/17.
Critchley, Macdonald (1934) *Lancet*, **i**, 68–72.
Critchley, Macdonald (1935) *Med. Ann.*, 53rd year, 120–3.
Dalziel, C. F. (1943) *Electrical Engineering Trans.* **62**, 739.
Dalziel, C. F. (1960) *AIEE Elect. Engineering*, **79**, 667.
Dalziel, C. F. (1962) *Trans. Amer. Inst. Elect. Engrs.*, **81**, 978.
Dalziel, C. F. (1963) *AIEE Elect. Engineering*, **82**, 978.
Dalziel, C. F., Lagen, J. B. and Thurston, J. L. (1941). *Elect. Engineering Trans.*, **60**, 1073.
Dalziel, C. F. and Lee, W. R. (1968) *IEEE Trans.*, Vol. I. G. A. **4**, 467; *ibid.*, p. 676.
d'Arsonval, (1885: 1887) *C. R. Acad. Sci. (Paris)*; cited Jex-Blake (1913).
Dérobert, L. and Grèzes-Rueff, Ch. (1958) *Ann. Méd.-lég.*, **38**, 182.
deVille, E. (1955) *Electricity*, 414–16 Penguin Books Harmondsworth
Dickson, W. E. C. (1947) *J. Path. Bact.*, **59**, 359–65.
Dill, A. V. (1942) *Brit. Med. J.*, **ii**, 426.
Dürwald, W., Holzhausen, G. and Hunger, H. (1964) *Arch. Kriminol.*, **134**, 164.
Ennis, J. E. (1967) *Med. Sci. Law*, 7, 142.
Ennis, J. E. (1968) *Med. Sci. Law*, **8**, 53.
Ferris, L. P., King, B. G., Spence, P. W. and Williams, H. B. (1936) *AIEE Electrical Engineering Trans*, **55**, 498–515.
Fitzsimmons, J. O'C. (1924) *Brit. Med. J.*, **ii**, 932.
Fry, J. F. (1962) Personal communication and copy of Fire Research Note No. 976. (R. E. Lustig).
Furman, S., Schewedl, J. B., Robinson, G. and Harwitt, E. S. (1961) *Surgery*, **49**, 98.
Gey, R. (1926) *Arch. Orthop. Unfall-Chir.*, **24**, 137–50.
Glaister, John and Rentoul, E. (1966) *Medical Jurisprudence and Toxicology*, 12th ed. Edinburgh: Livingstone.
Goldie, R. H. and Lee, W. R. (1976) *IEE*, 123, 1163–1180.
Gordon, A. S. (1968) *I.EE. Trans.* Vol. I.G.A., **4**, 676.
H. M. Chief Inspector of factories (1946) *Ann. Rep.*, 1945; Cmd. 6992, London; H.M.S.O.
H. M. Chief Inspector of factories (1951) *Ann. Rep.*, 1949; Cmd. 8155, London; H.M.S.O.
H. M. Factory Department (1954) Form 1705; Nov. 1954.
Hassin, G. B. (1933) *Arch. Neurol. Psychiat.* (Chicago), **30**, 1046–60.
Hassin, G. B. (1937) *J. Nerv. Ment. Dis.*, **86**, 668–73.
Hirth, L. (1959) *Dtsch. Z. ges. gerichtl. Med.*, **49**, 109–12.
Holzhausen, G. and Hunger, H. (1963) *Arch. Kriminol.*, **131**, 166.
Humphreys, F. R. (1940) *Lancet*, **ii**, 154.
Jaeger, H. (1921) *Schweiz. med. Wschr.*, **ii**, 1251–61.
Jaffé, R. H. (1928) *Arch. Path.*, **5**, 837–70.
Jellinek, S. (1927) *Der Elektrische Unfall*, 2nd ed., Leipzig and Wien; Deuticke.
Jellinek, S. (1932) *Die Elektrischen Verletzungen*, Leipzig; Barth.
Jellinek, S. (1957) *Triangle*, **3**, 104–10.
Jex-Blake, A. J. (1913) Goulstonian Lectures, *Brit. Med. J.*, **i**, 425–30, 492–8, 548–52, 601.
Knickerbocker, G. G. and Kouwenhoven, W. B. (1961) *Elect. Engng. (N.Y.)*, **80**, 761–6.
Kotagal, S., Rawlings, C. A. Chen, su-chiung, Burris, G. and Nouri, S. (1982) *Pediatnis*, **70**, No. 2, 190–192.
Kouwenhoven, W. B., Chesnut, R. W., Knickerbocker, G. G., Milnor, W. R. and Sass, D. J. (1959) *Elect. Engineering*, **78**, 163.
Kouwenhoven, W. B., Knickerbocker, G. G., Milnor, W. R. and Jude, J. R. (1960) *Elect. Engng. (N.Y.)*, **79**, 800.
Langlois, J.-P. (1922) *Bull. Acad. Med.*, **87**, 158–60.
Langworthy, O. R. and Kouwenhoven, W. B. (1930) *J. Industr. Hyg.*, **12**, 31–65.
Langworthy, O. R. and Kouwenhoven, W. B. (1932) *Amer. J. Hyg.*, **16**, 625–66, bibliography.
Lee, W. R. (1961) *Brit. J. Industr. Med.*, **18**, 260–9.

LEE, W. R. (1964) *Brit. J. Anaesth.*, **36**, 572.
LEE, W. R. (1965a) *Med. Sci. Med. J.*, **2**, 616.
LEE, W. R. (1965b) *Med. Sci. Law*, **5**, 23.
LEE, W. R. (1970) *Post. Grad. Med. J.*, **46**, 355.
LEE, W. R. and MCNAMEE, R. (1982) personal communication.
LEE, W. R. and ZOLEDZOIWSKI, S. (1964) *Brit. J. Industr. Med.*, **21**, 135.
LEE, W. R., ZOLEDIOWSKI, S. and FORDYCE, I. D. (1965) *Brit. J. Industr. Med.*, **22**, 43.
L'ÉPÉE, P., LAZARINI, H. J., N'DOKY, TH. and DOIGNON, J. (1965) *Annls. Méd.-lég., Crimin. Police Scient*, **45**, 550.
LONG, M. H. E. (1935) *Med. Pr.*, **191**, 150–6; *ibid.*, 172–8.
LUSTIG, R. E. (1961) Fire Research Note No. 467/1961.
LYNCH, M. J. G. and SHORTHOUSE, P. H. (1949) *Lancet*, i, 473–78.
MACLACHLAN, W. (1930) *J. Industr. Hyg.*, **12**, 291–9.
MEDICAL DEFENCE UNION (1961) *Annual Report*, pp. 35–36.
MEDICINE AND THE LAW (1963) *Lancet*, **1**, 1155.
MODY, S. M. and RICHINGS, M. (1962) *Lancet*, **2**, 698.
MOORHEAD, J. J. (1910) *J. Amer. Med. Ass.*, **54**, 1127–32.
MOYLE, V. Southern Electricity Board (1961) *The Times*, 24 Oct.
MUNCK, W. (1934) *Dtsch. Z. ges. gerichtl. Med.*, **23**, 97–109.
NIPPE, M. (1921) *Vjschr. gerichtl. Med.*, **61**, 211–13.
NIPPE, M. (1942) *Dtsch. Z. ges. gerichtl. Med.*, **36**, 307–10.
NOORDIJK, J. A., OEY, F. T. I. and TEBRA, W. (1961) *Lancet*. **1**, 975.
OLIVER, T. and BOLAM, R. A. (1898) *Brit. Med. J.*, **1**, 132.
OLLIVIER, H., VUILLET, F. and BASTARET, M. (1961) *Annls Méd.-lég. Crimin. Police Scient.*, **41**, 585.
PANSE, (1930) cited Critchley (1935), also Langworthy and Kouwenhoven (1932).
PAYNE, R. T. (1940) *Brit. Med J.*, i, 819–22.
PETIT, G.-J., PETIT, A. G. and CHAMPEIX, J. (1962) *Ann. Méd.-lég.*, **42**, 343.
POLSON, C. J. (1955) *The Essentials of Forensic Medicine*, pp. 193–4. London, E.U.P.
POLSON, C. J. (1959) *Med.-leg. J. (Camb.)*, **27**, 121–35.
PREVOST, J.-L. and BATTELLI, F. (1899) *J. Phys. Path. gen.* **1**, 399; *ibid.*, p. 427.
PRITCHARD, E. A. B. (1934) *Lancet*, i, 1163–7.
RANDALL, K. J. (1966) *Med. Sci. Law*, **6**, 45.
RAVITCH, M. M., LANE, R., SAFAR, P., STEICHEN, F. M. and KNOWLES, P. (1961) *New Eng. J. Med.*, **264**, 36.
REES, W. D. (1965) *Brit. Med. J.*, **1**, 103.
ROBERTS, H. J. (1966) *Arch. Environ. Health*, **13**, 125.
ROSSANO, M., VUILLET, F. and OLLIVIER, H. (1964) *Annls. Méd.-lég* Crimin. Police Scient., **44**, 275.
SCHÄFFNER, M. (1965) *Dtsch. Z. ges. gerichtl. Med.*, **56**, 269.
SCHNEIDER, H., SCHONTAG, A. and KREMLING, G. (1962) *Arch. Kriminol*, **130**, 34.
SCHOLLMEYER, W. (1959) *Dtsch. Z. ges. gerichtl. Med.*, **49**, 213–17.
SCHRIDDE, H. and BECKMANN, A. (1924) *Virchow's Arch.*, **252**, 774–82.
SCHWERD, W. (1959) *Dtsch. Z. ges. gerichtl. Med.*, **49**, 218–23.
SELLIER, K. (1966) *Dtsch. Z. ges. gerichtl. Med.*, **57**, 161.
SESTIER, —. (1880) *Brit. med. J.* (1888) **2**, 242, annotation.
SILVERSIDES, J. (1964) *Canad. Med. Ass. J.*, **91**, 195.
SIMONIN, C. (1955) *Médicine Légale Judiciaire*, 3rd ed. Paris: Librairie Maloine.
SIMPSON, K. (1953) *Modern Trends in Forensic Medicine*, p. 62, London: Butterworths.
SKAN, D. A. (1949) *Brit. Med. J.*, i, 666.
SMITH, Sir SYDNEY and FIDDES, F. S. (1955) *Forensic Medicine*, 10th ed., p. 241. London: Churchill.
SPENCER, H. A. (1932) *Lightning; Lightning Stroke and its Treatment*. London: Baillière.
STRASSMANN, G. (1933) *Dtsch. Z. ges. gerichtl. Med.*, **20**, 239–59; abstr. *Méd.-lég. Rev.*, **1**, 221–2.
TABBARA, W. (1962) *Annls Méd.-lég. Crimin. Police Scient.*, **42**, 340.
TAYLOR, A. S. (1948) *Principles and Practice of Medical Jurisprudence*, 10th ed., p. 471, ed. Sydney Smith. London: Churchill.
TAYLOR, A. S. (1956) *Ibid.*, 11th ed., ed. Smith and Simpson, p. 415. London: Churchill.
TAYLOR, A. S. (1965) *Ibid.*, 12th ed., ed. K. Simpson, Vol. I, London: Churchill.
TIDY, C. M. (1882) *Legal Medicine*, vol. i, pp. 510 et seq. London: Smith Elder.
URQUHART, R. W. I. (1927) *J. Industr. Hyg.*, **9**, 140–66.
URQUHART, R. W. I. and NOBLE, E. C. (1929) *J. Industr. Hyg.*, **11**, 154–72.
WAGNER, C. F. and MCCANN, G. D. (1941) *Electr. Eng.* **60**, 374–384.
WEIMANN, W. and PROKOP, O. (1963) *Atlas der gerichtlichen Medizin*, Berlin: Volk und Gesundheit.
WHICHELLO, H. (1899) *Lancet*, i, 1490.
WOOD, J. L. (1965) *Med. Sci. Law*, **5**, 19.

CHAPTER 7

Thermal Injuries

I. The Ill-Effects of Heat

Heat Exhaustion: Heat Hyperpyrexia

Exposure to excessive heat, whether it be that of the sun or in an enclosed place such as the engine room of a ship, can cause severe symptoms and signs which were formerly designated "sunstroke". It was realised, however, following investigations by Morton (1931–2), Ladell *et al.* (1944) and others, that the effects of excessive heat present in one of two quite distinct forms, namely, "heat exhaustion" and "heat hyperpyrexia". The former is a result of salt-depletion and dehydration, whereas the latter is due to a temporary failure of the heat-regulating mechanism. A classification was given by the Medical Research Council in 1958. The clinical features of each were studied by Ladell *et al.* in healthy soldiers, while serving in the African desert during the summer of 1943.

Heat exhaustion claimed its victims during the first half of the summer. Its manifestations were due to salt-deficiency and dehydration, which were promptly relieved by replacement of salt and water. Severe cases were treated with intravenous saline with excellent results. The patients were those who normally excreted much chloride in their sweat and whose salt intake was inadequate to counter excessive excretion. The symptoms included vomiting, cramps and profuse sweating. The pulse pressure and, possibly, the blood pressure were reduced. In consequence, the men were liable to faint and fall when standing. Their plasma and whole-blood content of chloride was grossly reduced, the haemoglobin and plasma protein content was raised and the blood urea content was very high; extracellular fluid and plasma volumes were diminished. Urine was scanty, of high specific gravity and almost devoid of chloride. The body temperature is normal or only slightly raised. Infection, especially of the gastro-intestinal tract, is frequently a precipitating factor.

Cases of heat exhaustion are unusual in this country; the occasional victims of heat exhaustion are usually elderly persons. In June 1950, for example, a man aged 80 and a woman aged 70 collapsed in the street and were dead on arrival at hospital; another man aged 78 collapsed and was detained in hospital. The temperature at that time was between 86° and 88°F; in one sweet factory it was so hot that the chocolate would not set and the girls had to be sent home; a sea breeze at an East coast resort kept the temperature down only to 76°F (*Manchester Guardian*, 6 June 1950).

Heat hyperpyrexia was observed in the second half of the summer. These patients suffered from a breakdown in their defence mechanism against heat. They were cured by transfer for a few days to cooler conditions. They sweated little but had polyuria; prickly heat was more or less severe; there was no vomiting, cramps nor any cardio-vascular changes. Although there was some salt deficiency it was not as severe as in the first type and these patients were not dehydrated. During convalescence their sweat had a high salt content. The essential diagnostic sign is hyperpyrexia; the body temperature tends to rise to that of its surroundings and attains 107°F, or over. When a level of 108°F is maintained, even for a short time, death will occur. At necropsy petechial haemorrhages are then present in the viscera. As with type 1, minor infections favour the development of heat hyperpyrexia and they must be recognised and treated.

The pathology of deaths due to acute heat stroke was described by Chao *et al.* (1981). Ten subjects studied were young men aged between 18 and 29 years who collapsed during prolonged physical exercise, death occurring up to 99 hours later. All had died from disseminated intravascular coagulation. The most striking autopsy finding was large areas of pulmonary haemorrhage. Their brains were congested and oedematous and there were petechial haemorrhages in the white matter. Haemorrhages were found elsewhere in several of the bodies, for example in the stomach and intestines, the myocardium, renal pelvis and adrenals. Microscopically there were microthrombi in small blood vessels of many organs, with small foci of necrosis of parenchymal cells.

When hyperpyrexia was due to the combined effects of high environmental temperature and excessive intake of amphetamines the autopsy revealed excessive congestion of organs, especially brain and lungs, with microscopical evidence of haemorrhages into the sub-pial space, and into the atrioventricular bundle and branches, as well as elsewhere in the myocardium (F.M. 14,082 A).

Other drugs which may be associated with hyperpyrexia, in addition to amphetamines, are D.N.O.C., and atropine. The possibility of heat hyperpyrexia occurring in operating theatres must not be overlooked. This may be due simply to high ambient temperature and humidity in the theatre as described by Harris and Hutton (1956). One of their cases became affected 2 days after operation. More often, these days, the condition is likely to be that of malignant hyperthermia. This is a relatively new medical syndrome, first reported in 1966, which is associated with, and possibly caused by, general anaesthesia induced with halothane in conjunction with suxamethonium.

It is characterised by a rapid rise of temperature and signs of increased muscle metabolism, e.g. tachycardia, tachypnoea, sweating and a blotchy cyanosis. The one distinctive sign appears to be rigidity immediately after the administration of suxa-methonium, as seen in the majority of patients, but it can develop insidiously during halothane anaesthesia. In about one fourth of the patients rigidity does not develop at any stage until after death. This condition is discussed in more detail in Chapter 19, in connection with anaesthetic deaths.

Overheated Cots

Heat hyperpyrexia may occur if an infant be kept in an overheated cot. A child aged 6 weeks, of poor physique, had been left alone in its cot, heated by an electric blanket which could attain a temperature of about 54°C (129°F), for a period of about 3 hours. This temperature was too low to burn the skin, but it could cause heat hyperpyrexia if the heat-regulating mechanism was inefficient, as in an infant of this age and of poor physique. The child had been covered by an eiderdown and wore woollen nightclothes. Although this may have been the cause of death in this case, the evidence was conflicting. The doctor, who saw the child 2 hours after it was found ill in its cot, had found the child's temperature to have been normal. Moreover, death occurred within 12 hours. On balance it was decided, after a canvass of opinion of a group of experts, that this death was due to a fulminating, unspecified infection. The fact remains that it is distinctly dangerous to leave a small infant alone in a heated cot, lying on an electric blanket (F.M.6882A).

Burns

The term "burn" is applied more often in lay than in medical circles, to a variety of conditions, of which the local effects of dry heat are the commonest example. There are, however, differences in the circumstances and in the resulting destruction of tissue, which call for a separate account of the several kinds of "burns". The term "burn" is here restricted to the local effects of dry heat.

Burns Due to Dry Heat

Destruction of tissue by the application of dry heat, producing a burn, is usually the result of contact with a naked flame or the heated elements of an electric fire. It can also follow contact with hot metal or glass, a risk which is often apparent only after the accident, since these substances can be at a dangerous temperature although outwardly they appear to be cool or cold.

The worst burns in domestic circumstances—unfortunately they are still all too common—follow the ignition of clothing which has come into contact with a coal gas or electric fire or an oil stove. These are true tragedies because the loss of life or the serious disability, which may be lifelong, arising out of these accidents need not occur. There is also the further and serious problem of the occupation of hospital beds, often for long periods, by many of these unfortunate persons. The histories of these accidents show only too often that simple precautions or the exercise of a little forethought would have prevented them.

Failure to protect an open fire in a room where young children are at play, an obvious danger, is the subject of specific legislation, but its good intentions are nullified because proceedings cannot usually be instituted until injury or death of a child reveals a failure to observe the law. Even were it desirable, it is impracticable to inspect every household where there are children, to ensure that guards are used to protect fires. It is enacted, under s. 11 of the Children and Young Persons Act, 1933, and under s. 8 of the Children and Young Persons (Amendment) Act, 1952, that

> If any person who has attained the age of 16 years, having the custody, charge or care of any child under the age of 12 years, allows the child to be in any room containing an open fire grate or any heating appliance liable to cause injury to a person by contact therewith not sufficiently protected to guard against the risk of his being burnt or scalded without taking reasonable precautions against that risk, and by reason thereof the child is killed or suffers serious injury, he shall on summary conviction be liable to a fine not exceeding 10 pounds: Provided that neither this section, nor any proceeding taken thereunder, shall affect any liability of any such person to be proceeded against by indictment for any indictable offence.

Gas and electric fires of old pattern are a grave potential danger since the fuel or elements are not protected in a manner which prevents contact with clothing. It is now illegal to manufacture and to sell domestic gas, electric or oil stoves unless they are fitted with adequate guards. The Heating Appliances (Fireguards) Regulations, 1953, S.I., 1953, No. 526, made under s. 5 of the Heating Appliances (Fireguards) Act, 1952, require that . . . "any heating appliance of a type which is so designed that it is suitable for use in a dwelling house or other residential premises . . . shall be fitted with a guard which shall be robustly made . . . and the guard shall be so constructed that the guard when in use with the appliance shall be securely attached thereto". The schedule to the regulations describes the required standard of construction and fitting. The regulations apply to gas fires, electric fires and oil stoves, which, without a guard, create a risk of injury by burning. The regulations apply to all appliances manufactured after the coming into operation of the regulations.

Legislation to compel manufacturers to render fabrics used to make garments fire resisting has now been introduced in part. Regulations under the Consumer Protection Act (1980) Regulations, The Nightdresses (Safety) Regulations 1967, have now been introduced. These make it illegal to sell children's nightdresses unless they are in accordance with certain specifications or are marked as inflammable.

The Appearances of Burns

The appearances of burns can range within wide limits, depending, in the main, upon the intensity of the source of heat responsible and the duration of contact. Burns due to the ignition of clothing are less severe over the parts where the garments are tightly applied to the body.

The range of damage is from a negligible but acutely painful reddening of the skin, which resolves completely in a day or so, to gross incineration not only of the soft parts but also of bone. Six degrees of burns were recognised by Dupuytren but they were merged into three principal groups by Hebra, whose classification is now adopted.

Burns of First Degree (first and second degrees, Dupuytren)

Any burn which can resolve without leaving a scar belongs to the first degree. The changes, as already indicated, may be limited to reddening of the affected part. Commonly, the injury results in a blister which is covered by whitened, avascular epidermis and bordered by reddened, hyperaemic skin. Small blisters, e.g. not exceeding $^1/_2$ in. in diameter, may resolve by absorption of fluid but the raised epidermis is later shed and replaced by new growth from the periphery of the burn; large blisters may require evacuation. All burns of the first degree are distinctly painful but relief usually follows the application of cold dressings.

The blisters may become infected but, since the true skin is not injured, repair of all first degree burns is normally complete without scar formation.

When small, burns of the first degree are little more than a nuisance, although their site may interfere with full use of part of a limb. When they cover over one-third of the body surface, and more especially when the burns involve the head and neck, trunk, or the anterior abdominal wall, the patient's condition is always grave. It is generally held that involvement of a third or one-half of the body surface will prove fatal even when the burns are only of the first degree.

When situated on a hairy part of the body burns, unlike scalds, are accompanied by singeing of the hair.

Burns of Second Degree (*third and fourth degrees, Dupuytren*)

Burns of the second degree always heal with scar formation because the true skin is damaged. Contraction of the scar tissue, moreover, may produce disfigurement or impaired function, according to the site and size of the burn.

These burns present as shrivelled, depressed areas of coagulated tissue, bordered by reddened, blistered skin. In the course of a few days, usually within a week, the necrotic tissue separates to leave an ulcer which, in turn, heals slowly. Natural repair by scar tissue may often require correction by plastic surgery.

For the rest, the features are those of burns of first degree, except that pain and shock are greater.

Burns of Third Degree (*fifth and sixth degrees, Dupuytren*)

The burns are characterised by gross destruction not only of the skin and subcutaneous tissues but also of muscle and even bone. Destruction of nerve endings also occurs and this accounts for the relatively painless character of these burns. Devitalisation of tissues in the burnt area renders them prone to infection and slow to repair. There is also danger from shock, the onset of which is usually delayed for from 1 to 3 days. Until this period is past the prognosis is uncertain since the patient may pass into coma and die.

The assessment of the degree of a burn is made by reference to the area most severely damaged rather than to the over-all appearance of the burn. As already indicated, it is the extent of burning rather than the degree of the burn which determines the probable outcome. A third degree burn of an arm or leg, although it may result in grave disability, is unlikely to prove fatal, whereas burns of first degree involving one third or more of the body are always dangerous to life.

In most cases burns are caused by brief exposure to intense heat, such as a flame, or red hot object. However it should be remembered that for a burn of a given extent, the intensity of the heat is related to the duration of the exposure. Thus even temperatures as low as $44°C$ can produce burns if applied to the body for a period of several hours (Moritz and Henriques, 1947).

The Medico-Legal Aspect of Burns

The forensic pathologist is normally concerned only with fatalities due to burns or with circumstances in which bodies are recovered from burning buildings.

It is necessary first to determine whether the burns were received before or after death. If ante-mortem in origin, it must be determined whether the burns were of themselves the cause of death. There are also circumstances where disease (the primary cause of death) has led to collapse and unconsciousness and caused the victim to fall into a fire or against an electric stove. It is then necessary to determine whether the burns accelerated the death.

It is particularly important to ascertain the cause of death in circumstances where the burns are sustained after death, and the body has been recovered from the scene of fire, in a house or a motor-car, because there is always the possibility that death was due to violence followed by an attempt to conceal the crime by arson.

The clothing as well as the body of the victim should be examined. This task is more properly to be performed by the police or the forensic scientist but, whenever practicable, the medical examiner should make his own observations. The distribution of the burns on the clothing may throw light upon the manner in which it was ignited, the posture of the victim at the time, the path taken by the flames, and it may be possible, as in *R. v. Rouse* (see p. 337), to discover that unburnt cloth was still saturated with some inflammable material.

It must not be forgotten that burns may represent injuries inflicted on the victim by an assailant just as much as bruises or abrasions caused by a blunt object. Where such a deliberately inflicted burn has a particular pattern, it may indicate the shape of the object causing it; this is particularly relevant to the examination of a suspected "battered baby". Small rounded burns may be caused by the application of a lighted cigarette to the child's body. Professor Usher has described a case where the clear imprint of a knife blade was left as a burn on a child's body. We have seen burns on a child's buttocks caused by holding him on to the lid of a hot stove.

With the increasing number of reports of cases of torture from various parts of the world, instances of burns of the body surface are reported frequently as consequences of this practice. Examples have been described by Professor Marshall in Northern Ireland, of victims of the I.R.A.

Deaths in Burning Buildings

Although many of the victims of a conflagration die of burns, some of them are killed by falling masonry, timber or machinery. There are others who die of injuries sustained by a fall when a vain attempt has been made to escape from the fire by jumping from a window. Not rarely a victim may have been overcome by fumes, which usually contain carbon dioxide and carbon monoxide, produced by the incomplete combustion of wood or paint, etc. In consequence, the victim's collapse prevents his escape from the fire or, on some occasions, inhalation of fumes may cause death from carbon monoxide poisoning. The examination of bodies recovered from a burning building should always include an estimation of the carbon monoxide content of the victim's blood. Its presence in the blood, together with soot in the air passages which are usually acutely engorged, constitutes proof that the victim was alive at the time of the fire and, usually, that the death was due to the fire (Plate 5). In this manner it is possible to explain deaths which occur in a fire when no burns or other signs of violence are found on the body and there is no evidence of natural disease. In these circumstances it is usual to find that the blood of adult victims, especially the elderly, is about half-saturated with carbon monoxide; the results range from case to case between 30 and 80 per cent. Although other factors, for example shock, may play a part, this degree of saturation in an elderly person is of itself capable of causing death. Three elderly persons were dead when removed from burning premises in Leeds during April 1954. None was burnt or injured and all the victims were healthy. Examination of blood samples demonstrated saturation by 45 per cent in each victim and it was concluded that these deaths were due to carbon monoxide poisoning following the inhalation of the fumes. There was also soot in the air passages of each victim (F.M. 3583–5).

When children die in a fire from this cause it is to be expected that a higher saturation is necessary to kill, and this does occur. After the body of a baby had been recovered from a burning house, no trace of violence or disease was found at the necropsy. Its blood, however, was saturated to 80 per cent with carbon monoxide (F.M. 2390). In all eight of those who lost their lives in a mill-fire at Keighley, the blood was saturated to 75–80 per cent.

The fumes and smoke in a conflagration may contain cyanide. Although its concentration in the blood of victims is usually too low to have played a significant part as a cause of death, it must sometimes be a contributing factor. This occurred when a prisoner barricaded himself in his cell and set fire to his polyurethane mattress. The cyanide concentration of his blood was 295 μg per 100 ml (F.M. 27334).

Studies of the various gases inhaled in fires and their contribution to death has been carried out (Anderson and Harland 1980).

Hyperglycaemia in relation to burns was reported by Bailey (1960); four cases are recorded.

Belt (1939) found zonal liver necrosis in persons who had died of burns. It has long been held that acute duodenal ulceration may be found in these victims.

Although shock due to extensive burns is the usual cause of death, delayed death may be due to inflammation of the respiratory tract caused by the inhalation of smoke. Cox *et al.* (1955) recorded the deaths of thirteen infants in a fire at a maternity home; twelve died of bronchopneumonia within 3 days of the fire. Severe damage, at least to the extent of blistering of the tongue and upper respiratory tract, can follow the inhalation of smoke (Plate 5).

Other causes of death may be congestive atelectasis of the lungs, renal failure, and septicaemia (Sevitt, 1966). Pulmonary fat embolism has been reported in cases of death due to burns.

Ante-mortem Burns

Burns which are produced during life exhibit a vital reaction, which, even in its early stages, is recognisable by reddening or hyperaemia of the part. This is seen in the tissues in the floor and at the periphery of blisters. Doubt about the gross appearances is resolved by microscopical examination of tissue from the burn and the sample should include intact skin beyond its margin. Congestion of vessels, possibly small haemorrhages, and, more especially, an infiltration of polymorphonuclear leucocytes into the tissues and into blister fluid will not be found in burns sustained after death.

Mallik (1970) described conventional histological and also histochemical methods applied to burns, both in experimental animals and in human tissues. Similar results with enzyme histochemical techniques were obtained to those found when ordinary wounds were examined by these methods (see page 143).

Blister fluid should be collected for chemical and microscopical examination. If produced during life it will be rich in protein even to the extent of becoming solid on heating; polymorphonuclear leucocytes may be present even when there has been no infection of the burn.

Post-mortem Burns

Burns caused after death are never reddened by vital reaction; they are hard and yellowish in colour. Blisters may form after death but the fluid in them contains scanty albumen, yielding at best only a faint opalescence with heating or chemical test; polymorphonuclear leucocytes are absent, or scanty.

Blisters due to putrefaction, when they contain blood-stained watery fluid, are accompanied by an abundance of putrefactive changes elsewhere.

Distinction may also have to be made between blisters due to heat and those due to disease. This will be practicable, for example, by considering the size and distribution of the blisters and the presence or absence of other signs of burning.

Heat Ruptures

Heat ruptures occur when the body is exposed either before or after death to considerable heat. They are produced by a splitting of the soft parts, as by cooking (Fig. 5). These ruptures may be of considerable length, up to several inches, and superficially they may resemble lacerations or, at times, incised wounds. In view of the possibility that an attempt has been made to dispose by fire of the body of a victim of wounds care is necessary in the interpretation of these changes.

A distinction between heat ruptures and incised wounds is often simple. There is no bleeding in heat ruptures since heat coagulates the blood in the vessels. This is less important than the demonstration of intact vessels and nerves in the floor of the heat rupture; these structures are exposed and run across, or in the long axis of, the rupture. On close inspection its margins are not clean-cut but are irregular.

Distinction from lacerations is made by the absence of bruising or other sign of vital reaction in the margins of the heat rupture. Microscopical examination can usually establish the distinction beyond doubt.

Confusion may exist for a time if the heat rupture involves the scalp. In *R.* v. *Rouse* (see p. 337) the scalp of the victim presented appearances which resembled those of a laceration, and the prosecution submitted that the victim had been stunned with a mallet before his body was set on fire. The medical evidence, however, leaves no doubt that this was a heat rupture.

Post-mortem changes caused by heat include rupture of the skull, with herniation of the brain, as in *R.* v. *Rouse*. On occasion an extra-dural "haematoma" with or without rupture of the skull may be present.

"Heat Haematoma"

This condition has the appearance of an extra-dural haemorrhage, but it is unaccompanied by any signs of injury by blunt force. It occurs only in circumstances where the head has been exposed to intense heat, sufficient to cause charring of the skull. The appearances are characteristic and, once seen, there should be no difficulty in recognising them on a future occasion. Difficulty, if any, is only likely to arise if the victim of a fire had been struck on the head by a falling beam or masonry, or the death had been due to a head injury and there had been an attempt to conceal homicide by arson; heat rupture is unlikely to cause confusion.

The blood in the haematoma is converted into a soft, friable clot of light chocolate colour, to which there may be added a pink tint, if the victim's blood was appreciably saturated with carbon monoxide. The clot is not uniformly solid, but presents a honeycomb appearance; the spaces had been occupied by bubbles of steam produced when the blood was boiled by the external heat. The thickness of the clot varies from about 1.5 mm ($^1/_{16}$ in.) up to 1.5 cm ($^5/_8$ in.) and the volume of blood represented by the clot can be up to about 120 ml (4 oz).

The distribution of the clot follows closely the distribution of the charring of the outer table of the skull. In some cases, therefore, it is maximal in relation to the frontal lobes, but in others it lies elsewhere. In one of our cases it had an hour-glass shape, lying over the upper surface of both hemispheres (Fig. 113); charring of the skull had a similar distribution (F.M. 4655J).

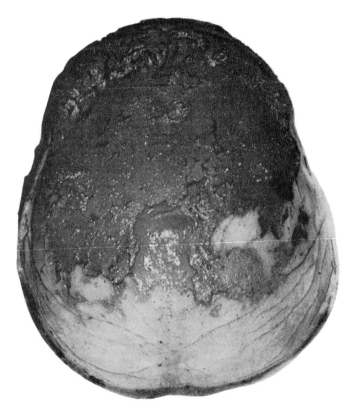

FIG. 113. "Heat haematoma": as seen within the frontal of the calvarium. Coagulated blood in the extra-dural space.

The mechanism of its development is obscure. Presumably there must still be circulation of the blood in order to permit the accumulation of up to 4 oz of blood in the extra-dural space. This quantity could scarcely be driven from the skull into the space by heat after death. It is not derived from the brain or meninges; the latter are intact; there is no evidence of obvious rupture of the superior longitudinal sinus, but this is a possible source.

For the comfort of surviving relatives, it may be presumed a post-mortem change; it is only likely to occur when the victim is already unconscious, either because of poisoning by carbon monoxide or shock due to severe burns.

I can offer no explanation, but I have no doubt that it is a phenomenon peculiar to exposure of the head to intense heat, normally in the circumstances of a conflagration.

In February 1956, with Dr. T. K. Marshall, C.P. had an opportunity to observe this phenomenon when seven women and one man lost their lives in a fire at a woollen mill near Keighley (F.M. 4655c–4655j). The heads of seven of these victims were severely charred and a heat haematoma was present in six of them. It is not an invariable finding; it was also absent in the head of a man who died from burns, when covered by a heap of blazing hay (F.M. 749).

The above description of heat haematoma is based on our findings in the Keighley victims. All eight had carbon monoxide poisoning; their blood had been saturated by 75 per cent or over by carbon monoxide. The part played by burning, although severe, was of secondary importance; much of it had occurred after death. The distribution of the clot and charring of the skull, especially in two cases (F.M. 4655d and 4655j), was similar. In one case (F.M. 4655d) the bilateral, frontal haematoma was up to 1.6 cm thick, directly behind the forehead, and the amount of clot present represented at least 4 oz (118 ml) of blood (Fig. 113). A cast of paraffin wax, made to reproduce the haematoma, required over 4 oz of molten wax.

Heat Contractures

The posture of a body which has been exposed to fire is often characteristic and the so-called "pugilistic attitude" is a well-known feature of the effects of heat. Coagulation of muscles often occurs and they contract, the flexor muscles more than the extensors, and, in consequence, the limbs, the arms in particular, are fixed in an attitude commonly adopted by boxers (Fig. 5). It is evidence only of exposure of a body to considerable heat because it occurs irrespective of life or death at the time of exposure.

The simulation of a strangulation mark may be observed on the body of a person who has sustained burns, when the skin of the neck is (imperfectly) protected by clothing. When a man aged 87 collapsed and died as the result of rupture of the heart, due to myocardial infarction, he fell against a gas fire and his clothing caught fire. The autopsy (by the late Dr. William Goldie) demonstrated, in addition to the disease of the heart, extensive burns of the body. A band of intact skin, $^1/_2$ in. to 1 in. broad, remained on the right side of the neck (Fig. 114; Leeds City Coroner, No. 839/50). In this case there was no question of strangulation, but the appearances of the neck resemble those depicted by Sir Sydney Smith and Dr. Fiddes (1955). In their case an attempt had been made to conceal murder by strangulation by arson.

SCALDS

The term "scald" is applied to tissue destruction by moist heat and is distinguished from a burn by the absence of singeing and, usually, by the distribution of the injuries, which, when due to scalds, are normally restricted to exposed parts of the body. It is possible, of course, for scalds to affect parts covered by clothing but usually the fluid or steam is cooled by passage through the clothing before it reaches the skin. Scalds often have a distribution which is consistent with splashing of the injured parts.

Scalds are commonly produced by boiling water, but water at a temperature above 50°C (120°F), is capable of scalding the face and other vulnerable parts (Plate 6). Steam when inhaled will scald the throat and air passages; the subsequent inflammatory reaction, especially in children in whom the airway is narrow, may lead to severe obstruction and its rapid development may call urgently for relief by tracheotomy.

Oils and molten metal also produce scalds. The absence of steam, smoke or other signs of boiling, when the substances are still at a temperature well above that of boiling water, creates special danger. A child may readily appreciate when water is dangerous but, in the absence of the usual warning signs, it can come to harm with hot oil, e.g. in the frying-pan or bowl of dripping. Adults would do well to remember that the outside of the bowl may be greasy and this can lead to a serious accident.

The appearances of a scald are not unlike those of a burn of first degree, except that when a hairy part is involved there is no singeing of the hairs. Coagulation and carbonisation of tissue, seen in second and third degree burns, do not follow scalding.

Scalding of the skin may be simulated by toxic epidermal necrolysis (Lyall, 1956), but it

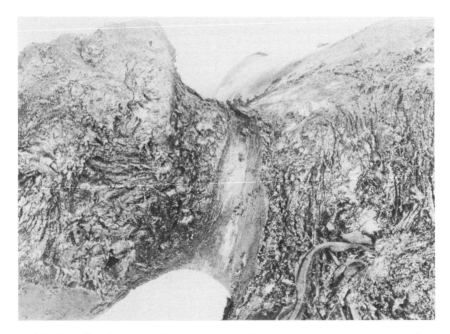

Fig. 114. "Pseudo-strangulation by a ligature." From a case of severe burns, at side of neck band of shirt (cf. the case of Smith and Fiddes in *Forensic Medicine*, 1955, 10th ed., Fig. 115. A case of attempted concealment of murder by arson.)

is doubtful that this skin condition will create any real medico-legal problem. It is a possibility which should be in mind, as suggested by Catto (1959), but an investigation of the circumstances should suffice to demonstrate or exclude scalding as the cause of the blisters. Moreover, Catto said that the syndrome of epidermal necrolysis is "well-defined, so that the diagnosis is fairly suggestive". The difficulty in differential diagnosis is much more likely to lie between it and other skin diseases or a drug eruption and not as between it and scalding. The danger of scalds lies in their superficial extent and situation.

The majority of scalds are the result of accidents. Suicide by scalding is rare and only the insane are to be expected to choose this mode. Donalies (1942) described a case of self-immersion in a soup cauldron, after attempted suicide by hatchet blows.

Boiling water may be thrown with intent to injure; a woman may punish a husband's unfaithfulness by pouring boiling water over his genitalia, as in examples cited by Tidy (1882). Murder by scalding is rare and the assailant is then likely to be an adult and the victim a child.

In February 1954 a woman was convicted of the murder of her daughter aged $3^1/_2$ years by throwing scalding water over her. The mother was jealous of the child because of her husband's devotion to it. Although, in the opinion of the prison medical officer, the woman was not certifiable, she was mentally defective; she had received treatment for mental illness in 1952. Her defence was that she had turned on the hot-water tap to prepare a bath for the child who struggled and fell in the bath, going under the water. The prosecution submitted that she had thrown scalding water over the child, and one-third of the child's body had been scalded.

When a child dies as a result of scalds the pathologist is likely to be pressed for an opinion on whether the findings are consistent with accidental or homicidal circumstances. In our experience children who have been accidentally scalded have the injuries on the lower limbs and waist, with a relatively clear cut upper limit. The position of the child in the water can sometimes be reconstructed by positioning the dead body so that the various scalds all lie below a level corresponding to the water level. However, in a case of homicidal scalding in our practice, of two young children by their schizophrenic mother the injuries were distributed in a bizarre fashion. In one of the children the scalds reproduced the pattern of water trickling across the face and down the neck and splashing on to the legs (F.M. 8634A).

Electrical Burns

Damage by electrical current is described elsewhere (see Chapter 6). A clear distinction must be made between the changes due to contact with an electrical circuit, i.e. the electric mark, and burns produced by the flash which usually accompanies a short circuit, i.e. a thermal burn. The latter are essentially the same as burns produced by any naked flame and their severity is assessed as to first, second or third degree. Burns which follow contact with a high tension circuit are often of the third degree, as described, for example, by Aldrich (1943).

Ultraviolet Light Burns

The sun or a mercury vapour lamp can readily burn the exposed skin. Sunburn in mild degree is a common experience, and, no doubt, mild burns are not infrequent amongst those who, without proper knowledge of the treatment, use ultraviolet-light lamps in the home. The speed with which exposure to these lamps can produce a "burn" is best realised by those who have experienced them. A few seconds exposure of parts normally protected by clothing may be sufficient to produce widespread hyperaemia and a distinctly uncomfortable irritation, which, although it subsides within a few hours, is a memorable experience. Personal test has not passed beyond that stage but extensive burns can readily occur, especially when the person is of fair complexion. Members of a canoe party on the Danube discarded their shirts during one hot summer. A redheaded Scot, who was a member of the party, was severely sunburnt and developed a blister which involved almost the whole of his back.

Overdosage with ultraviolet light can sometimes lead to severe and persistent dermatitis. A man of 22 was accustomed to take a "sun" bath lasting for 10 minutes. By mischance he fell asleep on one occasion and was exposed for 1 hour and 10 minutes. This led to severe dermatitis (MacCormac and McCrea, 1925).

Radiation and X-ray Injuries

X-rays

Grave injuries which result from prolonged exposure to X-rays were sustained by some of the pioneers of radiology, of whom the late Dr. Leo Rowden was a notable exception. One of them lost most of the digits of both hands and others had to sacrifice a hand because an epithelioma had developed in an X-ray burn. In the early days of deep X-ray therapy, during the 1920s, some of the patients sustained severe burns. One patient, for example, lost an appreciable part of the anterior wall of his chest; the recollection of seeing the movements of his lung and heart through this opening which was about 6 by 4 in., is still a vivid one. Pigmentation and telangiectasis may follow irradiation (F.M. 6176).

X-ray burns, other than mild erythema, are rare today since improvements in equipment, notably in protective screens, and precautions taken by the operators of the instruments, have reduced risk. There is no room, however, for relaxation in the care which must be exercised when using this potentially dangerous but essential diagnostic and therapeutic aid.

It cannot be said that X-rays have been rendered entirely harmless to patients because a "late reaction" to exposure, although a rare event, may still occur. This reaction may not appear until months or even years have elapsed since the last exposure to X-rays. It presents as a blue discoloration of the subcutaneous tissue, not unlike a bruise. This is followed by extensive and deep sloughing of the tissues and by delayed healing; severe atrophy of the skin may thereafter be permanent. Its cause is unknown and there is no known means of preventing its occurrence (Scott, 1931).

Mishaps which arise out of the clinical use of X-rays are likely at present to result in actions for damages for negligence. The complexity of modern X-ray procedures demand that only those conversant with them should express opinions to guide the courts on these occasions. It is terribly easy for the laity and the inexpert to allege negligence where none exists. It is not for the pathologist, unless specially qualified to do so, to assess these matters.

Another form of radiation likely to cause tissue damage is the laser beam (light amplification by stimulated emission of radiation). This form of radiation is now widely used in industry, and in scientific laboratories. The greatest danger to those using it is to the eyes; severe retinal burns can be sustained.

Radio-active Substances

The effects of large doses of radiation to the body produce the condition of the acute radiation syndrome, described in detail by Blakely (1968), to which the reader is referred for further information. An initial prodromal illness, with nausea and vomiting, is followed by a latent interval, the duration of which varies according to the size of the dose of radiation received. This may then be succeeded by epilation, signs of damage to the haemopoietic system, with haemorrhages and infections, and sometimes acute gastro-intestinal disorder with diarrhoea and dehydration, due to destruction of the lining of the small intestine. If the dose is high and the central nervous system is affected, convulsions and coma may be followed rapidly by death.

Apart from epilation, high dosage of radiation to the skin may produce lesions resembling slowly developing burns, with erythema, blistering, or dermatitis, or ulceration with delayed healing and ill-formed scars.

The long-delayed effects of radiation, occurring sometimes after many years, are chiefly malignant growths of various organs, such as lung or liver, or of the haemopoietic tissues. Premature ageing, cataracts, infertility, or congenital abnormalities in offspring have also been described.

There is a very extensive literature on the pathological effects of radiation on individual organs, e.g. on the heart (Fajardo *et al.*, 1968), the liver (Reed and Cox, 1966), kidney (Madrazo *et al.*, 1969, 1970), etc.

Injury ("Burns") by Corrosive Poisons

Certain chemicals, notably concentrated acids and alkalis, can cause extensive destruction of the tissues and even momentary contact may produce an injury which is slow to heal and its repair may call for treatment by plastic surgery. Concentrated sulphuric acid is probably the most dangerous of these agents not only because of its properties but because of its wide use in industry and in laboratories. The group also includes hydrofluoric acid, certain phenols, phosphorus, bromine, methyl bromide, and strong solutions of hydrogen peroxide and potassium permanganate. Petrol if spilt on to the skin will also produce severe blistering; this may occasionally produce unusual findings in victims of road accidents.

INJURY BY CORROSIVE ACIDS

Each of the three common corrosive acids, sulphuric, nitric and hydrochloric acids, can produce severe "burns" of the skin and clothing. The inhalation of the fumes of nitric and hydrochloric acids is highly dangerous because even short exposure to these fumes may cause severe inflammation of the air passages and bronchopneumonia. Those who have to deal with accidents where a quantity of fuming acid has been spilt must be alive to this danger and take suitable precautions. Prompt dilution or neutralisation of the acid is imperative, but those who take these steps should guard their mouths and noses and must not remain in direct contact with the fumes for more than a few seconds.

Injuries produced by corrosive acids may be recognised by certain colour changes. Sulphuric acid will leave dirty red stains on dark fabrics and may also be recognised by the sticky wetness of the stain. Precious time is not to be lost by applying chemical tests to confirm its nature. The skin and mucosae are at first whitened but soon become brownish and later black, and the affected tissue, e.g. of the stomach, becomes a pultaceous, blackened mass.

Nitric acid combines with organic material, whether skin or fabric, to produce yellow discoloration due to the production of picric acid. There is no charring. Hydrochloric acid stains do not have any specific colour; the tissues are whitened at first and later black areas, due to the production of acid haematin, appear and the tissues are severely corroded.

Sulphuric Acid Injuries

Sulphuric acid injuries merit more detailed consideration because they are the most serious. An account of them, which should be consulted in the original, was given by Cashell *et al.* (1943–4). Copies of their illustrations ought to be prominently displayed wherever sulphuric acid is kept in bulk, i.e. in amounts exceeding half a litre.

Injury of the skin by the acid is almost immediate but because there is no pain, unless the acid involves the eye, it may escape notice or be disregarded; there is no blistering of the skin. The danger lies in the fact that the acid devitalises the tissues and this predisposes to infection. The injuries are penetrating and deformity, following repair by scar tissue, may be incapacitating. A notable feature of the injury, well illustrated by Cashell *et al.*, is the distinctive *magenta* colour of the damaged skin, ascribed by them to the production of acid haematin. The case in our practice was one of gross, extensive burns (Hainsworth's Case) sustained when the driver of a lorry loaded with carboys of acid was in collision. The man was splashed with acid from broken containers (F.M. 10,330c) (Polson and Tattersall, 1969).

Murder or attempted murder by the external application of corrosives is rare. Tidy (1882) cites the case of a woman who died at the end of 6 weeks from the effects of nitric acid poured into her ear while she slept. In another case, cited by Tidy, molten lead was poured into a child's ear when he was asleep.

Treatment

Immediate dilution and neutralisation of the acid is imperative. Water or a solution of sodium bicarbonate are remedies likely to be at hand. Skin injuries should also be treated by the application of magnesium oxide or carbonate in powder or paste. Eye injury calls for prompt and thorough irrigation with a solution of sodium bicarbonate.

Workers should be warned of the dangers of the acid and instructed in the correct handling of vessels containing it. They should also be urged to take immediate steps to obtain treatment when splashed by the acid.

Prevention of Accidents

The obvious treatment of all corrosive injuries is essentially preventive. Precautions are taken in industry to limit accidents but there is still room in some laboratories and warehouses for the introduction of better safeguards. The principal danger arises with the Winchester quart, or 2-litre, glass bottles, because there is a "fatal" attraction for carrying them by their necks. The majority in use contain distilled water, normal saline, glycerine or other innocuous fluids, though formaldehyde and ammonium hydrate are notable and common exceptions. It is only too easy to extend this handling of these vessels to those filled with concentrated acid. Some of the acid may have escaped on to the neck to make the outside of the bottle slippery and, moreover, bottles filled with sulphuric acid are heavy. The moment the bottle falls and breaks there is a potential disaster.

Another practice which, fortunately, is uncommon, caused one victim to sustain burns on the abdomen and limbs which will leave lifelong scars. She had to carry some Winchester quarts of sulphuric acid in a warehouse. To speed up the process, she took one in each arm and held a third between them in front of her body. The inevitable happened; the central bottle, followed by the others, slipped and all were broken.

Stocks of corrosives, and sulphuric acid in particular, should be set apart in a storeroom away from the normal traffic of a laboratory. I have seen half a dozen of these Winchester quarts kept for days on the floor of a laboratory close to the pathway frequently used by technicians. The maximum amount to be kept on any laboratory bench, unless there is some exceptional need and special precautions are taken, should not exceed half a litre. This amount, moreover, should be kept in a bottle which is designed to collect drips after it has been used. Replenishment of the bench bottles should be performed only by those who have received specific instruction in the precautions to be taken in the handling of acid in bulk.

INJURY BY CORROSIVE ALKALIS

Ammonia

Ammonia, even in strong solution, does not usually cause serious injury to the skin but it can "burn" the eye. Its ingestion causes grave damage of the digestive tract; it was a mode of suicide not rare in my experience. The prime danger of ammonia, however, lies in the inhalation of the fumes. Fortunately few are unable to smell them and most, therefore, receive adequate warning to leave the scene forthwith, but a head cold may render a person insensitive to ammonia.

On 12 July 1938 several employees at an icecream factory were severely burnt and one of the injured, a woman aged 25, died of her injuries. It appears the accident was primarily due to excessive pressure in a refrigerating plant, due to an error in its manipulation. The front of the machine was blown out and, in consequence of the explosion, ammonia gas was set free (*Daily Telegraph and Morning Post*, 22 July 1938).

The use, which appears to be increasing, of ammonia to throw into a victim's face during a robbery carries the obvious risk of permanent eye injury.

Caustic Soda Injuries

The widespread use of caustic soda in industry creates a risk of injury to the skin and eyes. Prompt treatment, or preferably, preventive measures, are essential since these injuries, especially of the cornea, may have serious consequences.

Terry (1943) urged that caustic soda used in industry should be in a closed system whereby the workers cannot come into contact with it. Leaking pipes and collections of waste soda on the ground should be forbidden. The eyes should be protected by well-fitting goggles and although they are not infallible the wearing of them should be compulsory.

In the event of splashing with caustic soda the skin should at once be drenched with an antidote and for this purpose he recommends a 5 per cent solution of ammonium chloride. This should be available in 5-gallon containers sited near danger points. He describes a suitable container, namely, an aspirator fitted above with a bung carrying a thistle funnel as an air inlet and, below, a large glass outlet. The outlet is fitted with a 6-ft length of rubber tubing controlled by a spring clip. This apparatus allows an abundance of antidote to be flooded at once over the clothing and skin when contaminated by alkali. It immediately arrests the action of caustic soda and greatly reduces the incidence of "burns". Even when a "burn" has occurred, further penetration by caustic will be prevented if the area is treated for up to $1/4$ hour in a current, not a bath, of the antidote. Thereafter, the treatment is that of a burn produced by heat. Terry emphasises that the treatment "must always be carried out by irrigation, never by immersion in a static solution or by compresses".

Treatment of injury to the eyes by caustic soda is urgent. Even when goggles are used it is not always possible to avert these accidents. Their effects will be minimised if a generous supply of antidote, in 8-oz bottles, is at hand. The bottles should be designed so that they flush the eye by gravity flow when inverted. Terry emphasises, however, that "any attempt to modify the bottle so that it may be used like a wash-bottle, by mouth blowing, must be forbidden. It may be injurious."

The urgency of eye-splash by caustic soda is such that there should be whistles provided so that an injured man may immediately summon aid. After flushing the eye with the contents of a full bottle of antidote, the victim is to be taken to the surgery so that continuous flushing with antidote may be continued for 5 minutes and, thereafter, with boric-saline, "for one hour by the clock". This treatment "is of supreme importance and must be started at once". It must precede the dispatch of the patient to hospital. If the treatment is strictly observed, not only is the eye saved but recovery is hastened and incapacity is reduced from weeks to days.

Since caustic soda is in fairly wide use in laboratories the possibility of accidents exists and those in charge are well advised if they maintain a solution of antidote on the benches and other places where caustic soda is handled. One experience of an accident causing a caustic burn of the eye is sufficient to impress anyone of the wisdom of this precaution. A Winchester quart of 40 per cent caustic soda was handled carelessly and a spot of fluid splashed into the technician's eye. Fortunately, immediate irrigation with plain water served to limit the damage to the loss of a little conjunctiva; complete healing followed in a couple of days. This was an exception, and a distinctly lucky exception.

The rationale of treatment with ammonium choride is based on the fact that this is a neutral salt, which, therefore, does not react with the body tissues. It reacts only with the caustic soda, to form sodium chloride, with the liberation of ammonia. Objection to weak acids, e.g. citric, acetic or hydrochloric acid, arises from the fact that these can react with the body tissues and may do so instead of combining with caustic soda. The older treatment with sodium bicarbonate aimed at the production of sodium carbonate which, in turn, was removed by irrigation.

The Circumstances of Burns

The circumstances in which the majority of burns occur are those of accident. It is usual to have abundant collateral evidence which excludes suicide or homicide. The victims may be predisposed to these accidents by the effects of drink or drugs, or bodily disease, e.g. epilepsy or coronary disease.

Suicide by burning is rare since most people, unless bereft of their senses, are well aware of the terrible pain which must follow this course. It was once the custom for a widow in India to cast herself upon the funeral pyre of her deceased husband, but "suttee" has been prohibited for many years. Suicides may throw themselves into vats of hot liquid or they may saturate their clothing with inflammable liquid, notably petrol or paraffin, and set themselves on fire.

Self-Immolation by Burning

The deceased, a man aged 21, was awakened with difficulty at about 7 a.m. on 7 January. He appeared to be semi-drugged. His parents pleaded with him to travel to Leeds by public transport and leave his car at home. They feared that in his condition he might have an accident. He refused the advice and left by car. At about 8.15 a.m. a car, identified as that of the deceased, was seen parked outside a house. A man, alone, sat in it with both his hands holding his head. His conduct aroused the suspicions of the householder, who made a mental note of the kind of car and its registration number when she left the house to go to her work. At 9.15 a.m. a man, identified as the deceased, called at a petrol station. He asked for two gallons of petrol in a can, saying that he wanted it for a friend whose wagon, nearby, had run out of petrol. He was supplied with two separate gallons and did not wait for the caps to be applied; he kept them in his hand and put the open cans on the passenger seat. When warned that the petrol might spill inside the car, he said, "Well, it does not matter". He paid for the petrol and drove away in the direction of Swinnow Lane. Two cans, of a kind resembling those supplied to him, were later recovered from the deceased's damaged car.

At 9.55 a.m. a woman walking along Swinnow Lane saw black smoke coming from a car parked on a piece of spare land. When she and a neighbour approached the car they saw it was ablaze inside. The heat was intense and they could not approach nearer than 3 yards. They could not see whether there was anyone inside the car. They went away to summon the fire brigade and the police. Before they left the car was blazing fiercely and they saw that the driver's door was open, but when first seen they thought the door had been closed. They now also saw that a man lay on the ground about 3 ft. from the car, with his clothing ablaze from waist to neck. He was alive and his body moved. By the time the police arrived the fire had been brought under control. The driver's door was open and a man lay on the ground about 1 yard from the car. He was taken to hospital and died at 4.30 p.m. Subsequently the police recovered two tins and two tin tops from the car. The man was identified by documents in his clothing. The distribution of the burns on his body tallied with that seen in air pilots taken from blazing aircraft. This indicated that he had been seated when the fire began. The maximum intensity of the burns was found on the thighs and lower abdomen and on the unprotected part of his neck; his face and hands were severely burnt. By contrast the front of the chest, buttocks and back were spared. It did not appear that he had poured petrol over his clothing, but he had set fire to the petrol in the car.

It appears he had had a number of jobs, in none of which had he stayed for long. In 1956 he had been in trouble for alleged acts of gross indecency. Prior to his appearance at the Assizes he had attempted suicide by taking an overdose of drugs. He was eventually convicted and put on probation for 3 years; it was a condition of the order that he received psychiatric treatment for anxiety neurosis. In 1958 he was admitted as a voluntary patient to a mental hospital, suffering from hysterical psychopathy. It transpired that he had made several attempts at suicide: by an overdose of tuinal, by drinking rust remover, by injecting himself with a drug and, on one occasion, by swallowing a large needle. While in the mental hospital he chewed the ends of the third and fourth fingers of each hand. He received treatment for this elsewhere and on his return he attempted suicide by swallowing the rotary cutter of an electric shaver; the foreign body was removed by operation. After this episode he was reclassified as a schizophrenic patient. He showed some improvement under insulin-coma therapy. He eventually discharged himself against medical advice on 28 September 1958.

In January 1960, after visiting the probation officer, he told his father that he had been advised to see his doctor. He received a prescription for two boxes of tranquillisers. That evening, after apologising to his parents for all the trouble he had caused them, he retired to bed, apparently in his normal health, at 10.30 p.m. Next day he was found gravely injured by burns, of which he died, beside his blazing car.

Death was due to shock, due to extensive burns. Since he had survived for several hours, it is not surprising carbon monoxide was not present in his blood. There was blistering of the larynx and his trachea and bronchi contained mucus freely mixed with soot. Verdict: Shock due to burns, self-inflicted while of unsound mind (F.M. 6893A).

In the past few years we have seen three cases of suicide by burning. In one the deceased had driven his van to the end of a cart track, syphoned petrol from the tank, and immolated himself inside the van (F.M. 17,528A). A second case was of a schizophrenic male who went into the bathroom of his parents' house in the night and set himself on fire (F.M. 18,302). The third youth committed suicide in the garden of his house in the early morning, after soaking himself in petrol (F.M. 18,574). We have not seen a case of suicide by burning in a woman; but the late Lester James described such a case, the victim setting herself on fire in a galvanised bath.

Homicide by burning or scalding is also rare. On the other hand homicide in some other form, whether by wounding, strangulation or shooting, may be followed not infrequently by an attempt to destroy the body by fire, as in *R. v. Rouse*.

Causing death by arson has become less rare in the past few years. We have seen several deaths in one West Riding town, where members of one ethnic group have died after their houses have been set on fire, usually by pouring petrol or paraffin through the letterbox and igniting it by members of another ethnic group. Recently (*R. v. Lee*, 1981) a youth was convicted of the manslaughter in Hull of 26 people, in the course of 10 years, by setting fire to their houses, or sometimes directly to them.

Disposal of Bodies by Fire

From time to time attempts are made, nearly always unsuccessfully, to conceal crime by disposal of the body by fire. Practical difficulties are of a kind which preclude success with adults since this step requires conditions rarely to be found except in a crematorium. The body of the victim of infanticide may be destroyed in the household fire but even then the calcined bones may remain (Leeds University Forensic Medicine Museum).

Webster was unable to destroy evidence of his victim's identity when he attempted to dispose of the body of Dr. Parkman in a laboratory furnace. As described elsewhere (see p. 70) the dentures of the victim were sufficiently preserved to establish his identity.

The commoner mode of disposal is by arson. The body is left in a house or garage and the criminal then sets the place on fire. The fire may be promptly extinguished and there is no certainty that it will effectively destroy the body. In practice, even in the nearly successful attempt by Rouse, who left his victim in a car which he set on fire, arson fails to destroy all evidence of the major crime. It was not possible to determine the precise cause of death of Rouse's victim since the neck structures were destroyed, but Sir Bernard

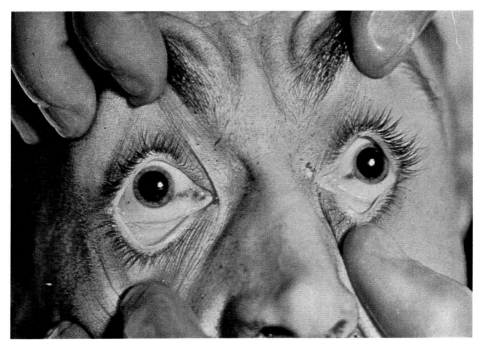

PLATE 1. Tache noire.

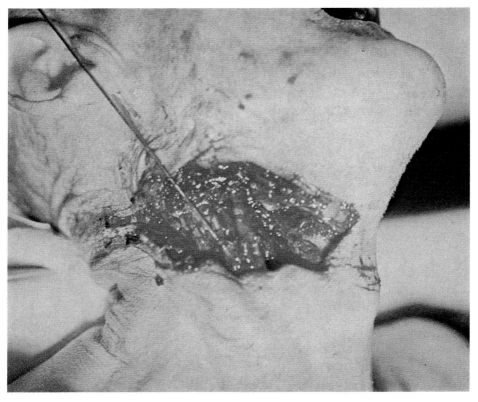

PLATE 2. Incised wound of neck (suicide).

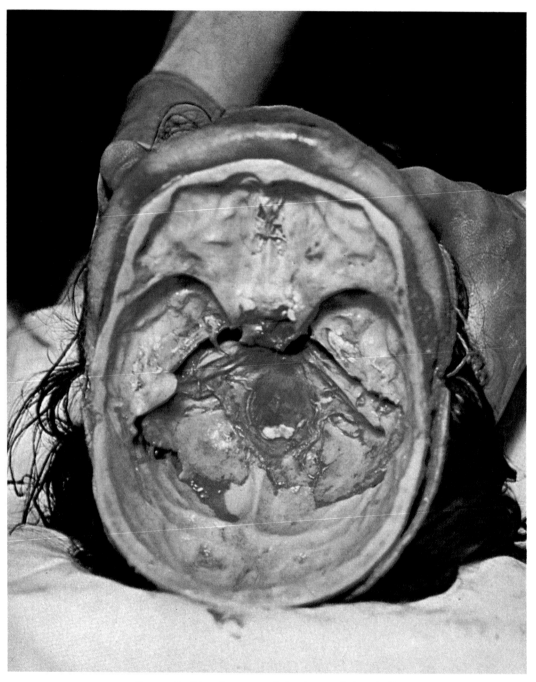

PLATE 3. Ring fracture of the base of the skull.

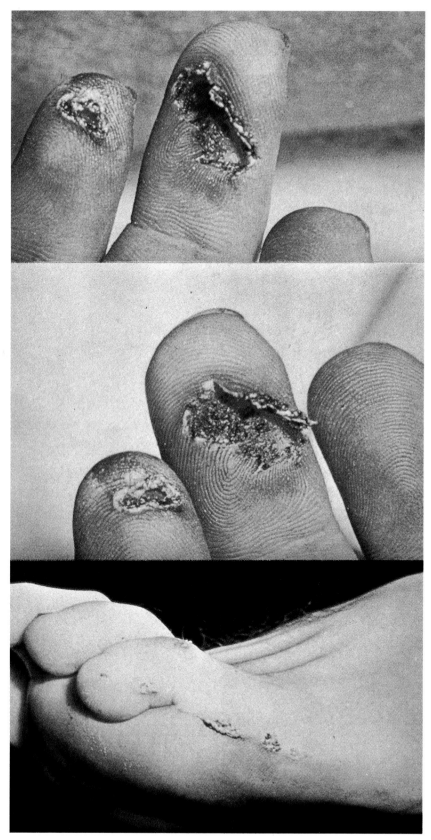

PLATE 4. Electrocution.

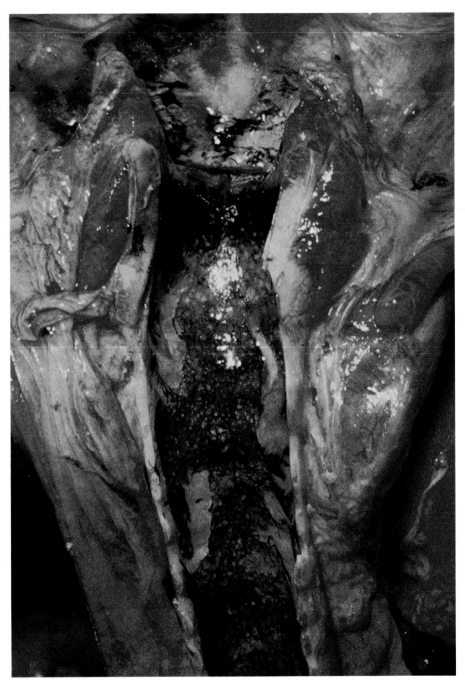

PLATE 5. Soot and mucus in the trachea after exposure to heat and
smoke in a fire.

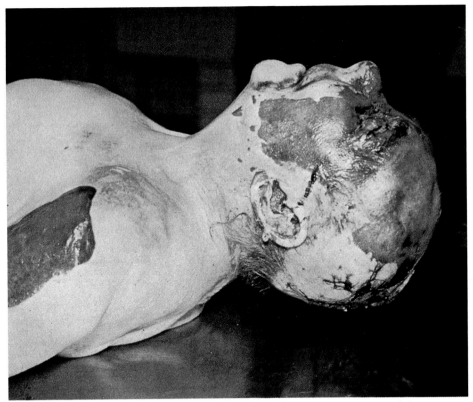

PLATE 6. Scalds and bruising. Victim killed by blows with a shovel; boiling water thrown over her in the course of the attack.

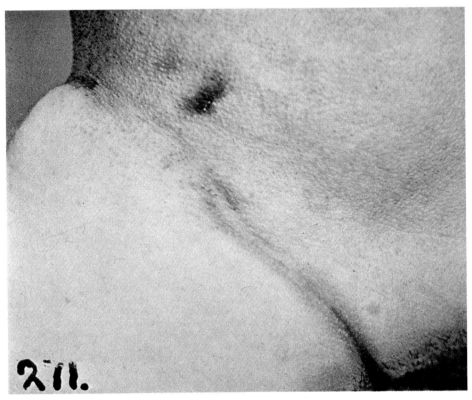

PLATE 7. Ligature mark; close view of the mark shown in Fig. 122 (at left side of neck).

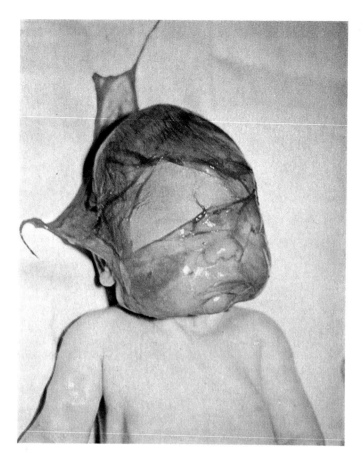

PLATE 8. Suffocation: born in a caul.

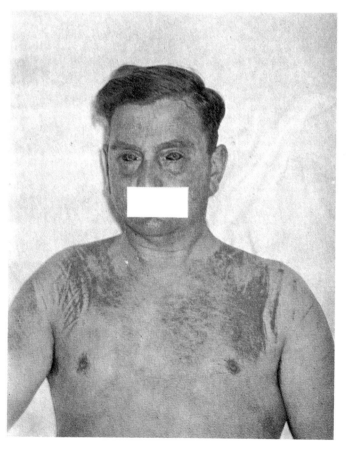

PLATE 9. Traumatic asphyxia.

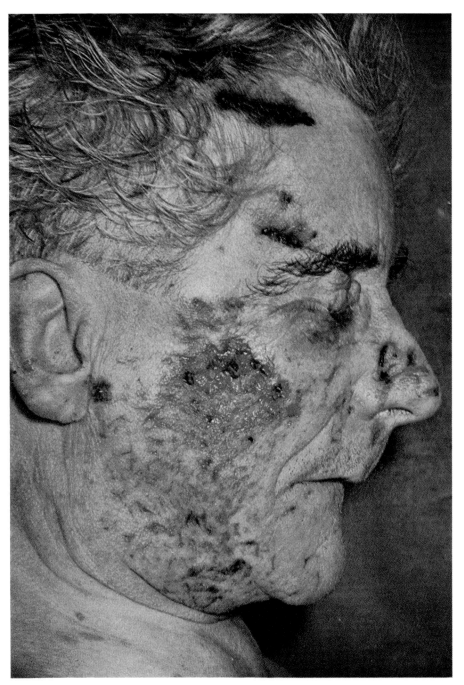

PLATE 10. Glass wounds.

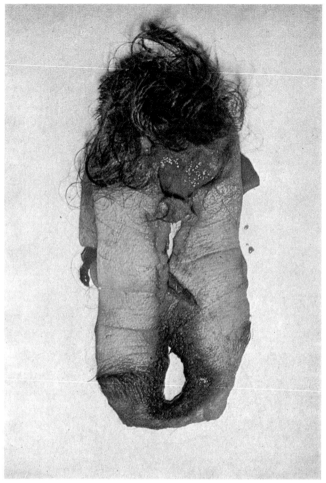

PLATES 11 and 12. Gunshot woun⟨

PLATE 11.

PLATE 12.

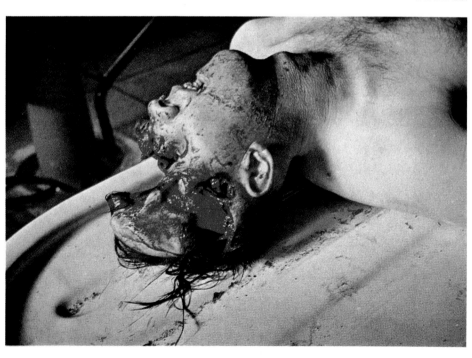

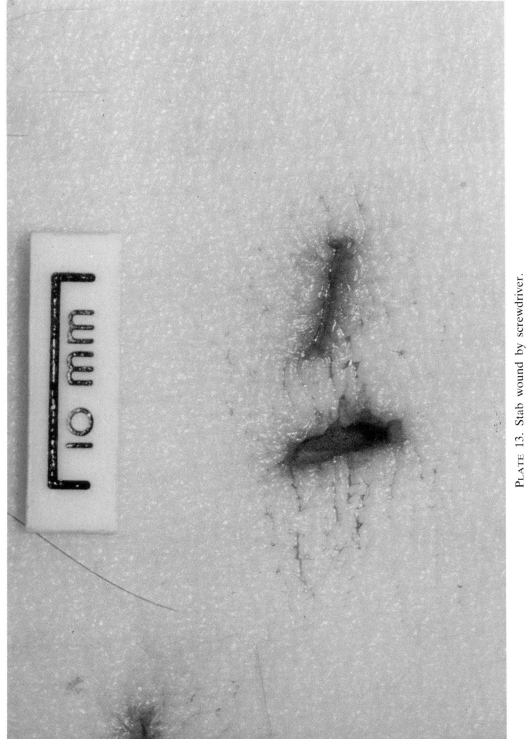

PLATE 13. Stab wound by screwdriver.

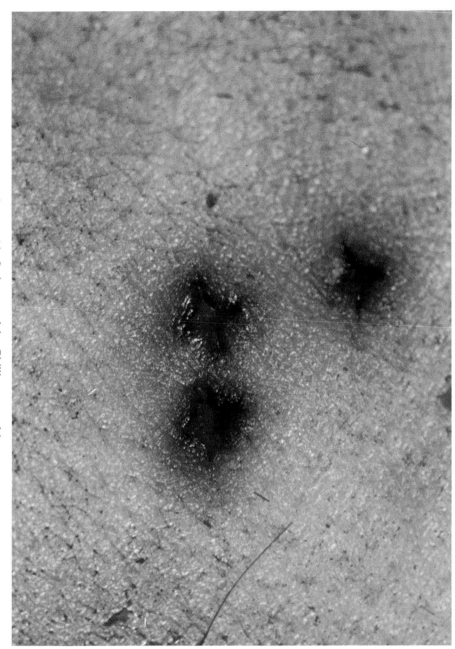

PLATE 14. Stab wound by Phillips screwdriver.

Spilsbury demonstrated soot in the air passages and carbon monoxide in the blood, and concluded that death was due to burns.

(This left open the question of how Rouse had been able to saturate his victim's clothing with petrol. It is probable that when the man was under the influence of drink he was throttled, but this was not disclosed until Rouse's confession was published after his execution).

R. v. Rouse

Two men, who were returning home from a dance in the early hours of 6 November 1930, noticed a fire in the distance. At that moment a hatless man, who appeared to have climbed out of a ditch, passed them; he seemed to be out of breath when he remarked "It looks as if somebody has got a bon-fire up there". They watched him for a time and noticed that he was uncertain of his direction; he hesitated and watched them run in the direction of the blaze. They found flames about 15 ft high coming from a motor-car. Unable to do anything at the scene they went to the village to call out the police officers. When the fire was partly extinguished, it was apparent that there was the body of a man in the car.

Rouse had planned that this body would be taken for his own. He had urgent need to be thought to have died in order to escape from the distinctly tangled circumstances in which he found himself. A man of limited means, he was responsible for the maintenance of a wife and two other women, by whom he had children; the birth of a second child to one of the women had occurred only a week before the crime. There was yet another woman who, at that time, was seriously ill during a pregnancy for which he was responsible. He had "married" her and on 6 November was due to take her to a house he had said he had bought for his bride. It did not exist and the girl's father and brother were calculated to create trouble when they discovered this deceit. Life had indeed become complicated for Rouse.

Although the police had no reason at first to believe the fire to have been other than an accident, they were anxious to trace the stranger who had been seen near the car that night. They saw Mrs. Rouse, who appears to have identified certain articles taken from the car; she thought they might have been his. The police no doubt received other information in the unpublished statement which she then made. Whatever it contained, the police were not long in realising that the body was not that of Rouse. He was traced to Hammersmith where he was detained at 9.20 p.m. on 7 November, when he arrived by bus from Wales. At the police station he was informed that the Northampton police wished to interview him. Rouse then said that, when in his car, he had picked up a strange man who was going to the Midlands. After they had travelled some distance, i.e. about 4 hours later, the engine began to spit and Rouse pulled up. He wanted to relieve himself and he told his passenger, meantime, to put some petrol, which was in a can in the car, into the tank. He showed the man what to do and left for a spot some distance away. He readjusted his trousers quickly and then ran to the car which he found in flames. He saw the stranger inside and tried to open the door but the flames repelled him. He lost his head and ran away to the place where he met two men. In due course, Rouse was charged with murder.

At the trial prosecution submitted that Rouse had stunned his victim with a mallet which was found some 14 yards in front of the car and had then poured petrol over him and set fire to the car. Evidence in support of this was slender. The mallet bore three hairs of which Sir Bernard Spilsbury said, "the longer piece . . . has the microscopic characteristics of a fragment of human hair . . . Of one of the other two, I am rather dubious as to whether it is human at all; but the other, which is a short fragment, may be human. That is as far as I think I can safely go." These three structures were embedded in mud on the mallet; there was no blood or any skin adhering to it.

The victim's skull was shattered but the appearances were entirely consistent with heat rupture; as Sir Bernard said, "That was due to bursting and splintering through the effects of heat, obviously". He had found no sign of any injury caused during life; the neck structures, however, had been destroyed by fire.

The evidence of stunning as the mode of overcoming the victim was negligible. Miss Helena Normanton (1931) drew attention to the difficulty of inflicting an effective blow with a mallet inside this small car; it would have had to have been delivered when he was at the road side. The man's bladder, however, contained half a pint of urine, an amount which is consistent with his having remained in the car during a journey which had lasted 4 hours, and until his death.

The cause of death was stated by Sir Bernard to be shock due to burns and the victim was "clearly alive" when the fire started. He had found that mucus from the air passages contained "large numbers of fine particles of carbon, such as would be deposited from smoke". Fluid lying free among the organs, a mixture of blood and water, was of bright colour. It contained carbon monoxide " . . . present in it in large amounts". But, Sir Bernard added, "I failed to find carbon monoxide in the other sample of blood" which he obtained from another part of the body. Sir Bernard explained this discrepancy on the ground that smoke from the fire "had not been inhaled for long because it had not had time to get into the blood in any appreciable amount, and that, therefore, the man had died shortly after the fire started". I find it difficult to believe that carbon monoxide which has been inhaled can be present "in large amounts" in one sample, a mixture of blood and water, but absent in a second from another part of the body. If the man had survived, as Sir Bernard believed, even about $^1/_2$ minute, it is possible, if not probable, that inhaled carbon monoxide would have been in both samples. The evidence that the man was alive at the time of the fire is accepted with hesitation.

The medical examiners were at a great disadvantage because the front portion of the neck was burned away. Had the neck structures been available they would probably have found that Rouse had throttled his victim. Had it been possible also to determine the alcohol content of the man's blood, it might have proved him to have been under the influence of drink; from time to time, throughout his last journey, which had lasted 4 hours, he had been sipping neat whisky, and in that event he could have been easily overpowered and throttled.

The only evidence of the precise course of events is Rouse's confession, which Miss Normanton assures us may be relied upon as authentic and substantially true. In it he said he had picked up this stranger, who during the journey "drank the whisky neat from the bottle and was getting quite fuzzled. . . . The man was half-dozing—the effect of whisky. I looked at him and then gripped him by the throat with my right hand. I pressed his head against the back of the seat. He slid down, his hat falling off. . . . He just gurgled. I pressed his throat hard. My grip is very strong. . . . He did not resist. It was all very sudden. The man did not realise what was happening. . . . After making a peculiar noise, the man was silent and I thought he was dead or unconscious." Rouse then went on to describe how he had poured petrol over the man, took the top off the carburettor and laid a trail of petrol from the car to enable him to fire it without danger to himself. This was as well since "the flame rushed to the car, which caught fire at once . . . the whole thing was a mass of flames in a few seconds".

It cannot be known whether Rouse had read a war spy story published in a newspaper in January 1929 or *The W Plan* by Mr. Graham Seton. Miss Normanton suggests, with hesitation, that he may have obtained his plan from one of those sources. Two men were executed on 2 May 1931 at Regensburg for similar crimes; both had killed motor-car passengers to obtain insurance money.

A woman murdered her husband by throwing spirit over him and setting it alight; she had, it appears, made an earlier attempt. Her defence was that he had poured spirit over her and chased her with a bowl of spirit; in the struggle the contents fell on her husband and were accidentally ignited. The woman, however, was neither burnt nor singed; the injuries on her fingers were bites made in self-defence by the husband. She was convicted and imprisoned for 3 years (Nippe and Mayer, 1933).

Severe damage to a body in a blazing garage did not prevent the late Prof. Sutherland from proving death by firearm injury. (Saxton Grange murder: *R. v. Brown, Leeds Assizes, 1935.*)

It is true that the bodies of these victims may be so badly burnt that it might seem a hopeless task to discover anything of note, but they must always be subjected to close examination.

Smith and Fiddes (1955) depict signs of strangulation in a badly burnt body. Keith Simpson (1943) was able to demonstrate a fracture of the great horn of the thyroid cartilage in the body of Mrs. Dobkin, although her burial, after an attempt to destroy the body by fire, had taken place over a year previously. When a victim of shooting was left in a garage and the garage was set on fire, the late Professor Sutherland was not prevented from demonstrating the cause of death. After strangling his wife, a husband set their home on fire in the hope that this would conceal the murder. He had, however, miscalculated because the fire was promptly extinguished, and the cause of death remained clear.

An elderly woman was found dead in her badly burnt house, and at first the cause was thought to be an accident. However, there was evidence that the gas meter had been forced, and at autopsy severe head injuries were found, with no soot or carbon monoxide in the blood, and no vital reaction to the burns. Death was found to have been caused by two young people whom the old lady had befriended (F.M. 13,664A).

On another occasion a woman was attacked and strangled in her home by a mentally disturbed intruder, who attempted sexual interference after death and then heaped cushions around the body and set them on fire. However, the body was only very slightly damaged (F.M. 15,975 A).

The body of another elderly lady found dead in the kitchen of her burning home was smoke soiled but otherwise unaffected by fire. Autopsy revealed head injuries, a broken neck, and other internal injuries; her scalp bore a patterned bruise which was ultimately found to match the buckle of her assailant's belt. Suspicion was raised initially when the fire brigade, called to the house fire, found clear evidence of five separate seats of fire, in the sitting room and a bedroom of the house (F.M. 25947 A).

Most recently the bodies of two women were recovered from a burning bungalow, one older woman lying on a bed, her daughter on the floor beside the bed. The fire was confined to a living room across the hallway. Initial thoughts that both had died when the daughter tried to save her mother, who was crippled, from the fire, were dispelled when, at autopsy, the daughter's clothes were found to smell of petrol, and she bore slight neck injuries, with no soot or carbon monoxide in her body. The mother's body had soot in the air passages and carbon monoxide in the blood, but also had marks of a gag, ligatures on the wrist, and a fractured femur, with far less carbon monoxide in the haematoma blood around the fracture than elsewhere in the body. The estranged husband of the daughter was later convicted of their deaths (F.M. 27457 A).

"Spontaneous Combustion": "Candle Effect"

Bodies are sometimes found in circumstances which initially suggest that attempts have been made to destroy the body by fire, in order to conceal a crime.

The body is almost always that of an elderly woman, found grossly incinerated in a room, the head being close to a source of ignition, such as a small fire in a grate. The body is so severely burnt that it is mainly reduced to ashes, but the damage ends at about the level of the knees, one or both lower legs remaining intact. If the floor beneath the body is boarded, these may be burnt through, and carpets are destroyed immediately beneath the body. The whole of the rest of the room, including combustible articles such as tea-towels close to the body, are undamaged apart from being soot soiled.

In the past such events were thought to be supernatural in origin, or else due to increased combustibility of the body in chronic alcoholics. One such description appears in Dicken's *Bleak House*. Recent reports (Thurston, 1961, Gee, 1965; 1974) have indicated that the cause is a "candle" effect, in which fat from the ignited head of the body saturates clothing, which acts as a wick. There are other authors who regard the phenomena as more likely to have a supernatural origin (Harrison, *Fire From Heaven*).

Vitriol throwing is a practice now happily rare. The crime had its origin in quarrels between workmen and masters over wages in Glasgow during the early part of the nineteenth century (Christison, 1836). Its frequency led to legislative action. The crime became a felony under The Offences against the Person Act, 1861, s. 29, and is punishable at the discretion of the Court by imprisonment for life. More often than not the motive, today, is spite or revenge. Proof of the crime turns upon proof of *wilful throwing of corrosive* on or at the victim and proof of intent to maim. It is not necessary to prove that injury resulted. If the intent was only to burn the clothing the offence seems to be outside the statute. Unless the contrary be proved, intention will be evidenced by the act of throwing vitriol.

The throwing or spraying of ammonia has been used to facilitate robbery by present day criminals.

II. The Effects of Cold

Human resistance to chilling and kindred adverse environmental conditions, providing the subjects are young and healthy adequately clothed and, more especially, if they have been subjected to severe tests of physical fitness in advance, is indeed remarkable. This is shown by records of polar exploration, such as *Scott's Last Expedition* (Scott, 1913), *South with Scott* (Evans, 1936) and *The Worst Journey in the World* (Cherry-Garrard, 1937), or of mountaineering, as in *Everest, 1933* (Ruttledge, 1934) and *High Adventure* (Hillary, 1955), or pot-holing, in *Ten Years under the Earth* (Casteret, 1933). It is true that Scott and his companions succumbed, but that most moving of all these records, the closing pages of Scott's diary, which he kept almost to the end, shows that there is a limit to human endurance. Another remarkable, unique record, of a negress aged 23, shows that even when chilled to the point almost of death, recovery is possible. Her rectal temperature had fallen to 64.4°F (18°C) yet, after a long convalescence, she recovered, but not without grave mutilation of her limbs by frostbite (Laufman, 1951).

It is otherwise when the subjects are at the extremes of life or are incapacitated by drink, drugs or disease. In the elderly and, perhaps, the newly born, severe chilling of itself may cause death, although in some cases, coincident factors also play a part. At a time when a number of elderly persons are living alone, the possibility of accidental hypothermia must be emphasised. It is only in recent years that it has received recognition, as by Rees (1958) and Emslie-Smith (1958); a detailed study of twenty-three cases was first published in 1961, by Duguid, Simpson and Strowers.

Neo-natal cold injury did not receive special attention until Mann (1953, 1955) gave an account of it, in the erroneous belief that it was a new syndrome. It had in fact been recognised, as "oedema of newlyborn children", by Henoch (1889), although his distinction between this condition and sclerema is now untenable. Even though this proved to be a "rediscovery", Mann (1955), with Elliott (1957), has properly drawn attention to the hazard and provided valuable guidance for its prevention.

Hypothermia as a result of alcoholic intoxication was first recognised by Reincke (1875; cited Rees, 1958). The liability of hypothyroidism to predispose to hypothermia, which may sometimes arise spontaneously, other than in chilling conditions, is now well known, but the first report of it appears to have been published as recently as 1953 by Le Marquand, Hausmann and Hemsted. In 1960 Angel and Sash, who added three more cases, were able to tabulate the records of twenty-five cases. Attention has also been drawn to the precipitation of hypothermia in hypothyroidism by the administration of chlorpromazine (Mitchell *et al.*, 1959) or an allied compound, Imipramine hydrochloride (Tofranil), by McCrath and Paley (1960). In the latter case, hypothermia occurred when the patient was in bed in a warm ward. Irvine (1966) recorded hypothermia pre-disposed to by Diazepam (Valium). Mental illness, depression, is another factor, as in the cases of Emslie-Smith (1958) and Duguid *et al.* (1961).

(a) ACCIDENTAL HYPOTHERMIA

Deaths due to chilling, or where chilling is the predominant factor, are uncommon but, in present times, they are not as infrequent as might be believed. The number of elderly people who live alone increases and many of them have slender incomes, while food and clothing and coal or other sources of heating are expensive. In winter, therefore, these persons are liable to severe prolonged chilling because their homes are inadequately heated and they get insufficient food. Some then develop hypothermia.

The victims are normally aged 70 years or over and the majority are women. The two described by Rees (1958) were males aged 71 and 86 respectively, but most of the other reports were of females, e.g. Rowlands and Rao (1962), Hardwick's first case (1962), seven of Emslie-Smith's eight patients (1958) and seventeen of the twenty-three Dundee/Perth series (Duguid *et al.*, 1961). In the latter series, the ages ranged from 56 to 86, but those of under 70 years had coincident disease, e.g. myxoedema, cerebral thrombosis or chronic alcoholism. Similarly, two of the four cases recorded by Rees (1958), women in their 40s, had coincident illness—in one, paraplegia due to fracture dislocation of the spine and in the other, diabetic coma.

Three phases of chilling were recognised by Duguid *et al.* (1961). The first, which has no clinical significance, is one in which the rectal temperature is between 98.4° and 90°F. There is a feeling of being cold and shivering. It represents the normal reaction to chilling and promptly responds to simple measures.

In the second phase, where the rectal temperature is between 90° and 75°F, the subject is depressed; there is a progressive fall in pulse and respiration rate and in blood pressure. Shivering ceases at about 90–85°F.

The third phase is that in which the rectal temperature falls below 75°F. The temperature-regulating centre ceases to function and there is progressive cooling of the body until it attains the level of the atmospheric temperature. Survival from this phase is rare and the case of Laufman (1951), where the rectal temperature was 64.4°F, remains unique. The depth of hypothermia, state of consciousness and survival are closely related.

The course of events during chilling is normally of this order:

The patient is pale, feels cold and begins to shiver. Shivering continues until the body temperature falls to between 90° and 85°F; it is absent at 81°F. Meantime, the muscles become increasingly stiff; consciousness is clouded at about 86°F. The blood pressure falls and falls rapidly at about 77°F. If untreated, death may then be due to cardiac failure (Rees, 1958). Torpidity and an intense desire to sleep is another feature. Those who are still ambulant may suffer from giddiness and impaired vision so that, to the onlooker, they appear to be drunk (Tidy, 1882; Seton Merriman, 1946).

When seen in hospital, the patients are "strikingly pale". The body as a whole, including the genitalia, is cold; no warmth is retained even by the relatively protected parts. Muscular rigidity is general and resembles rigor mortis. Shivering is rare and was seen in only two cases in the Dundee/Perth series, when the rectal temperature was 88°F in one and 89°F in the other. Peripheral oedema is common (over 50 per cent). The pupils are usually constricted and the light reflex, if present, is sluggish. In Laufman's patient the reflex was absent and to the touch the eyeball felt as if of glass. Bradycardia is common, the rate being below 60; in Laufman's patient it was only 12 to 20 at the outset. The systolic blood pressure is less than 100 mm Hg. Respiration is slow and shallow, but not often less than 12 per minute. (It was only 3 to 5 per minute in Laufman's patient.)

The Dundee/Perth patients were subjected to an extensive *biochemical investigation*, the details of which are given by Duguid *et al.* (1961). Plasma-bicarbonate was distinctly low in six out of fourteen patients tested. The most significant finding was a high serum-amylose level, as seen in eleven out of fifteen patients; five of these patients had pancreatic necrosis.

Electro-cardiographic changes occur in hypothermia and these were regarded by Emslie-Smith (1958) as pathognomonic. They resembled those seen in induced hypo-thermia and in experimental animals. This was confirmed by the Dundee/Perth series. There is lengthening of the PR and QRS intervals and a distinctive "J" deflection in leads to the left ventricle. Emslie-Smith advised the use of adequate leads, especially left chest leads, if these changes are to be detected.

Prognosis. Prolonged, severe chilling of the elderly, with or without coincident disease, is an emergency and the victims must receive prompt, skilled treatment in hospital. Even when this is done, the prognosis is grave if the rectal temperature had fallen to 80°F or less. Only one of six of these patients survived; all were unconsicous when admitted to hospital (Duguid *et. al.*, 1961).

The prognosis depends on the duration of chilling, degree of hypothermia and the occurrence of unconsciousness. Only seven of the twenty-three cases in the Dundee/Perth series survived, but three made a complete recovery. Thirteen of those who died did so within 24 hours of admission to hospital. The outlook, although grave, is not by any means hopeless. One of the patients who remained hypothermic and unconscious for 7 days made a complete recovery; it would appear, however, that she was, at 68, one of the youngest of the patients; it was estimated she had suffered hypothermia for 24 hours; her rectal temperature on admission to hospital was 82°F (27.5°C). Some may survive for a few days and then die of coronary thrombosis. Read *et al.* (1961) have suggested that repeated estimation of the serum-amylose content may be a guide to progress.

The post-mortem findings of hypothermia, as found in the Dundee/Perth series of thirteen examinations, are sometimes obscured by changes due to senility or coincident disease, because of the age of the subject. The immediate cause of death is circulatory failure, central and peripheral. Infarction of the myocardium, when small, may be a hypothermic lesion. Specific changes are to be found in the digestive tract, pancreas, parotid gland and brain. Acute gastric erosions or mucosal haemorrhages occur. A necrotising parotitis was seen in one case. Perivascular haemorrhages in the region of the third ventricle, with chromatolysis of ganglion cells, or petechial haemorrhages in the leptomeninges may occur. Multiple visceral infarcts, caused by stagnation of the blood by tightly packed red cells, should be sought for. Venous thrombosis may also be found. Perhaps the most striking change, related to the high serum-amylose levels, is pancreatic necrosis. This was severe in two cases and focal necrosis with fat necrosis occurred in three others. The association of pancreatitis with hypothermia was discussed by Read *et al.* (1961) when they reported two cases. It may be the cause of death in patients whose initial progress after hypothermia had been satisfactory. Mant (1964) described local necrotic lesions.

Pre-existing disease, e.g. myxoedema, will present its usual features.

Treatment. There appears to be a consensus of opinion that the elderly patient, suffering from hypothermia, must not be reheated artificially. He should be covered with blankets and kept in a warm room, but hot baths, heat cradles or electric blankets, etc., are dangerous. All six patients actively reheated, in the Dundee/Perth series, promptly died. Active reheating abolishes peripheral vaso-constriction, which is a natural compensation for the reduced blood volume in chilling; it predisposes to circulatory failure. The other steps in treatment include a prophylactic dose of an antibiotic, the administration of cortico-steroid hormones and intravenous infusion. The latter is no doubt valuable in countering dehydration and semi-starvation and to augment blood volume. Duguid *et al.* (1961) preferred 5 per cent dextrose to glucose saline, since they saw no specific need for saline. They advise caution where there is reduced urinary excretion, in the presence of hypotension.

They obtained no clear benefit with vaso-constrictor drugs.

In short, these patients, who are usually in a critical condition and for whom there is no specific treatment, should be treated in ways that are "harmless and as rational as our understanding of the altered physiology of hypothermia would permit" (Duguid *et al.*, 1961). Blankets and a warm room are, therefore, the first and principal therapeutic agents.

The importance of accidental hypothermia received fresh emphasis by the setting up of a committee on accidental hypothermia by the Royal College of Physicians. The report of this Committee, in October 1966, found hypothermia common, and confirmed its gravity; the mortality rate is high when the body temperature is less than 80° F and 73.3 per cent of the patients died. Those at special risk are infants aged under 1 year, especially if they also suffer from congenital malformations; and, at the other end of the scale, persons aged 75 years or over. The condition is not exclusive to these groups because the Committee found that accidental hypothermia was common amongst patients aged 35–65 years. The lowest temperature recorded in this series of 126 cases was 76.2° F. The patient was a tramp found unconscious at his home; his temperature rose to 92.4° F before he died, 3 days after admission to hospital.

Those who have charge of patients at risk should be provided with low-reading clinical thermometers, the scale of which registers between 75° and 105° F; these are cheap and adequate for ordinary clinical examination. In a large hospital it would be well to have, in addition, a thermistor for the control of treatment and for use in clinical studies of these patients.

Two other practical findings are important. It was clear that the transport of infants by ambulance was a factor in the production of hypothermia. Steps should be taken to ensure that there is adequate heating of these vehicles. The Committee also drew attention to the practice of nursing infants under a cradle covered by a blanket, whereby the patient is surrounded by a fairly cold air space; this should cease.

It is regretted that the Committee were unable to give authoritative guidance in treatment. The survey left them with the conclusion that "the efficiency of methods of treatment remains uncertain, while the relative advantages of slow or rapid warming of such patients remain unknown".

Treatment is one of the problems in this field which calls for urgent study. Previous reports (reviewed by Polson, 1965) suggested that rapid reheating of the elderly is dangerous. The young adult, on the other hand, suffering from immersion in cold water, is likely to respond satisfactorily to rapid reheating. Neonatal hypothermia is best prevented by avoiding exposure to cold, because the onset of "cold injury" is insidious and, therefore, its occurrence may not be appreciated until it is too late to save the patient. Midwives should also be provided with low-reading clinical thermometers.

(b) HYPOTHERMIA IN LONG-DISTANCE SWIMMERS OR THE SHIPWRECKED

This is a variant of accidental hypothermia which no doubt differs because the subjects are normally healthy young adults and they are resuscitated at an early stage. The case of Miss C . . . is a good example (Hardwick, 1962). This lady became hypothermic after swimming for 11 hours and 47 minutes, when she had almost accomplished the 21-mile crossing of the Irish Channel in 1957. She resisted rescue, but collapsed on deck. She was then as cold as a body in a mortuary and her death was thought to be impending. She was wrapped in blankets and, with that treatment alone, she made a complete recovery in 48 hours. In October 1960 she again became hypothermic after swimming for just over $7^1/_2$ hours. This time she gave up her attempt because she thought she was about to lose consciousness. Her rectal temperature was 90.4°F. On this occasion she was promptly immersed in a bath of warm water at 102°F. Within 40 minutes she "felt fine" and her rectal temperature was 97°F. It was suggested that acute hypothermia of this kind, likely to occur in the shipwrecked, should be treated in like manner. The present experience showed that a suitable bath could be taken on board even a small boat (38 feet long). In Hardwick's opinion, rapid reheating was the method of choice, providing there was no frostbite.

Hypothermia due to Exposure: Mountaineering, Pot-holing and
Polar Exploration

Mountaineers, polar explorers and pot-holers may be exposed to extreme conditions of cold and biting wind. Survival depends in large measure on skilful planning of the expedition, not least with special attention to appropriate clothing.

Attention was sharply focused, in 1971, on the disaster which can occur when a party is suddenly faced with adverse weather conditions in the mountains; this resulted in the death of six people: four schoolgirls, a schoolboy and a 19-year-old teacher. They had set out in clear weather from a centre near Aviemore to climb the Cairngorms. They were due to stay overnight in a mountain hut and return next day at 4 p.m. They were overtaken by a blizzard before they reached the hut; high wind, with gusts of up to 70 miles an hour, and low cloud base over difficult and dangerous terrain added to their danger.

Weather conditions of this kind are dangerous to healthy, uninjured adults, but if they are adequately clothed to face such conditions they can survive. On the other hand, if they are not thus protected and have no chance promptly to gain shelter, their chance of survival is remote and death can occur within a few hours. Protection against wind and conservation of body heat are all-important. In these circumstances it is better for the party to huddle together in such shelter they can find or devise and await help than to continue to walk on in the hope of finding shelter in a hut. Walking is safe only so long as it is possible to walk well. The first signs of flagging are a danger signal of utmost importance; shelter must be found within minutes. Otherwise, movement becomes rapidly slower and clumsy, muscles stiffen and the victims begin to stagger as if drunk. They experience weariness; speech is slurred and slow; vision is impaired. They stumble and fall and may be too weary to get up. Consciousness is lost and they may die within an hour.

There is an excellent account of the clinical features in Seton Merriman's account of the retreat from Moscow, when Napoleon's army suffered terrible loss from exposure to intense cold.

Excellent descriptions of the clinical features and circumstances of accidental hypothermia are also given by Pugh (1964, 1966); he also described experimental findings in cold stress and muscular exercise (1967). The difficulties in determining what the person suffering from accidental hypothermia has actually died of are pointed out by Munday (1967).

Death due to accidental hypothermia, from exposure to adverse weather conditions, is not only to be found in the wilder parts of the countryside. We had an example of a middle-aged woman who died from hypothermia while attempting to walk home from a party across a golf course in the middle of an urban area; in another, hypothermia was a contributory factor in the death of a boy trapped in thick mud in a quarry near his home.

Distinctive post-mortem findings in these cases are scanty, but one striking feature is the bright pink colour of the blood in the tissues and the fact the blood is fluid at autopsy, often clotting after being placed in a receptacle for analysis. The lungs may show slight oedema, and on microscopical examination of the tissues the degree of preservation is striking. Another feature likely to be of note are superficial abrasions of the limbs, possibly caused by stumbling and falling in a state of confusion, or during terminal convulsions.

Another feature which we have found to suggest the diagnosis on external examination of the body is prominent patchy purple discoloration of the limbs. This discoloration takes the form of areas up to 3″ in diameter, dark reddish purple in colour, over the knees and elbows in particular, though also to be found elsewhere on the limbs. These may be associated with irregular superficial abrasions. On one or two of the cases we have seen, where the deceased lay on a hard rough surface, these abrasions had penetrated through the full thickness of the skin, and appeared to have been caused by localised friction, possibly during shivering. These features are particularly noticeable in older victims of hypothermia, as in one old lady seen by us, who fell on the concrete yard behind her house, sustained a fracture of a very thin skull, and at death had large areas of bruising over the prominences of her limbs. The appearances may lead to the erroneous conclusion that the elderly person had been a victim of an assault (F.M. 13553 B).

Hirvonen (1976) described a series of 22 cases of fatal hypothermia. He considered the best diagnostic signs to be purple skin and oedema in face and ears, stomach erosions, degenerative foci in the myocardium, and high concentrations of catecholamines in the urine. The myocardial foci consisted of small groups of broken or curly homogeneous fibres with extravasation of red cells; or acid fuschin staining of solitary muscle fibres.

(c) NEO-NATAL COLD INJURY

Although the clinical appearances of hypothermia in newly-born infants were described by Henoch (1889), current interest in this condition was not aroused until Mann (1953, 1955) re-described it in the belief it was a new syndrome. Henoch termed it oedema of the newly-born and distinguished it from sclerema. He gave a detailed account of the nature and distribution of the oedema, which lacks the "board-like hardness" of sclerema. "The body temperature in oedema is usually very low, and in cases which end unfavourably may reach 86° F or even lower." He had recorded a terminal temperature of only 71.6° F. Later in his account he acknowledged certain similarities between the two conditions, but in his view they did not concern the skin condition but the symptoms which accompany it. The children prematurely born or those who from the beginning were placed under the most unfavourable conditions (cold, bad air and wretched nourishment). "Hence illegitimate foundlings, particularly during the cold time of the year, are especially liable to this condition, while in private practice, and even in that of a polyclinic, we have far less opportunity of observing it."

The modern experience is that neo-natal cold injury is not confined to premature infants; indeed, the special care which they now normally receive protects them from it. It is almost exclusively confined to infants born at home during the winter months.

The newly-born are prone to chilling for a variety of reasons. Their surface area in relation to body mass is considerable; their vaso-motor reflexes are undeveloped and the heat-regulating centre is inefficient for at least several hours after birth. The infant cannot produce heat by physical means; muscular exercise is restricted and it cannot shiver. The infant's production of heat by chemical means is restricted. It is at least theoretically possible that for these reasons a perfectly healthy new-born infant may suffer cold injury, even when born at full term. Mestyan (1962) doubts the risk in these circumstances, but in expressing his doubt he postulates not only perfect health but adequate clothing. It may well be that adequately clad, healthy infants, born at full term, are spared.

There is evidence that newly-born infants under disability, e.g. prematurity, birth injuries, infection, congenital heart disease, latent hypothyroidism (Gordon, 1962), mental retardation, etc., are indeed prone to cold injury. It can occur in circumstances where chilling is excluded. Mestyan (1962) saw cold injury within a few hours of birth in two premature infants in the absence of chilling.

Mann (1967) has given an extensive review of the condition with a discussion of the physiological mechanisms underlying the clinical picture. Three varieties of hypothermia were described by Ameil and Kerr (1963); babies who became hypothermic at birth; those who developed the condition during the neonatal period, and who are likely to have pulmonary haemorrhages; and those whose hypothermia is associated with marasmus, and where it develops insidiously and is likely to be overlooked in the presence of the more obvious wasting condition. This last variety may be of particular relevance to the forensic pathologist, as the hypothermia may be the final cause of death in a child whose marasmus is due to neglect by the parents. It is important that the pathologist excludes natural disease before diagnosing neglect; Mant (1969) has given a list of some associated predisposing conditions, such as hypothyroidism and cerebral malformations.

Whatever the precise mechanism may be in any particular case, there is little doubt that the chilling of newly-born infants can cause "cold injury", and when such injury occurs the principal factor, on most occasions, is chilling. This is potentially lethal, but, fortunately, it is eminently preventable. The mortality rate is not less than 26 per cent (Birmingham series) and may be as high as 50 per cent (Brighton series). It is most often seen during January to March, in homes where the bedroom of the infant is cold and without any form of artificial heating. The supply of fuel may have given out. Alternatively, the room may have been warmed by day, but at night a stream of "fresh", cold air may enter through an open window. There may be inadequate clothing for the child and its cot. The chilling occurred on the first day in a third of the cases and was especially common in babies born before the arrival of a midwife or doctor or, on other occasions, when the mother's condition was urgent. Delay in wrapping the baby promptly after delivery is a factor. As noted by Henoch, it occurs also in illegitimate babies where there is a desire to conceal birth or in circumstances of inadequate attention at the delivery.

Clinical appearance. The onset of cold injury is undramatic. These infants have a deceptive appearance, because their red cheeks and limbs suggest well-being. They become increasingly lethargic and apathetic; they refuse food. The outstanding feature is oedema of the extremities, which are cold to the touch. There may be bradycardia and oliguria. Sclerema may coexist and their skin and soft parts then feel as if made of wood or stone; the skin resembles thick leather and cannot be raised from the subcutaneous tissue, to which it appears to be firmly attached. The parts do not pit on pressure.

Post-mortem examination. It has been misdiagnosed as sclerema and, more often, as haemorrhagic pneumonia. There may be petechial haemorrhages in the lungs. The occurrence of oedema of the limbs and a frothy blood-stained secretion in the nose or mouth of a newly-born infant, coupled with a history of the circumstances of the birth, etc., should indicate the diagnosis.

Treatment

(a) *Preventive.* It is generally agreed that this is a preventable condition (Mann, 1955; Mann and Elliott, 1957; Bower *et al.*, 1960; Editorial, *Brit. Med. J.*, 1962).

Mann and Elliott (1957) stressed the importance of delivery in a warm room, free from draughts, and the maintenance of room temperature day AND night to be not below 65°F, and the room temperature should be at about 70°F during the bathing of the infant in winter. Adequate, loosely fitting clothing should be worn. The infant's rectal temperature should be taken daily during the first 14 days and should not fall below 96°F. Midwives should be supplied with low-reading thermometers to register down to 75°F. If the home conditions are inadequate, transfer to hospital must be considered. Bower *et al.* (1960) mention the importance of prompt wrapping of the infant after delivery.

(b) *Curative.* These cases demand skilled treatment in hospital, for the patient is in grave danger. They must be re-warmed, but it appears there is a difference of opinion as to the mode. Some favour rapid re-warming, but others, the majority, believe it should be gradual, taking days rather than hours unless, that is, chilling has been of only short duration. Mann and Elliott (1957) and Bower *et al.* (1960) recommend slow re-warming. Wallis (1962) drew attention to the medieval remedy for frozen limbs. *The Boke of Chyldren* (Phaire, 1545) states that the best remedy is "not to set them to the fire . . . but to put them in a pail of clean cold water". Wallis says that this principle is adopted by fruit farmers when late spring frosts threaten their trees.

Re-heating apart, it seems that glucose by intra-gastric drip and antibiotic prophylaxis is the sum of the curative treatment. Otherwise, it must be symptomatic.

In view of the attention now given to this hazard and the clear, simple instructions for its prevention, it should be a rare cause of death.

Local Effects of Cold

The local effects of cold are frostbite and "immersion foot", which are phases of the same process.

Immersion foot, so called because it is most often seen in shipwrecked mariners, who may have their feet immersed in the sea for many hours, is the result of long exposure to chilling which is short of freezing. (Its features have been described by Critchley (1943), Blackwood (1944) and Molnar (1946).) The condition, however, is not peculiar to seamen because, as Ungley and Blackwood (1942) pointed out, similar changes may be seen in the hands of persons exposed on land when the temperature is low but insufficient to freeze the tissues and thus to cause frostbite. These authors termed the changes "Peripheral Vasoneuropathy after chilling".

The body tissues freeze at about $-2.5°C$ and sea water freezes at $-1.9°C$; the body tissues cannot therefore be frostbitten by immersion. If, however, the tissues are chilled at temperatures between $5°C$ and $8°C$, for several hours, e.g. 14 hours, the nerve damage leads to "immersion foot" or "immersion hand". Ungley and Blackwood (1942) in their study of eighty cases found that the course of events begins with a short pre-hyperaemic phase; this is followed by hyperaemia and the limb becomes hot, red and painful; it is swollen and sometimes blistered; if gangrene follows it is always superficial. The inflammation subsides and vascular tone returns. Although the skin temperature falls, the vessels remain hypersensitive to cold. Swelling, pain and tingling cease and finally there is regeneration of the peripheral nerves. Injudicious warming of the affected parts accentuates the damage because it raises the metabolic demands of the tissues. The correct treatment is to keep the limbs cool but the body warm for several hours after rescue.

The changes in frostbite were the subject of experimental study by Greene (1943). The tails of mice were frozen, and samples, taken at predetermined distances from the tip, i.e. at 1, 4, and 8 cm, were submitted to microscopical examination. These experiments showed that prolonged degrees of mild cold, especially in the presence of water and factors which increase capillary pressure or permeability, caused an excessive transudation from the vessels into the surrounding tissues. Severe cold caused a more serious breakdown; the blood supply of the distal tissue was then cut off by the silting up of the afferent vessels by stranded red cells. This is to be distinguished from true thrombosis which, though it may occur, is a secondary change, and is no part of the process. Silting of red cells is due to escape of plasma into the tissues. The changes beyond this are not signs of tissue death but a reaction of the living body to a part which has become a foreign body. It is concluded that these and the corresponding changes in man, both in frostbite and immersion foot, are the result of a breakdown in the physiological adaptation to cold.

References

ALDRICH, R. H. (1943) *Ann. Surg.*, **117**, 576–84.
AMEIL, G. C., and KERR, M. M. (1963) *Lancet*, **2**, 756.
ANDERSON, R. A. and HARLAND, W. A. (1980) in *Forensic Toxicology*. Proceedings of the European meeting of the Internat. Assoc. of Forensic Toxicologists. Ed. Oliver, J. S. London, Croomhelm Ltd.
ANGEL, J. H. and SASH, Z. (1960) *Brit. Med. J.*, i, 1855–9.
BAILEY, B. N. (1960) *Brit. Med. J.*, ii, 1783–5.
BELT, T. H. (1939) *J. Path. Bact.*, **48**, 493–8.
BLACKWOOD, W. (1944) *Brit. J. Surg.*, **31**, 329–50.
BLAKELY, J. (1968) *The Care of Radiation Casualties*. London: Heinemann.

Bower, B. D., Jones, L. F. and Weeks, M. M. (1960) *Brit. Med. J.*, **i**, 303–9.
Cashell, G. W., Shay, H. B., and Bodenham, D. C. (1943–4) *Brit. J. Surg.*, **31**, 373–7.
Casteret, N. (1933) *Ten Years under the Earth*, trans. B. Massey, ed. 1952. Harmondsworth: Penguin.
Catto, J. V. F. (1959) *Brit. Med. J.*, **ii**, 544–5.
Chao, T. C., Sinniah, R., and Pakiam, J. E. (1981) *Pathology*, **13**, 145–56.
Cherry-Garrard, A. (1937) *The Worst Journey in the World.* Harmondsworth; Penguin Books.
Christison, R. (1836) *Treatise on Poisons*, 3rd ed., p. 138. Edinburgh: Adam and Charles Black.
Cox, M. E., Heslop, B. F., Kempton, J. J. and Ratcliff, R. A. (1955) *Brit. Med. J.* **i**, 942–6.
Critchley MacDonald (1943) *Shipwreck-Survivors* Bradshaw Lecture. London: Churchill.
Donalies, G. (1942) *Dtsch. Z. ges. gerichtl. Med.*, **36**, 49–52.
Duguid, H., Simpson, R. G. and Strowers, J. M. (1961) *Lancet*, **ii**, 1213–19.
Emslie-Smith, D. (1958) *Lancet*, **ii**, 492.
Evans, E. R. G. R. (1936) *South with Scott.* London: Collins.
Fajardo, L. F., and Stewart, J. R. (1970) *Amer. J. Path.*, **59**, 299.
Fine, S. Edlow, J., MacKeen, D., Feigen, L., Ostrea, E. and Klein, E. (1968) *Amer. J. Path.*, **52**, 155.
Gee, D. J. (1965) *Med. Sci. and Law*, **5**, 37.
Gee, D. J. (1974) *Police Surgeon*, **5**, 63.
Ghidoni, J. J. and five others (1967) *Arch. path.*, **83**, 370.
Gordon, R. R. (1962) *Lancet*, **i**, 460–1.
Greene, R. (1943) *J. Path. Bact.*, **55**, 259–67.
Hardwick, R. G. (1962) *Brit. Med. J.*, **i**, 147.
Harris, T. A. B. and Hutton, A. M. (1956) *Lancet*, **ii**, 1024–5.
Harrison, G. G. (1971) *Brit. Med. J.*, **3**, 454.
Harrison, M. (1976) *Fire from Heaven.* London, Sidgwick and Jackson.
Henoch, E. (1889) *Lectures on Children's Diseases* trans. J. Thomson, vol. 1, 53. London: New Sydenham Soc.
Hillary, E. (1955) *High Adventure*, London: Hodder and Stoughton.
Hirvonen, J. (1976) *Forensic Sci.*, **8**, 155–164.
Irvine, R. E. (1966) *Brit. Med. J.*, **2**, 1007.
Ladell, W. S. S., Waterlow, J. C. and Hudson, M. F. (1944) *Lancet*, **ii**, 491–7, 527–31.
Laufman, H. (1951) *J. Amer. Med. Ass.*, **147**, 1201–12.
Leading Article (1971) *Brit. Med. J.*, **3**, 441.
Le Marquand, H. S., Hausmann, W. and Hemsted, E. H. (1953) *Brit. Med. J.*, **i**, 704–6.
Lyall, A. (1956) *Brit. J. Derm.*, **68**, 355.
Lyburn, F. F. St. J. (1954) *Lancet*, **i**, 731.
Lyburn, F. F. St. J. (1956) *Lancet*, **ii**, 1160.
MacCormac, H. and McCrea, H. M. (1925) *Brit. Med. J.*, **i**, 693–4.
McGrath, M. D. and Paley, R. G. (1960) *Brit. Med. J.*, **ii**, 1364.
Madrazo, A., Suzuki, Y. and Churg, J. (1969) *Amer. J. Path.*, **54**, 507.
Madrazo, A., Suzuki, Y. and Churg, J. (1970) *Amer. J. Path.*, **61**, 37.
Mallik, M. O. A. (1970) *J. For. Sciences*, **15**, 489.
Mann, T. P. (1953) *Proc. Roy. Soc. Med.*, **46**, 883.
Mann, T. P. (1955) *Lancet*, **i**, 613–14.
Mann, T. P. and Elliott, R. I. K. (1957) *Lancet*, **i**, 229–34.
Mant, A. K. (1964) *Med. Sci. Law*, **4**, 414.
Marriott, H. L. (1947) *Brit. Med. J.*, **i**, 245–50, 285–90, 328–32.
Medical Research Council (1958) *Brit. Med. J.*, **1**, 1533.
Merriman, Seton (1946) *Barlash of the Guard.* Harmondsworth: Penguin Books.
Mestyan, J. (1962) *Lancet*, **i**, 690.
Mitchell, J. R. A., Surridge, D. H. C. and Willison, R. G. (1959) *Brit. Med. J.*, **ii**, 932–3.
Molnar, G. W. (1946) *J. Amer. Med. Ass.*, **131**, 1046–50.
Moritz, A. R. and Henriques, F. C. (1947) *Am. J. Path.*, **23**, 695.
Morton, T. C. St. C. (1931–2) *Proc. Roy. Soc. Med.*, **25** (2), 1261–71.
Munday, M. C. (1967) *Brit. Med. J.*, **2**, 372.
Nippe, M. and Mayer, R. M. (1933) *Dtsch. Z. ges. gerichtl. Med.* **21**, 120–31; *abstr. Med-leg. Rev.*, 1934, **2**, 100–1.
Normanton, H. (1931) *Trial of Alfred Arthur Rouse*, Notable British Trials Series, Edinburgh; Hodge.
Polson, C. J. (1965) *The Essentials of Forensic Medicine.* 2nd ed., p. 267. Oxford: Pergamon.
Polson, C. J. and Tattersall, R. N. (1969) *Clinical Toxicology* 2nd ed., p. 43. London: Pitman medical.
Pugh, L. G. C. E. (1964) *Lancet*, **i**, 1210.
Pugh, L. G. C. E. (1966) *Brit. Med. J.*, **1**, 123.
Pugh, L. G. C. E. (1967) *Brit. Med. J.*, **2**, 333.

R EG, V. LEE (1981) Hull.

R. V. ROUSE (1931) *Trial of Alfred Arthur Rouse*, Notable British Trials Series, ed. Helena Normanton. Edinburgh: Hodge.

READ, A. R., EMSLIE-SMITH D., GOUGH, K. R. and HOLMES, R. (1961) *Lancet*, **ii**, 1219–21.

REED, G. B. Jr. and COX, A. J. Jr. (1966) *Amer. J. Path.*, **48**, 597.

REES, J. R. (1958) *Lancet*, **i**, 556.

ROWLANDS, I. P. and RAO, H. M. J. (1962) *Lancet*, **i**, 745–6.

Royal College of Physicians, London (1966) Report of Committee on Accidental Hypothermia. London: R. C. P.

RUTTLEDGE, H. (1934) *Everest 1933*, London: Hodder and Stoughton.

SCOTT, R. F. (1913) *Scott's Last Expedition*. London: Smith.

SCOTT, S. G. (1931) *Radiology in Relation to Medical Jurisprudence*. London, etc.: Cassell.

SEVITT, S. (1966) *Med. Sci. and Law*, **6**, 36.

SIMPSON, K. (1943) *Med-leg. Rev.*, **11**, 132–44.

SMITH, SIR SYDNEY and FIDDES, F. S. (1955) *Forensic Medicine*, 10th ed., p. 234. London: Churchill.

TERRY, H. (1943) *Brit. Med. J.*, **i**, 756–7.

THURSTON, G. (1961) *Med-leg. J.*, **29**, 100.

TIDY, C. M. (1882) *Legal Medicine*, vol. 1, p. 494. London: Smith Elder.

UNGLEY, C. C. and BLACKWOOD, W. (1942) *Lancet*, **ii**, 447–51.

WALLIS, H. (1962) *Lancet*, **i**, 534.

CHAPTER 8

Mechanical Asphyxia

The term mechanical asphyxia is here applied to circumstances in which mechanical interference either (a) impedes access of air to the lungs or (b) reduces the blood supply to the head and neck or (c) causes sudden cardiac arrest, due to stimulation of the carotid sinus-vagal reflex mechanism.

On many occasions the circumstances of the death and the external appearances of the body are strong, if not conclusive, evidence of death by mechanical asphyxia. All of these deaths, however, should be subjected to the same thorough investigation as that necessary to ascertain the cause when it is obscure.

Obstruction of the air way, e.g., choking by a foreign body, a common experience but fortunately an uncommon cause of death, may be obvious as is also flooding of the air passages by water in drowning. Perfunctory examination can result in failure to observe a massive foreign body in the throat. A female prisoner, found dead in her cell, was deemed to have died of cerebral haemorrhage and her body was passed to the local school of anatomy. Some time later, when the neck structures were to be dissected, a relatively large rolled piece of blanket was found wedged in her throat; she had thus committed suicide (Handyside, 1842). On the other hand the keen eyes of an experienced examiner were needed to discover a tiny down feather, which, when inhaled, had caused death by acute cardiac arrest when it made contact with the vocal cords (Spilsbury, 1934).

Death following submersion is usually due to flooding of the air passages but, when submersion be sudden and unexpected, "dry lung" drowning may occur, since the immediate cause of death is then acute cardiac arrest and little fluid enters the lungs.

The characteristic appearances of death due to mechanical asphyxia are most likely to be seen when there is compression of the veins, causing their engorgement. This is usually a feature of manual strangulation, self-strangulation by a ligature, hanging from a low point of suspension, e.g., the kneeling, sitting or prone positions, or choking but not when the foreign body has caused acute cardiac arrest, the so-called "Café Coronary" death. Nor are the appearances a feature when death is by hanging from a high point of suspension, e.g. the standing position or whenever there is complete suspension of the body, e.g. from the bough of a tree. The signs may be present and pronounced without external trace of injury as in mugging, when the neck of the victim is held in the crook of the assailant's arm or the neck is compressed by an unshod or naked foot.

Crush or traumatic asphyxia is in a class apart; its striking features (see page 468), once seen, are promptly recognised on subsequent occasions. These are the victims of grave,

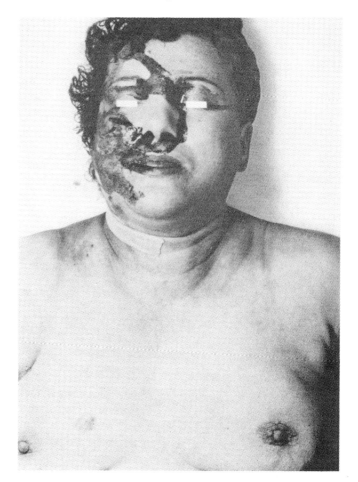

FIG. 115. "Classical" asphyxia. A case of homicidal throttling.
(There was a bite mark on the right breast (see Fig. 18) and the
dressing on the right of the neck concealed another bite mark.)

massive bodily compression, e.g. by the fallen roof of a mine or the sides of a trench. The
greater part of the blood in the body is forced into the relatively incompressible part, i.e.
the head and upper fourth of the trunk. Violent compression of the chest prevents
breathing, which becomes impossible.

The Signs of Mechanical Asphyxia

Cyanosis

The skin of the head and neck above the level of obstruction is blue and intensely
discolored if survival had been prolonged, which, in these circumstances is a matter of
only seconds or, possibly, minutes. Examination of the body, whenever practicable, must

be made under satisfactory lighting; otherwise slight degrees of cyanosis may be overlooked.

Ocular signs

The eyes may bulge; the pupils may be dilated. The conjunctivae are suffused and there may be sub-conjunctival haemorrhages, varying in size from pin-head petechiae to large blood blisters. The tongue may protrude and may have been bitten. Foam or saliva, sometimes blood-stained, may be seen at the mouth and nose and this may be the one notable external sign of death by drowning when a body is recovered from water.

Petechial Haemorrhages

These are usually of pin-head size but they vary in size and number. They may be scanty and are to be detected under low magnification or they may be so numerous that the appearances resemble those of a measles rash. They occur in the skin of the face and eye

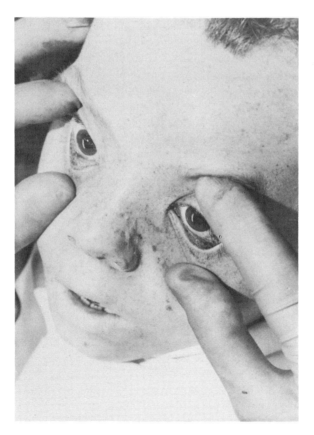

FIG. 116. Mechanical asphyxia; petechial haemorrhages
beneath the conjunctivae and in the skin on the face.

lids and beneath the conjunctiva. They are the result of venous stasis leading to capillary congestion and rupture. Although they may be seen in circumstances other than those of mechanical asphyxia, and in deaths from natural causes, they should alert the examiner to the possibility of mechanical asphyxia as the cause. This is especially important when the haemorrhages are confined to the head and neck, i.e. above the level of any obstruction.

Internal Examination

Petechial haemorrhages beneath the pleura and pericardium were regarded by Tardieu (1866) as pathognomonic of death by mechanical asphyxia and they became known as Tardieu's spots. Although this view was widely accepted for many years their validity was doubted at an early date e.g. by Liman and Gordon (1944) also questioned their significance because he had seen them in other forms of death. Gordon, Turner and Price (1953) had seen them in deaths from secondary shock as well as in many deaths from natural causes. Gordon and Mansfield (1955) questioned not only their specificity but also their ante-mortem origin. They commonly developed after death and often during the autopsy. Shapiro (1955) pointed out that some of these spots were spontaneous post-mortem artefacts and some, seen at autopsy, disappeared in a short period. This disappearance was confirmed and depicted by Zaini and Knight (1981) who considered them to diminish *when intra-venous pressure is reduced in the major pulmonary vessels at autopsy*. They also drew attention to the difficulty of distinguishing between false and true petechiae by naked-eye inspection alone. Microscopical examination demonstrated that some of these spots were haemorrhages but the majority, about two-thirds, were false: they were either intra-pleural venous channels or air blisters or thickened pleural plaques and some were dust pigment. In 100 consecutive autopsies apparent petechiae were present in 33, mostly unrelated to mechanical asphyxia and, of these, only one third were proved to have been haemorrhages.

Clearly the time has come to disregard these haemorrhages as diagnostic of mechanical asphyxia. But they still should recall this possibility and cause it to receive due consideration.

Stasis Haemorrhages

Fine pin-head haemorrhages may be seen beneath the mucosa of the larynx, especially in the sub-glottic space, above the level of constriction by a ligature; it is likely in homicidal strangulation. These haemorrhages are the result of venous stasis and subsequent capillary rupture.

Haemorrhages due to natural disease are likely in coronary deaths; there is the possibility that, sometimes in the final moments the patient's condition is asphyxal. In any event, there is then no room to doubt the diagnosis. Haemorrhages when due to disease tend to have large size, greater number and wider distribution, within as well as externally. They tend to coalesce. A blood film, appropriately stained, may disclose an unsuspected blood disorder. But let it never be forgotten that laboratory findings may sadly mislead. A substantial leucocytosis and the presence of immature white cells is not necessarily evidence of leukaemia; it once, temporarily, obscured the diagnosis of smallpox (F.M. 3056).

Sudden Cardiac Arrest

In a considerable proportion of deaths from mechanical asphyxia in the Cardiff area, the immediate cause of death was sudden cardiac arrest. Knight found that slightly more than 50 per cent of cases of constriction of the neck (manual and ligature strangulation, choking and hanging) showed no congestive, cyanotic nor haemorrhagic stigmata. These deaths were thus ascribed to rapid death from cardiac arrest. Karate blows to the neck, mugging and some cases of drowning also may cause sudden death from acute cardiac arrest.

An accurate history of the circumstances of the death is important. Sudden collapse and loss of consciousness is an outstanding feature but cessation of breathing, or pulse and the heart beat may not occur until 15–30 seconds have elapsed. There may be ventricular fibrillation, e.g. when electrocuted. If defibrillation be prompt it is possible to restore the patient. Slowing of the heart beat may occur within 90 seconds and this may continue for even a few minutes, with a few bouts of tachycardia before death. Prompt intensive care at least theoretically might restore the patient but on most occasions the interval is too long to allow success or the circumstances are such that the last thing the assailant desires is recovery of his victim.

An important feature which supports the diagnosis of acute cardiac arrest, especially in death by drowning manual or ligature strangulation and karate blows is evidence of surprise, or emotion or apprehension or fright. Alcoholic intoxication is another factor.

A thorough examination of the body is directed especially to signs of injury and its degree of severity. If signs of injury be absent or slight this supports the diagnosis of acute cardiac arrest and a submission that the death was the result of an accident. Normally grave injury favours the allegation of criminal intent. But Knight has examined a number of fractured hyoid bones and horns of the thyroid cartilage, accompanied by haemorrhage, laryngeal mucosal bleeding and skin bruising with no congestive/petechial signs, and yet the history was consistent with rapid death. There is a time interval of from 15–30 seconds available for trauma before there are signs of asphyxia.

The "cafe coronary" circumstances are perhaps the easiest in which to diagnose sudden cardiac arrest with certainty. One of our subjects was enjoying a mixed grill when he suddenly collapsed and died. His larynx was obstructed by a piece of kidney. But the object does not have to be large; a tiny down feather or a nail clipping, suddenly making contact with a vocal cord, can trigger off acute cardiac arrest.

Pulmonary Oedema in Relation to Mechanical Asphyxia

It is often maintained that the presence, and amount, of pulmonary oedema is a guide to the time which elapsed between injury and death. This is a view which must be adopted with caution. It is not a reliable guide. When there is sufficient oedema of the lungs to permit its naked-eye detection, it may well be that an appreciable time, measurable in hours rather than minutes, has elapsed between the injury and death. At the same time, examination of the bodies of those who died shortly after road accidents has shown us that an appreciable amount of fluid had accumulated in their lungs. Moreover, as Camps and Hunt (1959) pointed out, this can occur in the posterior and dependent parts of the lungs after death and may be misinterpreted by the inexperienced as pulmonary oedema.

When only moderate, and certainly when its demonstration requires microscopical study, it is necessary to be cautious in offering an opinion on the probable time interval between injury and the occurrence of pulmonary oedema. Even in those whose deaths were virtually instantaneous, following aircraft accidents, pulmonary oedema was present in histological preparations of their lungs (Mason, 1962). See also Swann (1964).

It has come to our notice that a pathologist was prepared to estimate the interval, and in his view, one of hours, not only on the presence of oedema but also the intensity of its coloration by eosin in the histological preparations. This we are unable to accept. If twelve consecutive sections from a series be given to twelve technicians it would be a miracle if they produced preparations in which the eosin intensity was precisely the same.

References

CAMPS, F. E. and HUNT, A. C. (1959) *J. Forens. Med.* **6**, 116.
GORDON, I. (1944) *Brit. Med. J.*, **2**, 337.
GORDON, I. TURNER, R. and PRICE, T. W. (1953) *Medical Jurisprudence*. 3rd ed. pp. 462: 467. Edinburgh and London: Livingstone.
HANDYSIDE, P. D. (1842) *Edin. med. J.*, **57**, 391–4.
KNIGHT, B. (1982) Personal communication and commentary on this chapter.
MASON, J. K. (1962) *Aviation Accident Pathology*, London: Butterworths.
SHAPIRO, H. A. (1955) *J. Forens Med.*, **2**, 1–4.
SPILSBURY, B. (1934) *Med.-Leg. Rev.* **2**, 340–4.
SWANN, H. E. Jr. (1964) *J. Forens. Sci.* **9**, 360.
TARDIEU, A. A. (1866) Ann d'hyg. Publ et de Mèd-Lèg. **2**, 357 and in his text book: *La Pendasion, la strangulation et la suffocation*. Paris. Baillière. [First ed. 1875; our copy is of the 2nd. ed., 1879].
ZAINI, M. R. S. and KNIGHT, B. (1982) *J. Forens. Sci. Soc.* **22**, 141–5.

CHAPTER 9

Hanging

HANGING is due to constriction of the neck as a result of suspension in such a manner that the weight of the body, or a part of the body, of the victim pulls upon the ligature. Hanging is thus distinguished from strangulation by a ligature. This distinction has practical importance because hanging raises a presumption of suicide, whereas strangulation is usually homicidal.

It is still true, as found by Dixon Mann (1908) in respect of the period 1885–1904, that the majority of deaths due to hanging are suicidal. Latterly the proportion of accidental deaths has increased somewhat because hanging as a concomitant of sexual deviation is now recognised as accidental; formerly these cases were returned as suicides. Homicidal hanging, and suspension of the victim of murder, to simulate suicidal hanging are rare. Radian and Radovici (1957) recorded a case of homicidal hanging, and the case of Emmett-Dunne (Camps, 1959) was one of suspension after murder by a blow to the neck.

The Scene of Hanging

The well-known fact that the majority of these deaths are suicidal, indeed the proportion is of the order of 90 per cent or over, is calculated to condition the mind of the observer with a preconceived idea of the situation. It is necessary, therefore, to give special attention to the details of the scene if an accurate interpretation is to be made. The place, the posture of the body, and the manner in which it is clothed should be noticed. Several details concerning the ligature also require attention. It may be necessary to know something of the antecedents of the victim and to discover whether he had in his possession pornographic literature or photographs. Injuries, other than those due to hanging, require explanation.

The Ligature in Hanging

(a) *Composition.* Since many of the victims are suicides, and it seems there is little premeditation, it is to be expected they will use something at hand in the home or place where they are found suspended. This is borne out by the fact that many use the household clothes-line, which is either knotted to make a fixed noose, or if, as is not infrequent, it carries a metal ring at one end, the line is arranged in a running noose by passing it through the ring.

Articles of dress are also a common choice, for example the cord of a dressing-gown or pyjamas, belts, braces, ties, scarves or handkerchiefs; a bootlace or piece of string may be used. Unusual ligatures arouse suspicion. One man, who hanged himself from a small pine tree, used its roots passed over a low branch of the tree as a ligature (Gulbis, 1939) Hanging in an unusual place also arouses suspicion, for the choice of the suicide is usually in his home or place of work.

When the point of suspension chosen by the suicide is a high one, he or she may use a composite ligature. Braces may be joined to a belt or, as in one of my cases, the victim may tear curtains into strips and join the strips to provide a ligature of suitable length.

Hanging Without the Use of a Fixed or Running Noose

Occasionally death in a vehicular accident is due to hanging, when the victim is suspended by the steering wheel of his car. Similarly, a cyclist who collides with the rear of a lorry or cart, may be suspended on the edge of its tail-board. A person who slips when descending a ladder may be suspended by one of its rungs, or a slip on a staircase may result in suspension on the edge of one of the treads. In one of my cases a baby slipped out of its high chair and was suspended on the edge of its table; others have been suspended by their harness.

Another form is illustrated by the death of an adult woman who, when drunk, fell across the sharp edge of a sofa in such a manner that the weight of her body was exerted on her neck as she lay incompletely suspended (Keiller, 1855–6). As in all of these cases, the mark of hanging on this victim was restricted to the front of her neck.

A similar case of hanging occurred when a man aged 60 was incompletely suspended by the arm of a chair. He was found dead in a kneeling posture with his chin resting on the arm of a chair (Fig. 117) His arms were extended and a handkerchief lay on the floor below his right hand. There was a broad compression mark on the skin of the neck, of up to $1\frac{1}{2}$ in. broad, and $\frac{1}{10}$ in. deep, crossing the front of the neck to the region of the carotid arteries on each side. The skin of the face above the mark was reddish purple in colour but petechial haemorrhages were absent both from the skin and eyes. No bruising of the neck muscles nor any fracture of the hyoid bone or thyroid cartilage was found. A little glairy material, having an acid reaction, was present in his trachea. A small area of consolidation, 1 in. in diameter, was present on the upper lobe of the right lung, an early carcinoma. It would appear he had had an attack of choking and violent coughing had caused him to gain a crouching position, so as to bring his neck on the arm of the chair, and he had failed to regain the erect posture. There was no natural disease to account for this death nor was there any evidence of injury, alcoholic intoxication, nor poisoning. Either the coughing had been brought on by regurgitation of a little gastric contents or he had one of the bouts of severe coughing which he was known to have (F.M. 5757B).

(b) *The mode of application of the ligature.* Any departure from a running noose or a noose fixed by a granny or reef knot calls for special care in interpretation, e.g. the artificer's knot used in the case described by Tardieu (1875). Usually the ligature is arranged in a simple loop but the suicide may wind a cord with more than one turn round his neck; this is unusual in murder. When, however, there are two or more knots, their kind and firmness should be noted. A ligature which is knotted firmly at the first turn and then knotted again after a second turn is unlikely to have been applied by a suicide; it is possible but rare.

(c) *The position of the knot.* The common sites are the right or left side of the neck, or at the occiput; suspension by a knot below the chin is rare; a good example was depicted by Tardieu (1870), with a legend which described the victim as being "*dans une position extrêmement remarquable*". It is not easy to retain the knot beneath the chin.

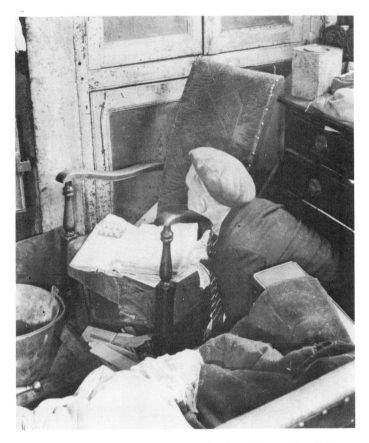

FIG. 117. Hanging: accidental; suspension from the arm of a chair.

A man aged 57 was hanged by a ligature of which the knot was in front of the face at about eyebrow level. The grooving produced by the ligature was deepest at the nape of the neck and at the sides of the face, on the cheeks; on the right side the upper end of the mark was directed towards the right eye and on the left side it was traced from an inch below the left ear to a point on the cheek midway between the nose and eye. The precise mechanism of this death was obscure; there were no signs of asphyxia but the left arm of the ligature could have obstructed the carotid artery; the death could have been due to vagal inhibition. Other causes, i.e. natural disease, injury elsewhere and poisoning, were excluded (F.M. 7935A, Figs. 118, 119).

The level at which the loop lies is also of importance in making the distinction between hanging and strangulation by a ligature. Since the loop is likely to rise up to the limit set by the lower jaw at the moment of suspension, the ligature lies above the thyroid cartilage in at least 80 per cent of hangings; it may be at the level of the cartilage in about 15 per cent but it is below this cartilage in only about 5 per cent of hangings. In one series of 279 cases it was above in 215, at the level of the larynx in forty-three and below it in nineteen; the site was not stated on two occasions (Tardieu, 143 cases, and Minovici, 136 cases, cited by Étienne Martin, 1950). The low position is likely only when a running noose tightens rapidly; the weight of the body can drag the loop above the thyroid cartilage; a thyroid cartilage of unusual size occasionally prevents the ligature running up beneath the chin. In strangulation, by contrast, the ligature is usually over or below the thyroid cartilage.

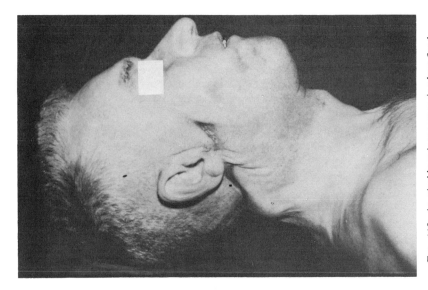

FIG. 119. Atypical hanging: suspension by a fixed-loop with the knot in front of the face (right side of the face).

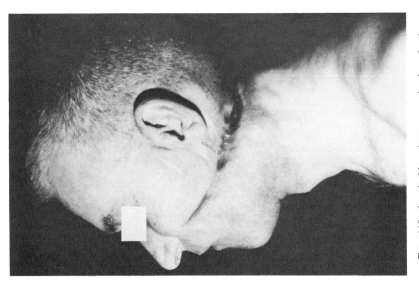

FIG. 118. Atypical hanging: suspension by a fixed-loop with the knot in front of the face (left side of the face).

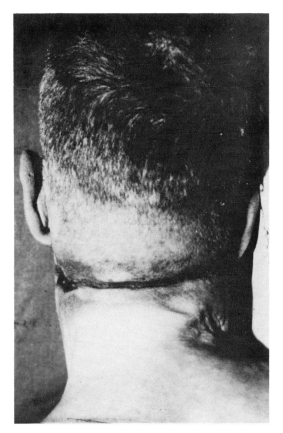

FIG. 120. Atypical hanging: suspension by a fixed-loop with the knot in front of the face (nape of the neck; see also Figs. 118 and 119).

(*d*) *The course of the ligature around the neck.* The usual appearance is that of a groove which is deepest opposite the position of the knot, although this is modified to some extent when the knot is in front, because the firmer muscular tissues at the back of the neck rarely groove as clearly and deeply as those at the front or sides of the neck.

It is important to trace the course of the ligature as indicated by the mark on the neck (Fig. 121). The body may be found after the ligature has been removed and it will then be necessary to determine whether the death was by hanging or by strangulation. When a man found his wife suspended, he cut her down, hid the rope, and reported that he had found her collapsed on the floor. This was a foolish step because, if the mark had not been clearly one due to hanging, he might have found himself in serious trouble.

When the loop is arranged with a fixed knot, the course of the mark is deepest and more or less horizontal on the side away from the knot, but as the arms of the cord approach the knot the mark turns upwards towards it. This produces an inverted "V" at the site of the knot (Fig. 122, 123). The apex of the "V" may lie over intact and unmarked skin, because the head tends to fall away from the knot. Occasionally, however, the course of

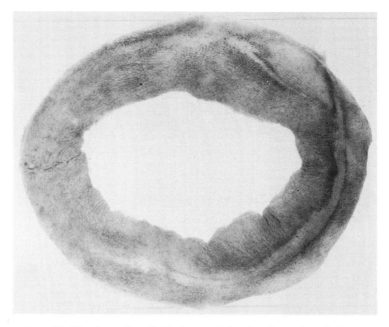

Fig. 121. Hanging: collar of skin from neck bearing the mark made by a fixed loop, knot at left of neck; clothes line (method of museum preservation).

the cord may be directly traced up to the knot, which may have left an abrasion or indentation of the skin at the point of apposition. The mark of strangulation might simulate that of hanging, when the victim is thrown to the ground, strangled, and then his body is moved by pulling upon the ligature. No instance of this has yet occurred in our practice nor has an authentic record of it been traced.

When hanging is effected from a low point of suspension, the mark on the neck closely resembles that of strangulation; it may take a horizontal course round the neck at about the level of the upper border of the larynx (F.M. 1548, Fig. 124, and F.M. 1566, Fig. 125).

The running noose can tighten at the time of suspension and may then produce a mark which takes a horizontal course, resembling that of a ligature used in strangulation, except that is likely to lie above the level of the thyroid cartilage. If a running noose fails to tighten, as for example when the ligature is of thick electric flex, the mark may resemble one produced by a fixed loop (F. M. 840).

Cords may impact a herringbone or diagonal pattern to the mark (Fig. 126). Ligatures which are other than of cord, for example a chain or leather belt bearing an embossed pattern, may leave a mark which reproduces the pattern of the material.

A ligature which is wound more than once round the neck will impart a corresponding complexity to the grooving, usually with red linear bruising between the grooves, where the skin has been pinched between the strands. If a complex ligature is used, for example one which is composed of knotted pieces of twine, the mark will at first sight suggest that a ligature has been wound more than once round the neck. The distinction may be made by the demonstration of abrasions in the course of the mark denoting the site of the knots

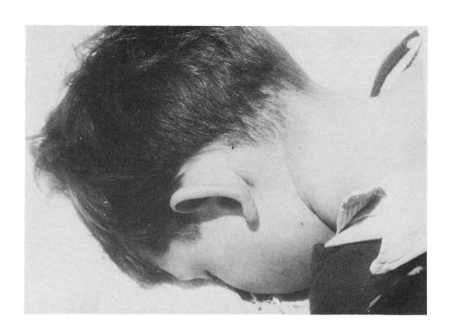

FIG. 123. Hanging: characteristic mark when the loop is closed at the nape of the neck. (The scene is shown in Fig. 131.)

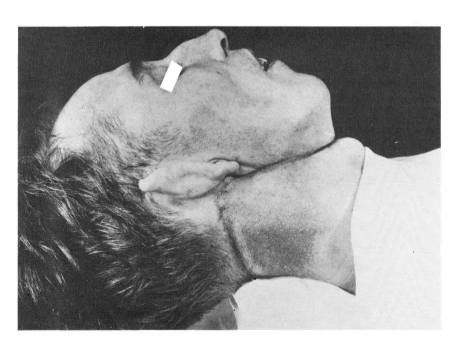

FIG. 122. Hanging: characteristic inverted "V" mark of the ligature, when the loop is closed with a knot behind the ear.

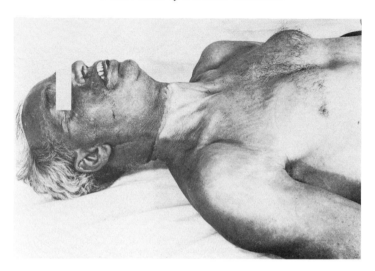

Fig. 124. Hanging from a low point of suspension: simulation of strangulation by a ligature. (The scene is shown in Fig. 128.)

which united the pieces of the ligature (*R. v. Jolly*, Leeds Assizes 1947, Figs. 133, 134, F.M. 86).

Occasionally, especially if the body is promptly cut down and a soft broad ligature has been used, there may be no external mark. Nobiling (1884), cited by Dixon Mann (1908), described the suicide of a man aged 24, who used his pocket handkerchief as a ligature and it was attached to the latch of a door, at a point 3 ft 7 in., from the floor; he was found in a kneeling posture. The broad, folded ligature had left no mark.

It is not essential that the ligature surrounds the neck; it is sufficient if it be applied beneath the chin so as to compress the sides of the neck. Persons have hanged by suspension by the chin, e.g. by the steering wheel of a motor-car, the tail-board of a cart, edge of a sofa, or the arm of a chair. A man was found suspended by a cord attached to the rafters of a granary or loft. He had passed his cotton scarf over the cord and tied the ends under his chin; the front part of the neck was alone engaged. His toes rested on the floor in a heap of corn; the knees were flexed and were a few inches above the floor. (This case was originally published by Wegler (1812), cited and redrawn by Marc (1851) to form one of his illustrations of a paper on the suicide of the Prince de Condé. It was redrawn and included by Tardieu (1879) in his monograph on hanging, plate 2, which was also used by Brouardel (1897); others have since reproduced it. The rest of Marc's illustrations, which he published in 1851, have also been reproduced, usually without acknowledgment).

Webb (1852) recorded a case of hanging where a man was found in bed, lying on his stomach, with his head inside a leather strap, tied to the bed post to make a loop 21 in. long; he was suspended by his chin.

(*e*) *The point of suspension.* The point of suspension chosen by the suicide is normally one which is within easy reach, with or without the aid of some kind of platform, e.g. a chair, stool or table. A hook or nail on a door is an obvious choice. Sometimes the ligature is passed over the top of a door and fastened to a hook on the other side. In that event

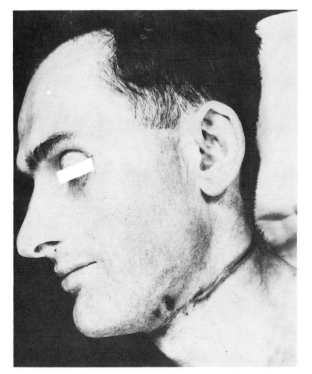

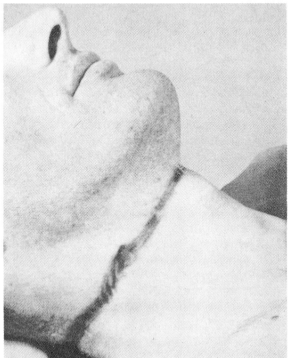

Fig. 125. Hanging from a low point of suspension; mark on neck simulating that of strangulation by a ligature. Site of knot at gap in mark (see also Plate 7).

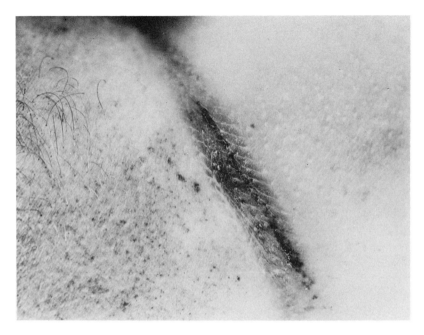

FIG. 126. Hanging mark: groove made by the ligature, diagonal imprint of strands
in the rope.

some platform, e.g. a stool or chair, will have been used by the victim to reach the point
suspension, as in the example depicted by Mant (1960).

The majority of the victims choose a point of suspension which permits hanging from
the standing posture, with the feet, or at least the toes, on the ground. Complete
suspension, to provide a "long drop", approximating to the circumstances of judicial
execution, is uncommon and occurred in only five of the Leeds cases. One man suspended
himself from the fourteenth rung of a 30-ft ladder, having used the rungs as his
"platform". In that case coincident head injury occurred when his body swung back
against the side of the ladder. Another suicide suspended himself from the bannister of a
staircase and had used the stair treads to reach the point of suspension. Both of these
victims sustained a fracture-dislocation of the neck. Complete suspension from the bough
of a tree occurred in two other cases (F.M. 161 and 4978A).

Example. A man, aged 39, had been left alone in his home for about $2^1/_2$ hours. When
his son returned, the man was found hanging in the well of the stairs between the first and
second floors. He was suspended by a length of rubber-covered flex, which was looped
once round the neck and tied to the bannister rail. The man was completely suspended,
with his feet on the level with, but in front of, the lower treads of the stairs. He was naked
but his head and shoulders were covered with a bedspread. It appears that the bedspread
had been inserted between the noose and the neck. As is not unusual in cases of auto-
erotic practices, the members of the family had no knowledge of his indulgence in them.
There was no motive for suicide. Marks on the bannisters indicated that he had practised
suspension in this manner on prior occasions. There was a mark in the skin of the neck

consistent with the application of a noose with its knot at the back of the neck; the mark was red when he was cut down but the colour had faded at the time of the autopsy. There was no injury to the neck muscles nor fracture of the larynx and hyoid bone. This indicated that he had not jumped from the stairs, as in suicide; it was consistent with miscalculation during an autoerotic practice (F.M. 10,660).

Hanging can be accomplished only too readily from low points of suspension, e.g. a door knob, the leg of a table, a bed post or rail, or the hand rail of a staircase (as depicted by Brouardel, 1897). These are points of suspension within 3 ft or less of the ground. It is even possible to hang oneself when supine in bed, as described and depicted by Harvey Littlejohn (1925) and by Brouardel (1897).

The point of suspension in Hurpy's (1881) case was only 17 in. from the floor. The victim, a woman aged 77, hanged herself by a ligature 40 in. long attached to the leg of the kitchen table; she was found lying on her chest on the floor.

Failure to find a platform at a scene of hanging by complete suspension must arouse suspicion but attention to detail may lead to its recognition. When a woman was found completely suspended, in the apparent absence of a platform, her husband came under suspicion. Fortunately for him, footprints, identified as those of the victim, were found on the table of a sewing machine near the body (Söderman and O'Connell, 1947).

The Posture and Clothing of the Victim

Hanging in the standing posture is readily effected by the simple act of flexing the knees. In a series of 261 cases of incomplete suspension, 168 or 64.3 per cent had both feet on the ground; 42 or 16.1 per cent were kneeling, twenty-nine or 11.1 per cent were recumbent and 19 or 7.3 per cent were seated; the other three were in a huddled or squatting posture (Tardieu, 1879).

The suspended body of a male clothed in female attire, or when nude, raises the presumption of accidental hanging, as also any complex arrangement of the ligature, especially if it involves the genitalia. The presence of padding between the ligature and the neck is distinctly unusual in suicide.

The "gondola" posture in Pontoni's case (cited Brouardel, 1897) is outwith the normal range of suicidal hanging but this seems the correct interpretation. It is deemed otherwise in respect of the unusual case depicted by Simonin (1955). A nude male lies prone, with a complex ligature around the neck and ankles, suspended by a second ligature to a bed post; the wrists were tied by a third ligature. The legend, with which I respectfully disagree, is "Suicide par pendaison incomplète compliquée de ligotage".

It is by no means certain that the case depicted by Gordon Turner and Price (1953) was a case of suicide. A complex arrangement of cord not only involved the neck but also the trunk and the perineum. Unfortunately their excellent pictures are not supported by details of this case.

Some of the victims secure their wrists and "walk through" their arms, as depicted by Tardieu (1879, Fig. 11), or as described by Filippi *et al.* (1889; cited Dixon Mann, 1908). The late Dr. Grace once examined a man, found suspended from the bracket of a street lamp; the victim's head was covered by his shirt, and his wrists, fastened by his own necktie, were behind his back. In my case (F.M. 1548, Fig. 124) the victim was blindfolded and had his wrists, fastened together with a strap, behind his back.

The case reported by Neugebauer (1937) still appears to be unique. Suspension had been effected by a fixed loop of a rope passed over a pulley to a peg on the right of the door. The victim was found in a standing posture with one foot on a chair. She held a knife pointing towards her vulva; she wore no knickers and held up her clothing with her left hand.

Suicide Pacts and Hanging

Suicide pacts, effected by hanging, are rare. Szekely (1924) described the case of two lovers who were found hanged by the same ligature which was fastened to the bough of a tree beneath which they were seated. Having fixed the ligature it remained only to incline their bodies backwards. In another case each victim stood on a chair, on the opposite sides of a door. When the male victim had fixed the ligature to his neck he passed the free end over the top of the door to enable his partner to fix it round her neck. When this was done, they jumped simultaneously and were hanged (Brouardel, 1897).

The Mechanism of Hanging

The effects of applying the weight of the body to a ligature round the neck are complex. The veins, arteries and the air-way may all be obstructed; there may be injury to the vagus nerves or their branches and there may be injury to the spine, spinal cord and the base of the skull. In any given case, however, only certain of these effects are produced and, in any event, it is rarely possible to demonstrate the degree of involvement of the vagi. Fracture of the spine, injury to the cord and to the base of the skull is likely only in judicial hanging or similar circumstances, i.e. when there is a long drop, e.g. equal to the height of the victim, an unusual event.

The effects are modified by the kind of ligature used, whether it be a fixed or running noose and, if fixed, by the position of the knot, but the effects depend more upon the degree of suspension, whether complete or incomplete.

Many people, even medical men, are surprised when they learn of the case with which it is possible for hanging to take place from low points of suspension, no more than a few inches from the floor. This, however, is readily understood when it is appreciated how little force is required to occlude the vessels of the neck and the airway and how much force is applied when, in a semi-reclining posture, only a fraction of the total body weight is exerted upon the ligature.

Brouardel (1897) estimated that the pull then exerted was of the order of 20–40 kg (44–88 lb). I have confirmed by experiment that the head and shoulders of a subject whose body weight was 10 stones exerted a pull of 30 lb on a ligature. The subject adopted a semi-reclining posture and a fixed loop was placed round his neck; the free end of the rope was passed over a pulley and weights were then tied to the rope until they equalled the weight of the head and shoulders.

Experiments by Hofmann, confirmed by Brouardel (1897), showed that the jugular veins are closed by a tension in the rope of 2 kg (4.4 lb) and when this was raised to 5 kg (11 lb) the carotid arteries were closed. An increase to 15 kg (33 lb) closed the trachea and at 30 kg (66 lb) the vertebral arteries were closed.

Reuter (1901) repeated these experiments and found that even less tension was required to produce the effects. The carotid arteries, for example, were closed by a tension of only 3.5 kg (rather less than 8 lb) and the vertebral arteries were closed by a tension of 16.6 kg (about $36^{1}/_{2}$ lb).

By experiment I have confirmed that the carotid artery is appreciably obstructed by a ligature under low tension. Having first established free flow of fluid between the common carotid artery, exposed in the upper chest, and the internal carotid artery, seen inside the skull after removal of the calvarium, I then applied a ligature with a running noose round the neck. Weights were added and injection was repeated, below the level of the ligature. The tests showed that a pull of as little as 7 lb (3.2 kg) was sufficient to reduce free flow through the artery to a mere trickle.

Severe obstruction of the carotid arteries, which requires only a tension of about 3 kg (6.6 lb), will rapidly induce cerebral anoxia and unconsciousness. This accounts for the failure of these suicides to save themselves, if they changed their minds, by a simple movement to ease the tension on the ligature. Once launched upon suicide by hanging there is no retreat. Unconsciousness is almost instantaneous although death may not ensue for some minutes after the body is suspended.

Slow asphyxia is the exception in hanging and is likely to occur only when the point of suspension is a low one, or the ligature exerts pressure below the chin and does not encircle the neck. It occurred, for example, when the loop was within 4 in. of the floor and the greater part of the victim's body lay prone, in contact with the floor (F.M. 1548, Fig. 124). It can also occur if the ligature breaks between the knot and the point of suspension, then slackens a little, but still remains tight round the neck.

Modification of the Mechanism by the Position of the Knot

When a fixed loop is used with the knot at the back of the neck, sometimes termed "typical hanging", the weight of the body bears principally on the front of the neck and a force, of almost equal amount, is applied also to the sides of the neck. The result is that the loop draws the base of the tongue upwards against the posterior pharyngeal wall and folds the epiglottis over the entrance to the larynx to occlude the air-way, as shown by the experiments of Langreuter (1886). Using the bodies of persons who had died of natural causes, he cut away part of the skull and prepared the parts in a manner which permitted direct inspection of the effects of applying a ligature as in hanging. He found that only moderate tension was necessary to close the air passages and this was due to the ascent of the tongue and displacement of the pharynx, folding back the epiglottis. When, however, the ligature was applied over, or below, the thyroid cartilage, the vocal cords were not closed by an upward and backward pull of great force. Experiments with a rolled handkerchief yielded similar results but they required greater force than did a cord (Dixon Mann, 1908). Ecker (1870) examined the frozen body of a man found hanging from a tree in winter. When he sectioned it in the vertical plane, it was shown that the tongue was doubled up and had ascended to the naso-pharynx. Hofmann (cited by Tidy, 1883) confirmed this observation by section of bodies which were first frozen to preserve the position of the parts.

Even so, it was his opinion that closure of the large vessels was the more important factor in hanging. The result is immediate arrest, or severe reduction, of cerebral circulation. Unconsciousness must be rapid and death is not long delayed, i.e. between 10 and 20 minutes. It has been found in judicial hanging that the vertebral arteries may remain patent and the heart-beat continue for from 5 to 20 minutes (Kalle, 1933).

The victims usually present but slight evidence of asphyxia, when suspension is complete or in the standing posture.

Closure of the air-way is not an essential ingredient of hanging. Reineboth (1895) described the suicide by hanging of a man who had had a tracheotomy for relief of cancer of the throat. Although he had died from hanging, the ligature was above the tracheotomy (Bertelsmann, cited Puppe, 1908, described another example).

When hanging has occurred in the sitting or semi-reclining posture, it is then likely that the tension exerted on the ligature has been insufficient appreciably to reduce cerebral circulation. Obstruction of the jugular veins, while the arteries remain patent, leads to severe engorgement of the head and neck. Obstruction of the air-way is the main result and these victims die of asphyxia rather than cerebral anoxia. At the same time, obstruction of the cerebral circulation is then sufficient to cause rapid loss of consciousness.

Cord or medulla injuries are unusual events in suicidal hanging. The inexperienced should be mindful of the possibility of false fractures of the cervical spine. These can be produced either by rough handling of the body or forced flexion of the head when reflecting the scalp. They present as transverse splits in the spinal column at the level of the discs between C4/5 and C5/6 and, *note*, they may be accompanied by slight oozing of the blood in their vicinity. Genuine fractures of the spine are unusual in suicidal hanging.

Hanging in the semi-reclining or sitting posture, especially when a running noose is used, may cause asphyxial phenomena to dominate the picture and, the mark, taking a horizontal course, may resemble that of strangulation. Collateral evidence is then important, notably a reliable description of the scene before there has been any interference.

Although the ligature in hanging makes contact with the region of the carotid sinuses, it appears that death from vagal inhibition in hanging (as in F.M. 7935) is the exception and not the rule. Kalle's observations, in particular, suggest that the cause of death is other than vagal stimulation. In death by strangulation, on the other hand, and, in particular, manual strangulation, a proportion of the deaths are due to vagal inhibition alone.

The Symptoms of Hanging

There are few survivors, and fewer still amongst them give an account of their symptoms. Experimental observations, such as those of Minovici (1905, cited by Martin, 1950), are exceptional; indeed, his experiments are apparently unique, which is as well in view of the risks involved.

A woman, who attempted suicide by hanging herself from the foot of her bed, was saved by a fellow prisoner. She told Marc (1851) that she had attempted to strangle herself whilst kneeling at the foot of the bed. She experienced severe pain and then lost consciousness. She could remember nothing of what happened afterwards and was unaware of the length of time she had been suspended from the bed. Marc believed she had been found soon after the event or she would have died. She made a complete recovery, although for a time she had symptoms of cerebral congestion.

Petrina (1880), cited Dixon Mann (1908), described the recovery of a victim of attempted suicide by hanging. The man remained unconscious for 24 hours and during that time had violent clonic convulsions of the whole body, followed by generalised muscular rigidity. When he became conscious he had a crossed paralysis, involving the right side of the face and the left side of the body. This passed but was followed by ataxia on the right side of the body, extending later to both sides. In Terrien's (1887) case, epileptiform convulsions were accompanied by tetanic spasm; the victim remained unconscious for several days after the hanging. In his second case, Terrien found the convulsions accompanied by opisthotonus. When the victim recovered consciousness he made movements as if walking. Wagner (1889), cited by Dixon Mann (1908), described another case in which acute dementia was said to be due to attempted suicide by hanging.

Experimental hanging was described anonymously in the *Medical Times and Gazette*, 1882, **ii**, 729. The symptoms then experienced were a feeling of heat in the head, flashes of light in the eyes and a deafening sound in the ears; there was also a benumbed feeling in the legs. Pain was not acute. Commenting on this, Tidy (1883) said loss of consciousness was sudden. The event may be noisy or noiseless; there may be no convulsive phase. A man had hanged himself in a sitting position in bed and yet two children who shared the bed were not awakened (Ogston, 1878).

Recovery from hanging occurred when one Harnshaw, accustomed to suspend himself for public entertainment, mistimed his act. He said he had lost consciousness almost at once. He could not get his breath and felt as if a great weight was attached to his feet; he had been unable to move his hands to save himself. The power of thinking was quickly lost (Tidy, 1883).

Another victim, aged 33, who hanged herself when drunk, was rescued within a few minutes; the precise duration of suspension did not exceed 10 minutes. She was unconscious, her face was pale and her breathing was slow and laborious; a dusky red mark, $^1/_4$ in. wide, was present on her neck. She had used a silk handkerchief with the knot at the right side of her neck (Tidy, 1883).

Loss of consciousness in hanging, when not instantaneous, is rapid. Minovici became unconscious almost at once when a maximum tension of only 5 kg was exerted on the ligature. When suspension was incomplete, i.e. when he leant on the cord, his face at once became reddish-violet, his sight was blurred and he had whistling in his ears, all within 5 to 6 seconds. When the knot was at the nape of the neck the ligature rapidly closed the blood vessels and air-way. Tolerance of the ligature when its knot was at the side of the neck was more prolonged but only for about 8 or 9 seconds.

Minovici, a man who weighed 79 kg, also experienced the effects of complete suspension, his feet being raised a metre above the ground. From the first moments, until he descended, he experienced pain at the site of the knot; the pain to the right of his hyoid bone was so intense that he could not continue the experiment. As soon as his feet left the ground, his eyelids contracted violently and closure of the air-way was complete so that he found it impossible to breathe. He could not hear the voice of his assistant, who was holding the cord, as he counted the number of seconds. Whistling in his ears and inability to breathe compelled a prompt conclusion of the experiment. When he was released he had watering of the eyes and increasing difficulty in swallowing, the pain being especially severe in the neighbourhood of the great horns of the hyoid bone. These signs persisted for 10 to 12 days. There was congestion of his pharynx and dryness of the throat; great thirst persisted for 1 or 2 days. The mark of the cord presented as a groove accompanied by many small haemorrhages which were confluent especially to the right of the hyoid bone and near the mastoid process. These haemorrhages appeared at about 5 to 10 minutes after his release and persisted for 8 to 11 days.

Minovici also tried the effects of a running noose but, despite his courage, after experiencing effects similar to those already described, he stopped the experiment within 5 seconds.

Some of those who have attempted suicide by hanging have described the pain as mild. They may, however, experience a retrograde amnesia and their accounts are unreliable. If suspended for a longer time than that endured by Minovici, the victim passes into a convulsive phase, during which he is unconscious. He may then drum on a door with his feet or overturn and break furniture nearby.

> A man aged 20 made a noose with a silk stocking and hung it on a hook behind the door of his room. He climbed on to a chair, put his head through the noose, and stepped off "to see if his feet would touch the floor". He found his feet were a few inches short. The slip-knot tightened and he was unable to release the pressure on his throat. During his struggles he kicked a chair over and, when his mother heard the noise, she went to discover the cause. The man was then unconscious but she had the presence of mind immediately to cut the stocking. After a brief stay in hospital he was able to return home (*The Yorkshire Post*, 1 May 1948).

It is possible that when found some of these victims are in a state of suspended animation. It is at least a sound policy to assume they may yet be alive and therefore to be prompt to cut them down and institute resuscitation forthwith.

Those who are rescued will retain signs of the mark on the neck for several days. This was Minovici's experience, confirmed by that of the man of 20 already mentioned, and by one of the illustrations in Hofmann (1927), which shows a well-defined mark on the neck 8 days after suspension. There has been one instance of survival in our own records. This was a youth who slipped and got his neck entangled in the cord of a window blind. He was promptly rescued. A photograph in colour shows a clear congested mark round the neck, still pronounced several days after the accident. (Unfortunately the clinical notes were lost.)

As soon as the ligature is relaxed, blood returns to the region of the groove but, because vessels have been injured by the ligature, haemorrhage occurs in the neighbourhood. This was apparent in Minovici's neck within 5 to 10 minutes after his descent.

Pain on swallowing is usual and was a pronounced feature in Minovici's experiments. There may be aphonia.

Late results may include delayed shock and bronchopneumonia. Cerebral anoxia during suspension may cause permanent cerebral damage, the extent of which may not be apparent for some time after rescue. A guarded prognosis should be given until a few weeks have passed and recovery appears to be complete.

Death delayed for several days after hanging is indeed rare. Thomas and Kluyskens (1962) recorded the case of a woman aged 63, a neurasthenic, who had suspended herself during a short absence by her husband. She was promptly cut down and resuscitated but she died 15 days later, not from respiratory complications, but from cerebral damage due to cerebral anoxia following compression of her carotid arteries during suspension. Her hyoid bone was intact but both superior horns of the thyroid cartilage were broken. Histological preparations demonstrated reparative changes in the fracture sites. (The authors traced one other report, that of repair of the left horn of the thyroid cartilage of a man aged 60, whose death was also a delayed result of suspension.)

The External Signs of Hanging

The mark on the neck is the principal external sign of hanging. It requires detailed inspection, bearing in mind, meantime, the possibility of coincident signs of strangulation. Strangulation must be excluded when information concerning the circumstances of the death is incomplete or unsatisfactory. Difficulty can arise when the ligature breaks at a point between the knot and the point of suspension. The victim may be found, for example, at the foot of a tree in circumstances which at first suggest strangulation by a ligature. The other end of the ligature may still be tied to a branch high up in the tree. Comparison of the free ends of the ligature will show them to coincide and that a break had occurred, at, or shortly after, the moment of suspension. On these occasions the ligature round the neck may relax sufficiently to permit limited circulation of the blood to the head and, in consequence, the victim may present the appearances of slow mechanical asphyxia.

The mark of a fixed loop takes the form of a groove which is deepest opposite the knot. Here the width of the groove is about, or rather less than, the width of the ligature. The skin in the groove is pale or it may be yellowish-brown, and is not infrequently hard, like parchment. Any well-defined pattern in the ligature is likely to be reproduced in the groove; even when the cord is comprised of strands, the latter may produce a faint diagonal marking in the groove (Fig. 126). If suspension is during life, it is likely that a thin red line of congestion or haemorrhage will be seen above and below the groove at some points, if not throughout its course.

The groove nearly always lies above the larynx and its course is to be traced round the neck, although the mark is rarely as clear as the nape as at the front or sides of the neck; in the region of the knot the mark takes an upward course to form an inverted "V"; the apex of the "V" corresponds with the site of the knot (Figs. 122, 123).

Scratches or abrasions on the neck of the suspended victim at once excite suspicion. It is remotely possible that a victim might pluck at the ligature and, if he had long nails, he could then abrade his skin. As a rule, however, any definite scratches and, certainly, crescentic nail-marks point to manual strangulation prior to hanging; if associated with bruising of the neck structures and fracture of the larynx, the probability of murder is strong. Care is necessary, however, since the upward movement of the rope at the time of suspension may scratch the skin. Low magnification may permit the distinction, since there is then unlikely to be any vital reaction, e.g. no bruising of the skin (Walcher's case, 1935).

A third possibility is that scratches, indeed nail marks, on the neck may be produced by another, not in an attempt to throttle, but in attempted resuscitation. A man aged 42 was found suspended in his cell. He had died of hanging but, in addition to a ligature mark round the neck, there were several scratches on the skin. Some could have been "tentative" marks of cut-throat but three curved scratches, directed downwards, under the chin were identified as nail marks. Inquiry showed that these had been made by a prison officer during his attempt to cut the ligature prior to applying artificial respiration (F.M. 3036).

Differential Diagnosis of the Mark

When present, the mark on the neck is distinctive, but certain possibilities, if overlooked, may erroneously suggest hanging (or strangulation). A "mark" may appear on the neck of an obese subject, particularly a fat baby, as a result of hypostasis. The skin in the natural folds of the neck remains pale by contact flattening and hypost asis ends abruptly on each side of the fold. When the neck is extended the resulting appearances superficially resemble those produced by a ligature. The "mark" however, can easily be shown to coincide precisely with folds in the neck.

Tight neckwear, through contact flattening, may also yield a mark which superficially resembles that of a ligature. The helmet-like hats, modelled on airmen's helmets, worn by children produce contact flattening which may mislead, as in the case of a boy found drowned in 1951. The true cause of the mark was at once apparent when he was known to have worn this kind of hat; it was replaced on his head and shown precisely to fit the mark.

The use of soft ligatures, especially broad ones, applied only for a short time, may lead to difficulty in the diagnosis of hanging as well as of strangulation, since the resulting mark may be faint or there may be none. In hanging, however, it is usual but not invariable to have collateral information which leaves the fact of suspension beyond doubt.

Other External Appearances in Hanging

The face of the victim is usually pale or of leaden hue. Severe cyanosis is likely only when hanging is effected from a low point of suspension or the ligature has broken between the knot and the point of suspension (Fig. 124). In contrast to other circumstances, notably strangulation, choking or smothering, the faces of those who were hanged were placid, as seen in twenty-one of forty cases (Ogston, 1878). Whilst suspended, or shortly after the body has been cut down, puffiness of the face may be apparent but it has usually disappeared by the time the body comes to autopsy. There may also be evidence of excessive salivation, more likely to be noticed at the scene of suspension than in the post-mortem room. The tongue may be swollen and protrude between the lips or it may be behind the teeth; protrusion occurred in fourteen of forty cases (Ogston, 1878). Blood-stained froth at the lips or nose is uncommon. The right eye may remain open and the left closed with the left pupil small and the right dilated, i.e. "le facies sympathique" (Étienne Martin, 1950); it is an ante-mortem phenomenon and therefore important. Lopes (1945) believes it is a result of unequal tension on the neck structures.

Petechial haemorrhages, as in any other asphyxial death, may be present in the skin of the face and forehead and beneath the conjunctivae. They are, however, infrequent, being absent in nine out of every ten victims; they are normally present when hanging has been from a low point.

Haemorrhages of post-mortem origin, in the dependent parts, e.g. Harvey Littlejohn's case (1925), are uncommon since it is usual to find the victim within a short time of suspension.

Internal Signs of Hanging

The Neck Structures

Bruising, and occasionally rupture of the muscles, notably the sternomastoid, may be seen, but it occurs in only from 2 to 12 per cent of bodies. There may be bleeding between the pharynx and the spine, a feature emphasised by Brouardel (1897), by other French authors and by Lopes (1945), but in my experience, it is an uncommon event. The carotid arteries may be injured by the ligature whereby there is slight bleeding into their walls or a horizontal breach of the intima at the level of the ligature (Amusat, 1828, cited Brouardel, 1897); this is seen in only about 5 per cent of hangings. This may be a "traction" injury.

The hyoid bone may be broken. The fractures involve the great horns, which are likely to break at about the junction of their outer third and inner two-thirds (Fig. 127). Although this can be a traction or "tug" fracture (Camps and Hunt, 1959) it is more likely to be a direct result of the application of the ligature to the neck.

There is lack of unanimity of opinion concerning the frequency with which fracture of the hyoid bone occurs in hanging. Reuter (1901) held this fracture to be relatively common, present in 60 per cent of "typical" and 30 per cent of atypical hangings, i.e. where the knot is at the side of the neck. Étienne Martin (1933) had made a collection of these fractured bones and describes the event as "assez fréquente" in hanging. Smith and Fiddes (1955) said that "the hyoid bone is practically never injured".

This discrepancy is in part explained by a consideration of the ages of the victims; those under 40 years of age are unlikely to have a fracture of the bone. The incidence in any particular series also depends upon the extent of the search. Our experience coincides with that of Martin, who rightly stresses that the fractures can be easily overlooked unless a detailed dissection is made.

Fracture of the hyoid bone is a probable finding in a seventh of all hangings and in a fifth of victims aged over 40 years, irrespective of the mode of hanging. Weintraub (1961) found the hyoid bone fractured in nine or 27 per cent of thirty-three cases.

In our experience the thyroid cartilage was the most susceptible to fracture in hanging. In a series of eighty consecutive cases, of which the age range was from 18 months to 81 years, the great horn or horns of the thyroid cartilage, with or without coincident fracture of the hyoid bone, was found in thirty-seven, or almost 50 per cent, of the cases.

Fracture of the hyoid bone was only half as frequent; it occurred, alone or with fracture of the thyroid cartilage, in twenty or 25 per cent. In seven of these persons the hyoid bone was alone fractured; although uncommon, this, therefore, is not rare. Camps and Hunt (1959) found fracture of the hyoid bone comparatively frequent and suggested it was due to downward traction on it.

The series confirmed the fact that fracture of the thyroid cartilage and hyoid bone was appreciably more frequent in persons of over 40 years of age, i.e. in those in whom the hyoid bone is likely to be ankylosed and the thyroid cartilage ossified. These fractures were present in thirty-eight of those aged 40 or over but in only nine of those who were under that age, i.e., a ratio of over 4:1. Absence of fractures in those over 40 was also accounted for in some of the cases by the fact that they had chosen a low point of suspension; one had arranged the knot in front of his face (F.M. 7935; Figs 118, 119) and another had a congenital absence of the great horns of the thyroid cartilage (F.M. 1008).

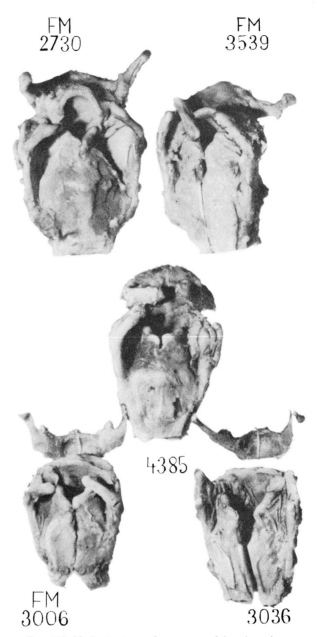

FIG. 127. Neck structures from cases of hanging: demonstrating fractures of hyoid bone and great horns of the
thyroid cartilage.

Fracture of the body of the thyroid cartilage was distinctly uncommon; there was one instance of fracture of an ala (F.M. 560).

A man, aged 64, who had a fracture of the right ala of his thyroid cartilage had hanged himself by tying the ligature to the bannisters; he then climbed over the top with the rope round his neck and jumped into the well of the stairs. The knot of the ligature was on the left side of the neck (F.M. 560).

Injury to the trachea is unusual; the only instance accompanied a fracture-dislocation of the neck, following hanging by a jump from a ladder, with complete suspension of the body (Leeds City Coroner, No. 76/47). Fracture-dislocation of the neck was also rare; the only other example followed hanging from bannisters, with a fall into the well of the hall, there being complete suspension (Leeds City Coroner, No. 386/47). These are the only two in a series of 188 hangings (other than judicial hangings) in Leeds during 1926–60. This coincides with the experience of Lopes (1945) who had only two instances of such fractures, each following a long drop, in a series of 242 hangings.

On two occasions alone was it not possible to demonstrate bleeding in the line of fracture of the great horns of the thyroid cartilages. There was, however, no doubt about the circumstances, which were proved to be those of suicide. One victim, a woman aged 28, was found completely suspended from a hook behind a door by a fixed loop of which the knot was at the occiput. The hyoid bone was intact but both horns of the thyroid cartilage were broken. No bleeding was detected at the lines of fracture. The other victim, a man aged 44, was found at the foot of a tree with the loop round his neck. The ligature was broken and the other end was tied to a branch of a tree, 14 ft above the ground. Although it was a running noose, it was still tight round his neck, closed on the right side. The left horn of the thyroid cartilage was bent backwards by a fracture-dislocation but bleeding was not apparent at the line of fracture. He had three lacerated wounds of the scalp at the back of the head and these showed vital reaction. Whether they occurred as he swung from the bough against the tree or whether they had been inflicted by his wife during an altercation at his home before he went to hang himself was not determined. As a result of her injuries the widow was too ill to attend the inquest (F.M. 161).

Fractures of the hyoid bone were divided by Weintraub (1961) into (a) those caused by inward compression, (b) those due to antero-posterior compression and (c) avulsion fractures. The latter are sometimes called "tug" or "traction" fractures, the result of muscular pull and not direct injury to the bone. In inward compression fractures, the distal fragment should be bent inwards; the periosteum may be torn on the outer side but on the inner side it may be intact. Conversely, antero-posterior compression displaces the distal fragment outwards and the periosteum may be torn on the inner side alone. Weintraub stresses the importance of the injury to the soft parts since the fracture line itself gives no clear indication of the mechanism of its production. In our experience hanging has produced both inward and outward fractures of the hyoid bone, or, as Weintraub found, one horn may be fractured on the inner side and the other on the outer side. Deductions from the position of the fragments are to be drawn with caution, but his experience that outward fracture of the bone did not occur in throttling is likely to be general.

Accidental Hanging

Cases of accidental hanging are divisible into two distinct groups. One includes the cases where hanging occurred during play or when at work, in circumstances which were essentially accidental. The other group is of hanging as a concomitant of sexual deviation or accidents arising out of experiments with ropes, cords or chains, etc., i.e. auto-erotic accidents.

The first group requires no detailed description and the examples given below are self-explanatory.

Accidental hanging in the course of some abnormal sexual practice has certain characteristics which are virtually specific. The victims are exclusively males. No authentic instance of a female victim has yet been recorded. [The case of Neugebauer (1937, see p. 368) might have had a sexual element.] Some are nude, some are attired in female garments, and others, if normally clothed, may have opened their trousers and there is evidence of manipulation or bandaging of the genitalia. Protection of the neck is by soft material, a handkerchief, vest or other cloth, interposed between the ligature and the skin of the neck. (An excellent example was depicted by van Hecke and Timperman (1963) and our case F.M. 10,616A.) This is a rare step in suicidal hanging.

A complex arrangement of the ligature which involves the genital area also points to accidents of this kind; the wrists may be fastened and, as in one of our cases, the victim may blindfold himself. Some arrange mirrors in which to watch events (Koopmann, 1938; Mann, 1960) or arrange a camera to record them (Reuter, 1938). The victim may have in his possession, at the scene or elsewhere, pornographic literature or obscene photographs.

Even in the absence of positive evidence of some abnormal sexual practice, these accidents often occur in circumstances which involve more preparation than that made by suicides. The more bizarre and unusual the circumstances, the less likely are they to have been those of suicide.

Sexual deviation not infrequently leads to the performance of sexual acts in circumstances of partial asphyxia which may enhance sexual sensation. Some have inhaled coal gas, others suffocated themselves, e.g. in plastic bags, and yet others suspended themselves. There is no intent to commit suicide; the victims do not realise the grave danger of these practices or miscalculate the safety margin which is indeed narrow. It can be, also, that having successfully evaded a fatal accident on one or more occasions, they grow careless. It does not follow that each fatality is the result of a first attempt; there may have been repeated incidents prior to the fatal one. The case reported by Thomas and van Hecke (1959) was most unusual.

Some of these cases are described as accidents resulting from experiments with ropes, etc. When the victim is very young, say under 12, it is difficult to believe the basic cause is sexual deviation. An example cited below concerned a boy aged 11 years. It could be that he had been conducting an "experiment" with the noose. In such cases this is perhaps the fairest interpretation. Something he had read about or seen may have prompted his acts. Suicide has occurred in children at the age of 10 years.

The manner in which the rope or cord is tied requires attention. If of a kind unlikely to be known to the deceased and one used in some special circumstances, the possibility of murder arises, e.g. the use of a sailor's knot; see the case in Beck and Beck (1836).

Accidental Hanging at Play

Case 1. A boy, aged 6 years, was found suspended from the finial of a garage by a lasso which was part of a cowboy's outfit he had been given; the rope was about 2 ft long. He had walked along the top of the wall at the rear of the garage and thrown the loop over the finial. He then lost his balance and slipped between the wall,

5 ft 6 in. high, and the garage, 8 ft 6 in. high, i.e. out of sight and became suspended by the lower part of the loop which was round his neck. Injuries to his forehead and face, and scratch marks on the wall by his shoes, showed that he had struggled in vain to escape from his predicament (Leeds City Coroner, 336/1937).

Case 2. A girl aged 3 years was found suspended by her chin in a loop of curtain material, the ends of which were tied to a clothes post. The older children had used the loop as a swing. The victim had reached the loop by standing on an overturned pram nearby and, it seems, had slipped and passed her head into the loop. She was alive at the time of suspension. She had been playing with a boy aged 6 years, who had gone away to buy a balloon, and when he returned he found her "asleep on the line". The loop was 2 ft 6 in. from the ground (F.M. 498).

Case 3. This female infant, aged 10 months, had slipped out of a swing in which she had been fastened by a scarf. When her mother returned to the room a few minutes later the child was found suspended by the scarf (F.M. 1327).

Case 4. An epileptic was found dead in bed. His body lay over the side of the bed so that his face and chest rested on the floor. His nightshirt was held between his body and the bed and its collar was thus tightly drawn around his neck, where there was a shallow mark, $^1/_2$ in. broad, bordered by haemorrhages. Lesser (1890), who reported the case, was unable to exclude homicidal strangulation. It was also possible that the real cause of the asphyxia was obstruction of the nose and mouth by the carpet. Carry-cot or pram harness has also been the agent of accidental hanging (F.M. 11,889A).

Another variation of accidental hanging occurs when boys climb trees or railings. They lose their foothold and, in falling, their coat or some other garment is caught by a bough or spike and is drawn tight round the neck. Zulch (1894, cited Dixon Mann, 1908) recorded a case; others are reported from time to time in the Press.

Auto-erotic Hanging

Case 1. This was a man aged 64 who was found lying face down with his head in a noose which was suspended from a beam in his cellar. The noose was within 6 in. of the floor. His fly was open and the genitalia were bound with a handkerchief; ejaculation had recently occurred. His wrists were bound with khaki webbing and its clasp was against his body; he was blindfolded. He was an "escapologist" and was known to practise tying himself and his wife with ligatures; a doll in the bedroom had been similarly treated. He had books on escapology and pornography in a locked bookcase. Death had been by slow asphyxia (F.M. 1548, Figs, 124, 128).

Case 2. A university undergraduate aged 20 was found nude in the bathroom, suspended by a length of climbing rope attached to a point inside the airing cupboard; he had placed underclothing between the loop and his neck. He was incompletely suspended, his feet being on the floor. Attention was drawn to the accident by the fact that the water was running and the bath was emptying by the overflow. His parents had retired but the father heard the water and went to find the cause; the bathroom door was not locked. The victim was found slumped near the airing cupboard. He was interested in rock-climbing and had experimented with ropes about the house. Some evidence of an interest in pornographic matters was found amongst his effects (P.M. by Dr. John Benstead, 1950).

Case 3. A man, aged 30, was found nude, lying face down with his elbows resting on the top step of stairs to the landing near his bedroom; the rest of his body lay on the stairs, directed downwards. A ligature, a soldier's lanyard, had been tied to the newel of the bannisters, passed round his neck and down his back, to end in a slip knot which enclosed his penis and scrotum. A second cord, a short length of twine, was fixed, also with a slip knot, round the root of his penis; the free end of this cord was in his left hand. Suspension was incomplete and he had died of asphyxia. Petechial haemorrhages were plentiful in the skin of his face where they had a rashlike distribution; his tongue was indented but not bitten. Haemorrhages were present in the submucosa of his larynx, both behind the epiglottis and in the sub-glottic space. The root of the tongue, pharynx and tonsils were engorged. The hyoid bone and larynx were intact. The mark on the neck took a horizontal course at about the level of the upper border of the larynx; it was incomplete on the left side; it was up to $^1/_4$ in. broad and $^1/_8$ in. deep.

It is probable that this incident began on the landing but he had moved and his body had slipped downstairs. If this had been other than a first attempt, his wife was completely unaware of his practice. There was nothing to suggest that he would have intended suicide (F.M. 1822).

This case resembled that recorded by Weimann (1935) except that on that occasion the victim had used a relatively high point of suspension; an overturned stool was near his feet. It also resembles the case reported by Mann (1960). The victim, a student aged 19, was found nude in his locked bedroom. He was seated before a mirror. A cord was looped round his penis; the free ends had been passed backwards below the perineum to the top of his bedpost and from there the ends had been brought round his neck and fastened with a large bow in front of it. He had used a towel to pad the ligature round his neck.

Case 4. In another of our cases the victim was a well-developed boy aged 15 years. He was suspended by a length of plastic clothes line from a beam in the attic of his home. He had inserted a handkerchief between the ligature and his neck. He was clothed in a shirt and trousers but the fly of the trousers was open. The attic overlooked adjacent houses and some binoculars were near the body. There was no motive for suicide and, despite his age, the evidence pointed to sexual deviation (F.M. 7932).

Case 5. A man aged 26 was found hanged in his hall. He had tied a long cord to the newel post of the bannisters and had then gone downstairs and arranged a loop with a running noose around his neck; a nylon stocking had been inserted between the loop and the skin of his neck. He was in the standing posture with his knees flexed (Fig. 129). Had he not lost consciousness it would have been a simple matter to stand up and relax the pull on the loop.

He was wearing female underwear, earrings and a necklace; he had women's shoes on his feet. He had also donned one of the wigs at that time popular amongst young women (Fig. 129).

The circumstances were those of an erotic practice and his death was due to miscalculation of its hazard. Hanging was effected by the simple step of flexing the knees.

Case 6. A boy, aged 13, was found suspended with his chin in a loop of cloth fixed to a clothes rail inside a wardrobe. His feet were on the floor of the wardrobe and his knees were flexed. He had recently viewed a television programme in which a girl had attempted suicide by hanging (F.M. 10, 611). (This case may have been purely imitative, without any sexual content and may more properly belong to the former group of accidents.)

Case 7. A boy aged 16 was found fully suspended by a roller towel, looped over a central heating pipe in the toilet in a remand home. His trousers were lowered to his ankles and his penis was erect. There was no bruising of his neck muscles; the hyoid bone and thyroid cartilage were intact. Suicide was not excluded but this was less probable than death during an auto-erotic exercise (F.M. 12,477).

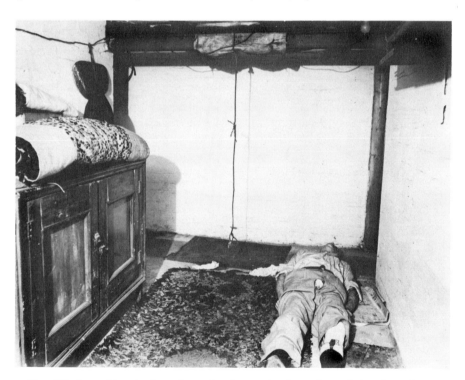

Fig. 128. Scene of hanging from a low point of suspension: knotted rope tied to a beam; loop within inches of the ground. Victim, when found, had his head in the loop, face and body to floor.

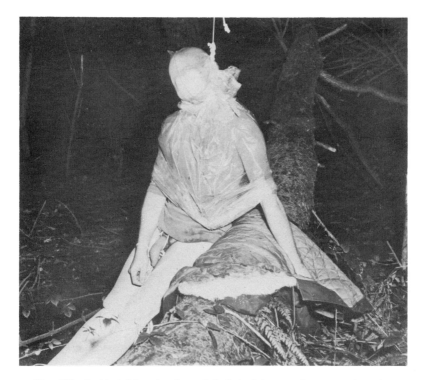

FIG. 129. Accidental hanging (sexual deviation) by a male transvestite, who inhaled a volatile substance from a pad inside the plastic bag over the face. Note ligatures around wrist and penis (F.M. 18363A).

Accidental Hanging: "Experiments" with Ropes

Case 1. The victim was a boy aged $11^3/_4$ years. He was found, slumped forward and incompletely seated on the toilet, with his head in a noose suspended from the outlet pipe of the cistern. He was fully clothed but his trousers and underpants were lowered, as if he had intended to use the toilet. The rope had been tied with several knots to a tap on the nearby wash basin and passed twice round the bend of the cistern piping; the free end had been made into a running noose, suspended at a level which coincided with that of his head and neck when seated on the toilet. The rubber mat on the floor in front of the toilet was partly displaced; he could have skidded on it.

Although suicide is not unknown even at this age, there was no motive for suicide and his religious faith discourages suicide. There was no doubt that care and thought had been used in arranging this noose. Was the case one of sexual deviation? Even at his age it is not impossible. There was slender evidence to show that he had played with a rope in the woods with one of his friends. The case was undoubtedly one of accidental hanging but with insufficient evidence to indicate sexual deviation (F.M. 6041, Fig. 130).

Case 2. The victim was a boy aged 16, an illegitimate child, who had been put on probation by a Juvenile Court on conviction of an offence, the nature of which was not disclosed at the inquest. It was a condition of his probation that he resided at a Home. He was employed as a page boy at a hotel. Those at the Home described him as a jolly boy, not depressed; he had never threatened suicide. His mother, on the other hand, maintained he was unhappy, there were domestic troubles and he disliked the Home.

On the evening of his death he had watched the television until 9.30 p.m. and then appeared normal. He went out to the garage of the Home ostensibly to clean his shoes. Another boy went to the garage and saw him standing on a chair, manipulating a rope which he had passed over a beam 8 ft from the ground; he was pulling it backwards and forwards and said he was making a swing.

The deceased's brother returned to the Home at about 9.55 p.m. and looked for his brother to wish him goodnight. He could not find him. He was told to go to the garage and, when he switched on the light, he saw

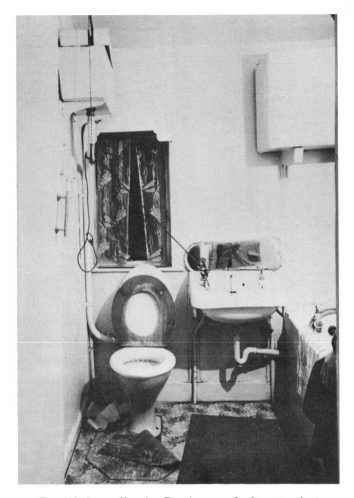

FIG. 130. Scene of hanging. Running noose fixed to water pipe to toilet. Deceased half-seated on toilet. (Either a sexual deviation or "experimental" accident or suicide.)

his brother completely suspended from the beam. It appears he had arranged the rope with a big loop which was not tight all around his neck. The loop was so big that the witness, the Welfare Officer of the Home, wondered that he had not slipped out of it. There was a handkerchief inserted between the rope and the deceased's neck. He confirmed that the boy was completely suspended but there was a chair nearby. The mark on the neck was of a kind produced by a loose loop and forward inclination of the body on to it. The face was blue.

The brother's evidence was unsatisfactory. To his mother he repeated that he and the deceased used to truss each other up with ropes but to the coroner he denied that they had ever played with ropes of string, either in the garage or elsewhere. Their mother, however, alleged she had seen them tie each other up; they had done so quite a lot.

The depositions, of which the foregoing is a summary, occasion no surprise that the coroner returned an open verdict. There might have been some motive for suicide—a recent conviction and, if the mother had been correct, the boy was unhappy. Those at the Home maintained he was not depressed or unhappy. The brother, who appears to have been an unreliable witness, had made a statement to the police in which he said that, when he asked where the deceased was, he had been told he had gone to the garage with a piece of string to strangle himself. At the inquest he said he did not know why he had said this to the officer. "I was brought out of bed and did not know what I was saying." The boy who was alleged to have mentioned strangling denied that he had said such a thing or anything like that—that he could remember. On the other hand there is evidence, notably that of the mother, that the deceased and his brother used to practise trussing each other with ropes or string. It is also not unimportant that he had protected the skin of his neck with a handkerchief, a step rare in suicide but a well recognised feature of sexual deviation (accidental) hanging. Although no conclusion can be drawn about this case, the balance of probability favours the latter explanation of the death (F.M. 7081).

Exclusion of suicide on the ground of age alone is not justified since it is in our experience that unequivocal evidence of suicide was obtained when the subject was only 10 years of age. Intent could be at an even earlier age. On one occasion, a boy, aged 8, who had hanged himself from the branch of a tree, was deemed to have been conducting an experiment or playing with a rope; there were special circumstances which called for the avoidance of an erroneous verdict of suicide. To this end the pathological findings were augmented by the opinion of a psychiatrist (at the request of the pathologist). About a year later his mother was killed in a road accident and her handbag contained a letter, which had been written by her dead son, but which she had suppressed. It contained an unequivocal threat of suicide. The father, and not the mother, gave evidence at the inquest on the boy.

If error is to occur on these occasions it should be in favour of misadventure; a verdict of suicide requires clear evidence of intent, notwithstanding that suicide was absolved from criminality by the Suicide Act, 1962.

Auto-erotic hanging is not to be excluded on the age of the victim alone. Today sexual development is advanced in children at an earlier age than formerly. Maturity is possible at 15 years of age and even at the age of ten or even earlier, the child may show an undue interest in sex.

Homicidal Hanging

There has been no instance of homicidal hanging in Leeds during 1928–82. A few are recorded in the literature, for example six cases by Reuter (1901) and single reports by Klauer (1933), Weidemann (1940) and Mayne (1942). During 1885–1904 there were seven homicides by hanging and six of the victims were each under a year old (Dixon Mann, 1908).

Unless the victim is an infant or an adult person incapacitated by drink, disease, or drugs or, perhaps, sleep, the murder is difficult to accomplish single-handed. There must be a notable disproportion between the assailant and his victim to make the crime possible, unless there are several assailants. It is a form of murder, however, which two persons, acting in concert, can readily achieve. The affair Bompard, a murder which occurred in Paris in 1881, is a good example. A noose and cord worked over a pulley were concealed in an alcove and, as Bompard sat on the victim's knee, she playfully put the noose over his neck. Eyraud, her accomplice, then hauled him up from the sitting position and he was hanged. Robbery was the motive (Dixon Mann, 1908).

Murder Presented as Suicidal Hanging

There are several instances recorded of murders staged to appear as suicide by hanging. As a rule the true cause is to be discovered by a satisfactory examination of the body.

Moreover, in his anxiety to obscure the crime, the murderer is likely to exaggerate the circumstances of hanging or, through unfamiliarity with the process as followed by the suicide, he may make errors which are revealed by a detailed examination of the scene.

It is usual on these occasions for the body to be completely suspended. Although that of itself does not preclude suicide, complete suspension in the absence of a platform whence a suicide can reach the point of suspension, at once raises a presumption of murder.

Distinction between murder and suicide by an examination of the body is not always easy, especially when suspension follows murder by strangulation or by throttling. It could be, although I doubt it, that nail-marks on the neck were made by a suicide by hanging, in an endeavour to slacken the ligature. Gross injury to the neck structures can occur in suicidal hanging but it is more likely to follow strangulation by a ligature and, especially, throttling.

Even in persons under 40, when it is likely that the larynx is still elastic, extensive bruising of the neck muscles is evidence of throttling rather than strangulation; it is rare in hanging. The course of the mark, when clear, may at once indicate hanging, but such marks can be simulated by suspension of the body shortly after death. In that event, however, signs of violence responsible for the death will also be present and will call for explanation.

This kind of problem is well illustrated by the case of Rooks (1935). A man threw a looped strap over his mother's head from behind and strangled her. He took the body to a loft and suspended it from a rafter. He then placed the ladder he had used to reach the point of suspension against the wall to suggest that it had been the victim's platform.

The Dundee murder of 1899 concerned a woman who was strangled by her husband. He went to the police and alleged he had found his wife on the floor with a ligature round her neck. There was nothing at the scene, however, to indicate that she had hanged herself and the injuries in her neck were consistent with violent manual strangulation. The husband was found guilty of her murder but the jury at first added a recommendation to mercy on the ground that there had been a difference of opinion between the medical witnesses. The judge refused to accept this and sent the jury back to reconsider the matter. An unqualified verdict was then returned (*Lancet*, 1889, **i**, 696).

When a nurse had murdered a woman by strangulation she arranged the body to suggest suicide by hanging. The victim was found in a sitting posture, suspended by a tape which was wound round her neck and attached to a small brass hook about 3 ft above her head. Her clothing was smoothly arranged beneath her and her arms were beside her body and the hands were open. Examination showed, however, fracture of the tracheal rings and a deep circular mark round the neck consistent only with complete suspension or the application of a ligature with great pressure by an assailant. She had a recent severe bruise of her right eye. The tape was arranged in such a manner that the maximum pressure was at the back of the neck and least in front, where there was the major injury. There was fresh blood on the tape where it passed over the hook but none on the hands of the victim. It was believed that death was due to manual strangulation and the victim's body was subsequently suspended by a double tape. The assailant, being a nurse accustomed to lay out bodies, appeared to have placed the corpse in a "becoming attitude" (*R. v. Pinckard*, Northampton Lent Assizes, 1852, cited Tidy, 1883).

A young woman was found suspended from a beam in a restaurant. A stocking was wound twice round her neck and knotted. The rope was between the stocking and her neck and had been skilfully knotted. The end of the rope passed over the beam to form a kind of pulley used to haul up the body. When the assailant was discovered he confessed that he had attempted to stop her screaming by closing her mouth. He then found she had died and suspended her in a manner to simulate suicide by hanging (Klauer, 1933).

Examination of the rope may help to distinguish murder from suicide. Does it bear paint marks? This was relevant in Klauer's (1933) third case. When a woman was found dead in bed with a rope round her neck, her husband maintained she had hanged herself. Suicide was excluded by the absence of paint on the rope and of any marking of the paintwork on the top of a door over which it was alleged the rope had been drawn.

The direction of the fibres on a rope may also serve to tell the direction in which it was pulled across the top of a door and, accordingly, whether the victim had suspended himself or had been pulled into position by another.

Emmett-Dunne, with the aid of an accomplice, suspended the body of his victim in order to simulate suicide. Killing had been by a blow with the side of the hand, delivered on the front of the neck, in the manner of unarmed combat. A vertical fracture of the thyroid cartilage, just to one side of the middle line, and vertical tears in the carotid arteries were the material findings as post-mortem examination. Suspension of the body was from the balustrade of some stairs in a block in an army depot. If, as it appeared, these were stairs not infrequently used by troops, it would have been an unusual place for a suicide to have chosen. Dunne was convicted of murder but, for technical reasons, sentence of death was commuted to one of imprisonment for life. He was released in 1962 after serving about 7 years in prison. [The case was reported by Camps (1959).]

Suicidal Hanging Simulating Murder

It may be that for motives of revenge, fraud or, for some other reason, a victim wishes his suicide to appear to have been a murder and though it is rarely the case with hanging, an interesting example is recorded by Heinrich (1867). A married woman aged 30 left home to get some flour and took with her a bag and some cord. That evening she was found suspended from a branch of an oak tree. The branch was 6 ft 6 in. from the ground and the victim's height was 5 ft 1 in.; her body was completely suspended by a cord arranged in a running noose round her neck. A pencilled note was pinned to her right shoulder saying "Three of us have committed this murder. We found one thaler and fifteen gros; she prayed only for her two children." Examination showed marks on the trunk of the tree and a branch, 6 ft long and the thickness of an arm, taken from elsewhere, was propped against the tree. This branch was a convenient platform from which to reach the point of her suspension. There was a new path in the grass to the road but no signs of any struggle. The wording of the note was scarcely that of a murderer and the reference to her children was deemed to have been prompted only by the mother love of the woman herself. It was suicide and the motive would appear to have been avoidance of an impending prosecution.

Tardieu (1855) also described the suicide of a woman in circumstances which were at first believed to be those of murder committed by her husband. Tardieu's lengthy, but masterly discussion is worthy of study in the original text (*The Affair Durolle*).

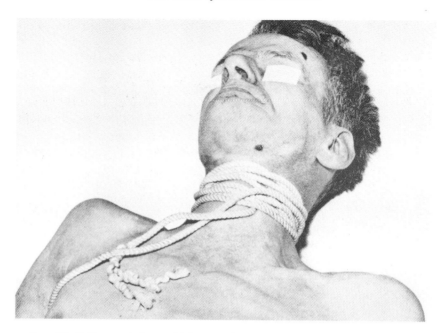

FIG. 131. Self-strangulation: multiple turns of rough cord; held in place by its texture: no knots. (Simulation of Professor Keith Simpson's case in Taylor's *Medical Jurisprudence*, 1965, 12th ed.)

Hanging as the Last Choice of an Impatient Suicide

Several cases of hanging as the last resort of an impatient suicide are on record. It may be that, having taken poison, the effects of which may be unexpectedly prolonged, the victim turns to hanging. In one of my cases a man drank some ammonia and then hanged himself from the trunk of a tree (F.M. 492). Extensive damage had been caused by the ammonia, but no doubt it had not killed as swiftly as had been anticipated and he must also have suffered intense pain.

More often, the victim has failed to kill himself by incised wounds, for example, the man who incised the inner side of his left forearm and then his wrist, severing the radial artery, before he died of hanging (Dixon Mann, 1908).

Attempted suicide by head injury is, in any event, uncommon and is rarely fatal; it may be followed by hanging. A woman aged 53 was found suspended in a loft. Much blood was present not only immediately below the victim but also elsewhere at the scene. She had lacerated wounds of the scalp and a localised depressed fracture of the skull. Investigation showed that she had first attempted to wound herself with a knife found in her pocket. She then struck herself with the butt of a hatchet. Streaming with blood from her head wounds, she searched for a cord, and, despite her injuries, she was able to arrange a running noose and hang herself (Riembault, 1867).

Stabbing may occasionally precede suicide by hanging. When the body of a woman was found suspended in a barn it was at first thought hanging alone was the cause of death. Examination showed, however, that she had a small stab wound beneath her left breast;

the heart had been transfixed. This case of Deveaux (cited by Dixon Mann, 1908) differs from another reported by Vrolik, where murder by stabbing was followed by suspension of the body, which had been washed and dressed in a clean shirt.

Hanging may follow attempted suicide with a firearm. Maschka described a man who first shot himself in the mouth and then resorted to hanging. This is possible when the injuries, due to a firearm, are of a minor kind, for example, when restricted to a laceration of the soft parts at the point of entry and fracture of the palate (Dixon Mann, 1908).

Another remarkable case concerned a man aged 48 who first attempted suicide by cutting his throat and his left wrist. The wrist tendons were severed but the throat wounds were all superficial. He then shot himself in the right temple and left hand. One bullet had passed through the palm but the other did not penetrate the skull. He then suspended himself from the bannisters (Harvey Littlejohn, 1925).

Hanging Followed by Interference to Suggest Natural Death

When a man returned home to find that his wife had committed suicide by hanging, he cut her down and hid the rope. When the police arrived he said he had found his wife on the floor, where she had collapsed and died.

He had hoped that he could thus avoid publicity. Fortunately for him Professor Sutherland indentified the mark on her neck as that of hanging. He was thus innocent of her death but the coroner censured the husband for his foolish conduct which had caused a good deal of unnecessary trouble to all concerned (*The Yorkshire Post*, 7 May 1948).

Injury Inflictea on the Body of a Suicide

A woman aged 60 was found suspended. When a man found the body he cut it down and then cut her throat (Maschka, cited Dixon Mann, 1908). This behaviour seems explicable only on the ground that it was the act of a masochist. The case appears to be unique.

References

BECK, T. R. and BECK, J. B. (1836) *Elements of Medical Jurisprudence*, 5th ed. Edinburgh: Longmans.
BROUARDEL, P. (1897) *La Pendaison, la Strangulation, la Suffocation, la Submersion*. Paris: Baillière.
CAMPS, F. E. (1959) *Med.-leg. J.* (*Camb.*), **27**, 156–61.
CAMPS, F. E. and HUNT, A. C. (1959) *J. Forens. Med.*, **6**, 116.
ECKER (1870) *Virchow's Arch.*, **49**, 290–1.
GORDON, I., TURNER, R. and PRICE, T. W. (1953) *Medical Jurisprudence*, 3rd ed., p. 492. Edinburgh and London: Livingstone.
GULBIS, E. (1939) *Dtsch. Z. ges. gerichtl. Med.*, **31**, 246–7.
HEINRICH (1867) *Vjschr. gerichtl. Med.*, N.S., V, No. I; abstr. *Ann. Hyg. publ., Paris*, 2nd ed., **27**, 460–1.
HOFMANN, E. R. (1927) *Lehrbuch d. gerichtl. Med.*, 11th ed., A Haberda, Berlin: Urban u. Schwarzenberg. (First edition 1878.)
HURPY, A. (1881) *Ann. Hyg. publ., Paris*, 3rd series, **6**, 359–67.
KALLE, E. (1933) *Dtsch. Z. ges. gerichtl. Med.*, **22**, 192–203; also abstr. *Med.-leg. Rev.*, 1934, **2**, 119.
KEILLER, A. (1855–6) *Edinb. Med. J.*, **1**, 824–30 (828).
KLAUER, H. (1933) *Dtsch. Z. ges. gerichtl. Med.*, **20**, 375–85; also abstr. *Med.-leg. Rev.*, i, 284–6.
KOOPMANN (1938) cited in abstr. of Reuter, K. (1938); in discussion.
LANGREUTER (1886) *Vjschr. gerichtl. Med.*, cited Dixon Mann (1908).
LESSER, A. (1890) *Vjschr. gerichtl. Med.*, **32**, 219.

LITTLEJOHN, HARVEY (1925) *Forensic Medicine*. London: Churchill.
LOPES, C. (1945) *Portugal Médico*, **29**, 361.
MANN, DIXON (1908) *Forensic Medicine and Toxicology*. London: Griffith.
MANN, G. T. (1960) *J. Forensic Sci.*, **5**, 169–72.
MANT, A. K. (1960) *Forensic Medicine*, p. 115. London: Lloyd-Luke.
MARC (1851) *Ann. Hyg. publ., Paris*, **5**, 156–224.
MARTIN, F. (1933) *Rev. méd. Franc.*, **14**, 123; also abstr. *Med.-leg. Rev.*, **1**, 248.
MARTIN, É. (1950) *Précis de Méd. Lég.*, 3rd ed., Paris: Doin.
MAYNE, H. (1942) *Beitr. forens. Med.*, **16**, 80–99.
MINOVICI, N. S. (1905) *Étude sur la pendaison*, Paris, cited Dixon Mann (1908).
NEUGEBAUER, W. (1937) *Dtsch. Z. ges. gerichtl. Med.*, **28**, 111–31.
OGSTON, F. (1878) *Lectures on Medical Jurisprudence*, ed. F. Ogston, Jr. London: Churchill.
PUPPE, G. (1908) *Atlas u. Grundriss*, vol. i. Munich: Lehmann.
RADIAN, I. and RADOVICI, L. (1957) *Annls. Méd-Lég.*, **37**, 232–6.
REINEBOTH, L. (1895) *Vjschr. gerichtl. Med.*, **9**, 265–84.
REUTER, F. (1901) *Ztschr. Heilk.*, **22**, 145–72.
REUTER, K. (1938) *Dtsch. Z. ges. gerichtl. Med.*, **29**, 186; also abstr. *Med.-leg. Rev.*, **6**, 218.
RIEMBAULT, A. (1867) *Ann. Hyg. publ., Paris*, 2nd series, 27, 164–74.
ROOKS, G. (1935) *Arch. Kriminol*, **27**, 104–9.
SIMONIN, C. (1955) *Médecine Légale Judiciare* 3rd ed., p. 210. Paris: Maloine.
SMITH, Sir SYDNEY, and FIDDES, F. S. (1955) *Forensic Medicine*, 10th ed., p. 252. London: Churchill.
SÖDERMAN, H. and O'CONNELL, J. J. (1947) *Modern Criminal Investigation*, p. 128. New York and London: Funk and Wagnalls.
SZEKELY, K. (1924) *Beitr. gerichtl. Med.*, **6**, 133–6, cited Hofmann (1927).
TARDIEU, A. (1855) *Ann. Hyg. publ., Paris*, 2nd series, **4**, 132–46; 371–441.
TARDIEU, A. (1870) *Ibid.*, **33**, 94.
TARDIEU, A. (1875) *Ibid.*, 2nd series, **43**, 140–69.
TARDIEU, A. (1879) *La Pendaison*, etc., 2nd. ed., Paris: Baillière.
TERRIEN (1887) Phenom corse à deux pentative de pendaison, *Gaz. Med. de Nantes*, 1886–7, **5**, 130–4; also *Progrès Méd.* (Par.), 1887, 2S, **6**, 212–14.
THOMAS, F. and KLUYSKENS, P. (1962) *Dtsch. Z. f. ges. gerichtl. Med.*, **52**, 253.
THOMAS, F. and VAN HECKE, W. (1959) *Internat. Crim. Police Rev.*, **14**, 173; abstr. *Med. Sci. Law*, **1**, 120.
TIDY, C. M. (1883) *Legal Medicine* vol. ii, pp. 409–45, 336 et seq. London: Smith Elder.
VAN HECKE, W. and TIMPERMAN, J. (1963) *Ann. Med.-leg., Criminol., Police Scient.*, **43**, 218.
WALCHER, K. (1935) *Dtsch. Z. ges. gerichtl. Med.*, **25**, 141–6; also abstr. *Med.-leg. Rev.* 1936, **4**, 64–65.
WEBB, F. C. (1852) *Med. Times*, London. N. S. **5**, 137.
WEIDEMANN, M. (1940) *Dtsch. Z. ges. gerichtl. Med.*, **33**, 163–70.
WEIMANN, W. (1935) *Arch. Kriminol.*, **97**, 62; also abstr. *Med.-leg Rev.*, 1936, **4**, 317–8; also abstr., *Dtsch. Z. ges. gerichtl. Med.*, 1936, **27**, 157.
WEINTRAUB, C. M. (1961) *Med.-leg. J. (Camb.)*, **21**, 209–16.

CHAPTER 10

Strangulation

ASPHYXIA by strangulation is caused by the application of a ligature to the neck in such a manner that the force acting upon it is exerted solely by the ligature; the weight of the victim's body plays no part. It is thus distinguished from hanging.

Strangulation is divisible into two groups, namely, strangulation by a ligature and manual strangulation or throttling; the features of the two are distinctive and require separate description. Mugging (the strangle-hold) is also described.

The Circumstances of Strangulation

Homicidal Strangulation

Many of the victims are adult women and not infrequently strangulation is then associated with sexual interference. The victim is likely to be found strangled by her stocking or scarf, but any other handy ligature, e.g. necktie, handkerchief, string, cord, electric or telephone flex may be used. Unusual ligatures may be of material used by the assailant at his work. A luggage strap, an elastic cord 18 in. long and $^1/_2$ in. in diameter, with metal at each end, which required force to expand it, was used to strangle a woman (F. 15,075A). Although the ligature may be round the neck more than once and knotted at each turn, it more often has a single turn, fastened firmly by a knot.

Removal by the examiner should be effected by cutting the ligature at a distance from the knot, which should not be undone. Undue emphasis must not be placed upon the kind or position of the knot, since the homicide and suicide, as found by Glaister and Rentoul (1966), are equally likely to make either a granny or a reef knot, at the right or the left of the neck. If, however, it is of an unusual kind, this merits attention since it may suggest that it was made by one with special knowledge of knots (e.g. scaffolder's knot). When there are two or more firm knots, each on separate turns of the ligature, homicide is almost certain.

Soft ligatures applied with skill and removed promptly after death may leave no external mark. It was imperceptible when a woman applied her husband's necktie to the neck of her child; she had held the ends until death occurred and then removed the ligature (F.M. 39, Fig. 132). A rough ligature, on the other hand, applied without skill and, as is not unusual, with more force than is required to kill, may produce extensive abrasions and bruising. A knotted piece of rough cord, when applied to the neck of a boy aged 2 years, produced a mark which clearly reproduced its pattern, which simulated multiple turns

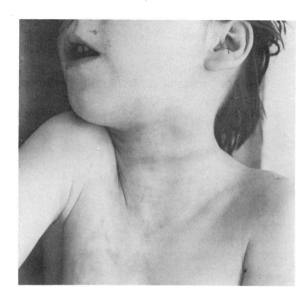

Fig. 132. Homicidal strangulation: a "mercy killing".
Faint mark, without abrasion, made by necktie, held in
place by the hands of her assailant.

(F.M. 86, Figs. 133, 134). Belts, chains, etc. may also leave a clear imprint of their pattern.

Infanticide by strangulation is sometimes accomplished by winding the umbilical cord round the infant's neck. The distinction between accidental and homicidal strangulation will then rest largely upon the condition of the cord. If it presents appearances indicative of rough handling, with displacement of Wharton's jelly, the death is probably homicidal, especially if the child has been injured.

If the victim is aware of the attack there is likely to be a struggle, its duration and extent depending upon the physique of the victim. In consequence both assailant and victim may bear abrasions and bruising. Sexual interference, when present, will be indicated by injuries to the genitalia, and the presence of semen on the body or clothing of the victim, although either of these signs may be absent, according to the circumstances. In one case, recent bruising of a ruptured hymen was accompanied by spermatozoa in the vagina (F.M. 1516) in another, the fact of interference was shown by a recent tear in the hymen, produced in all probability by digital interference; spermatozoa were absent (P.M. 1326A, Fig. 159). Signs of interference are not conclusive proof of rape since injury may result in sadistic circumstances where consent had been given by the victim. On rare occasions injuries intended to simulate rape and to divert attention from the murderess may be inflicted, as in *R. v. Donald* (1934).

Homicidal attempts are not exclusively made by adults. In 1949 a boy aged 10 years, of a bullying nature, attempted to murder a boy aged 3 years by applying a belt to his neck, meantime kneeling on the child. Fortunately the mother of the victim, searching for the child, arrived in time to save him; her screams caused the older boy to release the belt. He had applied considerable pressure, it would seem, since the report states that the victim did not revive until artificial respiration had been practised for about 20 minutes. The

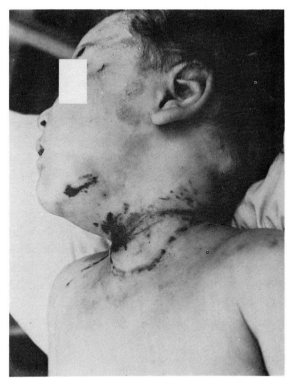

FIG. 133. Homicidal strangulation with a rough ligature—a combination of pieces of twine applied once round his neck. Simulation of multiple turns (see also Fig. 134).

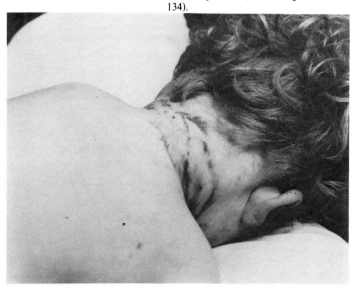

FIG. 134. Homicidal strangulation: a complex rough ligature of twine applied once round neck. Simulation of a "crossover" of the ligature at the nape of the neck.

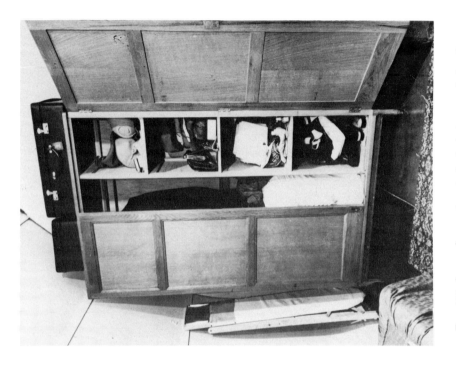

Fig. 136. Scene of concealment of a body in a wardrobe after homicide by strangulation (see also Fig. 145).

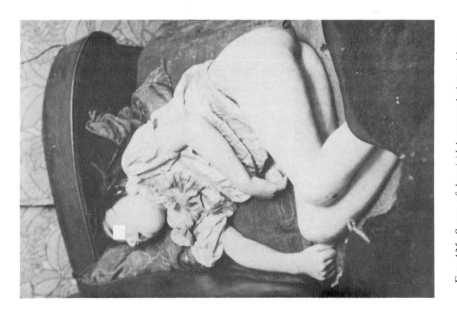

Fig. 135. Scene of homicidal strangulation with a necktie. External injuries negligible; a "mercy killing" by her mother (see also Fig. 132).

medical evidence was that but for this, he would have died. The assailant alleged he was only playing a game, and it was pleaded on his behalf that his act was foolish and unthinking conduct; probably influenced by the pictures and wireless. The Bench, however, found the boy guilty of causing grievous bodily harm and ordered him to a remand home for 21 days for examination by a Home Office psychiatrist (*The Yorkshire Post*, 25 Aug. 1949).

"Palmar strangulation". When a man was accused of throttling a woman in 1954 he insisted that at no time had he gripped her throat. Both horns of her thyroid cartilage, however, were broken and there was bruising of the neck muscles. He said she had threatened to scream to attract the attention of passers-by. He had placed his right hand horizontally across her mouth and had then reinforced the pressure by placing his left hand on top, at right angles to the other. In this manner the heel of the palm would have been in front of her neck (Fig. 137).

It did not seem feasible for pressure applied in this manner to be sufficient to fracture the thyroid cartilage. This was tested on suitable bodies prior to necropsy, i.e. persons of about the same age as the victim, a woman aged 52, and whose deaths were later shown to have been due to natural causes. It was impossible to reproduce the bruising but, contrary to expectation, a fracture of one or both horns of the thyroid cartilage was produced by

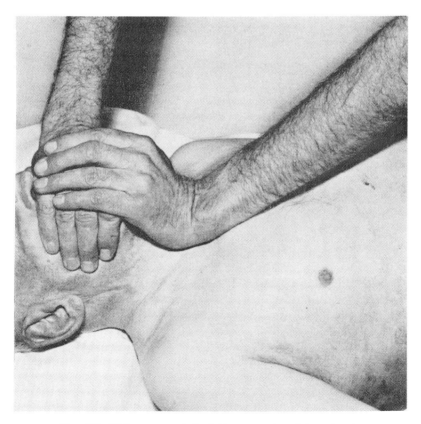

FIG. 137. "Palmar strangulation" (demonstration of the cadaver).

pressure, applied in the manner described by the accused, in six of eight tests. The two failures were explained by the fact that one was a male with a large thyroid cartilage and the pressure had forced the horns along the sides of the spinal column; the other was a woman whose chest was arched forward unduly and it was anatomically impossible to exert much pressure on her larynx.

The mechanism resembles that used in some experiments by Keiller (1855–56). He placed a block of wood across the larynx and applied a steady force to it to compress the larynx against the spine and fracture the cartilage. Two children were killed by their father when he pressed his palms, one on the front of the neck of each child, as they lay asleep. There was no injury to the skin or the neck structures (Gonzales *et al.*, 1954).

Garrotting. When a victim is attacked from behind, without warning, it is possible silently to overpower and kill a robust and vigorous male; robbery is the usual motive. The throat may be seized or a ligature is thrown over the head and quickly tightened. This results in abrupt loss of consciousness and collapse; there need be no struggle. The assailant is then able, single-handed, to tie the ligature with one or more turns. These are the circumstances of the crime of garrotting which was especially prevalent during 1862– 1863 and which called for specific legislation. It is a crime still practised abroad; in India, for example, the agent is usually a loin-cloth or lasso, thrown over the victim's head (Beck and Beck, 1836); a supple branch of a tree or a bamboo cane is also sometimes used.

Garrotting as a mode of execution is practised in Spain and Turkey. In Spain the prisoner is seated with his back to a post, to which he is secured; a metal collar is then applied to the neck and tightened. The apparatus may include a spike which is forced into the nape of the neck during the execution. The bowstring is used in Turkey.

When Dr. Clench was murdered in 1692 in a hackney-coach, the two assailants used a handkerchief with which they bound a piece of coal over his windpipe. This was done during a journey which lasted an hour and a quarter. The coachman was unaware of the murder until he found the doctor seated inside, apparently under the influence of drink. He called the Watch and they found that the doctor had been strangled (cited by Beck and Beck, 1836).

Mugging. The strangle-hold strangulation is sometimes effected by holding the neck of the victim in the bend of the elbow; this hold is no longer permitted in wrestling, because of its danger. Alternatively, the foot or knee may be applied to the victim's neck.

Example 1

A woman aged 35 was found dead beneath a bed. She lay face down but the intense dusky blue of her face was deeper than the colour of hypostasis elsewhere on the body. The face was puffy and there were numerous petechial haemorrhages in the skin of her face and beneath the conjuctivae. Some foam and a little blood had escaped from her left nostril. There was no trace of injury to the face or neck; the injuries at the back of her body had occurred after death and were due to contact with springs beneath the mattress.

Internal examination showed that almost all of the neck muscles had been bruised. The left great horn of the thyroid cartilage was broken and bent inwards; the cricoid cartilage was broken in two places so that the central anterior part, 0.8 inch long, had been displaced backwards for a distance of about 0.1 inch.

Clearly, considerable force had been exerted on the front of the neck by a relatively broad, smooth and firm agent, either a forearm or foot.

In due course a man informed the police that he was responsible for her death. They had gone to his house and retired to bed. When she learnt he had no money she made to leave. He put his arm round her neck to restrain her. This made her all the more determined to leave and he applied his arm a second time. According to the man, she then suddenly went limp. Realising she was dead he took fright, hid the body under the bed, and ran away (F.M. 11,042).

Example 2

An epileptic girl was found dead in an alcove, in an upper room of a derelict house. There was some upward displacement of her upper garments but no disturbance of the lower ones. There was a wooden plank on the floor beside the body. Her face was purple and puffy. She had a rectangular abrasion, 3 in. long across the front of her neck, centred over her thyroid cartilage. The abrasion was well-defined on the right side of her neck but on the left side it terminated in three narrow diverging scratches. The upper and lower margins of the mark were irregular.

Several of her neck muscles were bruised and the pharynx and root of her tongue were congested. There was no injury of the carotid arteries; the hyoid bone was intact but there was recent bleeding in the neighbourhood of its joints.

The left great horn of her thyroid cartilage was broken close to its base and displaced outwards; there was bleeding near the fracture and also behind the larynx, between it and the spine. Her lungs were congested and oedematous and there was blood-stained mucus in her bronchi and trachea. She had the scars of an operation on her head and old softening in her left frontal lobe.

Her death was due to asphyxia and the findings were deemed consistent with the application of a narrow, rough agent, e.g., the plank, to her neck and held there by hands. Although there were no injuries to her genitalia, semen was present inside her knickers and on a newspaper near her body. It was just possible that the plank had been applied in an attempt to control her during a fit (F.M. 12,941c).

Self-strangulation

Self-strangulation has been effected by one of several modes. A cord may be firmly applied with multiple turns, as many as 18 seen in one of Simpson's cases (Taylor, 1965), without knotting of the free ends. This is presumptive evidence of suicide, similarly when a ligature is firmly applied with one or more turns and a final tying of the free ends with a half-knot or half-hitch. This is the "hallmark" of self-strangulation but it is not proof of it. We have examined the bodies of two women, both of whom were murdered by strangulation but the ligature was left incompletely knotted. The circumstances of their deaths, however, left no doubt that they were wholly inconsistent with suicide or accidental death.

One victim was a girl whose body was found beneath a quantity of bricks and concrete rubble near a building site. The ligature round her neck was left in a half-knot. This was alleged to have been applied by two youths, each of whom held one of the ends until she died. Handkerchiefs had been stuffed into her mouth (F.M. 12,141c).

The second victim was a woman aged 42 whose body was exhumed from a relatively deep grave in the garden of the house where she lived. A length of clothes line was wound twice round her neck and fastened with a half-knot. It was described by the defence as more like a "lover's" knot than that of strangler. This was inconsistent with the fact that she also had a substantial piece of cloth forced into her throat and she had suffered other injuries, including a head injury. It was alleged that she had died of injuries sustained during a violent quarrel. The accused failed to report her death to the authorities and decided to conduct his own funeral arrangements. He buried the body in a plot where she was accustomed to sun bathe; it was well screened by fencing. His suggestion that he had wanted to give her a Christian burial was regarded by counsel for the Crown, and, apparently, the jury as one of the worst pieces of hypocrisy they had ever heard. He was convicted of murder (*R. v. Franklin*, York Assizes, March 1971; F.M. 15,124A). His appeal was dismissed.

Example 1. Self-strangulation with a Lisle Stocking

A woman aged 73 was lying full length on the floor of a bedroom, which she shared with another patient in a nursing home (Fig. 138). The bedclothing had been thrown back in a manner consistent with getting out of bed. There were no signs of any struggle. She was dressed in a nightgown and a brown stocking was round her neck; the fellow of a pair was seen suspended over the head of the bed. The stocking was applied with a half-knot at the nape on the first turn and with another half-knot at the front of the neck (Fig. 139). The first turn was tight, but the second, although close to the first, was easily released. There were no other signs of violence, but a little bleeding, which produced a small stain 1 in. in its diameter, had occurred from the nose; the stain was directly below her nose. Her face and neck, above the ligature, were congested and of purple colour. Bleeding had occurred beneath the conjuctivae, but petechial haemorrhages were not seen in the skin of the forehead and face. The tongue protruded, but was not bitten; she had dentures, but these were on her bedside

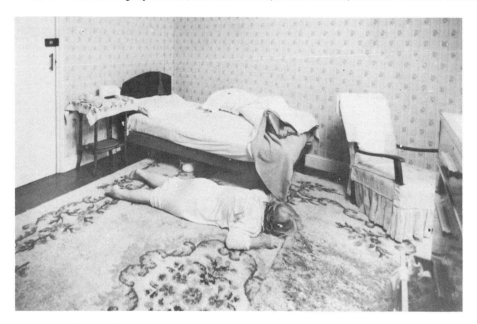

FIG. 138. Scene of self-strangulation with lisle stocking (see also Fig. 139).

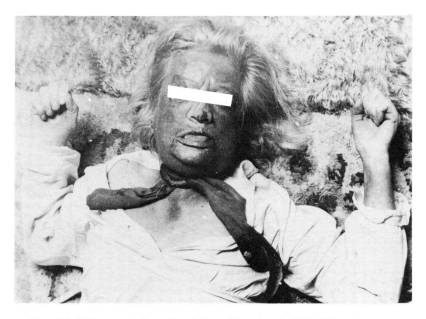

FIG. 139. Self-strangulation with a lisle stocking; closed with half-knot below chin. (Note also gross engorgement and puffiness of face.)

table. The ligature had compressed the neck to produce a shallow, broad groove of pale skin, in line with the upper border of the larynx. The groove was not more than $^1/_{10}$ in. (2.5 mm) deep, notably at the sides and nape of the neck. It was up to an inch broad in front, but only $^1/_2$ in. broad at the sides of the neck. There was no abrasion of the skin in the groove—or elsewhere. Nor was there any bleeding into the skin at either margin of the groove. Bruising of the neck muscles, left sterno-mastoid and the bellies of the digastric muscles, was slight. Although the laryngeal cartilages were calcified, they were intact, being neither fractured nor bent. Severe engorgement, with bleeding into the tissues, was apparent in the tonsils and adjacent pharyngeal wall, the base of the tongue and the left pyriform fossa. There were a few small haemorrhages beneath the mucous membrane at the back of the epiglottis and one other in the left half of the sub-glottic space. There was no natural disease to account for death. The mild grade of atheroma present was consistent with her age. The cause of death was asphyxia, following the application of a relatively broad, soft ligature to the neck with sufficient force to obstruct the veins and, to a lesser degree, the arteries of the neck; there was also obstruction of the air passages. The mode of application of the ligature was consistent with self-strangulation, as was all the other evidence.

She was a retired midwife, who had been under treatment for depression, but who had not indicated any inclination to suicide. Two days after her admission to the nursing some she was obviously ill in mind. A doctor prescribed a sedative and preliminary steps were taken to transfer her to a mental hospital. Next day she was found dead beside her bed; her room-mate was fast asleep (F.M. 6614A) (Polson, 1961).

Example 2. Self-strangulation with Stockings

The deceased was a widow aged 61, whose body was found on moorland near Halifax on 5 October 1957. It lay in a hollow, visible only to someone passing close to it and was discovered by a boy aged 12, who was searching for a watch he had lost on the moor. He realised her posture was unusual, but at first thought she was asleep. When he returned later she had not moved, so he picked up a small stone and threw it at her feet. When she did not move the boy went to tell the police. He met a doctor who went to the scene and, having found the woman was dead, he summoned the police. The body was fully clothed in outdoor dress and lay as shown in Fig. 140, the shopping bag was just under her left arm and not lying on the body. It was at first thought she had died of a heart attack, but when the body was lifted slightly, the top button of her coat was undone and a stocking was seen round the neck. There was no sign of any struggle or interference and, as first

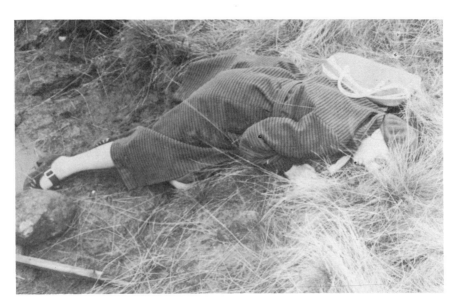

Fig. 140. Self-strangulation: a scene which at first suggested collapse and death from natural disease—ligature obscured (see also Fig. 141). (By courtesy of the late Dr. H. V. Phelon.)

noticed by the boy, her spectacles were in their normal position. Her handbag contained a little money and a receipt bearing a number, by which she was identified in the first instance.

It was later shown that two lisle stockings had been tightly applied, crossed at the back, drawn tight and fastened by a half knot in front of the neck (Fig. 141). Stockings of similar size and material were found in the bedroom of the deceased.

When the ligature was removed, it was seen that it had produced a broad, shallow furrow round the neck,

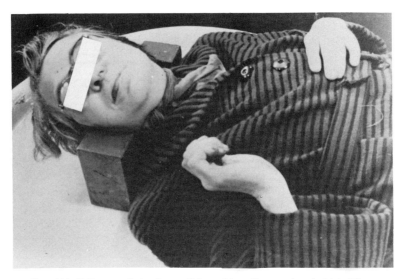

Fig. 141. Self-strangulation by two lisle stockings; ligature closed with half knot below the chin. (By courtesy of the late Dr. H. V. Phelon.)

being slightly higher at the nape than in front. Bleeding had occurred into the base of the tongue, but the larynx was intact. There was no natural disease to account for this death.

She had been depressed since the death of her husband 3 years previously and had been worried by defects in the new house to which she had moved. After giving her son his breakfast, she left her home at 10 a.m. on 5 October, ostensibly to shop. She had left a note which indicated her intention to commit suicide. (By courtesy of the late Dr. H. V. Phelon.)

Another variation, also presumptive of suicide, is by a tourniquet mechanism. The ligature is applied with one rather than several turns and knotted with a complete granny or reef knot. A stick or rod is inserted beneath the ligature, or tied to it, and twisted to tighten it. When consciousness is lost the stick unwinds, but only to a limited extent, one end being held under an angle of the jaw (F.M. 2827, Fig. 142). Compression of the neck is thus maintained and the victim dies of asphyxia. Guy and Ferrier (1895) described a case in which a poker was used to tighten the ligature; see also Mant (1960), who depicts another example, and Brouardel (1897): the case of General Pichegru.

The foregoing modes are well recognised and should create no difficulty in interpretation. Keith Simpson (1960) and Thurston (1971) have recorded another variation in this category. The victim applied a running noose to her neck and wound the free end three times round her right hand. She pulled hard and strangled herself. The weight of the hand and forearm acting on the cord could have maintained sufficient compression to kill after she had lost consciousness—see also Mant (1960).

This woman had applied a double loop of cord with a running noose round her neck and fixed it with a half-hitch; the end was wound round her right hand. She was found with her right arm flexed as if the forearm and hand were pulling on the cord. She held a

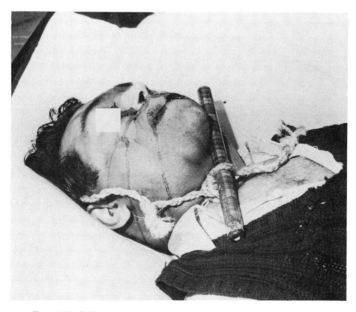

FIG. 142. Self-strangulation: wooden stick inserted to tighten the ligature; locked beneath left angle of the jaw after loss of consciousness.

stocking in her left hand. The stocking was grasped so tightly as to simulate cadaveric spasm (Simpson, 1960; Mant, 1960; Thurston, 1971).

Von Karger (1969) reported a similar case in which a woman who had effected self strangulation with a belt, was found with her hands holding the ends of the belt.

When the deceased is found with a cord forcibly applied to the neck and held with a firm, complete knot, it must not be regarded as proof of homicide. Simpson (1960) has recorded two cases of persons found dead with a stocking or piece of string wound twice round the neck and tied with a double knot beneath an ear in circumstances which, viewed as a whole, were those of suicide. At no small personal risk Keith Simpson and another doctor demonstrated that it is possible personally to apply a tight ligature, firmly knotted, to the neck, in the manner normally employed by another person, before losing consciousness. It is obvious that a correct interpretation can be made only after the whole of the facts are considered. Attention must also be given to the possibility of a coincident attempt at suicide by poisoning, notably barbiturate. The demonstration of the ingestion of a lethal dose of barbiturate in these subjects points to "impatient" suicide. Simpson also drew attention to the distinction between these cases and homicidal poisoning with barbiturate, hastened by strangulation of the victim when unconscious; it turns on a careful assessment of the whole circumstances of the death.

Another variation is occasionally recorded (e.g. Puppe, 1908; Glaister and Rentoul, 1966). Strangulation is here by means of a running noose; after this is applied to the neck, the free end of the rope, to which a weight is attached, is thrown over the end of the bed or couch on which the victim lies.

When the victim is known to have had injury to one hand and is found strangled or hanged, the death would appear to be homicidal. It is possible, however, for a one-armed person to commit suicide by strangulation. A girl committed suicide by strangulation in spite of the fact that her right hand was useless following injury by burns. She had rolled her scarf and shawl into a cord and wound them two and a half times round her neck. The cord was fastened with two knots on the left side, the first knot being tighter than the second (Tardieu, 1879).

As already mentioned, the kind and site of the knot is unlikely to be of assistance in distinguishing between homicide and suicide. In their experiments, Glaister and Rentoul (1966) found that whether made by a male or female, the kind of knot and its position in relation to the neck was likely to be the same. A granny knot, tied at the right side of the neck, was by far the commonest choice in "suicide" as well as in "homicide"; a central knot was an unusual choice.

The largest series yet recorded is one of twenty-six cases of self-strangulation, reported by Weimann and Spengler (1956). Two excellent reports were by von Karger (1969).

Accidental Strangulation

Accidental strangulation may occur *in utero* when the movements of the foetus cause the umbilical cord to be wound round its neck. Tightening of the cord may occur, then or during labour, and the constriction can be sufficient to asphyxiate. (The ability of the cord to tighten *in utero* is remarkable. If wound round a limb, it may amputate it, as in one infant I examined; a lower limb was attached only by soft parts of the body, following constriction by the umbilical cord.)

Example. The body of a new-born child was found wrapped in sheeting in a wardrobe. The body weighed $8^1/_2$ lb; it had not been washed. Its face was puffy, slightly purple and there were many fine petechial haemorrhages in the skin of the face. The cord was tightly wound twice round the neck and passed from the right side to the front of the neck, over the chest to the left armpit, thence over the right shoulder to the front of the right side of the chest. The free end had been cut. When unwound, the cord measured 32 in. and another 3 in. were attached to the placenta. There was no evidence whatsoever of injury to the cord. It had not been damaged by gripping or pulling on it.

There was a broad band of pallor in the skin of the neck beneath the site of the cord but there was no abrasion nor any bruising. The lungs were only part-aerated. It was concluded that the infant had died of asphyxia during delivery due to strangulation by the cord and, in all probability, it had been still-born (F.M. 10,895B).

This accident, however, may be raised as a defence to a charge of infanticide or murder. Examination of the cord will include search for disturbance of its constituents, especially Wharton's jelly; if damaged, the cord has probably been used in the perpetration of crime, especially when other signs of violence on the body of the infant, notably bruising and scratch marks, are present.

Accidental strangulation can also arise in the course of a person's occupation, when a necktie or scarf is caught in moving machinery or belts. A boy of 14 was nearly strangled in such circumstances (Taylor, cited Tidy, 1883). On another occasion a man was strangled by a loop of wire rope which controlled a scraper, drawn by a motor tractor. The winch operating the wire drew it tight round his neck and strangled him (Forbes, 1945). The danger of wearing neckties with long, loose ends near moving machinery is indicated by the following case. A boy aged 18 was engaged in passing sheets of paper through rollers in a glazing operation. A sheet slipped and he stooped to catch it. The ends of his necktie were caught between the rollers and he was drawn into the machine and strangled. (Anon., *Boston Med. Surg. J.*, 1845, **32**, 306).

The deaths of children restrained in their cots by harness may be either accidental strangulation or hanging. This depends on whether or not the weight of the body plays any part in constricting the neck. Dumont and Dérobert (1962) reported an example as one of strangulation. The child was suspended by its straps (Attache-bébé).

The circumstances of accidental strangulation may be simple but obscure. Gonzales *et al.* (1954) report the case of a man found on his back in bed; death was due to asphyxia. He was blue in the face and foam was present at the mouth. He was fully dressed when he had gone to bed drunk. He wore a necktie, which, however, was tied in a normal manner and, although it fitted the neck snugly, it was not drawn tight. There was no furrow in the skin of the neck nor any other signs of undue constriction. The circumstances were considered to be those of strangulation, in the belief that the degree of constriction by the necktie, although insufficient to a leave a mark, was sufficient to cause strangulation of a person depressed by alcohol.

It may be that strangulation is sometimes an accident in the course of a game or practical joke but, as shown by the case mentioned earlier, the circumstances will have to be clearly and convincingly distinguished from homicide or attempted homicide.

The External Signs of Strangulation

(*a*) *The ligature.* Close attention must be paid to the ligature and care taken when removing it to leave the knots intact and to cut it, as far as is practicable, so as to permit satisfactory reconstruction. Photographic record, the victim being dead, should precede removal of the ligature, and really good photographs at close range are required. Those taken of the army matron mentioned were of a quality which permitted accurate reconstructions of the circumstances of the death (F.M. 4484A, Fig. 145).

On most occasions the ligature is something handy and often some garment belonging to the victim, e.g. her nylon stocking or her scarf. It may be the flex of an electric fire or kettle (Fig. 143) or it has been, as in one of Professor Glaister's cases, the telephone flex. Unusual ligatures may narrow the search for the assailant since they may be material of a kind used in a particular occupation.

The mode of application is also important. The construction of the loop, notably the number of turns and the kind of knots, requires detailed study. Normally the ligature is applied with a single or double turn and fastened with a simple knot, like a granny or a reef knot, at the front or side of the neck. Departure from this is at once important. An unusual knot may be a knot used in some particular occupation, e.g. scaffolder. The application of a ligature with several turns, even up to 18 times as depicted in Taylor (1965), whether closed with a half knot or even a complete knot, is consistent with suicide. Similarly, a single turn of a broad ligature of rough cloth, closed with a half knot (Fig. 139) indicates suicide.

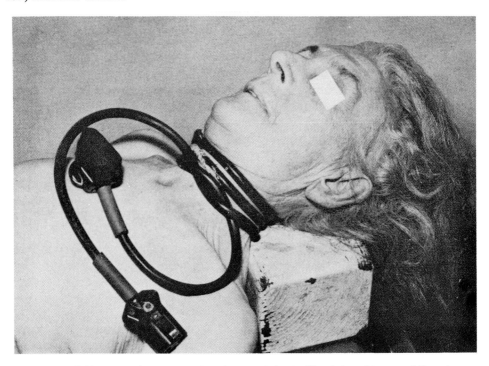

FIG. 143. Self-strangulation: agent the flex of an electric kettle. (Simulation of the case of Gonzales, Vance, Helpern and Umberger in *Legal Medicine*, 1954, 2nd ed.)

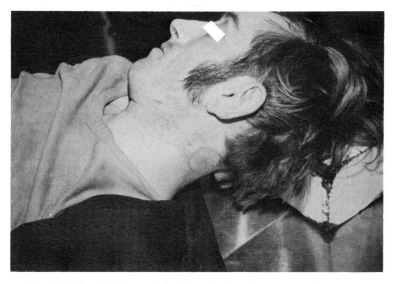

FIG. 144. Homicidal stangulation by a telephone flex; note mark of earpiece
(F.M. 20569).

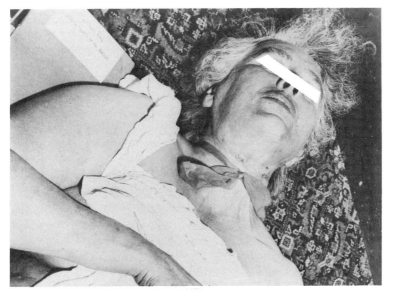

FIG. 145. Homicidal strangulation: nylon stocking wound tightly round neck
and knotted tightly in front of the neck. (Self-strangulation in this manner is
possible but rare.)

(*b*) *The mark on the neck* (see Polson, 1957, 1961). There are occasions when the ligature has been removed by the assailant. When the mother already mentioned strangled her daughter she used her husband's necktie and, it appears, held the ends tightly until the child died and then threw the tie on the kitchen table (F.M. 39). On these occasions, especially, a scrutiny of the neck is important. Normally the mark is a groove, of about the same width and about half the thickness of the ligature in depth, which takes a horizontal course round the neck, more prominent at the front and sides than at the back, at a level which lies on or below the Adam's apple; it is not usually, as is the case in hanging, above that structure. The occurrence of a narrow zone of engorgement or of bruising immediately above and below the groove confirms that the victim was alive at the time the ligature was applied. In addition, the course of the mark may be interrupted and an abrasion in the gap indicates the position of the knot. The groove is normally lined by pale, parchmented skin but at times there is a pattern which may point to the agent, e.g. a woven belt, an embossed belt or a chain, etc. Rough material, e.g. twine, is likely to abrade the skin in the course of the mark, or to leave an imprint of its strands (Fig. 126).

Multiple turns produce a complex mark in which it may be possible to trace the number of turns but it must be remembered that a complex ligature, composed of several pieces knotted together, may yield a mark which suggests multiple turns when in fact there was only one (Figs. 133 and 134). This child was strangled by a man without any discoverable motive; it was subsequently found that the assailant, aged 21, suffered from juvenile general paralysis (F.M. 86).

Putrefaction, by causing swelling of the tissues, can yield appearances which simulate strangulation by a ligature, if the deceased wore a shirt or blouse at the time of death. Obviously, in such cases interpretation must be guarded. In my opinion, if putrefaction be of sufficient degree to produce a false "strangulation groove", dissolution would continue by putrefaction and mummification would be most unlikely, if not impossible. If death had in fact been due to strangulation, the mark on the neck is not necessarily obliterated by putrefaction. On the contrary, the compressed skin in the mark tends to be better preserved than the skin beyond it and, even when obscured, subcutaneous haemorrhages in relation to the mark may still be found. At the same time, the presence of established putrefaction compels caution in an interpretation of the findings.

It is alleged that mummification can also produce a false groove round the neck in relation to the band of a shirt collar or blouse. Retraction of the soft tissues in mummification, in my opinion, would be general, without the production of a distinct, false groove. A deep groove would indicate one produced prior to the onset of mummification. A false groove in relation to the collar was seen on the neck of a person who had died of coronary thrombosis in a fire (Fig. 114); compare this with the case of Sir Sydney Smith and Fiddes (1955), one of murder by strangulation followed by an attempt to conceal the crime by arson.

Both in hanging and strangulation there may be additional marks by way of bruising and abrasion. These may be the result of manual strangulation, or attempted manual strangulation, prior to hanging or strangulation by a ligature, or they may be produced by the victim in an attempt to slacken the ligature, an event more likely in strangulation by a ligature than in hanging. In both they may rarely be a result of unskilled attempts at resuscitation.

Bruising of the forehead or face points to a homicidal attack, although bruising, usually a single bruise, could result if the suicide by strangulation had fallen upon his face. It could have been accidental (see below, F.M. 11,149B).

Internal Examination

The neck structures. Bruising of the neck muscles is commoner in strangulation than in hanging although in neither is it necessarily a notable feature.

In strangulation by a ligature the bruising is likely to be on the same level as the ligature whereas, in throttling, the bruises tend to be at different levels, owing to shifting of the grip or a reapplication of the hand or hands. Blows to the neck are likely to produce greater and more extensive bruising. Conversely, a ligature which is tightly applied and left on the neck until death occurs may fail to produce any bruising (Camps and Hunt, 1959).

In our experience, strangulation, whether by a ligature or by hand, produces severe engorgement, with haemorrhage into the tissues in and above the area compressed. This is absent in hanging unless, by low suspension and relatively mild constriction of the neck, the effects are comparable to those of strangulation.

There is usually severe engorgement of the oro-pharynx, tonsils, and the root of the tongue above the level of construction (Fig. 146). These tissues have a dull red colour and bleeding into them, if not apparent at their surface, is obvious when they are sectioned. The limits of the change, both above and below, are relatively well-defined.

Example. A woman aged 27 was strangled by a soft chiffon scarf which her assailant had applied to her neck and held the ends until she lost consciousness. He then removed the ligature and threw it away. The mark of a ligature was apparent on the left side and nape of her neck as a shallow, copper-coloured band of skin, $^1/_4$ in. broad. As its course was traced round the neck the mark broadened and became fainter on the right side where it was up to $^1/_2$ in. broad. The skin in the mark was neither abraded nor parchmented. Immediately to the right of the mid-line of her neck there was a linear abrasion, $1\,^1/_2$ in. long and about $^1/_{16}$ in. broad, situated $^5/_8$ in. above the ligature mark. She had a recent bruise and a shallow split in the inner lining of her lower lip. Her face was dusky (the body was on its back) and there were several petechial haemorrhages in the skin of her eye lids and forehead. There was no evidence of a struggle.

There was no subcutaneous bruising nor was there any bruising of the neck muscles. As might be expected in a young subject, the hyoid bone and larynx were intact. The outstanding feature was an abrupt change in the colour of the tissues in a horizontal line immediately above the level of the site of the ligature. The pharynx, tonsils and base of the tongue were plum coloured by severe engorgement. The injury to her mouth was due to a blow with a fist (F.M. 11,080).

Damage to the intima of the carotid arteries, unusual even in hanging, is exceptional in strangulation. It is seen as transverse splits in the intima. It may occur following a blow to the neck as in the case of Emmett-Dunne (Camps, 1959) or after hanging by a long drop.

Injury to the *hyoid bone* is uncommon since the level of constriction is relatively low and well below the bone; traction on the thyro-hyoid membrane also is negligible. In one of our cases, however, the left great horn of the hyoid bone was broken and the larynx was spared; the ligature had been applied at the level of the upper border of the thyroid cartilage (F.M. 2958). Fracture of the bone will depend also on the breadth of the ligature; when it is broad, the hyoid bone may be compressed. It is more usual to find fracture of the

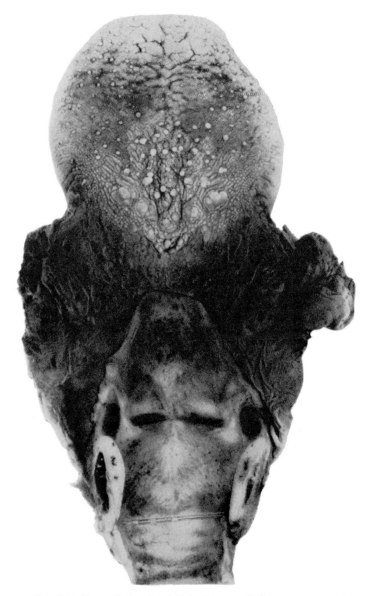

FIG. 146. Strangulation, homicidal, with a scarf. Gross engorgement
of structures immediately above level of constriction ("Stasis" haemorrhages in larynx). (See also Fig. 159 sexual interference, probably
digital.)

thyroid cartilage, especially of one or both superior horns. Fracture of the wings of the
cartilage or of the *cricoid cartilage* is less common and is likely only when considerable
force is used, or if some solid object is incorporated in the ligature and applied over the
front of the neck. Even in such circumstances, considerable force is required to fracture
the thyroid cartilage in the middle line, separating its wings, or to fracture the cricoid

cartilage. Camps and Hunt (1959) had experience of only two instances of fracture of the cricoid cartilage; one was the result of a blow to the front of the larynx and the fracture was associated with a mid-line fracture of the thyroid cartilage; the other was due to compression of the neck, probably by a forearm.

Fracture of both great horns of the thyroid cartilage occurred in the two cases of self-strangulation recorded by von Karger (1969).

It is rare for the trachea to be torn or broken.

Fractures of hyoid bone and larynx are almost exclusively due to homicidal strangulation but, if the structure be ankylosed or ossified, it is possible for the suicide to fracture them. When strangulation is suicidal the force exerted is usually less than that required to cause a fracture; in homicide, on the other hand, the assailant is likely to use more force than is required to kill. Fracture of the hyoid bone can be a result of accidental strangulation (Forbes, 1945). In that case, however, collateral evidence established that the circumstances were those of an accident. Such fractures may be found when the wheel of a motor passes over the neck. The injuries are then gross, with outward bending of the fragments; the appearances could only be simulated by someone trampling on the neck or inflicting blows with a heavy, blunt instrument. Our experience confirms that of Weintraub (1961). The soft parts at the front of the neck may be lacerated (Mitrani, 1962).

Example. A woman aged 66 was found dead in a room which was in apparent disorder. There was a pile of letters and papers in front of the hearth. She was clothed and wore a fur coat; she lay face down beneath a pair of household steps. She was separated from her husband, who lived in the neighbourhood. She had sustained a recent laceration of her forehead; the wound was an inch long and up to $^1/_4$ in. broad, situated across the forehead. It had penetrated to the bone but the skull was intact. She also had a faint recent bruise across the front of her neck, just above the thyroid cartilage.

There was recent bleeding into the subcutaneous tissues at the front of her neck in a band $1^1/_4$ in. long at the level of the upper border of the thyroid cartilage. Both great horns of the cartilage were fractured at their bases and there was recent bleeding in the tissues; the right horn had been broken on its outer side but the left horn was completely separated from the cartilage. The appearances were consistent with the cartilage having been crushed against the spine. The hyoid bone and the cricoid cartilage were intact. There was no evidence of throttling; there was no evidence of anyone having entered the house; and the husband's movements were checked and he was in no way responsible.

She had severe atheroma of her coronary and cerebral arteries; there was evidence of old-standing cerebral softening. It was found that the distance between the injury to her forehead and that of her neck was precisely the same as the distance between two treads of the steps. It was concluded that she had become dizzy and probably had a heart attack. This had caused her to fall against the steps which were kept against a wall in this room. After contact with two of the treads she had collapsed and died; the steps had fallen across her body (F.M. 11,149).

Haemorrhages beneath the inner lining of the larynx may occur and are the direct result of compression and due to stasis of blood rather than asphyxia. These haemorrhages are usually larger than the petechial haemorrhages of asphyxia (Fig. 146).

Laryngeal and hyoid fractures may be recognised at a late date, months or even years after death (*R*. v. *Dobkin*) but, of course, the longer the delay, even a few days, the more difficult it becomes to determine whether the fracture was inflicted before or after death. These fractures always raise a presumption of homicide.

Signs of Asphyxia Associated with Strangulation

These deaths are usually slow and are therefore accompanied by the presumptive signs of asphyxia. A dull red, violet or black colour of the skin above the ligature, with petechial haemorrhages into the skin of the eyelids, face and forehead are common findings. In many of the victims the face is puffy, the eyeballs bulge and the tongue protrudes. Petechial haemorrhages are often widespread, i.e. beneath the conjunctivae, in the scalp, beneath the pleura and epicardium, and elsewhere. Their number and extent, however, will be determined by the duration of the asphyxial process, there may be bleeding from the nose or ears. Pulmonary oedema is probably present. The signs are usually greater in self-strangulation than in homicide (Camps and Hunt, 1959).

Vagal inhibition. In the event of death from vagal inhibition, unusual in strangulation by a ligature, the signs of interference may be negligible both internally and externally.

It is generally accepted that gross changes, e.g. an obvious mark on the neck, bruising of neck muscles, fracture of the neck structures and obvious signs of asphyxia, are inconsistent with death by inhibition.

Evidence of sexual interference. Signs of sexual interference are detailed elsewhere (see p. 390). Murder of women by strangulation or throttling is not rarely the culmination of rape or attempted rape. In one case a consenting party demanded a higher fee during intercourse. When this was refused she threatened to scream. The man then strangled her. The ligature must be examined for the presence of blood or hairs or other suspicious material.

Pseudo-strangulation

The presence of bands of "contact flattening" in the skin of the neck of an obese person or well-nourished infant may at first suggest strangulation. They will be shown, however, to be of limited extent and to coincide with folds in the skin; there is no bruising, abrasion or parchmenting of the tissues in the area.

Where strangulation by the umbilical cord is suggested as the cause of asphyxia it is important to know the length of the cord. Littlejohn (1925) thus disproved this explanation of the death of an infant, found in a closet. There was a compression mark on the neck but the cord was too short to have been the agent.

Strangulation, after Death from Other Causes

The assailant may sometimes apply a ligature after death, e.g. after throttling. A man, charged with the murder of his wife, successfully pleaded that he had applied the ligature to her neck after death, with the intention that he should be found guilty of murder. He had a struggle with his wife who was accustomed to become violent when in a temper. During his attempts to quieten her by gripping her throat she died. He was so distressed at this that he too wished to die and therefore staged the death to appear to have been a murder. The prisoner was acquitted.

THROTTLING OR MANUAL STRANGULATION

Asphyxia produced by compression of the neck by human hands is termed throttling or manual strangulation.

The Circumstances of Throttling

Suicidal Throttling

It is generally accepted that suicide by throttling is well nigh impossible. When pressure by his or her own hands is sustained for a sufficient time to cause unconsciousness, they relax and the victim recovers. The only report traced of suicide by this means, for what it is worth, is that of Binner (1888).

> The victim was the wife of a policeman, in her late thirties. She suffered from articular rheumatism and, in September 1887, she developed mental symptoms. She became violent and had to be removed to hospital. She was anxious, excited and suffered from delusions. She tore and scratched her body and made repeated attempts to hang herself. She ate little and had loss of sleep. She returned home in October but towards the end of the month she had to be re-examined, with a view to certification. She was now quieter and rested a good deal. She had not attempted suicide whilst at home. On 26 October she was found by the daily help crouching in her bed and squeezing her throat with both of her hands. Her elbows were supported by her knees, her back was supported against the wall. Her hands were pulled away from her throat and she was laid on the bed. Binner arrived soon afterwards and found the patient so deeply unconscious that her corneal reflex was absent. Breathing was slow and irregular, convulsive in character, accompanied by rattling in the throat. She was pulseless at the wrist. The skin of the face and the mucous membranes were cyanosed, the tongue, also blue, was firmly clamped between the teeth. Numerous irregular and, in places, abraded marks were present on both sides of her neck. After 2 hours of resuscitation, mainly by artificial respiration, her breathing became regular and she recovered consciousness.
>
> The foregoing experience was followed by a notable improvement in her mental health. It was no longer believed necessary or advisable to send her to a mental hospital. Binner, however, warned the husband to take care and to retain the daily help. The patient was anxious to dismiss her and said she could manage the housework herself. The woman was dismissed at the end of November. When the husband left his home to go on duty early on 3 December he left his wife in the best of health and spirits. Their child went to school and the patient was left alone in the house. The husband returned at 10.30 a.m. and found his wife dead in her bedroom. She was in a crouching position beside her unmade bed. She had both of her hands round her throat and her elbows were supported by her knees and thighs; her head had fallen forwards so that her face lay on the bed. Artificial respiration was unsuccessful. When the body was seen by Binner at noon the same day, he found a number of bluish spots and impressions of finger-nails on both sides of the neck. (Binner regretted he could not describe them more exactly because the relevant notes had been lost.) There were no other injuries on the body and no sign of a mark on the neck of any ligature. There was no post-mortem examination of the body.

Binner said the husband might have killed her, but he was on good terms with his wife and the neighbours had heard no sounds of violence. Yet, had there been a struggle, the noise would have been heard through the thin walls of the house. When the body was examined at 12 noon, i.e. $1^1/_2$ hours after the husband returned home, it was noticeably cooling and rigor mortis was in its beginnings. Binner believed, therefore, that she must have died some hours before he saw the body and at a time when the husband could prove he was on duty far away from his home. No one else had entered the house during his absence. She had nearly killed herself in a similar manner in the previous October.

Accidental Throttling

A sudden application of one or both hands to another person's throat is capable of causing sudden death from vagal inhibition, in circumstances which are essentially innocent. The act may be done in jest, or during intercourse, demonstration of affection or it may be part of a physiological experiment. Its dire results are abrupt and injury to the parts is negligible; it is other than accident when death is by asphyxia and there are obvious signs of injury.

This mode of death received attention especially by French medical jurists, notably Tardieu (1879) and Brouardel (1897), who described several examples. The cause of death from inhibition in these circumstances was first recognised by Brown-Séquard.

> An early, excellent example is that related by Tardieu (1879). A young boy was sent by his father to a neighbouring shop to buy some tobacco. The shopkeeper was an elderly, thin woman whose neck was wasted. The boy, amused at the sight of her larynx ascending and descending with each movement of swallowing, wished to take hold of it *"comme il attraperait un papillon qui vole"*. He sprang forward and struck the woman's larynx and she fell dead.

Another variation of this mode of death was the subject of a murder charge in the United States. A couple were dancing and the man, either playfully or erotically, squeezed the neck of his partner. She went limp in his arms and is alleged to have died instantly. The accused was acquitted of her murder.

Homicidal Throttling

In general, a death from manual strangulation raises the presumption of homicide, whenever the death is due to asphyxia. The victims are usually infants, children or women. Robust adults can be throttled but not unless they are under the influence of drink or drugs, or stunned, or the attack is sudden and by stealth. Throttling is a common mode of homicide, as might be expected, since the agent is immediately available.

It is a method of choice in infanticide. Throttling of women is not rarely preceded by rape or attempted rape. Homicide by throttling, in circumstances of manslaughter, rather than by murder, may occur during an altercation, when, in a temper, one of the parties seizes a person, usually a woman, by the throat, to quieten or prevent her cries but without intent to kill or cause grievous bodily harm.

Occasionally the victim may be throttled to end suffering from natural disease. The son of a woman who had severe cardiac asthma, throttled her because he could not bear to see her suffer any longer (F.M. 477).

External Signs of Throttling

Most assailants who throttle probably use more force than is necessary to kill and it might be thought therefore that there will be obvious signs of injury, and of a kind which leave little doubt about the manner of their production. Sometimes, as depicted by Littlejohn (1925) clear crescents are cut in the skin by the nails; most are less clean-cut crescents. There are, however, not a few cases where the injuries are indefinite grazes which can readily escape notice by the less experienced and even by the experienced, if the body is seen under poor lighting. It is a prerequisite of clear crescents that the assailant has well-manicured fingernails, but most who embark on throttling are careless of their nails.

Irregularity of the nails may leave a signature on the skin of the victim. This occurred when the assailant had a projection on the nail of his thumb; the mark made on the lobe of the victim's left ear was angled as by such a nail (F.M. 6727).

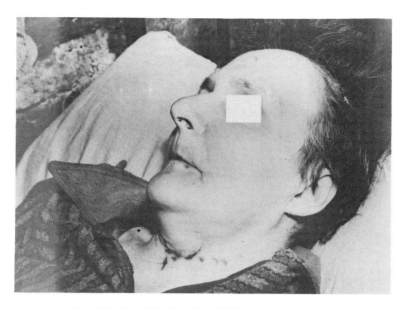

Fig. 147. Homicidal throttling. Nail marks in skin of neck.

Some bite them and in the case of an army matron the assailant had bitten his nails to the quick. There is no doubt about the pressure he had exerted with his hand on her neck before he applied her stocking, because when examined he had a severe sprain of his thumb. Yet the only external mark left was an indefinite circular abrasion on the front of her neck (F.M. 4484A).

There are occasions when the marks of throttling are clear, yet, at the trial, the result may be wholly unexpected. The defence invited me to examine the body of a woman alleged to have been throttled and I came to the conclusion that there was little doubt that this was homicidal throttling; the report of the Crown pathologist was more favourable to the defence than mine would have been. Needless to say I was not asked to give evidence. I was allowed to know the accused's explanation, which was something like this: He and his wife had had an altercation and she moved forward as if, he thought, to attack him. He moved to stop her, lost his footing, and clutching at the nearest support to break his fall, his fingers closed accidentally on her neck. He was acquitted.

In the absence of crescents or irregular abrasions or, for that matter, accompanying them, there may be round or oval bruising on the neck or near the mouth and nose. A second hand may produce marks on the face. Round, and more especially oval, bruising of recent origin in these regions is almost always produced only by the pads of fingers (Fig. 148).

Shifting of the grip, or its reapplication, usually increases the bruising and inflicts it at different levels. The direction of the scratches may be significant. This was important in the case of Cook. He had four parallel scratches running diagonally across his face (Fig. 16). He ascribed them to injuries due to handling rambler-rose canes but the jury preferred to regard them as scratches made by the girl whom he drowned in a flooded ditch (*R. v. Cook*, Dr. Gerald Evans.). The study of the scratches may determine whether they had

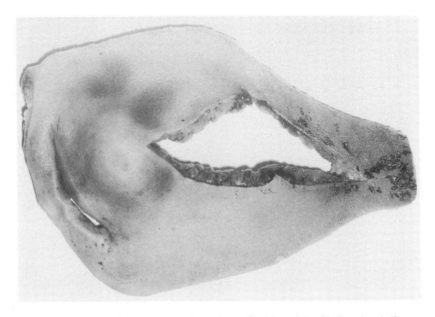

FIG. 148. Homicidal throttling and cut-throat. Bruising of the skin by a hand. (See also Fig. 149—scene of death).

been inflicted by the assailant or were self-inflicted when attempting to release a ligature, or were made on the assailant in self-defence.

Once abrasions or bruising of the neck have been noticed a closer scrutiny may discover coincident tiny cuts made by the nails. The external appearances are not rarely undramatic. The bruises may be only "tiny faint bruises" which, e.g. when five in a line at upper level of the larynx, have grave significance, providing they are proved microscopically.

If the assailant interposes soft material, for example the scarf of the victim, between his hand and the throat, external marking may be absent. Bruising may also be absent if the assailant maintains pressure upon the neck until after the victim has died, but this is an unusual event (F.M. 4391A). This is likely if pressure is maintained at one point until circulation ceases (Camps and Hunt, 1959).

Abrasions or scratches made by the fingernails of the assailant are usually multiple, at each side, or, in infants, towards the back of the neck, i.e, in an area likely to be covered by the fingers of a contracting hand or hands; these marks must attract close attention and receive adequate explanation. Occasionally, when the assailant's nails are long and well-trimmed, the marks are almost unequivocal evidence of throttling. Pressure of the nails then produces crescentic indentations with or without actual incision of the skin. They are more likely to be seen at the site of the thumb than the fingers because, when the throat is gripped, the thumb exerts more localised pressure and is likely to move less than the fingers during the struggles of the victim; it has a better purchase on the neck.

An interesting reconstruction of a left-handed throttling was reported by Mackintosh (1965); he found the injuries were accompanied by thrombosis of the common carotid artery.

If one hand alone was used, there may be more extensive abrasion on the side of the neck to which the fingers were applied; the thumb makes fewer scratches. If, therefore, the scratches are more numerous on the left side of the victim's neck, it may be inferred that throttling was by the right hand of the assailant, and vice versa.

On some occasions the attack is two-handed and this may be shown by the distribution of the scratches (see the case of Walker, below). It could be, of course, that the attack was from behind.

The range of external changes in throttling is almost unlimited. In some cases there may be no external signs, whereas, at the other extreme, there may be multiple abrasions, and obvious bruises. It is relatively a simple matter to interpret the latter but when the changes are slight or absent, it may be necessary to consider the evidence as a whole before reaching a conclusion as to the circumstances of the death. It is important to bear in mind that minor changes, or their absence, do not exclude a deliberate assault.

Although abrasions and bruises may be absent in throttling, they are present in most victims. Gonzales (1933) found them absent only once in a series of twenty-four cases of throttling. Even when absent externally it is almost invariable to find bruising of the neck muscles beneath.

Although attention is primarily directed to the neck, a complete examination of the body surface may demonstrate confirmatory signs. There may be abrasion and bruising, or other signs of pressure, over the shoulder blades, when the victim has been held down on the ground (Spilsbury, 1939, also F.M. 6727). Abrasion and bruising of the arms, in particular, and of the face and breasts of adults, may be sustained during the struggle which is usually a feature of homicide by throttling. The assailant may also sustain injury, notably scratches and bruising of the face and arms, or his hand or fingers may be bitten.

It is also imperative, in each case, to examine a female victim for signs of sexual interference. The victim may have been held down by the throat during intercourse or throttled to stop her cries. The signs of rape are considered separately (see p. 390).

Internal Signs of Throttling

The external signs may be equivocal but internal changes, when present, as they almost always are, can be of material assistance in determining the mode of death. The internal signs may be slight; e.g. bruising restricted to the subcutaneous tissues, a single neck muscle, accompanied by a recent complete or incomplete fracture of a great horn or of a thyroid cartilage (F.M. 16,050).

Bruising of the tissues deep to the skin, e.g. the fascia and muscles, is generally present, even when there are no external marks. Muscles, notably the sternomastoid, may be torn. This, however, can be the result of inexpert artificial respiration; a man who collapsed at a football match received first-aid and, in consequence, both sternomastoid muscles were ruptured. Bruising may be restricted to one or two of the smaller muscles.

Bruising of the tongue, also, is not infrequent, either a long the anterior border or elsewhere. The tongue may or may not be bitten; it is often protruded and thus exposed to injury by the teeth.

The body of the thyroid cartilage can be broken by a karate blow to the front of the neck (as in the case of Emmett-Dunne (Camps, 1959)), or by contact with the handlebar of a bicycle or the edge of a chair or similar ledge.

Fracture of the cricoid cartilage is almost exclusively the result of antero-posterior compression of it against the spine, e.g., by the thumbs or the forearm of the assailant. The central portion of the cartilage may be completely separated and displaced inwards, as in Gonzales's case (1933). When the cricoid breaks only in one place it is usually at the back (Thomson and Negus, 1948).

The horns of the hyoid bone may be fractured by a grip high up in the neck under the angles of the jaw or, possibly, as a result of traction on the thyro-hyoid membrane. The bone is drawn up and rigidly immobilised by muscles. Alternatively, it may be broken by a violent downward or lateral movement. (Camps and Hunt, 1959.)

In some of the victims the horns of the hyoid bone and thyroid cartilage may be broken (F.M. 2663A). Avulsion of the thyro-hyoid membrane with fracture of the right great horn of the hyoid bone was seen by Gonzales (1933).

It is to be expected that lateral compression, causing fractures of the hyoid bone and/or horns of the thyroid cartilage, will drive the distal fragments inwards. Weintraub (1961) saw no outward displacement of the fragments of the hyoid bone in fourteen cases of throttling. He attached more importance to an examination of the periosteum than the bone when an attempt is made to ascertain, in a case of fracture of the hyoid bone, whether the fragment was driven inwards or outwards.

Fracture of the neck structures in persons under 40 years of age or, more accurately in those whose laryngeal cartilages have not become ossified or whose hyoid bone still has mobile joints, is uncommon. The application of much more force than is required to kill usually leaves these elastic structures unbroken in the young. It is otherwise when the parts are ossified. The great horns of the thyroid cartilage are then especially vulnerable and deviation from the vertical is at once significant. It must not be concluded too hastily that throttling has occurred. A man who committed suicide by inhaling coal gas was found also to have a fracture of the right great horn of his thyroid cartilage. There were no external marks of throttling and this was an unequivocal case of suicide. It appears his neck had rested on a ledge; forcible removal from this position by his rescuer had caused the fracture. He was still breathing when released and bleeding occurred into the line of fracture and into the adjacent tissues (F.M. 5448). A similar injury occurred in a man whose body was found in a culvert where contact with its rocky floor could have caused the fracture (Dr. F. D. M. Hocking's case, see below).

Engorgement of the tissues, in a band the area of compression, is usual. The pharynx, tonsils, base of the tongue and upper part of the larynx are often involved and the degree and duration of compression may lead to extensive bleeding into these parts (Fig. 146). Haemorrhages may also appear beneath the capsule of the thyroid, submaxillary and carotid glands; they may occur in the lymphatic glands of the anterior triangle of the neck.

Injury to the hyoid bone or laryngeal cartilages, although inconstant, is of first importance. Since many of the victims are young, fractures do not occur but, in those over 40 years of age, and in others below that age when there is appreciable calcification of the structures, fractures are common and more frequently present than in persons of like age whose death is due to hanging or strangulation by a ligature.

The thyroid cartilage is the most vulnerable, as might be expected from the mechanism of throttling. The hand or hands are likely to apply the maximum force to this structure. The superior horns are often broken near their base but the extent of the damage varies. Only one horn, oftener on the side to which the thumb was applied, may be broken. The injury line may involve only the outer side of the horn. The fracture is then discovered by close search and gentle pressure upon the horn to reveal the fracture line. The occurrence of fracture is often apparent by bleeding beneath the periosteum and into the adjacent soft tissues, rarely, however, involving an area of above an inch in diameter. On other occasions the fracture line is recognised by a thin red line of bleeding restricted to its immediate neighbourhood, with or without limited bleeding into the substance of the cartilage. Such fractures are easily overlooked. Radiological examination of the larynx and hyoid bone, when practicable, is advisable prior to the direct investigation of obscure fractures, but may be disappointing, i.e. negative when dissection subsequently proves the occurrence of a fracture.

Fracture of a horn, even when associated with a little bleeding, is not proof of injury during life. It can be produced after death (Camps and Hunt, 1959; we have confirmed this). Such a fracture, unaccompanied by bruising of the skin and or muscles, can be caused by rough handling of the body, e.g. by hyperextension of the neck, and possibly by unskilled resuscitation—we once found rupture of the sternomastoid muscles which, on investigation, were the result of an unskilled attempt to resuscitate a man who had collapsed at a football match.

The demonstration of these fractures and bruised muscles calls for delicate handling and careful dissection of the parts. The technique described by Gordon, Turner and Price (1953) is the only proper one for the investigation of cases in which interference with the neck structures is suspected. That is to say, the dissection must always be a delicate removal of the structures, *layer by layer*. The block removal of the neck structures prior to dissection must never be done, because it is thus easy to produce artificial changes, difficult to distinguish from bruising. (The late Mr. Herbert Battison, our Chief technician, was highly skilled in detecting obscure fractures of the hyoid bone and larynx.)

Injury to the trachea is rare but was found in the case of *R. v. Pinckard* (see p. 384).

Although haemorrhage into the carotid sheath and thrombosis of the carotid artery may be seen, visible injury of the arteries, veins or nerves is unusual.

Sub-mucosal haemorrhages in the larynx are common and are to be distinguished from those directly due to asphyxia. They are larger and tend to coalesce and they are situated usually beneath, or in, the mucosa over the back of the epiglottis. Gonzales (1933) considered them the result of blood stasis rather than a direct result of local pressure because they lie above, rather than under, the point of pressure. Camps and Hunt (1959) ascribed these haemorrhages to overdistension of the venous plexuses of the pharynx and upper oesophagus and they are not then evidence of local injury to the larynx.

Signs of Asphyxia in Throttling

Throttling, except in deaths by vagal inhibition, is likely to give rise to well-developed signs of asphyxia. Lividity and puffiness of the face, and petechial haemorrhages in the "asphyxial" sites are common. Subarachnoid haemorrhages and possibly haemorrhages in the brain may occur. Gonzales reported their occurrence in a fourth of his cases but of the brain haemorrhages he said, "Rarely, areas of *small* haemorrhages occur in the brain substances and its membranes" (Gonzales *et al.*, 1954). This should be compared with the evidence in the trial of Ley and Smith (1947) and Camps and Hunt (1959).

Pulmonary oedema may be present. Its amount may be an index of the duration of the application of force to the neck but any assessment based on the presence or absence of oedema, or on its amount, must be made, and accepted, with considerable caution. It is well established that pulmonary oedema can occur in circumstances of immediate death and its amount may be appreciable, seen even with the naked eye, within minutes (Mason, 1962).

Survival after Throttling

Survival will depend, of course, upon the degree and duration of compression of the neck. It does not follow that minor fractures of the larynx will prove fatal. Fractures of the larynx, of all kinds, were formerly held to have a grave prognosis but "the more prompt relief of obstruction has in all probability reduced the previous death-rate to smaller figures" (Thompson and Negus, 1948). In their view, which relates only to accidents but is likely to be true also of criminal injuries, fractures of the thyroid cartilage are more serious than those of the hyoid bone; fracture of the cricoid cartilage proved fatal in every recorded case.

In throttling, however, the results are not those of injury to the larynx alone. As a rule the intent is to kill, and therefore, compression is continued, until or after, death takes place. If the grip seriously interfered with the cerebral circulation, and recovery occurs, it may be incomplete; the victim may then have permanent disability arising out of cerebral damage following cerebral anoxia.

Survival after collapse from vagal inhibition is unusual, but prompt resuscitation is capable of success and should be more often undertaken. Unfortunately, these incidents almost invariably occur when no one present is familiar with their treatment or desires to save the victim.

Throttling at About the Moment of Death from Other Causes

When throttling has been attempted at about the moment of death, it may be difficult to say with certainty whether the deceased was alive or dead at the time. Nail marks, in particular, can appear much the same whether inflicted just before or just after death. Is this also true of small bruises of the skin of the neck? In my opinion, such bruises are only produced during life, but the possibility that they could be produced after death merits experimental investigation. Tests so far made failed to yield such skin bruises after death.

A woman of 72 died after she had been severely assaulted. She had nail marks on her right cheek and neck; these could have been produced after death. She also had mild bruising of the skin in the neighbourhood of the right angle of the jaw and below the middle third of the left side of the lower jaw. There were no signs of asphyxia. She had severe coronary disease and fibrosis of her heart. The accused, who was found unfit to plead, made a statement in which he admitted that he had attacked his mother and thrown her to the ground. She got up and gained her armchair. He resumed his attack and put his hands round her neck; she died almost immediately (F.M. 6727A).

In searching for nail marks and small bruises on the neck, it is imperative that the examination, whenever practicable, is made under good conditions of lighting. The scrutiny of coloured subjects must be especially close, since slight skin injuries can readily be overlooked in them (Polson, 1961). Asphyxial petechiae are to be sought for beneath the conjunctivae.

The Time Taken to Kill by Throttling

Again and again the pathologist is asked to estimate the duration of fatal throttling. If the interval be brief, i.e. virtually instantaneous, this lends support to a defence of accidental death. Conversely, if it be long, a matter of minutes, the assailant must surely have been aware of the danger to the victim and intended to harm.

Unfortunately, unless present at the time, it is rarely, if ever, possible to give an accurate assessment of the interval. Even when the assailant himself gives an estimate, as I heard one do in the witness box, it cannot be relied upon. That man said he held the woman's neck for 30 seconds; it may have seemed like "a minute or more" to him but, when counsel timed 30 seconds in court, it seemed an eternity. An attack may continue for a period of 5 minutes but there are few who are capable of a sustained grip of the neck for that inordinate length of time.

The Amount of Force Used by an Assailant

This is a question which the pathologist must expect to be asked whenever it is alleged that death was due to throttling. Of course a violent and sustained attack is indicative of intent to injure, if not to kill. Conversely, a brief and minor contact with the neck would be consistent with restraint without intent to injure; it could be an accidental contact.

Unfortunately it cannot be stated as a rule that minor damage, or absence of damage, to the neck structures is proof of innocence. It may be presumptive of innocence, but, it is well established that deliberate interference with the neck structures can kill and leave little evidence of damage; the karate blow is an outstanding example. In the presence of slight changes in the neck structures the pathologist can only offer a guarded opinion on the probable degree of force used; he should err, if at all, in favour of the defendant. The interpretation of the circumstances must rest with those who hear and weigh the evidence as a whole. On the other hand, when there is abundant damage to the neck structures, it is reasonable to say that appreciable, or even, in some circumstances, considerable, force was used. This must be related to the physique of the assailant; men with a powerful grip can do far more damage than those with a weak grip and this may bear on the question of intent. A man under the influence of alcohol may also use greater force than he might have done when sober. If there is fracture of the larynx or hyoid bone, the grip used must have been such that the person was aware of doing this; it is scarcely an accidental touch or momentary grip.

EXAMPLES

1. *The Booth Case* (*F.M. 4391*A). The victim was a well-nourished woman aged 40. Her face was dusky and puffy and petechial haemorrhages were present in the skin and beneath the conjunctivae of the lower eyelids. Bleeding had occurred from the right nostril. The tongue protruded by about $^1/_4$ in. but it was not bitten. No nail marks were detected but an elliptical bruise, a love bite, was present in the right side of the neck; a second was on the right breast. Two other bruises were found but they were small, $^1/_8$ in. $\times$ $^1/_{16}$ in., and of indefinite character. The muscles at the front of the neck, including both sternomastoid muscles and those directly related to the larynx, were bruised and there was also some recent bleeding into the connective tissues

near the larynx, especially on the right side. A small bruise was present in the tongue, on its left side at about the midpoint of the margin of the tongue. The hyoid bone, although ankylosed, was intact. The larynx was still wholly cartilaginous; it was intact but there was congestion of the mucosa and twelve pinhead haemorrhages were present in the mucosa of the subglottic space. The cricoid cartilage and trachea were normal. Bleeding had occurred into lymphatic glands in the right anterior triangle of the neck. The tonsils were engorged and haemorrhage had occurred in their substance. Petechial haemorrhages were plentiful and had a wide distribution in the deeper layers of the scalp; more were found in relation to both temporal muscles and there was a small haemorrhage within the right temporal muscle. The rest of the examination disclosed no abnormality. There were no internal petechial haemorrhages.

The appearances were consistent with manual strangulation, pressure being applied until death occurred, or strangulation by a soft, broad ligature.

The accused admitted he had killed the deceased and had gripped her throat for several seconds. This incident was the culmination of an affair which had become too onerous. He was a married man, a taxi driver, who made a practice of taking the deceased for journeys in his taxi-cab. He had found himself unable to meet the demands of both women. He had taken the deceased to a quiet place and a quarrel arose. He was tired and she resented his reluctance to have intercourse. She upbraided him, he lost his temper, and in an attempt to end her tirade he pulled her towards him and gripped her throat with his left hand. He held on to her throat "for a minute or more." "I held on until she was dead." He had strong hands. He then attempted suicide by cutting his wrist; it was only a shallow cut. He eventually gave himself up and told the police he had strangled the deceased.

An attempt was made by the defence to suggest that death in this case could have been due to vagal inhibition. It was also suggested that the absence of internal petechial haemorrhages negatived death by throttling. The prisoner was convicted of manslaughter and sentenced to imprisonment for 4 years.

2. *The Walker Case* (*F.M. 2959*). A woman, aged 45, was throttled by her husband. Abrasions were present on the throat and face. One principal area of abrasion, an inch square, with local minor scratches, was present on the right side; several abrasions, of up to $^1/_2$ in. long, one of which was crescentic with the convexity directed backwards, were present on the left side of her nose and her left cheek; bruising was not apparent. The interpretation was that it had been a two-handed attack, the right hand at the throat and the left on the face, the assailant being in front of, or above, the victim as she lay in bed. There had been no struggle and, since it was shown that she had taken a barbiturate in medicinal quantity, she may have been asleep at the time of the attack. There was fracture of both superior horns of the thyroid cartilage; the cricoid cartilage and hyoid bone were intact.

3. *The Massey Case* (*F.M. 1516*). A girl, aged 18, was murdered by throat-cut but, prior to that, she had been partially asphyxiated by throttling. Abrasions were negligible, but recent bruises, of the lips, beneath the chin and on the left cheek, were oval and could have been made by the pads of the fingers (Fig. 148). Three small abrasions, each oval, were present on the left side of the neck, just below the angle of the jaw; these may have been made by the fingernails of the assailant.

4. *The Hessler Case* (*6 Feb. 1952*). The victim was a woman aged 38 years, who was throttled by a man of good physique, when he attempted to stop her shouting and screaming. There were marks on the neck and the cricoid cartilage was fractured. The interest of this case lies in the fact that the assailant described how he had acted. According to the report he said he did not put a hand over her mouth. "I got hold of her with both my hands round her throat. I pressed on her throat and she still made a little noise. I just pressed again and she stopped shouting and screaming . . . I knelt down in front of her . . . I put both my hands round her neck, with my thumbs to the front." (Here he demonstrated to the jury.) "My hands were not too tight. They were just placed round her neck. I applied very slight pressure with my thumbs and then I took my thumbs away. She was still making a noise and I pressed again with my thumbs and I took my thumbs away and there was no noise." He had done this "just to quieten her and to stop her making such a fool of herself; she was under the influence of drink". The assailant was found guilty of manslaughter (*R. v. B.*, Durham Assizes, February 1952).

5. *The Wills Case*. This unusual and interesting case is one about which the reader may like to draw his own conclusions.

The deceased was a farmer aged 39, who was dominated by his mother. Some years previously, he had married a local girl at her instigation. She told him he should get married and that "Maggie down the road" would do. It would appear to have proved a workable arrangement; there was one child.

Several members of his family had committed suicide. The day before his death he had been fined for an offence in relation to the affairs of the farm which he shared with his brothers. He had been much upset by this conviction and the family only learnt of it from the Press report. There was no evidence of a quarrel over the matter and there was no other motive for murder.

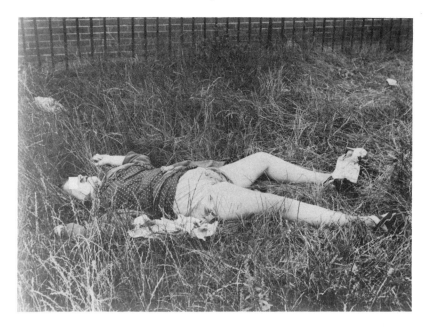

Fig. 149. Scene of homicide by throttling and cut-throat (see Fig. 148).

On the day of his death he arose at 7 a.m. and, as was his custom, went out to feed the chickens. When he had not returned at 8 a.m. for his breakfast, two of his brothers went to find him. A track made by his hob-nailed boots was followed and, eventually, his body was found in a shallow pool, concealed by a steep bank, tree loppings and vegetation. This pool, however, could be reached by at least two other paths and it was unusual for only one set of footmarks to be on the path he had followed; it was one used by farmers and foresters.

The body lay outstretched, face down, with the head inside a culvert through which a fair volume of water was then running. The shoulders had probably been either just inside or just outside the opening which was rectangular and about two feet in size. The rest of the body lay in a shallow pool, fed by the culvert. His brothers, who found him, said they had had no difficulty in lifting the body to the bank. They had lifted him by the shoulders, arms and, perhaps, legs. They had not handled his neck. The water in the pool which was muddy was only 2 to 4 in., but in the mouth of the culvert it was about 12 in. deep.

External injury was limited to fairly severe grazing, with recent bruising, of the whole of the bridge of the nose. Submersion was quite recent. Signs of asphyxia, external and internal, were absent but there were a few small haemorrhages inside the larynx. There was a little bloodstained froth in the trachea; no water was found in the air passage or lungs. There was about $1/2$ pint of water in his stomach; this contained diatoms but was not muddy.

The neck structures were injured: a recent bruise, $3/4$ in. in diameter, was present at the anterior border of the right sterno-mastoid muscle just above the sternum, and a similar bruise, 2 in. higher, was associated with mottled bruising of the whole thickness of the adjacent muscle. Two more recent bruises, one $3/4$ in. and the other $1/8$ in. were, respectively, above and below the left side of the hyoid bone. Recent bruising was also seen at both margins of the tongue. Although no bruising of the skin was seen over the deep bruises, it was subsequently shown by microscopy that bleeding had occurred in some areas of the skin at the front of the neck.

The great horn of the hyoid bone was broken on the left side at about $1/2$ in. from its tip. The appearances were entirely consistent with fracture after death. (Although absence of bleeding in these fractures is usually conclusive of post-mortem origin, it was absent in two cases of unequivocal suicide by hanging (see p. 377).

He had been a healthy man. There was no evidence of disease.

There were other places near the farm where suicide by drowning could have been accomplished with greater ease and convenience. The water in his stomach, in the culvert and the house, had the same microscopical appearances, i.e. diatoms were present in all three, but the pool water was muddy and that in his stomach was not. His widow said he had not had a drink before leaving the house.

It is difficult in a summary to present all the relevant facts or, in any event, to know the full details. There may be enough evidence, however, to permit the reader to form an opinion on the probable cause of death and the circumstances in which it occurred.

Some of the questions which might be considered are these: did he die of homicidal manual strangulation, causing shock and was the pressure increased, after death, to cause fracture of the hyoid bone? Did he commit suicide by attempting to jam his body in the culvert and thus sustained the neck injury? (The culvert was lined by jagged rocks with sharp edges likely to cut the face and neck of a person struggling in the culvert but, on the other hand, the flow of water may have had a cushioning effect.)

(I am indebted to Dr. F. D. M. Hocking (1953) for a report on this case and permission to make use of it.)

References

BECK, T. R. and BECK, J. B. (1836) *Elements of Medical Jurisprudence*, 5th ed. Edinburgh: Longmans.

BINNER (STETTIN) (1888) *Z. Med.-Beamte*, **1**, 364–8; trans. provided by Professor J. R. Wilkie.

BROUARDEL, P. (1897) *La Pendaison, la Strangulation, etc.*, p. 228. Paris: Baillière.

BROUARDEL, P. (1904) *Ann. Hyg. publ.* (*Paris*), **2**, 193–227.

CAMPS, F. E. (1959) *Med.-Leg. J.* (*Camb.*), **27**, 156.

CAMPS, F. E. and HUNT, A. C. (1959) *J. Forens. Med.*, **6**, 116.

DUMONT, G. and DÉROBERT, L. (1962) *Annls. Méd.-lég. Crimin., Police Scient.*, **42**, 475.

EVANS, G. (1961) *Med. Sci. Law*, **1**, 33. R. v. COOKE (1955) Flintshire Assizes.

FORBES, G. (1945) *Police Journal*, **18**, 27–32.

GLAISTER, J. and RENTOUL, E. (1966) *Medical Jurisprudence and Toxicology*, 12th ed., Edinburgh: Livingstone.

GONZALES, T. A. (1933) *Arch. Path. Lab. Med.*, **15**, 55–66.

GONZALES, T. A., VANCE, M., HELPERN, M. and UMBERGER, C. J. (1954) *Legal Medicine and Toxicology*, 2nd ed., pp. 467, 469. New York: Appleton Century.

GORDON, I., TURNER, R. and PRICE, T. W. (1953) *Medical Jurisprudence*, 3rd ed., pp. 481–5, Edinburgh: Livingstone.

GUY, W. A. and FERRIER, D. (1895) *Principles of Forensic Medicine*, 7th ed., W. R. Smith, London: Renshaw.

HOCKING, F. D. M. (1953) Personal communication and file of his case.

KEILLER, A. (1855–6) *Edinb. Med. J.*, **1**, 527–34; 824–30.

LITTLEJOHN, HARVEY (1925) *Forensic Medicine*. London: Churchill.

MACKINTOSH, R. H. (1965) *Med. Sci. Law*, **5**, 117.

MANT, A. K. (1960) *Forensic Medicine*, p. 139. London: Lloyd-Luke.

MITRANI, J. (1962) *J. Forens. Med.*, **9**, 20.

POLSON, C. J. (1957) *Med.-leg. J.* (*Camb.*), **25**, 101–8.

POLSON, C. J. (1961) *J. Forensic Sci. Soc.*, **1**, 79–83.

PUPPE, G. (1908) *Atlas u. Grundriss*, vol. 1, Munich: Lehmann.

R. v. DONALD (1934) *Trial of Jeannie Donald. Notable British Trials Series*, vol. 79, ed. J. G. Wilson, Edinburgh, etc.; Hodge.

R. v. LEY and SMITH (1947) *Notable British Trials Series*, ed. F. Tennyson Jesse. Edinburgh, etc.; Hodge.

SIMPSON, C. K. (1960) *Int. Crim. Pol. Rev.*, **138**, 137.

SMITH, Sir SYDNEY and FIDDES, F. S. (1955) *Forensic Medicine*, 10th ed., p. 234. London: Churchill.

SPILSBURY, Sir BERNARD (1939) *Med.-leg. Rev.*, **7**, 215–23.

TARDIEU, A. (1879) *La Pendaison, la Strangulation et la Suffocation*, 2nd ed., p. 206, Paris: Baillière.

TAYLOR, A. S. (1965) *Medical Jurisprudence*, ed. K. Simpson, 12th ed., vol. 1. London: Churchill.

THOMSON, ST. C. and NEGUS, E. (1948) *Diseases of the Nose and Throat*, 5th ed., p. 543. London: Churchill.

THURSTON, G. (1971) in a lecture to the Harrogate Medical Society; also reported by SIMPSON, C. K. (1960) *Int. Criminol. Pol. Rev.*, **138**, 132.

TIDY, C. M. (1883) *Legal Medicine*, vol. 2. London: Smith Elder.

VON KARGER, J. (1969) *Arch. Kriminol.*, **144**, 95.

WEIMANN, W. and SPENGLER, H. (1956) *Arch. Kriminol.*, **117**, 29, 75 and 145; *Ibid.* **118**, 71, 110.

WEINTRAUB, C. M. (1961) *Med.-leg. J.* (*Camb.*)., **29**, 209–16.

CHAPTER 11

Drowning

DROWNING is the result of submersion or partial submersion in a fluid. Although the precise mechanism of drowning is complex and is modified by the medium and other factors, in the majority, the inhalation of fluid, thereby obstructing the air passages, is the essential cause of death. When fresh water is inhaled in quantity there may be rapid and considerable dilution of the blood. When a quantity of salt water is inhaled, there may be haemoconcentration and grave disturbance of the electrolyte balance. In some cases, admittedly a minority, when little water had been inhaled, neither mechanical obstruction nor absorption of the fluid medium caused death. In these cases death was due to abrupt cardiac arrest, due to vagal inhibition. There are also a few reliable reports which compel the view that death was then the result of immediate, sustained laryngeal spasm. The post-mortem appearances of each of these variations of death by submersion are also modified if, prior to submersion, the victim had been rendered unconscious, as by a head injury or an epileptic fit.

In considering the post-mortem appearances of bodies recovered from water, it is also necessary clearly to distinguish between the changes which are due to drowning and those which are solely the result of submersion in water. The latter, of course, will occur in bodies immersed in water after death from causes other than drowning.

The Medium of Submersion

The medium is usually water but occasionally a victim may fall into a vat of beer, dye or some other chemical solution or paint (Gold and Ollodart, 1967).

The death may occur in a river, lake or canal, the sea, or in a household or public bath. James (1966) reported a case of drowning in a vat of beer. When endeavouring to ascertain the cause of death, the composition of the medium should be determined. If it contains substances peculiar to it, notably diatoms, similar substances may be demonstrated in fluid from the air passages or stomach of the victim. Samples of water from the place of submersion and from the body of the victim can be examined for the presence of, say, diatoms, sand, weeds or seaweed or some chemical substance which could have entered the lungs or stomach only as the result of inhaling or ingesting the water from which the body was recovered. Langton Hewer (1962) drew attention to the special danger of the inhalation of a thick suspension of sand in sea water. This may occur during surf bathing in shallow water, when knocked down by a large wave or hit in the abdomen with the surf board. "Death can then ensue with appalling suddenness."

The presence of chemicals in the medium may not contribute to the cause of death but their detection in the fluid and in the body of a victim confirm the fact of drowning in that fluid, i.e. pond, lake or river, etc. For example, a boy aged 7 years was drowned in a pond near a colliery tip. Phenol compounds were present in the water and in the boy's blood but the concentration was too low to have been a factor in his death. It confirmed the fact of submersion in that pond (F.M. 14,926A; analyses by R. A. Dalley).

The Extent and Duration of Submersion in Fatal Cases

Ordinarily the whole body of the victim is submerged but submersion of the nose and mouth alone for a sufficient period can cause death from drowning. A victim, therefore, can be drowned when the head and shoulders are submerged or even when the face alone is under water. Small children, of course, may be completely submerged in relatively little water, for example, an ornamental pond less than 2 ft deep. These are best omitted from gardens where small children may play.

Even pails can be dangerous (Scott *et al.* 1980).

Pearn *et al*, (1979) reported a study of childhood deaths from drowning in the bathtub. He and other authors (Nixon and Pearn, 1977) have drawn attention to the possibility of non-accidental injury in children masquerading as accidental drowning. Factors which are considered to be suggestive of the possibility of deliberate child abuse are an older age group (15 to 30 months) than the accidental immersion; a handicapped child who is the eldest in a small family; and the only child in the bath at an unusual time of the day.

A baby was killed by his father, who held his face under a water tap. The baby inhaled sufficient water to produce severe haemo-dilution and death within a few minutes (F.M. 12,126B).

The victims of drowning in shallow water, although usually children, may be adults, usually epileptics, who, during a fit, fall face down into shallow water, which may be no more than a puddle in the road. Adults under the influence of drink or drugs may also be drowned in similar circumstances. Another possibility is collapse due to coronary artery disease or dizziness due to essential hypertension. A man, when fishing on the bank of a river, suddenly pitched forward into the water and his head and shoulders became submerged. Although he was promptly removed by friends, he was dead. Examination of his body demonstrated severe disease of the coronary arteries and some evidence of drowning. It was believed, therefore, that he had collapsed as a result of a heart attack and that his death was accelerated by drowning (F.M. 308).

A farmer aged 61 was in the habit of putting his head into a bucket of cold water during hot weather. He was found dead, half-kneeling, half-crouching, in his wash-house. He had signs of death by drowning and also of severe coronary artery disease. It appeared he had had a heart attack and death was accelerated by drowning (F.M. 540).

A woman aged 50 intending suicide, drowned herself by thrusting her face into a bowl of water, the depth of which was only 6 in. She was found dead in her bed with the bowl still tightly held in her hands.

The Time it takes to drown varies within somewhat wide limits, which are determined by the circumstances, for example, the kind of victim, his reactions to submersion and above all, the volume of water inhaled. The time is reduced when submersion is unexpected and when the victim is of poor physique or unable to swim. Death may be immediate when due to cardiac inhibition. Those who give way to panic will succumb more readily than those who endeavour, even if but indifferent swimmers, to keep calm. The factors of cramp or injury sustained at the time of submersion will also play a part.

Hypothermia may develop rapidly in cold water (Keatinge, 1969). Skilled swimmers were unable to keep swimming for more than a few minutes since they were exposed to excessive activity, difficulty in breathing, and increased viscosity of the water. They were exhausted by the extra work and were suffering from panic. According to Keatinge the principal cause of death in shipwreck is hypothermia. A man aged 81, who did not wish to become a nuisance to others, sat in a bath of cold water with intention to end his life. A "suicide" note was left in the bathroom. His death was ascribed to hypothermia (*Yorkshire Post*, 19 Nov. 1971).

It is possible that *sudden* immersion into cold water can cause death from cardiac failure, due to rises in venous and arterial pressure. These were demonstrated after sudden immersion in water at $6°C$ ($43°F$) by Keatinge and McCance (1959). Alternatively, uncontrollable respiratory distress during cold immersion may cause the victim to inhale water (Keatinge and Nadel, 1962).

The principal cause of death in hypothermia due to immersion is cardiac arrest, since with decreasing body temperature, the cardiac output progressively declines. The other major hazard is ventricular fibrillation (Keatinge, 1977).

A case of sudden death, apparently due to ventricular fibrillation, occurring in a good swimmer immediately after getting out of a swimming bath has been described (Keatinge and Hayward, 1981).

Ordinarily, unconsciousness, if not death, ensues within from 2 or 3 to 10 minutes after submersion. Before death there may be a period of suspended animation during which it is still possible to resuscitate the victim, if promptly recovered from the water. Payne (1940) said success is possible even when the victim has been completely submerged for as long as 30 minutes and Kvittingen and Naess (1963) recorded recovery of a child after submersion for 20 minutes. Artificial respiration, therefore, should not be readily abandoned, even though submersion has continued for a matter of several minutes.

The popular and still prevalent belief that a person sinks and rises three times before he is drowned is not based upon fact. There is wide variation in the number of times he may sink before he remains submerged. The ordinary course of events, when a non-swimmer falls into the water, is that he first sinks and, shortly afterwards, through the natural buoyancy of the body, he rises to the surface. When he cries for help and struggles he is likely to inhale water, which induces coughing and this, in turn, leads to disturbance of the rhythm of breathing; his struggles increase and again he sinks. If this occurs at a moment of inspiration he will inhale more water. The process may occur once, thrice or oftener, until he remains submerged. There is then usually a brief convulsive phase, followed by coma or suspended animation and death. The body eventually sinks and remains on the bed of the river, sea or canal, until putrefaction sets in. The formation of gas then causes the body to float, which occurs in from 7 to 14 days.

Experimentally, Karpovitch (1933) found that animals, when submerged, made an immediate struggle for freedom and during this time there might be a surprise inhalation of water. A quiet period followed, when movement was suspended; a little air was exhaled and the animal swallowed frequently. The third phase was characterised by violent struggles for freedom. This was followed by the onset of convulsions, accompanied by expiratory and spasmodic inspiratory efforts; meantime, the mouth was open wide. The reflexes then disappeared and soon afterwards the animal died. Using coloured water, it was shown that it could reach any part of the lungs. Resuscitation was considerably hindered by the formation of froth and the presence of water in the air passages and lungs. The amount of water inhaled varied within wide limits, e.g. from 12.5 cm³ to 36.9 cm³ per kilo of body weight. The longer the water took to enter the body, the more of it was absorbed into the blood stream; the quantity inhaled might then exceed the amount ordinarily required to drown the animal. These experiments confirmed, with slight amplification, the results obtained by Brouardel (1897).

A film recording the results of experimental drowning was prepared by Professor F. Thomas of Ghent.

Voluntary submersion can normally be tolerated only for short periods. With training it is possible, for example, to swim the length of a swimming pool under water. The time limit to which even pearl divers can attain is only of the order of 2 to 3 minutes.

The risks of hyperventilation before swimming under water were brought to notice by the report of eight people who lost consciousness but survived while swimming under water and of five others who were drowned in similar circumstances (Craig, 1961). The dangers of "plunge" or underwater swimming competitions, where it is the standard practice to hyperventilate prior to entering the water, have been stressed. This practice can lead to sudden loss of consciousness and the drowning of supremely fit persons. Those in charge of children, in particular, should prohibit the practice and warn their charges of its dangers.

The Mechanism of Drowning

It is only within recent years that the mechanism of drowning has been recognised as something more complex than simple mechanical obstruction of the air passages by fluid. There is a danger, however, that in the enthusiasm for electrolyte imbalance and scientific medicine this factor in drowning may be overlooked.

Experiments have shown that small amounts of sea water of from 1 to 3 ml/kg body weight, when introduced into the air passages of lightly anaesthetised sheep, killed four out of eighteen; death was due to anoxia. Fresh water was found much less lethal (Halmagyi and Colebatch, 1961).

The inhalation of water can and does result in its absorption by the circulating blood; the ensuing changes in the blood contribute materially to death by drowning. It is, of course, presupposed that enough fluid has been inhaled and the victim has survived long enough for absorption and electrolyte exchange to take place, but this can occur within a few minutes following total submersion.

It could well be that this aspect of drowning would have been recognised much earlier, if more attention had been paid to Brouardel's experiments. From relatively early times, i.e. the mid-nineteenth century, if not before, the fluidity of the blood in the bodies of the drowned had attracted attention, e.g. by Devergie, Casper and Orfila. It was Brouardel, with Vibert, in 1880, who first sought an explanation. Their experiments with dogs demonstrated that drowning caused a notable reduction in the red cell count and, in their view, this was the result of haemodilution; they wrongly rejected haemolysis as a coincident cause of red cell loss. They also demonstrated that the route of absorption was the lungs and not the stomach and that it occurred only when submersion was relatively prolonged (Brouardel, 1897).

This problem was studied by Revenstorf (1903) and Banting *et al.* (1938). Experiments by Swann and his colleagues, notably Spafford during 1947–51, produced results on which the modern view of drowning is based. They confirmed that fresh water was rapidly absorbed in large, indeed enormous, quantities when dogs were submerged. Within 3 minutes the circulating blood could be diluted by as much as 72 per cent with coincident haemolysis. The heart muscle in consequence sustained what Donald (1955) in his review termed "a serious biochemical insult"; there was plasma potassium excess and sodium loss; there was also extreme myocardial anoxia. Haemodilution also overloaded the circulation. A rapid and considerable fall in systolic blood pressure occurred and within minutes there was ventricular fibrillation. Although the heart may continue to beat feebly for several minutes after rescue, there will have been severe cerebral anoxia, which is the immediate cause of death. It is not surprising, as Rushton (1961) has pointed out, that the mortality rate in drowning is high.

The mechanism of drowning in sea water is different. Swann showed that there is haemoconcentration; there may be up to 42 per cent withdrawal of water from the circulating blood into the lungs whereby massive pulmonary oedema is rapidly produced. Exchange of electrolytes from sea water to the blood also has its adverse effects; the haematocrit and plasma sodium levels rise steeply. Ventricular fibrillation is not a feature and heart failure is slower—it took from 5 to 8 minutes in dogs; its cause, however, is myocardial anoxia, and this, with increased viscosity of the blood, causes rapid weakening and failure of the heart. There is no haemolysis. The systolic blood pressure may be maintained for several minutes.

Modell (1968) has reviewed the mechanism of drowning. He suggests that 10 per cent of drowning victims do not aspirate water, but die of asphyxia due to laryngospasm. In animal experiments, if freshwater is aspirated there is an increase in blood volume proportional to the amount of water aspirated with decreases in serum sodium, chloride and calcium, and increase in potassium in arterial blood samples. In near-drowning victims the electrolyte levels returned to normal within an hour. The principal effect on all animals was that they suffered from acute asphyxia, whatever the volume of water aspirated.

In experimental drowning in sea water haemoconcentration occurs, and sea water drowning is twice as lethal as fresh water.

In human near drowned victims he found no significant alterations in electrolyte values, but severe hypoxaemia and acidosis. This is thought to result from atalectasis caused by loss of surfactant due to the effects of the water. Survival for a short period allows time from readjustment of electrolytes.

The Symptoms of Drowning

Authentic information is scanty but, such as it is, it does not confirm the popular belief that, while submerged, the victim is always preoccupied with a review of the incidents of his past life, but this is sometimes true. When a youngster, Admiral Beaufort fell overboard at Portsmouth. He recalled this experience in a letter to an acquaintance, some years later. He said he lost all hope of rescue and, "From that moment all exertion ceased, a calm feeling of the most perfect tranquillity superseded the previous tumultuous sensations. It might be called apathy, certainly not resignation, for drowning no longer appeared to be an evil. I no longer thought of being rescued, nor was I in any bodily pain." He likened his sensations to the state preceding sleep after fatigue. His senses were deadened but his mind remained active. His thoughts were of his home and family and then he passed on to recall his last cruise and former boyish adventures. All this took place in the space of about 2 minutes before he was rescued (*Brit. Med. J.*, 1894, ii, 823).

Another man described how he lay on the bed of a river in a semi-conscious condition. During this time he imagined that he saw his relatives and friends around him, showing their grief at his death; he visualised the circumstances of his own funeral, even to the point of the earth falling on the coffin. His other thoughts recalled past events in his life. There was no bodily pain but he had tinnitus and coloured vision; eventually he became unconscious. When he recovered consciousness he found himself on the bank of the river "being subjected to the disagreeable process of restoration of life" (*Brit. Med. J.*, 1894, i, 823).

A woman who was rescued when in difficulties in Morecambe Bay said that, having gone down twice, her only thought was that "she had only to go down once more and all would be over" (*Brit. Med. J.*, 1894, ii, 823).

Self-preservation was also the dominant thought in the mind of a woman who was in difficulties when bathing in the sea with her family. She experienced particular distress when, despite her cries, she saw the others apparently swimming away from her, leaving her to drown. Unlike the others mentioned, she found her experience one of acute suffering. "I sank again and gasped involuntarily. Then all other senses were overpowered by the agonising scorching pain which followed the rush of salt water into my lungs. From that moment I was conscious only of that burning suffocation, and the intense desire that the others might know what had become of me. Except for that one thought my brain was dulled." She complained of a roaring in her ears and a red mist before her eyes. Her general reaction was summed up by her statement "I only suffered". She was unconscious when rescued by her husband within 3 minutes of the time she first sank (Cullen, 1894).

Lowson (1903) said that he breathed in when apnoea became intolerable and immediately swallowed a large gulp of water. After about ten gulps he experienced increasing relief. This he later ascribed to the sedative effects of a rising CO_2 tension. He became unconscious but recovered when he regained the surface. He then took a few breaths and was able to swim to the shore, where he vomited a large amount of water. For some reason he suffered no signs or symptoms of the inhalation of water.

The Signs of Drowning

Although the bodies of those who die from drowning do not present infallible and constant signs peculiar to drowning, the opinion of Casper (1862) still holds, namely, that the difficulties in the recognition of a death from drowning have been much overrated, providing that putrefaction has not set in to obscure or obliterate the changes by which a death from drowning may be recognised. It is usually possible also to state with reasonable certainty whether the victim was alive or dead at the time of submersion. It is necessary, however, on all occasions to consider all the available information. The special difficulty in interpretation is to distinguish between accidental, suicidal and homicidal drowning. "In no other case is it of more importance for solving this riddle, to ascertain the combination of circumstances preceding or accompanying the death, and in no other is so little of these generally known, because very often the body is only found after a lapse of time so great as to prevent its being recognised, to say nothing of the impossibility of discovering anything regarding the previous history of a body found perhaps many, many miles away from its dwelling-place while alive" (Casper, 1862). Although in this country this is perhaps an over-statement of the difficulties, the fact remains that not infrequently the coroner is compelled to return an open verdict at an inquest on a body recovered from water.

It is imperative that all available information concerning the circumstances of drowning is given to the pathologist prior to autopsy. We have had experience of the consequences of delay, or possibly deliberate suppression, of information. Fortunately the examination was thorough and adequate. The death appeared, on first information, to have been an accidental drowning but, some months later, it was alleged that the man had either been pushed into the water or fell into it when chased. It was also alleged that he had been assaulted. The only evidence of injury was a trivial round bruise of his forehead; the skin and skull were intact. Although the body had been in the water for several days the diatom content of his lungs was consistent with death by drowning. The two persons charged with his unlawful killing were acquitted (F.M. 13,932) (Leeds Assizes, Nov. 1971).

The External Signs of Drowning

Although the external appearances of the drowned are of less importance than of those who die of other forms of mechanical asphyxia, a detailed record of them is essential. They will be apparent to best advantage only when putrefaction is absent.

In this country cooling of the body in water ordinarily occurs at about twice the rate of cooling in air and, therefore, most bodies of the drowned are cool or cold when recovered. It is only during the first few hours that observation of the rectal temperature is of value. The rate of fall of temperature is of the order of $5°F$ per hour and, therefore, the temperature of the body is usually likely to fall to that of its surroundings within 5 or 6 hours, and nearly always within 12 hours of submersion.

Post-mortem hypostasis may be confined to the head, neck and front of the chest and is frequently bright pink in colour, simulating the tint in carbon monoxide poisoning but distinguished from it by its distribution and, of course, the absence of carbon monoxide in the blood. The colour is due to exposure and oxygenation of the dependent blood and its distribution is determined by the position of the body as it floats in the water.

Putrefaction is often present and the skin may be of green or bronze colour, or it may be exceptionally dark, and the head and neck may then present the *tête de nègre* appearance. Only too often putrefaction has advanced to a stage when the bloated and discolored tissues preclude identification. It is then necessary to rely upon clothing or articles on the body, when available. Fingerprints or dermal prints may also be valuable for this purpose, even in the presence of putrefaction.

Goose-flesh, or cutis anserina, once believed an important external sign, is frequently present but this change can occur during the interval between somatic and molecular death, or it can be a post-mortem change due to rigor mortis of the arrectores pilorum muscles. It may be absent at the time of the recovery of the body but may become apparent next day (Sydney Smith and Fiddes, 1955). Goose-flesh can also occur in circumstances other than drowning. It has no value as a diagnostic sign.

The presence of foam at the mouth or nostrils, or both, is an important, although in no way a conclusive sign of drowning. It can occur when death is due to strangulation, in acute pulmonary oedema or during an epileptic fit, or, rarely, after an electrical shock (Jellinek, 1932). It is, however, usually possible to make a clear distinction between these causes by a consideration of the other findings and circumstances of the death. It is unusual for the nature and quantity of the foam to simulate that of drowning.

This foam presents as a small balloon or mushroom-like mass, *champignon de mousse* White or pinkish colour (Fig. 150). In one case the foam resembled a protruded tongue (F.M. 2190). It is tenacious and persistent; if wiped away, more may appear. It resists submersion for an appreciable time and it is usually estimated that in summer it will remain in position for 2 or 3 days or, even, 5 days; in winter, it may still be seen 3, 5 or, even, 8 days after submersion (Simonin, 1955). The mass of foam is composed of fine bubbles which do not readily collapse when touched with the point of a knife.

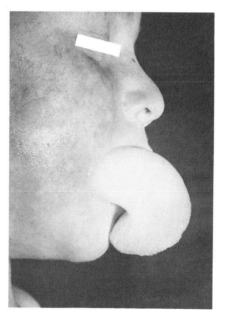

FIG. 150. Drowning: foam   in mushroom-shape at the mouth.

It is sometimes suggested that the appearance of the foam externally is a result of putrefaction. Simonin (1955) said, "*C'est la putréfaction qui la fait monter vers les orifices respiratoires et la détruit*". While this may be a possibility in some cases, it is clear from our experience that the foam, not only by the mechanism of its production but also by the time at which it appears externally, is essentially a vital phenomenon. Three illustrations must serve. Foam was present on the face of a barge inspector, aged 65, whose body was recovered a few minutes after he had fallen overboard into a canal (F.M. 1549); it was present also when the body of a boy aged 2 years was recovered within 2 hours (F.M. 2190); it was even present when a boy, aged 11 years, was still alive, but who died shortly after his rescue (F.M. 1397). The examination of each of these bodies was made within 24 hours of death and they had been stored meanwhile in a refrigerator; no signs of putrefaction were apparent.

The production of tenacious foam in drowning is, therefore, essentially a vital phenomenon. The entry of fluid into the air passages provokes them to produce mucus. This substance, when mixed with water, and possibly also surfactant from the lungs, is readily whipped into a tenacious foam by the violent respiratory efforts made by the victim (Manktelow and Hunt, 1967).

Putrefaction destroys the foam but it is then possible for a pseudofoam, a blood-stained fluid containing bubbles of gas, to be present. This has none of the persistent, tenacious qualities of that produced by drowning, and putrefactive changes elsewhere are likely to be obvious.

Foam may be absent externally if those who recover the body wipe it away. Pressure upon the thorax may cause more foam to escape or it may be found when the air passages are open to direct inspection. However, it is not uncommon for there to be no foam in the nose or mouth of a body recovered from water.

The conjunctivae are sometimes suffused. Occasionally scanty petechial haemorrhages are seen beneath the conjunctivae, especially of the lower eyelids.

The male genitalia may be contracted, erect or semi-erect. This sign has long ceased to have any importance. Ogston (1882) found that in rather more than half of the male victims, the genitalia were semi-erect.

The position of the tongue in relation to the jaws has no importance. "The tongue is just as often found behind the jaws as between them" (Casper, 1862). A bruised or bitten tongue, however, may point to a struggle during, or possibly prior to, drowning or to an epileptic fit, as a result of which the victim fell into water.

Instantaneous rigor, always uncommon, is sometimes a result of submersion and, in consequence, objects. e.g. weeds, sand, etc., may be held in the hands or feet and, when present, provide valuable evidence of life at the time of submersion.

Nail scrapings merit investigation, providing the findings are not given undue importance. It may be that sand or mud or other material from the place of submersion gets under the nails when the victim makes an unsuccessful attempt to struggle out of the water. The recovery of such material, however, provides only an indication that the body was in contact with it, either before or after death (Ogston, 1882; Scheider, 1931).

The external examination of the body will include, of course, a search for injuries which occurred prior to, during, or after, submersion. Abrasions on the fingers and tearing of the nails may occur when the victim grasps objects in an attempt to save himself. Other injuries may be sustained after death, especially in navigable waters, and there can be yet other injuries, which may have been the cause of death, when there has been an attempt to dispose of the body by submersion, for example, after infanticide; infanticide by drowning is uncommon.

Injuries may be sustained during the fall into the water or in some accident which led to submersion. The nature of the injuries and their distribution may be clearly consistent with these circumstances and examination of the scene may furnish confirmatory evidence. Some projection nearby or part of a boat, for example, may bear traces of contact with the victim. A barge inspector, aged 65, was walking along the gangway deck of a barge. When he stumbled and overbalanced, he made a grab at the mast to save himself but fell overboard, pulling the mast with him. There were recent bruises and abrasions on the face, in particular near the left eye, forehead and nose, consistent with a fall against the mast or deck. They had not caused death, nor in that case, unconsciousness because death was due to "typical" drowning (F.M. 1549).

On other occasions, especially when the body is recovered from navigable water, severe injuries including extensive laceration and multiple fractures may be present but, being without vital reaction, there is no difficulty in recognising them as of post-mortem origin. Injuries are sometimes inadvertently inflicted during the recovery of the body. Examination of a man aged 73 whose body was recovered from a canal, showed that the spine and several ribs were broken; there was also laceration, with a fracture dislocation, of the right ankle. There was no vital reaction in relation to any of these injuries (F.M. 835).

The appearances were somewhat complex in another man, aged 38, whose body was recovered from a canal. He had threatened to drown himself, but the manner in which his body came to be in the canal was not determined. It was discovered when a coal barge was found to have something fouling its propeller. The engine was stopped and, in due course, the body was recovered with a barge pole. His clothing had been torn by the propeller and there were grave injuries, which included extensive laceration of the scalp and ears, without any vital reaction. The spine was completely severed at the level of the seventh, and incompletely severed at the level of the third cervical vertebrae, again without trace of vital reaction. In the chest, however, the injuries had occurred during life; surgical emphysema was detected in the left armpit and there was a little recent bleeding into the left pectoral muscles. The thoracic cage was extensively damaged; the ribs two to nine on the left side were broken both at their convexities and also near to the spine. The ribs two to seven on the right side were broken at their convexities. Both scapulae were comminuted and there was a fracture in the outer third of the right collar bone. Slight bleeding had occurred beneath the pleurae and also into the soft parts near the scapulae. Despite these injuries there was evidence of death by drowning. The interpretation offered is that whilst unconscious, as a result of drowning, he came into contact with the propeller. This produced the chest injuries and almost within seconds renewed contact fractured the spine, after his death. There was no reason to believe they could have been sustained in any other way (F.M. 1119).

Bleeding may occur around injuries, especially of the head, even when they are inflicted after death. Children, seeing the crown of the head of a drowned man floating just above the water, fired at it with an airgun, thinking it to be a turnip floating on the water. The wounds produced by the pellets were surrounded by well-marked zones of bleeding in the scalp (F.M. 10,603A).

Injury which occurs during a fall into the water, and which is the primary cause of death, is illustrated by an accident which occurred in a public swimming bath. The deceased, a man aged 20, dived from a board at about 7 ft above the deep end. At the time another man was in the water below the board. He felt something strike his right thigh with considerable force but thought nothing about it. He said, "I turned to swim back to the side and I could see nothing of Foster (the deceased) so I looked round and saw him underneath the water in a doubled-up position with his head bent forwards". When the deceased was recovered from the water he said, "I can't move any of my limbs or feel anything". Death, from fracture of the cervical spine, took place in hospital a few hours later. Evidently his head had struck the thigh of his companion as he dived into the water (Leeds City Coroner, 475/46). Sometimes extensive injuries are present. (They may be sustained after death in navigable waters; as by injury from propellers.) Even if sustained during life, the immediate cause of death can be drowning. For example: When a woman aged 38 jumped from a height into a shallow stream she sustained a fracture of her cervical spine, right radius and ulna; she also had multiple lacerations, but her death was due to drowning. Her stomach contained a quantity of phenobarbitone, but there was none in her blood (F.M. 13,618).

The Internal Signs of Drowning

It is again assumed that putrefactive changes are negligible for, otherwise, the internal signs of drowning are abolished or obscured.

Attention is directed primarily to the respiratory system. Foam is usually apparent, in amounts which vary from body to body, in the air passages. They may be completely filled by it, or as is more usual the foam may be restricted to secondary bronchi and beyond. Its features are those already described. There is also a variable quantity of water in the air passages. This may be abundant and escape from the mouth when the body is turned on the operating table, a point worthy of note, because it is unusual for this to happen except after drowning.

The pleurae may be discolored by haemorrhages but those of the usual asphyxial kind are always infrequent, and indeed rare. This may be due to compression of the inter-alveolar septa, as suggested by Gardner (1942), or because the convulsive phase may be short and less violent in drowning than in, say, smothering. Rather larger haemorrhages, produced by tearing of the inter-alveolar partitions—originally noticed by Paltauf (1882)—are sometimes seen especially immediately beneath the pleurae. According to Hansen (1938) they are shining, pale bluish-red in colour, and may be minute or have a diameter of 3–5 cm and are usually present in the lower lobes of the lungs; they may be seen on the anterior surfaces of the lungs but they are more often seen on the interlobar surfaces; they are rarely seen (Simonin, 1955). The absence of haemorrhages in no way excludes death by drowning, but their presence is confirmation of it.

The *larynx* may be congested, a feature which Simonin (1955) considers a reliable sign.

The *lungs* are bulky or ballooned, often to a degree which causes them to overlap the pericardium; rib markings may be present. They have a doughy feel and pit on pressure; their weight is increased, not perhaps to the extent seen in severe pulmonary oedema but to about twice the normal weight, i.e. 700–800 g, or 25–29 oz. The heaviest as yet in our series weighed 2 lb 2 oz (960 g) right and 1 lb 14 oz (740 g) left but Simonin (1955) gives 1000–1700 g for men and 800 to 1000 g for women. The general appearance is one of pallor but there may be mottling with red areas amongst those of grey colour, i.e. alveoli which contain blood and those which are anaemic; many alveoli are visibly distended. Section of the lung sets free a quantity of watery fluid, which may be blood-stained and which usually contains fine bubbles. The over-all picture of the lungs in drowning has been described as *emphysema aquosum* or "emphysème hydroaérique" and, when present, as it is in about 80 per cent of cases, this is of itself presumptive evidence of death by drowning. The other conditions, notably severe pulmonary oedema, which may resemble it, are excluded, as a rule, by the collateral circumstances of the death.

In sea water drowning the lungs are typically very distended, full of water and froth, and very heavy, weighing up to 1000 g each, a finding which is much less common in fresh water drowning (Hendry, (1982) personal communication).

Pleural adhesions when extensive and dense will prevent the occurrence of emphysema aquosum. This was well shown in one of my cases when it was apparent in the right lung, where the pleura was healthy, but absent in the left lung, which was bound to the chest wall by old-standing pleural adhesions.

The degree of emphysema aquosum will also depend upon the time taken to drown. It is absent when the victim is unconscious at the time of submersion and when death is due to cardiac inhibition. On other occasions its degree will be influenced by the occurrence of laryngeal spasm; the more prolonged this is, or the more frequently spasm recurs, before the victim dies, the less will be the degree of emphysema aquosum.

The mechanism of the production of emphysema aquosum and of the foam in the air passages is peculiar to drowning. The inhalation of water irritates the mucous membrane of the air passages and stimulates the secretion of mucus. Respiratory movement of the air in the passages, piston-like in character, whips up this substance into a foam. Soon its amount and consistence are sufficient to create an effective check value. The more powerful inspiratory efforts carry air past the obstruction but expiratory efforts are insufficient to expel air, water and foam.

Emphysema aquosum is not a result, as it is sometimes said, of the entry of fluid pushing the air before it to distend alveoli. If this were true, the appearances of the lungs of those who die of drowning when unconscious would be like those of the conscious. On the contrary, there is a clear distinction to be drawn between the appearances in these two circumstances, i.e. as between oedema aquosum and emphysema aquosum. The latter results only when a conscious victim of drowning has made a prolonged attempt to survive. Experimental flooding of the lungs, although it distends them—and may do so greatly—does not reproduce the appearances of emphysema aquosum.

Further evidence of drowning is found in the circulatory system. Obstruction of the pulmonary circulation, due to the inhalation of water, results in distension of the right heart and the great veins, which are filled with dark red blood. The blood, also, is likely to remain fluid and free from clots. Dilution of the blood by inhaled water is responsible for the prevention of coagulation. The blood often has a watery consistence and does not tend to adhere to the hands. The aorta may have haemolytic staining of its intima.

Chemical Tests of Drowning

It was suggested by Gettler (1921) that a comparison between the chloride content of blood samples taken respectively from the right and left sides of the heart, would furnish a test of death by drowning. If submerged in river or canal water, the blood on the left side of the heart, being diluted by water, should have a lower chloride level than that on the right; conversely, if drowning takes place in salt water. It is a test of doubtful value; Soutter (1936) placed little reliance on it. The test will fail if either of the heart septa be patent. It is useless when the water is brackish, having a saline content of about that of blood and—most important of all—the test is vitiated by putrefactive change. Nevertheless its use was supported by Fisher (1966). The blood changes in man following death due to drowning were investigated by Durlacher *et al.* (1953). In their view the most reliable index was the determination of the difference in the plasma specific gravity from the two sides of the heart. On the other hand, Modell and Davis (1969) rejected both the chloride estimation and the specific gravity of serum as reliable tests on which to base a diagnosis of drowning; Timperman (1969) also considered these tests untrustworthy. Rammer and Gerdin (1976) studied osmolarity and sodium and potassium concentrations in serum from the right and left sides of the heart, cerebrospinal fluid and vitreous humour.

They considered that a lower osmolarity in the left heart blood than in cerebro-spinal fluid, and a substantially lower concentration of sodium and potassium in the left heart blood than in the cerebro-spinal fluid made the diagnosis of drowning in fresh water highly probable.

In our experience analyses of the sodium and chloride levels and the specific gravity of serum, from each side of the heart and a peripheral blood sample can, on occasion, provide confirmatory evidence of drowning, when recovery of the body has occurred within a few hours of submersion. On other occasions, when naked-eye evidence of drowning is obvious, there is no detectable difference in the electrolyte levels in samples of blood from different parts of the body.

It has been suggested that chemical compounds discharged as industrial waste into waterways might enter the body during the course of drowning, and after death act as another diagnostic feature. Rarely this has proved possible (see page 422; F.M. 14, 926 A). Further research in this area could be valuable, especially in an industrial country like Britain. Pleukhahn (1977) has recommended the use of the plasma specific gravity difference between right and left heart blood, and the magnesium concentration of vitreous humour in salt-water drownings.

Diatom Analyses

Fluid from the lungs should be examined microscopically in order to detect particulate matter derived from the submerging fluid. It is of even greater importance to demonstrate specific particulate matter in the blood stream and in enclosed organs. This mode of investigation was first attempted by Revenstorf (1903) who, using an acid digestion technique, demonstrated diatoms in the lungs of the drowned. Corin and Stockis (1909, cited Thomas *et al.*, 1960) conducted experiments, by which they demonstrated that lycopodium, yeast and starch entered the lung capillaries and were present in blood in the left side of the heart of drowned animals. The further development of the method in Hungary is described by Tamáska who, in 1942, assisted by Incze, demonstrated, by a haemolysing technique, that plankton entered the blood stream of the drowned. In 1949 Mueller, with Gorgs and in 1952 unaware of the earlier discoveries, demonstrated diatoms in the blood and organs of the recently drowned. The possibility of contamination, yielding false positive results, was appreciated at an early stage, but improvement in technique, by Weinig (cited Thomas, 1960) and, more recently, by Thomas, van Hecke and Timperman (1960) and Tamáska (1961) has gone far to exclude the source of false positives. Thomas and his colleagues take samples only from enclosed organs and they gave an excellent demonstration of their technique and results, recorded by films and lantern slides. Tamáska (1961) has conducted a systematic study of the bone marrow for diatoms and regards this as the best method in all circumstances of drowning, including those where the body is in an advanced state of putrefaction. It is now the routine procedure in Hungary. (Details of the technique are given). The femur is the bone of choice but, when practicable, a humerus also should be available. The doctor who makes the post-mortem examination, if he is not himself to undertake the diatom analysis, should send the bones, or a piece sawn out of each, to a laboratory where the examination can be made. Rushton (1961) used an acid digestion method for diatom analyses in his sixty-two cases of death by drowning. He confirmed the value of this procedure especially when the changes are atypical or the body is decomposed. In his view it is a very sensitive test but, because of the difficulty of total exclusion of contamination, the results are not conclusive evidence of death by drowning. The test, however, provides reliable, supportive evidence.

The demonstration of plankton and, more especially, diatoms in the submerging fluid and in the body of the victim, is of particular value as a confirmatory test. The test material is treated by acid digestion as a preliminary step in diatom analysis. In the case of decomposed bodies, the demonstration of diatoms in enclosed organs and especially in the bone marrow, due care being taken to exclude contamination, is strong if not conclusive evidence of death by drowning. This is the view of Tamáska (1961), of Thomas, van Hecke and Timperman (1960) and Rushton (1960, 1961). Further confirmation may be given by diatom counts of the submerging fluid as well as of specimens from the body of the victim (Mueller, 1959). Nevertheless, Timperman (1962) found none in 10 per cent of the drowned and only a few in another 10 per cent.

An examination of lung juice alone has limited value, although a high diatom content is then indicative of death by drowning. Rushton (1961) has confirmed that even the most favourable conditions, e.g. the application of artificial respiration to the submerged body of a dog, fail to flood the lungs with water in a manner normally seen in drowning. Timperman (1969) found that after death diatoms only penetrate as far as the main bronchi.

At the Third International Meeting in Forensic Medicine held in London in April 1963, W. V. Spitz, of Berlin, reported the results of researches which showed that diatoms were plentiful in the air of Berlin. His experiments threw considerable doubt on the validity of the finding of diatoms in the organs as a diagnostic sign of drowning.

This view had been challenged by Timperman (1969), who cited Mueller. We have endeavoured to assess the extent of air diatom pollution in Leeds by submitting papers, used by the Public Health Department to measure the amount of smoke pollution, to chemical digestion. Each day the paper bore the deposit from $70\,ft^3$ of air. The maximum number of diatoms for one month, in winter, derived from approximately $2100\,ft^3$ of air, was thirty; a control test with unused papers totalled only seven diatoms.

In ten cases of death due to causes other than drowning we found that the maximum number of diatoms in $100\,g$ of lung was twenty whereas 135 diatoms were present in a similar sample of lung taken from the body of a man recovered from a canal in the City of Leeds. The maximum diatom content of samples of liver, each of $100\,g$, was only thirteen. We conclude, therefore, that in this area the diatom content of samples of lung due to atmospheric contamination is unlikely to vitiate results which support a diagnosis of death by drowning; it might do so with results obtained from samples of liver.

Jaaskelainen (1967, 1968) has described techniques for the detection of diatoms in histological preparations. It is obvious that diatoms can only be found in the tissues if they are present in sufficient numbers in the water in which the body was immersed. In winter, and in waters which are heavily polluted by industrial effluent, they may be scanty. It is our experience to find relatively few diatoms in bodies taken from rivers in the industrial areas of the West Riding of Yorkshire, even when the naked-eye signs of drowning are prominent. We have also noted that some canals, which draw their water from reservoirs in geological areas which do not encourage the growth of diatoms, remain comparatively low in diatom content throughout much of their course.

Recently Peabody (1980) has compiled an extensive review of the published work on the detection of diatoms in drowning, and draws attention again to the controversy concerning the value of this technique in the diagnosis of drowning. His review should be consulted in the original. He points out the need for further research to resolve the controversy, by establishing with certainty whether non-drowned subjects do have diatoms in their organs in significant numbers, and to what extent results may be vitiated by contamination of reagents and glassware.

Terazawa and Takatori, (1980) and Fukui *et al.* (1980), have suggested newer methods for isolating diatoms from tissues, using colloidal silica gradients, and ultrasonic radiation.

The Stomach Contents in Drowning

The stomach may contain fluid, since some is usually swallowed during drowning. (It may have been ingested prior to the event: chemical analysis may assist if it shows the water in the stomach has the same composition as that of the submerging medium). Pond weeds or algae may be present. Stomach contents should be examined microscopically, and it may occasionally be worthwhile to subject them to chemical analysis. Do they contain chlorinated water, such as might come from a service supply thus treated, or water contaminated by animal excrement and therefore rich in nitrites? This point arose when a man was found dead with his head in a culvert. The possibilities were murder by strangulation, or suicide by drowning. Drowning was suggested by fluid in his stomach, and investigation on the lines indicated might have been able to show that the water in his stomach had either been drunk before he left home or swallowed by him as he lay in the culvert.

The absence of fluid in the stomach is noteworthy, because it may mean either that the death, if by drowning, was rapid, or that the victim was dead at the time of submersion.

The demonstration of alcohol and the estimation of its amount in the blood or urine should be undertaken whenever practicable, since a drunken person can readily fall into water and be drowned. Death may then occur rapidly (Giertsen, 1970; Jaaskelainen, 1968; Editorial, *Brit. Med. J.* 1979; Pleukhahn, 1977.)

Other changes directly associated with drowning are occasionally to be found in the locomotor system. The victim who makes a violent struggle to survive, may bruise or rupture muscles, especially those of the shoulder girdle. Paltauf (1882) found haemorrhages in the muscles of the neck and chest. The scaleni and pectoralis major are most often involved and the bleeding tends to follow the line of the muscle bundles. The haemorrhages may be bilateral. There may sometimes be bruising of the structures in the floor of the mouth. Muscular injury may be present in as many as 10 per cent of victims and, when present, the haemorrhages are an important sign (Wachholz, 1934).

We have also found small ruptures of the anterior border of the liver, close to the ligamentum teres, in some bodies. These injuries may be the result of attempted resuscitation.

Mueller (1969) and Sammut (1967) described bleeding into the middle ear and temporal bone following drowning but Haarkoff and Weiler (1971) found bleeding into the tegmen tympani in eighty of a series of 100 deaths from all causes. This, therefore, is not a reliable sign of drowning. In our experience it was not constant and was absent in cases where there were unequivocal signs of drowning.

Dislocation of joints is a rare event and is likely to occur only when the victim is precipitated from a height, in a posture which predisposes to dislocation. A man who, for a wager, jumped from London Bridge, entered the water with his arms horizontal. Examination of his body showed that both shoulder joints were dislocated (Beck and Beck, 1836).

Fractures may be the result of striking an object on the way to the water or, more likely, they are ante-mortem injuries inflicted by another person. Fractured ribs, with or without abrasion and bruising of the sides of the trunk, can result from well-meant but unskilled attempts at artificial respiration; they may occur also after death through contact with propellers, etc., in navigable waters, as already mentioned.

The Prognosis of Drowning

Although the biochemical changes differ according to the nature of the medium, the practical consideration is that, whether it be fresh or salt water, the duration of submersion or, more exactly, the volume of fluid inhaled, determines the prognosis. In any event the period is brief, a matter only of a few minutes. The prospect of successful resuscitation is slight when complete submersion has lasted for 6 minutes and death is almost invariable when the period exceeds 10 minutes. When, as is then likely, large amounts of water have been inhaled, the continued feeble beating of the heart for several minutes after rescue does not alter the gravity of the prognosis (Rushton, 1961). Even so, resuscitation after submersion for 20 minutes was successful (Kvittingen and Naess, 1963).

Although the asphyxial element is the dominant factor, the systolic blood pressure is also important; it may remain high for several minutes and prognosis is related to its level. According to Swann's experiments, 115 mm is the critical level; above it recovery is probable, if not certain, but when it falls to only 50 mm death will occur (Rushton, 1961).

The prognosis is also governed by the order in which respiratory and heart failure occur. If respiratory failure precedes heart failure, then immediate artificial respiration may succeed and is indeed valuable. Respiratory failure precedes heart failure in one third of the cases, it is coincident in one third and follows it in the other third (Rushton, 1961).

When resuscitation has been successful, the outlook is good, although a guarded prognosis is necessary for a few days, since there are certain possible complications. Some may develop pneumonia, especially after submersion in infected water. A temporary renal failure, caused by excessive red cell destruction, may be indicated by haematuria. Myocardial anoxia may cause delayed heart failure, which may not occur until a few hours after rescue.

Post Immersion Syndrome (Secondary Drowning)

Apart from death during submersion, the features of which are well established, it is now recognised that a person surviving the episode of submersion may subsequently suffer complications, or die, from the delayed effects of the inhalation of water. The matter was fully discussed by Fuller (1963).

Clinical signs in such cases included pyrexia, coma, and other symptoms related to the central nervous system. Respiratory signs included shallow respiration, pain in the chest, and the production of bloody, frothy sputum. X-rays of the chest in many cases showed mottled opacity of the lung fields. Cardiac arrythmias sometimes occurred. Vomiting was a frequent symptom. Electrolyte changes in the blood were not marked.

In fatal cases the early histological changes in the lungs are described as haemorrhage, desquamative and exudative reaction with early polymorph exudate formation. Subsequently changes are of inhalation pneumonitis with hyaline membranes in alveolar ducts, and foreign body reaction to inhaled particles; progression may be to broncho-pneumonia or abscess formation. Long surviving cases may show histological evidence of brain damage. The features in children have been described by Pearn (1980).

Such a condition may cause medico-legal problems. For example, a child, aged 2, died at home shortly after returning from the swimming baths where it had been taken by its sister and her boy-friend. The original story was that when they had taken the child home it had become sleepy, vomited, and died. It was anticipated that autopsy would show evidence of some undiagnosed natural condition. However, no such cause for death was revealed. Further enquiries then ellicited the fact that the two adults had been endeavouring to teach the infant to swim by putting it, unsupported into the water, splashing it, etc. It became distressed and other people in the baths remonstrated. When taken out of the bath the child vomited water, had difficulty in walking, and then died subsequently at home, as already described. Histological findings in the lungs showed changes consistent with secondary drowning, with desquamation of bronchial epithelium, early polymorph exudation, collapse, oedema and congestion. A subsequent charge of manslaughter at Crown Court failed (Jacobs, S. (1982) personal communication).

Treatment of Drowning

Although asphyxia due to obstruction of the air passages may no longer be the true explanation of death from drowning, the treatment of the submerged is unchanged. Artificial respiration remains the first, *immediate* step, irrespective of any injuries the victim may have sustained. The methods of performing artificial respiration are many, but the Holger-Nielsen method is now officially approved. This treatment must be begun at once—a delay of minutes precludes success—and it must be continued for at least 15 minutes.

Probably the most effective method is "mouth-to-mouth" respiration, commenced as soon as possible and, when practicable, before the victim is recovered from the water. Postural drainage and any other appropriate treatment must take second place to efficient artificial respiration. Examination of the patient can also await his recovery from submersion. Since a doctor rarely reaches the scene forthwith, members of the public should be instructed in the application of a safe, simple method of artificial respiration.

Obviously the best treatment is prevention, i.e. by taking precautions to avoid accidents.

In the event that a hospital competent to deal with the patient is at hand and he survives long enough to reach it, there are other steps which should be taken. Those drowned in fresh water could be submitted to an external defibrillation and later an adjustment of electrolyte balance. Those drowned in sea water can have tracheal intubation to permit repeated suction; they may require mechanical artificial respiration. Hypotonic infusion, controlled by appropriate laboratory investigations, will correct haemoconcentration. Correction of acidosis with bicarbonate, the administration of a "broad-spectrum" antibiotic and exchange blood transfusion are also advocated in appropriate circumstances (Keatinge, 1969).

Golden (1975) has described treatment, both first aid and subsequent measures, to be used in hospital, especially as regards treatment for hypothermia and the secondary drowning syndrome.

Atypical Drowning

This term is adopted to include deaths from submersion which are due to vagal inhibition or laryngeal spasm, and the submersion of the unconscious. It is convenient, also, to mention here those whose bodies are disposed of by submersion after death from some other cause.

1. Vagal Inhibition due to Submersion Deaths due to cardiac inhibition following submersion are uncommon but important. Their occurrence is now well recognised and, therefore, failure to find the changes normally present in the drowned does not exclude submersion as a possible cause of death. On the other hand, I should be reluctant to accept vagal inhibition as the explanation until all other possibilities have been considered and investigated. A woman was found dead in her bath, and when the doctor, who had been summoned by the police, arrived, he was invited to certify the death as due to drowning. He knew the victim and declined to do this; he told the police she had probably taken an overdose of phenobarbitone; this was subsequently confirmed. See also *R. v. Barlow* (1957): murder by insulin poisoning. (Polson and Tattersall, 1971).

Vagal inhibition results from stimulation of the vagus nerves and, in drowning, this can arise in one of several ways. A sudden inrush of water into the naso-pharynx or larynx may be responsible or it may be due to a blow on the abdomen. Falling or diving into the water, feet first, or "duck-diving" by the inexperienced, or any clumsy diving, involving horizontal entry into the water with a consequent blow on the abdomen, are examples of these accidents. Gardner (1942) described the circumstances in which a young man suddenly sank while swimming and did not rise again. It seems that when he had turned his head to make some comment to a friend, the wash of a passing steamer struck his face and he unexpectedly inhaled water.

Both Spilsbury (1934) and Gardner (1942) have instanced fatalities due to the sudden entry of fluid into the naso-pharynx as examples of cardiac inhibition.

A boy, aged $2^1/_2$ years, fell head first into a drum which contained some chalky, sooty water; the water level was only 6 in. above the bottom of the drum. The child was removed at once but prompt resuscitation was of no avail; the child was dead. It was readily possible to trace the internal distribution of the water by its sooty content. Soot was present in the nasal cavities, there was a little in the larynx and traces of soot adhered to the vocal cords and the wall of the trachea, but there was none in the lungs. The child had swallowed about an ounce of the water but there was no soot in his mouth. The level of water in the drum was too low for any of it to have entered except by the nose (Gardner, 1942).

Surprise or unpreparedness are so commonly factors on these occasions that there can be little doubt that they play an important rôle.

The second of Smith's victims (see p. 448) presented none of the usual signs of drowning and almost certainly had died of vagal inhibition; she had been suddenly submerged in her bath by the murderer, when wholly unprepared for his attack. A small boy, aged 2 years, who overbalanced and fell into a static water-tank was promptly recovered but he was then dead; signs of drowning were absent and his death was due to vagal inhibition (Leeds City Coroner, 261/43). A girl, aged 8 years, when sitting on the edge of a small tank of water, suddenly fell backwards into it. She had only to raise her arms to reach the sides to save herself, because its dimensions were only 24 × 17 × 17 in., but when her body was recovered she had died of vagal inhibition, and was still clutching her doll (Gardner, 1942).

Loss of consciousness is usually instantaneous on these occasions and death ensues soon afterwards, at most in a few minutes. Mobility, therefore, is then negligible and the victim is likely to be found in the position he was at the time of death. There may even be instantaneous rigor but on some occasions death may not be rapid.

Keatinge (1969) has found sudden rises in arterial pressure and vagal output in men exposed to ice-water showers. Bradycardia and ventricular ectopic beats have also been recorded by the ECG in volunteers during the first few minutes of their immersion in cold water.

Examination of the body discloses none of the usual signs of drowning. There is no foam at the mouth or nose; emphysema aquosum is absent, and the right heart and great veins, if not empty, are never engorged. The skin is pale and there are no asphyxial haemorrhages.

Since the findings are negative, it is obviously imperative to ensure that other possibilities, notably poisoning and especially by some non-irritant substance such as a barbiturate, are excluded. Search will also be made for injuries, bearing in mind the ease with which a head injury can escape notice.

2. Laryngeal Spasm due to Submersion It is probable that in all or most deaths due to drowning, laryngeal spasm is provoked at some stage by the entry of water into the larynx. It is usually only a transient or intermittent factor and of secondary importance. The amount of water inhaled and the degree of emphysema aquosum varies appreciably in the bodies of the victims of the same accident. There are, however, rare occasions when laryngeal spasm following submersion is the prime cause of death. A boy aged 8 years, who jumped into the water, sank and did not rise again; there were signs of death from asphyxia but there was only a minute amount of water in his air passages; emphysema aquosum was absent (Gardner, 1942).

When the death is due to laryngeal spasm, the appearances are those of asphyxia as by other forms of mechanical obstruction of the air passages. The body will be cyanosed and petechial haemorrhages are present beneath the conjunctivae, in the skin of the face, beneath the pleurae, epicardium and, possibly, elsewhere; the heart and great veins are engorged. The lungs, however, are not waterlogged or ballooned. There is no fluid, or only a small amount of it, in the air passages, and there is no foam in them nor at the nose or mouth. It is a rare mode of death from submersion and these asphyxial signs are prominent; the possibility of some other cause of asphyxia prior to submersion must be considered (Donald, 1955).

3. Submersion when Unconscious Submersion when unconscious is a possibility if the victim is an epileptic or suffers from heart disease, especially coronary atheroma or dizziness due to essential hypertension. It can also occur if the victim is drunk. The rupture of a cerebral aneurysm or the onset of cerebral haemorrhage may also cause abrupt collapse. A healthy victim may sustain a head injury, e.g. during the fall into the water, and be unconscious when submerged.

When there is organic disease of a kind likely to lead to collapse and a fall into the water, or when the blood or urine contain much alcohol, interpretation is relatively simple. The epileptic may be recognised when his body has been identified; his relatives will be able to give information about his disability.

Head injuries can create special difficulty and due note should be taken of their nature. It is imperative to exclude the possibility of homicide, which is to be presumed, until disproved. The injuries may be accidental and search should be made for a likely agent at the scene of the death; there may be some projection, for example the parapet of a bridge or tree stump.

As a rule, a complete picture of death by drowning is not found. Ballooning of the lungs may be absent and the formation of foam may be negligible.

Disposal by Submersion

Although infanticide by drowning is uncommon, disposal by submersion of the body of a newly-born infant, the victim of some other mode of infanticide, or the body of a still-born, is not infrequent. Submersion is rarely the means of disposal of the body of an adult who has been murdered. The Luton Sack Murder (*R.* v. *Manton*, 1943; Simpson, 1945) came to light through a clumsy attempt to dispose of the body in a stream. Nodder strangled a little girl and attempted to dispose of the body in the river (*R.* v. *Nodder*, 1937). If the murder occurs near water, disposal of the body by submersion is an obvious step. Almost inevitably, the plan will fail because it is difficult to ensure that the body shall remain submerged for a sufficient time to destroy evidence of the crime.

> The body of a woman was recovered from a canal, where the depth of water was only 20 to 24 in. There was extensive bruising of the scalp and the skull was fractured. These injuries could not have resulted from a fall into the water and they must have been inflicted prior to submersion. Her husband had told another woman, whom he wished to marry, that his wife would either commit suicide or he would kill her (Wachholz, 1934).
> A man's body was seen submerged in a river, beside a bridge. When recovered it was found to be attached by rope to a block of concrete. The pathologist noticed several small holes in the skin and had the body X-rayed. This revealed a corresponding number of bullets in the body (F.M. 24,907 A).
> A Pakistani male disappeared after an alleged fight in a shop. A river was situated nearby. The body was found in the water some weeks later and several miles downstream. There were moderate changes of putrefaction, but autopsy clearly showed a stab wound of the neck, transecting a major artery (F.M. 28,073 A).

We agree with Étienne Martin that in the absence of all traces of violence the medical presumption is that submersion is the result of suicide or an accident. This must be, because of the difficulty of proof of homicide when putrefaction is established. In the latter circumstances, changes which might be due to violence require most careful scrutiny and, unless the examiner is able to prove their nature, he should not attach undue importance to them. On one occasion, for example, it appeared that there were finger-marks on the front of the neck of an infant recovered from a canal. These, although suspicious, were indefinite and unaccompanied by obvious bruising; putrefaction was evident. They were therefore discounted and the infant, for other reasons, was presumed to have been stillborn.

Weighted bodies call for special care in investigation because a suicide, anxious to ensure success, may load his body with weights. It is then necessary to determine whether the weights could have been applied by the victim. He may fill his pockets with stones or tie weights to his legs or arms; the manner in which they are tied and their kind must be noted. A notable example is provided by the case of Tourdes, Étienne Martin (1950). This suicide had not only tied his ankles and wrists but also fixed a bag full of stones round his neck.

The possibility of flooding of the respiratory system when the victim is dead at the time of submersion was investigated by Liman (cited by Casper, 1862). He submerged the bodies of children in a morass. This medium was chosen because it would be easy to trace its entry into the air passages. In fourteen of his sixteen experiments mud had entered the pharynx, oesophagus and trachea and, in seven, the stomach also. Fagerlund (1890), who submerged animals in coloured water, although partially successful in his attempts to cause the fluid to enter their bodies, found it difficult to achieve. Hofmann (1887, cited by Guy and Ferrier, 1895) failed to introduce water into the smaller bronchi of the dead.

Rushton (1961) failed, even in the most favourable circumstances of all, namely, by artificial respiration of the dead body under water, to cause the passage of more than small amounts of water into the lungs; there was no evidence of penetration of water into the circulation after death. It was impossible to reproduce the flooding of the lungs normally seen in drowning. (Timperman (1969) agreed.)

The Diagnosis of Death by Drowning

The diagnosis of death by drowning, *providing putrefaction is absent* or is only at an early stage, may be relatively simple, but once putrefaction is established, and certainly when it is advanced, the diagnosis is a matter of inference, based upon the circumstances of the death and the exclusion of other possible causes.

The search for plankton and notably for diatoms, in the lungs and preferably in enclosed cavities, when successful, points to death by drowning and is good evidence even in the presence of advanced putrefaction. When persistent foam is seen at the nose or mouth and there is no external mark of strangulation, this is in itself presumptive of drowning. If, in addition, the victim had passed into instantaneous rigor at the time of death and material from the water, e.g. weeds, sand, etc., are firmly held by the hands or feet, there is proof of life at the time of submersion. Well-known though this phenomenon is, its occurrence is distinctly uncommon in any circumstances.

The Circumstances of Drowning

The majority of deaths due to submersion are either by accident or by suicide; the victim of accidental drowning is usually an adult male, or a child of either sex, whereas the suicide may as often be a female as a male adult. Suicide by any mode is unusual in children; but youth *per se* does not exclude the possibility.

Two women, one aged 47 and her mother aged 80, were found dead in the bath at their home. There were signs of drowning in both, but on neither were there any external signs of injury. There was no evidence of a struggle; the bathroom door was bolted on the inside. The overall picture was that of a suicide pact. Murder of both by a third party was excluded and there was no evidence of any kind to suggest the daughter had murdered her mother (F.M. 6865 A and B; Fig. 151).

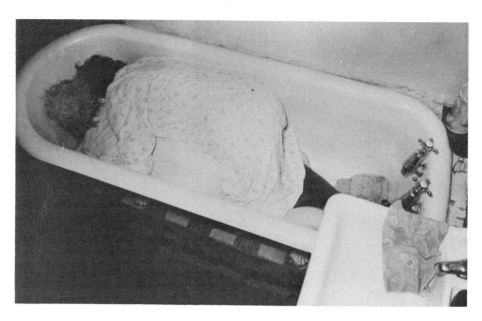

FIG. 151. Drowning: suicide pact between mother and daughter.

Geertinger and Voigt (1970) found, as we have done, that some of those found dead in a bath, presumed to have died of drowning, had taken an over-dose of drugs or had died of poisoning by carbon monoxide. It is necessary, therefore, that the investigation of these deaths should include screening for drugs and, when positive, a competent toxicological analysis.

All victims of drowning should be analysed for alcohol because of the likelihood of accidental drowning when drunk (see page 435). If early putrefaction is present comparison of the results of analysis of urine, if present, and of blood samples from several different sites, e.g. each limb, may show close approximation of levels in true intoxication, or wide variation of results if alcohol is being produced by decomposition.

Homicidal Drowning

The circumstances of accidental and suicidal drowning are familiar and do not require illustration but, because they are unusual, a few instances of homicidal drowning are cited.

Homicidal drowning, other than of newly-born infants or small children, is unusual because its accomplishment requires that there shall be appreciable physical disparity between the assailant and his victim or that the victim is incapacitated by disease, drink or drugs, or is taken by surprise. The suppositious circumstances of which Dickens gave a vivid account in *Our Mutual Friend* do not occur in reality, and the novel method employed by G. J. Smith, simple though it would seem, has not been used by any other known murderer in this country. The victim may be pushed or chased into the water and bear no sign of assault.

Case 1. In 1949 a girl aged 13 was murdered by drowning by a man aged 41. He had been drinking and met the girl, whom he knew, near a fish-and-chip shop in the town. She was promised a meal of fish and chips and, on that pretext, he got her to accompany him to the bank of a neighbouring canal, where, it appears, she let him carry her over the wall which guarded it. When they gained the towing-path he attempted to interfere with her but she was frightened and offered resistance. He told the police that "I got hold of her to shield myself and I threw her into the water. I watched her hands go down, she drowned." When charged with the offence he said he did this to prevent her telling her grandmother that he had taken her on the canal bank. At his trial, however, he alleged that, because she was frightened, she ran away and then fell into the canal. He had heard a splash but did not see her enter the water.

No signs of a struggle at the scene were found and the injuries on her body were slight. Certain of the small lacerations on her right forearm might have been caused by the finger nails of her assailant, but the prisoner's nails were bitten and were unlikely to produce characteristic marks. The death was due to drowning. Fluid in the lungs and stomach contained diatoms of the kind also found in the canal water; this showed she was alive at the time she fell into the water. (The examination of the lungs alone, of course, did not distinguish as between murder, manslaughter or accident. In each of these circumstances it is likely that the child would have made " a very determined effort to breathe whilst under water".)

The duskiness of her face and the fact that she had bitten her tongue were not inconsistent with attempted strangulation, prior to her death by drowning, but there were no marks on her neck, nor any injury of its deeper tissues. It seems unlikely, therefore, that considerable force had been applied to her neck. She did not wear a scarf which could have protected the tissues.

Precisely what took place is, of course, known only to the assailant. Disparity of size and physical strength could have permitted him to throw her into the water without any injury to her body and without signs of a struggle at the scene. He may also have minimised her resistance by partial strangulation.

The prisoner was convicted and sentenced to death, the sentence being later commuted to one of detention for life in a Broadmoor Institution (*R.* v. *Taylor*, 1949).

Case 2. On 1 October 1957 a girl aged 16 left her home with her brother aged 14 at about 7.30 p.m. About 10 minutes later they parted company; she said she was going for a walk and he returned to do his homework. They were then near the Chester-Queensferry Road. On one side of it there is a tarmac path, on the other a deep ditch, between the verge and the hedge. She went along the path. The next news of her was a report by the accused to the police that he had found a body in the ditch beside this road at about 7.50 p.m. The police went to the scene immediately and there found a body floating in the ditch. It was that of the girl, dressed in a duffel coat and jeans.

The accused's explanation of the circumstances was that, while travelling to work in his car along this road, he had seen something white at the ditch side of the road. He stopped his car and walked back to investigate. As he approached he heard sounds which suggested that someone was struggling in the ditch. He saw someone, apparently a boy, in the ditch and tried to get him out. It was slippery and he was unable to do this single-handed. In the course of his attempt, the "boy" grasped him and also scratched his face. The accused took fright and returned to his car where, he said, he sat for several minutes considering his position. He then went to the police to report the matter. In short, his version was that the girl's death was by accident.

The Crown alleged that this man had seen her walking along the road and had stopped and accosted her. She took fright and ran across the road and he pursued her. During this encounter a bus approached and, in order to avoid detection, he pushed her into the ditch and held her, face down, in the mud and thus caused her death by drowning. The scratches on his face were made by the girl in an attempt to escape; she had long pointed nails (Fig. 16).

The post-mortem examination by Dr. Gerald Evans proved death by drowning. The appearances were indeed remarkable because mud and leaves were present throughout the bronchial tree, even to the bronchioles, forming an almost solid cast of their interior; some fine foam and mud were present in the alveoli. The girl was a virgin and there was no sign of any sexual assault. Moreover, there was no evidence of injury as by a struggle; the only external signs of injury were a few trivial abrasions.

Dr. Evans and others carried out a series of experiments at the scene with an ingenious model, constructed to represent the body of the girl, and also had personal experience of the probable difficulties which would have prevented this girl from extricating herself from this ditch or making any effective resistance to an attack. It was a deep ditch, of "V" shape; one side was 3 ft. 4 in. and the other 2 ft. 8 in.; the base was 22 in. broad. The ditch contained water to a depth of $13^1/_2$ in. and, beneath it, there was a layer, $6^1/_2$ in. thick, of slimy mud. When wearing gum boots he rapidly sank in the mud and experienced considerable difficulty in extricating himself. This being the situation, if the girl had been thrust into the ditch, she would have found herself at once in difficulties. She could have been drowned with relative ease and without being able to attempt more than feeble resistance. The absence of signs of violence did not exclude homicidal drowning, because the circumstances had some resemblance to murder by drowning in a bath. The accused's suggestion that he had taken fright was countered by his record of war service. He had served in small armoured vehicles and, for a time, in Malaya. The jury were asked whether they thought a man with that record would go into a panic at finding a body in a ditch. The accused's account of stopping his car at the side of the road near to the ditch while he went to investigate the white object was disproved by several witnesses who saw him and his car in very different positions to that described by him. The accused was convicted of murder and sentenced to imprisonment for life (*R.* v.*Cook*, Flintshire Assizes, February 1958; Glyn-Jones, J.).

The murders committed by G. J. Smith depended on the element of surprise, and the victims were attacked in circumstances which permitted but feeble resistance. The details of these notable cases are related in *The Trial of George Joseph Smith* and it must suffice only to mention the method, which proved, for a time, an unqualified success. It would seem that Smith was not the first to employ the method because the Egyptian police in 1909 had reason to believe it had been used by a man to kill his wife (Watson, 1922); it is not known whether Smith knew of this.

Homicide by drowning may occur during the course of some other offence, or during reckless horseplay. Thus, in one of our cases a swimming bath caretaker surprised some youths who were intruding, and chased them around the bath. He appears to have slipped and fallen in, and, being fully dressed, and wearing Wellington boots, became submerged. It was later suggested that one of the youths had ensured his submersion by holding down his head with a foot (F.M. 10,704c).

On another occasion some young men, erecting temporary buildings beside a river, indulged in initiatory horseplay with a new employee. In spite of his shouts that he could not swim they threw him into the water, where he promptly sank and drowned, in full view of the police station and Coroner's Court on the opposite bank of the river.

Drowning is an occasional mode of infanticide, but the bodies of infants recovered from water are more usually those which have been disposed of by submersion after infanticide by some other means. Similarly, there are occasions, as for example the Luton Sack Murder, when the murderer of an adult attempts to dispose of the body of his victim in this way. Signs of injury are then important and may demonstrate the real cause of death. The body may be placed in a sack or weighted.

The Signs of Submersion and its Probable Duration

The fact of submersion is usually obvious but, unless recent, estimation of its duration presents difficulty which increases as the period lengthens. There is an undoubted and distinctive progression in the development of changes due to submersion but the rate of their development can be modified by one or more of several factors. These include clothing, the time of the year, and, maybe, the size and age of the body, and the composition of the submerging fluid. Difficulty in arriving at an estimate of the duration of submersion also derives from lack of reliable information concerning the probable time intervals which elapse between the successive stages. The original observations of Devergie (1829, 1831) still afford an approximate guide although present experience is that his estimates, especially for winter conditions in this country, are excessive.

In bodies immersed in waterways into which factories discharge effluent, caution must be exercised in interpretation as the water temperature in the region of the discharging effluent may be several degrees higher than in the rest of the waterway.

The changes found during the first 6 hours, in England, are limited to wetting of the clothing and the body, which may be soiled by mud, sand or weeds. In the event that the place of submersion is not known, material which soils the body can, by its character, indicate the probable medium.

The examination of thirty-five bodies, known to have been recovered within 6 hours of submersion, showed that, with one exception, irrespective of the time of year and other factors, no other changes indicative of submersion were found. The exception was provided by a boy, aged 8 years, who was drowned on 11 May 1948, in a disused quarry where the water contained a dye. Slight whitening and wrinkling of the skin was seen on the backs of his hands. According to Devergie, the earliest skin change, namely whitening of the skin, can appear in from 5 to 8 hours in summer or 3 to 5 days in winter.

Submersion causes progressive maceration of the skin, notably of the hands and feet and, in particular, the areas exposed to friction. As time passes the skin becomes whitened, swollen and wrinkled. Later still the epidermis is loosened, as are the nails, which are later shed from the body. If still present, the loosened tissues may be slipped off as if a glove (Fig. 152) or stocking, laying bare the underlying corium. Incidentally, if the body has not been identified, it is possible, by appropriate technique, to obtain impressions of the fingers either from the loosened skin or the bare corium, i.e. derma. Corresponding changes, which take rather longer to develop, include loosening of the hair and skin of the scalp.

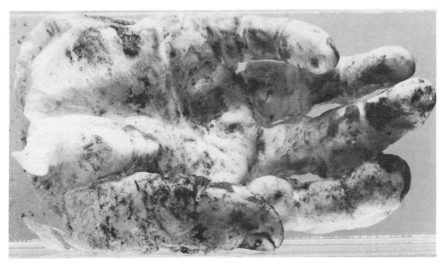

FIG. 152. Submersion: separation of skin of hand as if a glove.

Hands which show evidence of maceration have been likened to those of a washer-woman because relatively prolonged immersion of the hands, when washing clothes, produces similar changes. Probably the presence of soap, and more especially alkali, hastens the appearance of these changes in occupational maceration.

Maceration is usually first apparent in the skin of the pads of the fingers, and afterwards spreads to the palms, the backs of the fingers and the back of the hand, in that order. A corresponding progression is to be observed in the development of maceration of the skin of the feet but, when the deceased had worn shoes or boots, the changes in the feet are always less advanced than in the hands. It takes nearly twice as long for the skin of a clothed foot to attain the same degree of maceration as the unprotected hand.

With the exception already mentioned, early signs of maceration were not apparent in my cases until submersion had lasted for from 12 to 48 hours; moreover they were still absent even at the end of 46 hours in one case which occurred in March 1948. On the other hand, a body examined during the following December showed maceration of the palms, soles and the backs of the fingers, after submersion for 24 hours. It seems probable that slight changes are usual in from 12 to 24 hours or at the latest, 48 hours, even in winter. Devergie found the skin very white at 24 hours in summer but not until the end of 4 to 8 days in winter.

During the first week maceration of the hands, and the feet, if exposed, is likely to become general and well established. Towards the end of the week, early signs of separation of the skin of the digits, possibly limited to the thumbs, great toe and index fingers, may have appeared. Devergie estimated lifting of the skin to require 8 days in summer and 15 days in winter.

Loosening of the skin of the hands, and of the feet, when unprotected, progresses during the second week but, even then, detachment is still limited and the nails are likely to have remained firmly attached to digits, irrespective of the time of the year.

It is not until the third week, or thereabouts, that loosening of the skin and nails is sufficiently extensive to permit their removal as if a glove (Fig. 152) or stocking. By the end of one month this is usually the rule, irrespective of the time of the year. Devergie estimated that the glove-like change, the nails still being firm, took 10 days in summer or from 15 to 20 days in winter.

It is impossible to attempt any precise estimate of the duration of submersion when the period exceeds 1 month.

If the body be infested with fleas or lice at the time of submersion, note should be taken of their condition, since they may furnish additional information about its duration. Fleas can survive for up to about 24 hours, and lice for from 12 to 48 hours after submersion.

References

BANTING, F. G. *et al.* (1938) *Canad. Med. Ass. J.*, **39**, 226.

BECK, T. R. and BECK, J. B. (1836) *Elements of Medical Jurisprudence*, 5th ed. Edinburgh: Longmans.

BROUARDEL, P. (1897) *La Pendaison, La Strangulation, La Suffocation, La Submersion*, pp. 425, 453 *et seq.* Paris: J. B. Baillière.

CASPER, J. L. (1862) *Handbook of Forensic Medicine*, 3rd ed., vol. 2, English trans. G. W. Balfour. London: New Sydenham Soc.

CRAIG, A. B. (1961) *J. Amer. Med. Ass.*, **176**, 255–8.

CULLEN, W. L. (1894) *Brit. Med. J.*, **ii**, 941–2.

DEVERGIE, A. (1829) *Ann. Hyg. publ., Paris*, **2**, 160–96.

DEVERGIE, A. (1831) *Ann. Hyg. publ., Paris*, **5**, 429–57.

DONALD, K. W. (1955) *Brit. Med. J.*, **ii**, 155–60.

DURLACHER, S. H., FREIMUTH, H. C. and SWAN, H. E., Jr. (1953) *Arch. Path.* **56**, 454.

EDITORIAL (1979) *Brit. Med. J.* **i**, (6156), 70–71.

FAGERLUND, L. W. (1890) *Vjschr. gerichtl. Med.*, **52**, 1–42, 234–62.

FISHER, I. L. (1966) Abstracts of papers, 4th Int. Meeting in Forensic Medizine, p. 186.

FUKUI, Y, HALA, M, TAKAHASHI, S. and MATSUBARA, K. (1980) *Forensic Science Int.*, **16**, 67–74.

FULLER, R. H. (1962) *Proc. Roy. Soc. Med.*, **56**, 33–38.

GARDNER, E. (1942) *Med.-leg. Rev.*, **10**, 120.

GEERTINGER, P. and VOIGT, J. (1970) *J. Forens. Med.* **17**, 36.

GETTLER, A. O. (1921) *J. Amer. Med. Ass.*, **77**, 1650.

GIERTSEN, J. CHR. (1970) *Med. Sci. Law*, **10**, 216.

GOLD, M. I. and OLLODART, G. (1967) *J. Amer. Med. Ass.*, **200**, 645.

GOLDEN, F. ST C and RIVERS, J. F. (1975) *Anaesthesia*, **30** (3), 364–373.
GUY, W. A. and FERRIER, D. (1895) *Principles of Forensic Medicine*, 7th ed., ed. W. R. Smith. London: Renshaw.
HAARKOFF, K. and WEILER, G. (1971) *J. Legal Med.*, **69**, 62.
HALMAGYI, D. F. J. and COLEBATCH, H. J. H. (1961) *J. Appl. Physiol.*, **16**, 35.
HANSEN, G. (1938) *Munch. med. Wschr.*, **85**, 1103; abstr. *Méd.-lég. Rev.*, **6**, 410.
HENDRY, W. (1981) Personal communication.
HEWER, C. L. (1962) *Lancet*, **1**, 636.
INCZE, GY., TAMÁSKA, A. and GYONGYÖSI J. (1954–5) *Dtsch. Z. ges. gerichtl. Med.*, **43**, 517.
JAASKELAINEN, A. J. (1967) *Dtsch. Z. ges. gerichtl. Med.*, **61**, 41.
JAASKELAINEN, A. J. (1967) *Dtsch. Z. ges. gerichtl. Med.*, **64**, 29.
JACOBS, S. (1982) Personal communication.
JAMES, W. R. L. (1966) *Med. Sci. Law*, **6**, 164.
JELLINEK, S. (1932) *Die Elektrischen Verletzungen*, Leipzig: Barth.
KARPOVITCH, P. V. (1933) *Arch. Path.*, **15**, 828.
KEATINGE, W. R. (1969) *Brit. Med. J.*, **ii**, 623.
KEATINGE, W. R. (1977) *Practitioner*, **219**, 183–187.
KEATINGE, W. R. and Hayward M. G. (1981) *J. Forensic Sciences*, **26** (3), 459–461.
KEATINGE, W. R. and MCCANCE, R. A. (1959) *Lancet*, **ii**, 208.
KEATINGE, W. R. and NADEL, T. A. (1962) *J. Physiol.*, **162**, 56.
KVITTINGEN, T. D. and NAESS, A. (1963) *Brit. Med. J.*, **i**, 1315.
LOWSON, J. A., (1903) *Edinb. Med. J.*, **13**, 41.
MANKTELOW, W. F. and HUNT, A. C. (1967) *Med. Sci. Law*, **7**, 137.
MARTIN, É. (1950) *Précis de Médicine Légale*, 3rd ed. Paris: Doin.
MODELL, J. H. (1968) *Acta. anaesth. Scand. Suppl.* XXIX. Aspects of resuscitation.
MODELL, J. H. and DAVIS, J. H. (1963) *J. Amer. Med. Ass.*, **185**, 651.
MODELL, J. H. and DAVIS, J. A. (1969) *Anaesthesiology*, **30**, 414.
MUELLER, B. (1952) *Dtsch. Z. ges. gerichtl. Med.*, **41**, 400.
MUELLER, B. (1959) *Zacchia*, **34**, 1.
MUELLER, B. and GORGS, D. (1949) *Dtsch. Z. ges. gerichtl. Med.*, **39**, 715.
MUELLER, W. C. (1969) *J. Forens. Sci.*, **14**, 327.
NIXON, J. and PEARN, J. H. (1977) *Brit. Med. J.*, **i**, 271–272.
OGSTON, F., Jr. (1882) *Edinb. Med. J.*, **27**, 865–73.
PALTAUF, A. (1882) *Über den Tod durch Ertrinken*, Wien, cited Reuter (1901).
PAYNE, R. T. (1940) *Brit. Med. J.*, **i**, 819–22.
PEARN, J. H. (1980) *Brit. Med. J.*, **281**, 1103.
PEARN, J. H., BROWN, J., WONG, R. and BART, R. (1979) *Pediatrics*, **64** (1), 68–70.
PEABODY, A. T. (1980) *Med. Sci. Law*, **20** (4), 254–261.
PLEUKHAHN, V. D. (1977) *Med. Sci. Law*, **17**, 246–250.
POLSON, C. J. and TATTERSALL, R. N. (1971) *Clinical Toxicology*, 27 ed. Reprint, pp. 571–576, London.
R. V. BARLOW, (1957) Leeds Assizes 6 Dec.; see Polson and Tattersall (1971). Pitman Medical.
R. V. COOK (1958) Flintshire Assizes, per Dr. Gerald Evans; also *Med. Sci. Law* (1961), **1**, 33.
R. V. MANTON (1943) See Simpson (1945).
R. V. NODDER (1937) Warwick Winter Assizes and Nottingham Assizes, *Trials of Frederick Nodder*, ed. Winifred Duke, 1950, *Notable British Trials Series*, Edinburgh: Hodge.
R. V. SMITH (1915) *Trial of George Joseph Smith, Notable British Trials*, ed. E. R. Watson (1922). Edinburgh: Hodge.
R. V. TAYLOR (1949) Chester Assizes, 31 Oct.; police file, unpublished; lent by the Chief Constable of Cheshire, G. E. Banwell, Esq. O.B.E., M.C.; also *Manchester Guardian*, 27 Aug. and 3 Sept. 1949.
RAMMER, L. and GERDIN, B. (1976) *Forensic Sci.*, **8** (3), 229–234.
REVENSTORF, —(1903) *Vrtrljschr. f. gerichtl. Med.*, 3F, **26**, 31.
RUSHTON, D. G. (1960) 2nd Int. Meeting on Forensic Path. and Med., New York. *Program and Abstracts*, pp. 22–23.
RUSHTON, D. G. (1961). *Med.-leg. J. (Camb.)* **29**, 90–97.
SAMMUT, J. J. (1967) *J. Laryng.*, **81**, 137.
SCHEIDER, A. (1931) *Amer. J. Police Sci.*, **2**, 30–44.
SCOTT, P. H. and EIGEN, H. (1980) *J. Pediatr.*, **96** (2), 282–284.
SIMONIN, C. (1955) *Médecine Légale Judiciare*, 3rd ed., pp. 222–3. Paris: Maloine.
SIMPSON, C. K. (1945) *Police J.*, **18**, 263–73.
SMITH, Sir SYDNEY and FIDDES, F. S. (1955) *Forensic Medicine*, 10th ed., p. 265. London: Churchill.
SOUTTER, C. (1936) *Ann. Méd.-lég*, **16**, 217–44.

SPILSBURY, B. (1934) *Méd.-lég. Rev.*, **2**, 340–44.
SPITZ, W. (1963) *Dtsch. Z. ges gerichtl. Med.*, **54**, 42.
SWANN, H. G. and BRUCER, M. (1949) *Tex. Rep. Biol. Med.*, **7**, 511.
SWANN, H. G. and SPAFFORD, N. R. (1951) *Tex. Rep. Biol. Med.*, **9**, 356.
TAMÁSKA, L. (1949) *Orv. Hetil.*, 509 (Index Medicus).
TAMÁSKA, L. (1961) *Dtsch. Z. ges. gerichtl. Med.*, **51**, 398–403.
TERAZAWA, K. and TAKATORI, T. (1980) *Forensic Sci. Int.*, **16**, 63–66.
THOMAS, F., VAN HECKE, W. and TIMPERMAN, J. (1960) *Verh. kon. Acad. Geneesk. Belg.*, **22**, 9; English abstr. in Program and Abstracts, 2nd Int. Meeting on Forensic Path. and Med., New York, p. 23.
TIMPERMAN, J. (1962) *J. Forens. Med.*, **9**, 134.
TIMPERMAN, J. (1969) *J. Forens. Med.*, **16**, 45.
WACHHOLZ, L. (1934) *Arch. Kriminol.*, **40**, 45–46; abstr. *Méd.-lég. Rev.*, 1935, **3**, 229.
WATSON, E. R. (1922) *Trial of G. J. Smith, Notable British Trials Series*, Edinburgh; Hodge.

CHAPTER 12

Suffocation

THE term "suffocation" is commonly regarded as synonymous with "asphyxia", but it is here restricted to a group of circumstances, drowning excepted, in which asphyxia is due to causes other than constriction of the neck by a ligature, the hands, or a strangle-hold.

Suffocation here includes smothering, choking, overlying, traumatic or crush asphyxia, and burking.

General considerations

Although these several forms of suffocation differ in their circumstances, their effects upon the victims have much in common. It is usual for the asphyxial symptoms and signs to be severe since death is usually the result of slow asphyxia, often taking 2 to 5 minutes to kill. It is unusual, although possible, for unconsciousness to be immediate from vagal inhibition. Most victims present obvious external and internal signs of asphyxia. Cyanosis of the face, even of extreme degree, and petechial haemorrhages in the skin of the face and beneath the conjunctivae are usual. The tongue may protrude and may have been bitten; the eyes are prominent and staring. There may be bleeding from the nose and ears. Whilst external signs of injury are to be seen in some cases, the mechanism of asphyxia by suffocation is such that there may be no external injury. Alternatively, these injuries may be slight and can escape notice when the examination is perfunctory. Choking due to the insertion of a foreign body into the mouth, for example, is easily overlooked and may be difficult to prove when the agent was removed soon after the death of the victim. The ease with which it is practicable to kill by smothering without producing any external injury may create problems of great difficulty for the medical examiner. No detail is then too trivial to be disregarded if a correct interpretation is to be made.

The recognition of death by suffocation can be a simple matter but there are occasions when the most experienced examiner cannot go further than the conclusion that death was due to asphyxia. The distinction on medical grounds as between smothering, skilfully effected, and overlying may be impossible.

Smothering

Asphyxia by smothering is due to any circumstance which prevents breathing by obstruction of the nose and mouth. It is a possible but unusual mode of suicide, seen

449

almost exclusively amongst mental patients. Accidental smothering, especially of infants during the first three months of life, is not infrequent. It is a simple and common mode of infanticide. For obvious reasons, it is difficult to smother a healthy, robust adult; but one who is incapacitated by drink, drugs or disease may readily fall a victim. Selected examples of each group show the probable circumstances.

Suicide by Smothering

The reported cases of suicidal smothering concern, in the main, mental patients or prisoners. Suicide is practicable merely by burying the face in a flock mattress (Puppe, 1908) or even, it would appear, by lying against the bedclothing so as to obstruct the nose and mouth, especially when drunk.

More elaborate steps may be taken. A woman locked herself and her child in a bedroom. She lay under the bedclothes and instructed her child to pile cushions and clothing on the bed. Several hours later the woman was found dead of suffocation (Wald, cited by Étienne Martin, 1950).

A male prisoner committed suicide by stuffing his nostrils and mouth with pieces of cloth which were held in position by a handkerchief tied round his mouth. He was found lying dead, on his face (Taylor, 1956).

An epileptic was found dead in bed at a mental hospital. The body was on its back; a round pebble had been inserted into each nostril and the mouth was stuffed with a roll of flannel (Sankey, 1883).

Death by cut-throat may occasionally terminate by smothering. If the trachea be completely severed, the lower end is likely to be drawn down within the thorax by the weight of the heart and lungs; if the soft parts then close over the wound, they can obstruct the trachea and the victim is smothered.

Accidental Smothering

The circumstances vary according to the age of the subject.

(a) *Infants*, during the first month of life, especially when premature, may be suffocated merely by the weight of the bedclothes when they cover the nose and mouth. This, however, is an unlikely cause of death after the first month, and, in any event, it may be accepted as an explanation of asphyxia only when a thorough investigation, by the police as well as the medical examiner, has excluded the possibility of crime or disease.

Suffocation of the infant is also possible when it turns on its face in its cot and buries its face in a soft pillow or mattress.

Pillows of any kind are a potential hazard in a child's cot or pram. It is clear that even "safety" pillows are not necessarily safe. A boy, aged 4 months, died of suffocation in his pram. He was found with his face buried in a "safety" pillow. These pillows are designed with fifty-four ventilation holes in them so that breathing is still possible if the child buries its face in the pillow; they are covered with a loosely-knit cotton cover. If, however the pillow be covered with an additional nylon slip, through which air cannot pass, this defeats the object of the design. The mother of this child, desiring to make the pillow look more attractive, had fitted it with a nylon pillow slip. It appeared that no warning of the danger of this practice had been given by the manufacturers to the retailers, nor to the customers.

(Report of an inquest held by Mr. Ronald Lloyd, South West Lancashire Coroner: *Daily Telegraph*, 18 Aug. 1971.)

Suffocation by the mattress is rare. In October 1950 a boy aged 3 months was found dead in his cot. He was lying prone as was his custom when asleep. There was a mattress but no pillow in the cot. Death was due to asphyxia and there was no trace of violence or of disease to explain its origin. It seemed possible, therefore, that the child had suffocated by burying his face in the mattress. He may have had a convulsion although he was not known to have had any previously. The mother's evidence that he was "definitely teething" was not confirmed by necropsy. The case illustrates the difficulties in interpretation which these deaths can present.

A boy aged 1 month was found dead lying face down on a plastic-covered mattress with the head under the pillow in a carry-cot. Death was ascribed to asphyxia, with respiratory infection as a contributory factor ("Medicine and the Law", *Lancet*, 1961, i, 215).

Suffocation by a pillow is likely to occur only when an infant is aged 3 months or less. If, however, they are of poor physique, older infants may die in these circumstances.

Suffocation of an infant whilst in its pram may be caused by a cat which jumps on to the pram and settles on the baby's face or chest. A boy aged 1 month was asleep in his pram in the garden. An hour later the parents looked through the window and saw a large cat jump out of the pram. When they went to the child, it looked ill. A doctor was summoned at once but he failed to revive the child by artificial respiration. The necropsy demonstrated signs of asphyxia; some food had regurgitated into the air passages but this may have been a terminal event (Leeds City Coroner, No. 518/1945).

On another occasion it was possible to prove that the cat had sat on the baby's face because hairs, identical with those of the cat's fur, were present on the baby's face (F.M. 14,704).

A baby girl, aged 5 weeks, was found in her pram with a cat lying over her face. She was deeply cyanosed and gasping. Mouth-to-mouth resuscitation by her father restored normal breathing but her survival was brief; she died when aged 8 months from bronchopneumonia. The outstanding finding at the post-mortem examination was severe brain damage. There was bilateral, symmetrical dissolution of the white matter of the cerebral hemispheres and severe focal atrophy of the cerebral cortex. These neurological changes resembled those of severe anoxic birth injury and could only be explained by the smothering episode (Kearney, Dahl and Stalsberg, 1982).

(b) *Children and young adults*. Accidental smothering in this age group may be predisposed to by an epileptic fit but in our experience the victims of such fatalities are adults over the age of 21; we have examined only three of these subjects whose ages were below 21; they were respectively, aged 12, 15 and 20 years.

Another variety of accidental smothering, likely to involve children rather than adults, occurs in an air-tight place or one in which ventilation is negligible. A servant girl died of suffocation when shut in a trunk (Henke, cited Tidy, 1883). Two small boys, playing on a disused delivery van, lifted the lid of a locker which formed the driver's seat and climbed inside. The lid fell down and its hasp engaged with the staple on the front of the locker. They were thus imprisoned and asphyxiated in an almost air-tight space, $29^1/_2 \times 13 \times 20$ in. (Mr. E. G. B. Fowler, H. M. Coroner, City of Leicester; cited Glaister and Rentoul, 1966).

A boy, aged 3 years, died of asphyxia when locked inside a disused, empty refrigerator which had been left in a garden. Although the child could close the door from inside, it would then clip shut and he could not open it. The seal was tight and the internal dimensions of the refrigerator were 48 × 15 × 12 in., i.e. a capacity of 5 ft³ (*Yorkshire Post*, 5 June 1970).

> The song "The Mistletoe Bough" recalls the case of accidental smothering in a chest. It appears that Lord Lovell's bride hid herself in a large oak chest during a game of hide-and-seek on her wedding eve. Once inside, however, she was unable to escape because the lid closed with a spring lock. Her companions did not hear her cries and it was not until some years later that her remains were found. An oak chest preserved in Malmesbury Abbey is believed to be the original chest although there are several similar chests in the country. Mr. W. A. Brown, Organist to the Abbey, who kindly gave me the information about this matter, considers the Malmesbury chest likely to be the original one because it was presented to the Abbey by the late Mrs. Lovell. Her family lived in the neighbourhood and all of its deceased members are buried in the Lovell Chapel in the Abbey.

Dr. Roche had a case of smothering which occurred when a boy aged 10 hid in a disused refrigerator when playing hide-and-seek with his friends. He had not realised that when the door shut there was no handle on the inside and his friends did not suspect this hiding place. The result was that his body was not found until about 3 days later (Fig. 153).

(c) *Adults*. (i) *Accidental smothering at work*. Accidental smothering of adults by precipitation into a quantity of finely divided, solid material may occur in the course of their occupation. Substances such as flour, sand, coal-dust, cinders, grain or feathers are likely media. A man was smothered when he attempted to recover his fountain pen which had fallen into a large hopper of fine coal. On another occasion a man was buried by a quantity of barley. While the barley was being delivered into a ship's hold, the "feeder" which prevented the cargo from shifting suddenly collapsed and an avalanche of barley descended. Four men jumped clear but the fifth man was buried under about 190 tons of barley and was smothered (*The Yorkshire Post*, 29 Nov. 1949).

(ii) *Accidental smothering in epilepsy*. Accidental smothering of adults in domestic circumstances usually affects persons subject to epileptic or epileptiform fits. Most of these persons are over 21; with three exceptions, the range in the Leeds series was from 22 to 69 years. Several died of asphyxia from having buried their faces in soft pillows. One victim, a woman aged 43, was in the later months of her sixth pregnancy when she was found dead in bed with her face buried in the pillow. There were no marks of violence nor any reason to suspect foul play. It is possible that she had had an eclamptic fit, but this was not confirmed by signs of liver damage or urinary abnormality (H.M. Coroner for the Craven District, Mr. Stephen E. Brown, 8 May 1948).

The accident may occur out of doors when the victim, either in the course of an epileptic fit or when under the influence of drink or drugs, falls face down into mud, snow or thick grass.

PLASTIC BAG SUFFOCATION*

The synthesis of polythene and its manufacture in sheets and bags created a revolution in the packaging industry but it brought with it new hazards. Bags made of this tough, transparent, waterproof material are excellent containers but if placed over the head they

---

* This section was published by the Z. *Retsmed.—J. Leg. Med.* and its reproduction is by permission of the Editor in Chief and Springer Verlag, the publishers, See Polson and Gee (1972).

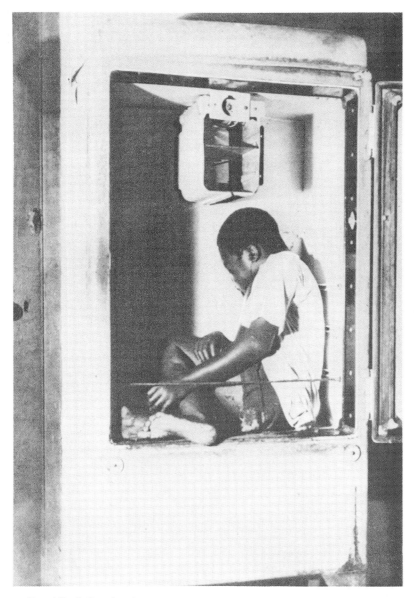

Fig. 153. Suffocation in a disused refrigerator. (by courtesy of Dr. Patrick Roche.)

are lethal. Children are at special risk, since in play they may put one of these bags over their own heads or over the head of a playmate; the bags have been agents of suicide and are potential agents for infanticide and homicide. Polythene sheeting is also dangerous as a covering of prams, cots, or cot mattresses.

The National Federation of Dry Cleaners adopted the printing of a warning notice under a red triangle, and some of the larger bags are also perforated.

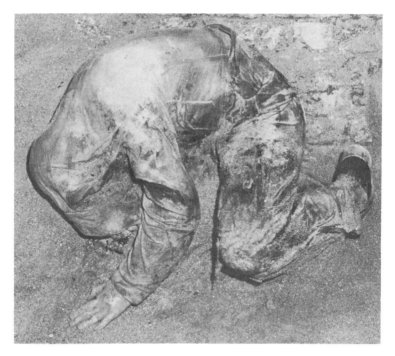

FIG. 154. Accidental suffocation of youth while hiding in a hole he had dug
in a sand heap (F.M. 15933A).

In the past, rubber sheeting was used by those who indulged in auto-erotic practices. They may still occur but its scarcity and ready access to polythene sheeting and bags has provided an alternative agent.

The Circumstances of Suffocation With Plastic Agents

1. *Accidental suffocation.* The majority of these victims are children and the circumstances are illustrated by the following cases: an illegitimate infant girl, aged 17 months, was dead when found on her back on the floor of her attic home. She was fully clothed and had a plastic bag over her head. There were signs of asphyxia but none of injury. Petechial haemorrhages were present in the skin of her forehead, eyelids and left temple but there were none beneath the conjunctivae; her lips were cyanosed; she also had petechial haemorrhages beneath the pleurae. No natural disease nor congenital malformation was present. Death was due to asphyxia. The mother came under strong suspicion but this accident occurred when she had left the child alone for several hours.

The bag was normally kept in a drawer near the child's body and the drawer was partly opened. It was at a level of 29 in. above the floor and the child measured 28 in. from the soles of her feet to the level of her eyes. It was possible therefore for her to have taken the bag from the drawer.

The bag had been made from polythene sheeting by tying it with four knots, three of which formed a handle. The aperture in the bag was 17 in. in circumference; it may have been a little smaller when first made. It was possible for the child to have pulled the bag over her head, although not without difficulty.

A consideration of the circumstances led to the conclusion that the child was alone responsible for the accident; the mother was exonerated (F.M. 15,935).

A boy of 3 years also died of asphyxia due to putting a plastic bag over his head. The child was perfectly normal but the mother had a long history of mental disturbance and was living apart from her husband. She told the police that she left the child in the house and went shopping and called at a fish and chip shop on the way home. When she got home she found the child with a plastic bread wrapper over its head. There appeared to be some doubt about the times which she gave in her story being correct, but she was very distressed and mentally disturbed when making the statement and there was no indication that she had done anything to the child.

There were no petechial haemorrhages in the eyelids, or the skin of the face, but a few fresh petechial haemorrhages were seen beneath the epicardium at the back of the heart, and there were a few more beneath the pleura. There was no evidence of injury of the kind seen in the "battered baby". The only other finding of note was the presence of a little regurgitated stomach contents and foamy mucus in the air passages. There was only incomplete obstruction of the main air passages but the bronchi within the lungs were filled with stomach contents. The tiny scratches and bruises on the child's face were consistent with injury caused by the hurried removal of the plastic bag and attempts to resuscitate the child.

2. *Auto-erotic (and narcotic) misadventures.* Plastic bags have been used in the course of auto-erotic practices for at least a decade and although the majority of reports have been in the continental journals, notably German journals, we in England have not been unaware of this practice. Plastic bags have also been used as an aid to intoxication by addicts to the inhalation of anaesthetics or narcotic vapours.

It is now widely accepted that the induction of partial anoxia, as by hanging, the most favoured mode, or other forms of mechanical asphyxia, accentuates sexual sensation during an auto-erotic exercise.

The mode of stimulation employed in auto-erotic practices was analysed by Schollmeyer (1966) and amongst 119 reported cases he found that sixty-two were by strangulation; twenty-two by electrocution, twenty by asphyxia (reine asphyxia) and fifteen by narcotic poisoning. We respectfully disagree with his term "strangulation", since the arrangement of the ligature in many, if not all, of these cases is such that the weight of the body or part of the body operated on the ligature and, therefore, these deaths were by hanging.

We formerly thought that the age range for auto-erotic accidents was between the ages of about 17–25 and 55–65 but it is now clear that the range is much wider, i.e. 11 to 80, and it may prove to be even wider still. One of our subjects, who was deemed to have died as a result of an experiment, but in circumstances which could have been those of an auto-erotic exercise, was aged $11^3/_4$ years (F.M. 6041; Polson, 1965).

An alternative explanation for the use of plastic bags was offered by Johnstone *et al.* (1960), who deemed it preferable to the less elegant and more superficial theory of partial anoxia. They suggested that enclosure represented an attempt to return to the womb. It might have been the motive of the man who was found dead, doubled up, inside a dustbin. We still prefer to believe that partial anoxia is the aim in the majority of these auto-erotic practices.

It is still true that all of the victims are males. No example or report of an example of a female dead in these circumstances is yet known to us.

Illustrative Cases

The earlier cases were reports of enclosure of the head in rubber sheeting, a sponge bag, or a diver's mask.

Rosselet (1927) reported the death of a young man aged 26 who had wrapped his head in layers of thick rubber sheeting which he had fixed firmly round his neck with string. His room was locked on the inside. There were no signs of a struggle. It was believed to have been suicide but we note that he was known to have exhibited signs of sexual abnormality and he was accustomed to carry rubber articles in his pocket and had a habit of touching rubber. This death could well have been the result of an auto-erotic exercise.

A man aged 41, when found dead in bed, was wearing a rubber swimming cap and his mouth and nose were obstructed by a rubber-lined sponge bag. His watch was nearby. The theory offered at the inquest was that he had been making an experiment. He had heard in India that it was possible to remain under water for long periods. He was believed to have been engaged in a test to see how long he could hold his breath, as if under water.

Another case concerned a man aged 25. When found dead in his bath, he was wearing a frogman's outfit; the clips were clamped to his nose. The body lay in only one foot of water. Death was ascribed to oxygen want; there was no evidence of drowning. Here also it was suggested that this accident was the result of an experiment. He was interested in under-water photography and he might have been engaged in tests to enable him to construct an under-water camera. His oxygen canister had been in use for some time. This was the second case of its kind within 4 months; the earlier victim, aged 27, was a neighbour of the deceased.

A boy aged 16 years and 10 months was found lying naked on the floor, near his bed. There was a plastic bag over his head, secured by a band. A second plastic bag enclosed his genitalia and it appeared ejaculation had recently occurred. His feet and legs were tied together and a second ligature was tied to one thumb as if he had also intended to tie his hands together. Death was due to asphyxia. (A report of this case was given to us by Mr. G. F. Goodman, Chief Constable of Halifax.)

A boy, or should we say today, a man, aged 16, when found dead in his kitchen had his head enveloped in a plastic mackintosh which he had fastened round his head with an elastic cord. On this occasion the explanation was that death was the result of an experiment. He was an assistant to a monumental mason and, aware of the danger of inhaling stone dust, he was believed to have been attempting to devise a dust mask (*Manchester Guardian*, 4 April 1950).

There are already a number of excellent and well-illustrated reports of these accidents with plastic bags, e.g. Holzhausen and Hunger (1960), Johnstone *et al.* (1960), Dumont *et al.* (1962), Weimann (1962), Weimann and Prokop (1963) and Schollmeyer (1966), and others. The following case in our practice occurred in circumstances as bizarre as any other yet reported:

Case 1

This man, aged 22, died in a hay loft, at his workplace, to which he had gained access by a ladder. He had placed a couple of blankets on the hay and his body was laid on them. It was encased in three large, thick plastic bags; one was over his head and loosely fastened round the neck with twine, a second encased his trunk and he had cut two armholes in the bag, through which his arms protruded. The third bag enclosed his legs and was fastened at the ankles and knees with twine. When the bags were removed it was seen that he had a large pad of cloth in front of his face; there was a strong odour of ether. He had encircled his body with several loops of twine and protected his shoulders with a large piece of cloth. Neither the neck nor the genitalia were included in these loops. The legs were enclosed in two large rubber inner tubes. The innermost was cut to the shape of an inverted U, the top of the U cut off, with the legs thrust down within each side of the tube, and with a flap fashioned from the upper part with a hole in it through which his genitalia were thrust. On top of this was a second inner tube, in the shape of a U, the legs thrust into the limbs of this tube.

There was a metal ring round his penis, a short length of chain was attached to each side of the ring, and the chains were fastened to twine which encircled his body. He had applied a metal clamp to his scrotum, above the testicles; the clamp was firmly bolted on the right side but the bolt on the left could be unscrewed with the fingers; the clamp had not exerted severe pressure on the scrotum; he had also fastened the clamp to his body with twine.

An aerosol, labelled "Quick Start", a ring spanner and a handyman's knife were beside the body. His clothing was in a neat pile about 15 ft. from the body. There was a pile of unused plastic bags in the loft and fragments of plastic, which he had cut from one of the bags on his body, were also found.

Death was due to the combined effects of asphyxia and the inhalation of narcotic vapour. There were no signs of injury and the freedom of his arms had enabled him to accomplish this fantastic situation. He had a few petechial haemorrhages beneath the inner surfaces of his eye lids and at the back of his heart. There was an odour of ether in his brain.

Analysis of the aerosol showed that it contained ether and toluene; these substances were present in his blood, brain and lungs (F.M. 15,828A).

Case 2. Narcotic (Ether) Addiction

This man, aged 27, was found in a state of advanced putrefaction but it was possible not only to establish his identity but also the circumstances of his death. He had a plastic bag over his head and had knotted the bag on the left side of his neck. A handkerchief was inside the bag, close to his chin. There was a bottle of dimethyl ether beside his bed. Dissection showed that the bag had been drawn into his mouth and naso-pharynx so as to effect complete closure of the airway; its apex reached the epiglottis. There was no evidence of sexual deviation; no signs of injury; no motive for suicide.

Analysis detected 1670 ppm of ether in the brain and 88 ppm in the liver; the alcohol level in the brain was 172 mg per cent and in the liver 130 mg per cent (F.M. 11,661A).

Case 3. Chloral Narcosis and Plastic Bag Suffocation

This woman of 40 was found dead, face down, with a plastic bag over her face. There were no signs of asphyxia; no signs of injury and no motive for suicide.

An 8-oz. bottle near her still contained a small quantity of fluid which was identified as chloral B.P., in a strength of 1.5 grains per ounce; the full bottle would have contained 12 grains of chloral (780 mg). Post-mortem changes destroy chloral and analyses are only approximate and are probably underestimates. The results showed that there were 600 mg (10 grains) of chloral in her stomach; 4 mg per cent in the blood; 5 mg per cent in the liver and 25 mg per cent in the urine. She had clearly taken a considerable amount but one which was below the average lethal dose, i.e. 10 g. She had taken enough to produce unconsciousness. The final factor was suffocation by the plastic bag (F.M. 12,447A).

Suicidal Suffocation with a Plastic Bag

This may be accomplished by use of the bag alone, or in combination with inhalation of carbon monoxide or other gas, as in the case of Tolnay (1963). Some are under the influence of alcohol.

Our practice has included the following cases:

A man aged 56 was found dead on the bank of a river. He had a plastic bag over his head and his death was due to asphyxia. His blood contained 209 mg per cent and his urine contained 255 mg per cent of alcohol.

A man aged 71, who died of asphyxia by a plastic bag, was under the influence of amytal. It was estimated that about 14 grains (900 mg) were circulating in his blood at the time of his death. His blood contained also 68 mg per cent of alcohol (F.M. 13,376).

Conversely, the death was due to asphyxia alone, in a woman, aged 41, who put a plastic bag over her head. The bag acted as a valve-like seal over her nose and mouth.

The first case in our practice occurred in 1961, when a male aged 22 died of asphyxia by putting a plastic bag over his head (F.M. 7801 C).

Homicidal Suffocation with a Plastic Bag

As yet we have had no instance of this form of homicide, nor does any appear to have been recorded. The following is an instance of attempted infanticide with a plastic bag.

An infant girl, when aged 5 days, had a plastic bag applied to her head by her mother, who, at the time, was suffering from puerperal insanity. A police officer was summoned and he promptly removed the bag and successfully resuscitated the child. Unfortunately, owing to prolonged cerebral anoxia, there was permanent grave cerebral damage. She suffered from quadraplegia; she could move her head and swallow. She had retained some mental faculty. Her intelligence quotient, measurable by special tests, was about 60, but because of her physical disabilities she was ineducable. The child was examined in 1970 at the age of 6 years and is still in the care of a national institution. (By courtesy of Dr. Mary Polson, School Medical Officer, and Mr. D. Pickles, Educational Psychologist, W.R.C.C.).

Asphyxia by the Amniotic Sac (Plate 8)

Asphyxia by the amniotic sac is a well-recognised complication of child birth but it is uncommon. To be "born in a caul" is, understandably, a lucky event if the child survives; there was a time when an amniotic sac from one of these cases would be bought as a charm against misfortune. A good example of asphyxia by a sac is depicted by Polson (1965) (F.M. 6684).

The Signs of Suffocation by Plastic Bags

These deaths occur in circumstances which are usually obvious and the majority present the signs of asphyxia; there are no external signs of injury. There may or may not be evidence of disease, which contributed to the death or predisposed to suicide. It is more important to bear in mind that there may be the coincident effects of alcohol or drugs and therefore the examination of the body should include a toxicological analysis. In some cases there is evidence of sexual deviation.

The presence of moisture inside the bag may mislead. It could be evidence of breathing inside the bag but it is more probable that this is due to condensation of moisture, dispelled from the body after death (Fig. 155). Organs conveyed to the laboratory in plastic bags frequently "breathe" and a cushion, enclosed in a plastic bag, also "breathed" when exposed to the warmth of the sun.

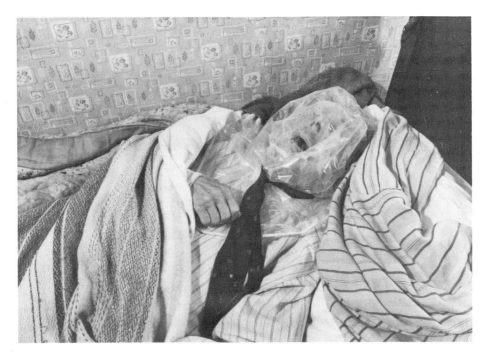

Fig. 155. Suffocation in plastic bag: no signs of asphyxia. Drops of moisture on inner surface of the bag.

When an old man was found dead with a plastic bag over his head, tied round his neck with a necktie, moisture was abundant on the inner surface of the bag. The first pathologist, having found severe coronary disease, ascribed the death to heart failure, i.e. natural cause; he discounted the bag as a factor in the death because he believed the deceased had breathed while it was over his head. The learned coroner was sceptical and sought a second opinion. There was evidence that the man had taken steps to prepare for death; he had given directions for the disposal of his deed box. A verdict of suicide was returned (Polson, 1965).

Some of the victims show no signs of asphyxia; three examples were reported by Hunt and Camps (1962); they were absent in two of our cases. The correct explanation of this difference from other cases of suffocation has yet to be ascertained. It is possible that the first inspiration may draw the bag into the back of the throat, as found in F.M. 11,661 A; Case No. 2 (see p. 457), and causes abrupt respiratory and cardiac arrest. On other occasions it may be that almost as soon as the bag is over the head the first inspiration sucks in the bag as an immediate, complete seal over the nose and mouth and this causes sudden cardiac arrest.

Homicidal Smothering

Homicide of an adult by smothering is practicable only when there is gross physical disparity between the assailant and his victim. Alternatively the victim must be relatively helpless by virtue of age, ill-health or incapacity from drink or drugs, but it is also practicable if the victim is first stunned by a blow. It is therefore a common mode of infanticide but is unusual in murder.

The simplest procedure is to hold a hand or cloth over the infant's mouth and nose, or a plaster may be applied. Masks of pitch were used in the early experiments on dogs.

It is usual for the assailant to use more force, far greater than is necessary to kill and, in consequence, finger-marks in the form of scratches and bruises or even more serious injuries may be found.

The victim's face may be pressed into the pillows as in the murder of a young girl depicted by Gonzales *et al.* (1954), or a pillow or cushion may be held over the victim's face. A small boy killed his baby sister by smothering her with a cushion; another pulled a plastic bag over the head of his brother.

The matron of a nursing home, apparently in a burst of temper, or in exasperation, placed a pillow over the face of a woman patient, aged 76, who was shouting, screaming and kicking, and asphyxiated her.

In 1953 a woman was acquitted of the murder of her husband who was dying of cancer. He had asked her to end his misery and it was alleged she had placed a pillow upon his face in an attempt to smother him.

The father of an infant aged 7 months was acquitted of its murder but found guilty of manslaughter when he suffocated it by applying the cot pillow to its face to stop it crying. He was left alone in the house with the child who, through illness, cried continually. Exasperated by this, the father lost his temper. At his trial he said he threw the pillow into the cot and it came to rest on the child's face. This left unexplained certain recent bruises on the right side of its forehead, of a kind which could have been made by the fingers of an assailant but which were not to be explained as due to accident. The cot pillow, also, was apparently intact when the mother left the house but it was badly torn when she returned (*R. v. Sheldon*, 1954, Leeds Assizes, F.M. 3630 A).

The External Signs of Smothering

In a proportion of the deaths from smothering there are no external signs of violence, especially when obstruction is by some soft material gently applied. Obstruction may then be by bedclothing, a pillow, a cushion, a mother's breast, or the hands of an assailant, applied with skill. On these occasions the only permissible conclusion from the medical examination is that death was due to asphyxia.

Even when there is collateral evidence of smothering it may be impossible to distinguish between it and overlying. A man was charged with the murder of his infant son aged 11 months by smothering it. The father said he had gone to bed with the child and lay with his arm round it. When he awoke he found the child dead. The death was due to asphyxia, without trace of violence on the body, and the only collateral evidence then available was the father's statement. It appeared to have been a death from overlying. Some weeks later, while he was serving a prison sentence, he made a confession, which he retracted almost at once, in which he then said he had smothered his son by holding him against his chest. He was acquitted of murder because it was impossible by medical examination to distinguish between these two modes as the cause of asphyxia in this case.

The Crown properly drew attention to the fact that this child was considerably older than those who die of overlying, because they are rarely over 6 months old. The victim, however, had hyperplasia of the lymphoid tissue, notably in the small intestine. The father was given the benefit of the doubt since this was believed to indicate that the child was less resistant to stress, e.g. of asphyxia. In any event, other considerations, notably absence of marks of violence on the child's body, precluded a precise diagnosis. An interpretation of smothering must rest on more substantial evidence than mere suspicion, for which, however, there was ample cause in this case (F.M. 1153, *R. v. Hunter*).

On other occasions the signs of violence are likely to include scratches, distinct nail-marks or even laceration of the soft parts of the victim's face. The lips, gums and tongue may be the site of bruising or laceration. Close attention must be given to the mouth and nose; the examination should include low magnification and section of the soft parts to detect bruising. The injuries may amount to nothing more than a mere ruffling of the skin, with or without slight bruising of the parts, to be confirmed by microscopy. When such changes are found, however slight they may be, they call for a satisfactory explanation from any person suspected of injuring the child.

Scratches and bruising due to violence but not those associated with disease, e.g. scabies, are unusual elsewhere on the bodies of infants but they may be present on the bodies of older children and point to resistance during a struggle with an assailant. The injuries are then most likely to be found on the arms, forearms and hands. When a boy aged about 3 to 4 years was found murdered by smothering, there were marks of violence on the body and several teeth had been dislodged from the upper and lower jaws.

Choking

Choking is the variety of asphyxia caused by an obstruction within the air passages. It is usually due to the inhalation of a foreign body, but it can be caused by the inhalation of the products of disease (or violence) or by anatomical changes due to disease. Death by choking is commonly an accident but occasionally it may be homicidal or even suicidal; in the latter event the victim was probably suffering from mental illness. Although, strictly, the cause of obstruction in choking is within the air passages, it is convenient here to include allied circumstances when, for example, a foreign body in the gullet may press upon and obstruct the trachea.

The usual mechanism of asphyxia in choking is simple mechanical obstruction; occasionally, however, the entry of foreign material may cause sudden death from vagal inhibition (the so-called café-coronary).

Accidental Choking

This usually occurs during a meal when food is accidentally inhaled, especially when, at the time, the victim is laughing or crying, or if someone, in jest, unexpectedly slaps him on the back. It is seen in mental hospitals where a demented patient may snatch food from another patient's plate and, in his haste to eat the stolen food, he chokes.

A man, aged 50, had been drinking and was put to bed; when next seen, he was dead. His respiratory tract was flooded with regurgitated stomach contents and his death was ascribed to asphyxia. His blood contained 325 per cent and his urine 342 per cent of alcohol, the equivalent of $5^1/_2$ pints of beer of 9 oz of spirits; it was deemed he had consumed an even greater amount (F.M. 11,117).

A Dutch drug pedlar choked to death at Karachi airport. He feared arrest and went to the toilet, where he swallowed 15 plastic bags each containing 250 grammes of opium. He collapsed and died immediately. It was a failed attempt to smuggle the drug out of Pakistan.

Choking is a common accident; most people have "swallowed the wrong way" and are familiar, at first hand, with the symptoms of a mild attack, but, fortunately, fatalities are infrequent.

The kind of foreign body inhaled may be one of a wide range, which includes food, collar studs, fruit stones, screws, pins or even partial dentures.

> The following illustration is cited because of its unusual and historical interest. Brunel, the engineer, had the misfortune to inhale a half sovereign on 3 April 1883. He experienced acute respiratory distress but it was of short duration. Two days later the symptoms returned. He caused himself to be strapped to a hinged platform, supported in such a manner that he could be inverted at an angle of 80° to the horizontal; his back was struck whilst in this position. The treatment caused a violent attack of choking but the coin remained in his air passages. When repeated on 27 April, this procedure dislodged the coin from his right bronchus and an unsuccessful attempt was made to retrieve it through a tracheostomy. The wound was kept open and, undaunted, he again submitted to treatment on 13 May, when the coin was successfully discharged through his mouth. He then made an uninterrupted recovery (Tidy, 1883).
>
> An unusual cause of choking, of which they saw two instances in close succession, is described by Smith and Fiddes (1955). Two men were fishing and suddenly one of them fell forwards into the water. His companion, who was arrested on a charge of murder, said that the man appeared to have died before entering the water; there had been no struggle. Examination of the body showed that "death was probably due mainly to inhibition" following the inhalation and impaction of a small fish in the air passages. It is a practice of some fishermen to use these as bait and to place them meantime in the mouth.

Choking due to disease may be the result of obstruction of the air passages by a bronchial growth. Such cases rarely come within medico-legal practice since the death results from a relatively slow illness, the cause of which has been definitely ascertained sometime beforehand. Occasionally, however, death may be sudden when due to erosion of a pulmonary artery by the growth, leading to severe haemoptysis and death by choking (P.M. 2023).

Pulmonary tuberculosis may terminate suddenly in like manner, although in these circumstances the presence of the disease has usually been recognised long before death. In some subjects, however, death may be sudden and wholly unexpected. A woman, aged 56, who was not receiving medical attention, collapsed and died in the street. Death was due to haemoptysis caused by pulmonary tuberculosis which was of moderate extent in both upper lobes (F.M. 3002). On another occasion a woman aged 66 was found dead at her home, where she lived alone. She had had an haemoptysis, due to rupture of a vessel in a chronic cavity, possibly an aneurysm, in the upper lobe of the left lung; there was no active disease, neither there nor elsewhere (F.M. 3023).

Rupture of an aortic aneurysm into the air passages may cause death by choking: erosion and rupture usually occur just above the bifurcation of the trachea.

Gauze packs inserted during an operation have been overlooked and caused fatal asphyxia (Fig. 156).

An abscess of the lung may empty rapidly and flood the air passages with pus and necrotic lung debris and thus choke the patient. A tuberculous gland may erode a bronchus and prolapse into its lumen to cause choking.

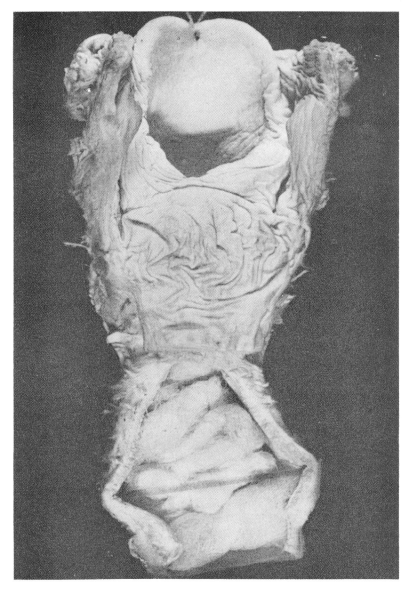

FIG. 156. Suffocation: impaction of gauze swab in the trachea.

Lesions of the larynx which can cause choking include oedema and tumours, in particular, papillomata. Oedema, sufficient to cause urgent obstruction, is most likely to result from the inhalation of steam or ingestion of irritant substances. The child who inhales steam from the spout of a kettle or the adult who drinks strong ammonia or corrosive fuming acids, are examples. Angio-neurotic oedema may develop with sufficient speed to cause fatal choking but this is a rare condition. Pharyngeal abscesses may cause sudden death by choking but they are likely to be recognised and treated before there is serious obstruction; it is important, of course, that proper steps are taken to ensure that the patient does not choke during surgical treatment of the condition.

Choking may terminate poliomyelitis or bulbar palsy, because disturbance of the swallowing mechanism in these patients permits accidental inhalation of food or secretion.

Injury leading indirectly to death from choking is illustrated by the death of a boy on the football field. During a game of rugby football, a boy aged 16 was tackled by an opponent and both fell to the ground. He remained in a crouching position and was obviously having difficulty in breathing; when he had been taken off the field, attempts to restore him by artificial respiration were unsuccessful. Examination of his body showed that some acid material, similar in appearance to that present in his stomach, had entered the air passages. Death was due to asphyxia. The interpretation was that the tackle, which was a perfectly proper one, had inadvertently caused him to regurgitate and inhale some of the gastric contents. Except for a minor graze on the left knee cap, the body bore no marks of injury (F.M. 734).

Choking by external causes is sometimes the result of impaction of a relatively large foreign body, a bolus of food or a denture, in the oesophagus. Compression of the trachea may then be severe.

Tolerance of Foreign Bodies in the Air Passages

Although the inhalation of a foreign body usually causes choking and, unless it is promptly removed, the victim may die, the circumstances of choking would be incompletely represented without comment on the remarkable tolerance which can be seen after the inhalation of a foreign body. Acute respiratory distress is immediate but, once this has passed, the victim may experience little subsequent discomfort. It may be that, weeks later, he develops a lung abscess or has other symptoms which lead to the discovery of the foreign body, but only after an appreciable latent interval. The records show that portions of chicken bones, pins, safety-pins and even partial dentures may lie within the air passages for relatively long periods without creating serious trouble. Jowett (1936) described an epileptic male, aged 34, who recovered after inhaling part of a bone paper-knife, which measured $24 \times 44 \times 3$ mm, and which he had retained for several days. He was unaware of having inhaled it; presumably it was between his teeth when he had had a fit. Another epileptic inhaled a partial upper denture, $1\frac{1}{4}$ in. in diameter, and it lodged in her larynx for 22 months (Lennox Brown, 1891). When Sir Morrell Mackenzie discussed this case he mentioned an amusing instance of supposed inhalation of a denture. The lady had been examined by several surgeons, who had felt it quite distinctly with their instruments; physicians, with their stethoscopes, had heard it move. After enduring 11 weeks of misery, the patient was at once cured when her maid found the missing denture hidden in a drawer.

An outstanding example of the long tolerance of foreign bodies is given by Ravenel (1891); this patient had retained a pin in his air passages for no less than 38 years. Its presence came to light when it was dislodged during a violent fit of coughing. Two inflamed, circumscribed areas, at opposite points on the posterior end of each ventricle were seen and, presumably, the pin had for long been impacted across the larynx.

A number of other cases are recorded, notably in the *Journal of Laryngology*.

Suicidal Choking

Suicide by choking, no doubt in view of its unpleasant nature, is rare. The victims are likely to be mental patients or, possibly, prisoners denied other more acceptable means of committing suicide. The case reported by Handyside in 1842 remains an outstanding example; it came to light in a dissecting room in Edinburgh. The subject was a woman, aged 29, who had been found dead in her room in the gaol and was thought to have died of apoplexy. Her body was handed to the anatomist and, a month later, when about to dissect the neck structures, Handyside found a foreign body fixed in the throat. It was a tightly rolled piece of blanket, of conical shape, fastened by a pin; it measured $3^{1}/_{2}$ in. in length and was $1^{5}/_{8} \times {}^{3}/_{4}$ in. at its base; a plaster cast of it was made and is still on view in the museum of the Department of Forensic Medicine in Edinburgh University. The lower end of this foreign body lay between the arytenoid cartilages; the pin had lacerated the throat to the left of the uvula (Handyside, 1842, also Littlejohn, 1925). Wagner (1834, cited Handyside) described a similar case; a prisoner had forced part of a woollen shawl into his mouth. A third case, also recalled by Handyside, was one of suicide by forcing a handkerchief into the throat.

A middle-aged inmate of a mental hospital, who suffered from delusions and was violently excited, was placed in a padded room. He was apparently asleep when observed at 9.0 p.m. Twenty minutes later when seen again, he had thrown off his bed clothing and was dead of asphyxia. He had torn a flannel blanket into strips and had forced three of them into his mouth and throat. A piece of flannel, 1 ft long and 1 in. broad, was removed from his mouth. Two similar strips were beyond, packed firmly into the throat (Renton, 1908).

A woman, aged 75, committed suicide by forcing a rolled handkerchief, followed by a wad of tissue paper, into her throat so as to block the air way. She had used some force since her tonsils were bruised. Prior to this she had attempted suicide, without success, by tying a scarf and lisle stockings round her neck (they were fastened with an incomplete half-knot). Since the mark of the ligature rose to an inverted V at the nape of her neck it was probable that, in her determination to commit suicide, she had followed self-strangulation by attempted hanging from the knob of her wardrobe. There was no other person involved (F.M. 12,921 A).

Homicidal Choking

Choking is a mode of infanticide but is an uncommon or rare mode of murder. Its accomplishment demands either appreciable physical disparity or that the victim is disabled by disease, drink or drugs.

Although the verdict was "not proven", the circumstances of the death of Jane Stewart, described by Littlejohn (1855–6), were strongly suggestive of murder, in part by choking. It may be that the confusion in the house at the time precluded a clear issue for a jury. When Littlejohn went to investigate this sudden death, all the adults in the house were drunk and he had to find the body himself; it lay in a coffin in a small bedroom. The victim was a woman of from 60 to 70 years of age. Her face was pale and composed, but slightly swollen. Palpation elicited the presence of surgical emphysema over the front of the body and in the arms and thighs. A hard, resisting mass was felt at the back of the throat. This was at first thought to be a piece of bone but it proved to be the cork of a quart wine bottle, impacted in the larynx, with the sealed end of the cork uppermost. Several ribs, on each side, were broken and the ends had punctured the pleura. There was also a laceration of the scalp. It appeared that she was drunk at the time of her death. A witness alleged that the accused had told the victim "I have broken your ribs on one side, turn round on the other side and I'll give you the same". The sealed end of the cork being uppermost did not confirm the suggestion that its impaction in the throat occurred when she had extracted the cork from a bottle with her teeth. Presumably her mouth had been open and someone had forced the cork down her throat; it was so far down as to be unlikely to have been pushed there by the victim.

On another occasion the victim was a boy who was choked by the stopper of a lemonade bottle. It was suggested that he had been opening the bottle with his teeth and the stopper had been forced into his throat by accident. This, however, was negatived by the fact that the base of the stopper was uppermost. It could not thus have been blown into his throat.

Choking due to regurgitation of food may occur during rape or violent sexual intercourse. A man was convicted of murder in 1899 when he had used brutal violence during rape. The cause of death was choking due to vomiting of a large meal (Taylor, 8th ed., cited in *R.* v. *Donald*, 1934, at page 194). It has occurred also in buggery (F.M. 3987A).

Choking, due to an accident, may sometimes occur in circumstances which suggest murder by other means. A married couple retired to bed when under the influence of drink. The man was able to get on to the bed and fell asleep. When he awoke he was horrified to find his wife lying dead on the floor with her face in a pool of blood. Investigation showed that the blood had come from her nose; it had drained directly below the face and none was found elsewhere. She had some recent bruises on her arms but no other injuries. A piece of onion had obstructed her air passages. Sir Sydney Smith (1948) interpreted the circumstances as those of accidental choking. It seemed that, having got on to the bed, the man had unsuccessfully endeavoured to help his obese and equally fuddled wife to join him. These attempts caused the bruising of her arms. Eventually she had fallen face down on the floor and this, possibly with congestion resulting from asphyxia, explained the bleeding from her nose.

Choking as a Cause of Vagal Inhibition (Sudden cardiac arrest)

Although choking usually causes death by mechanical asphyxia, there are undoubted occasions when the immediate result of choking is vagal inhibition and sudden death. The absence of overt signs on these occasions makes the diagnosis one of great difficulty, especially when the victim is an infant and the quantity of foreign material in the air passages is small. The fact that a terminal regurgitation of gastric contents, wholly unrelated as a cause of death, can also occur, adds appreciably to the difficulty. The determination of the cause of death may have to be a matter of exclusion of all other possible factors or a frank admission that the cause remains unexplained. There are occasions when vagal inhibition due to choking seems a proper interpretation of the circumstances.

A woman, aged 88, was lying in a hospital ward undergoing treatment for a fracture of the neck of her left femur. There was nothing in her condition to indicate impending death; she was in fact enjoying her lunch. Without warning she suddenly went pale, collapsed and died almost immediately. There were no asphyxial symptoms prior to her collapse. The post-mortem examination demonstrated a quantity of vegetable material, part of the lunch, obstructing the air passages downwards from the larynx to the intrapulmonary bronchi of both lungs. Similar material was present in the oesophagus and stomach. There were no signs of asphyxia and none of disease of a kind to cause sudden death. It was believed she had died of vagal inhibition due to the sudden entry of food into her air passage (P.M. 5182). This case resembles that of Perrin (1881), cited Dixon Mann (1908).

A female inmate of a mental hospital died of vagal inhibition when a bolus of bread $1^1/_4$ in diameter became impacted in her larynx; some of the bread had reached her secondary bronchi. Closed chest massage was responsible for fractures of ribs on each side of the chest (F.M. 11,500 B).

A woman, aged 22, a spastic patient, also died of vagal inhibition when she inhaled semisolid milky fluid; some of it had reached the smaller bronchi. There were no signs of asphyxia (F. M. 13,220).

A girl aged 3 years died of vagal inhibition following the inhalation of vomit. The circumstances were distinctly suspicious but they were consistent with neglect due to ignorance and no criminal charge was made. The case is discussed elsewhere as an example of the need for caution when making allegations of cruelty (F.M. 11,121A; see p. 542).

Syncope in such circumstances may be delayed. The first signs of trouble may be those of mechanical obstruction and syncope occurs later following re-impaction of the foreign material. This was illustrated by Sharman (1937). A mental patient, aged 37, while eating her breakfast, suddenly left the table and went to the lavatory. The nurse, who followed her, saw her cough and attempt to vomit, which yielded only a little saliva. The patient then walked about 30 yards, saying she wanted some air. A probang was passed, and the patient, apparently relieved, was able to return to the ward. She was laid on a bed and, shortly afterwards, she collapsed and died from syncope. The whole episode lasted about $^1/_2$ hour; there had been two separate attacks of choking, the second being due to re-impaction of a large bolus of food, which was later found impacted in the oesophagus, causing tracheal obstruction.

A man aged 78 choked and died because half a sheep's kidney, part of a mixed grill he was enjoying, became impacted and blocked the entrance to his larynx. Death was due to vagal inhibition (F.M. 3841).

A child aged 2 snatched a piece of tea-cake and thrust it into her mouth; she was a greedy child. She was seen to stumble and fall. When picked up she was dead. Her pharynx was obstructed by a mass of food; signs of asphyxia were absent. In these circumstances the death appears to have been due to vagal inhibition (F.M. 3862).

The diagnosis is simplified when there is a relatively massive obstruction. There are other occasions when the foreign body is small, yet the cause of death would seem to be cardiac inhibition. This is clearer when the foreign body is other than food. Spilsbury (1934) described the sudden death from syncope of an infant, who had inhaled a tiny feather from the eiderdown on its cot. The feather lay on vocal cords. The matter was discussed, with special reference to drowning, by Eric Gardner (1942). Sudden death may occur when regurgitation of food floods the post-nasal space or when only minute particles come into contact with the vocal cords; "unless it is realised how tiny inhaled foreign body may be, the cause of death may easily be overlooked". He suggested that these victims had an exaggerated protective reflex.

Operative procedures on the larynx, especially when the anaesthesia is light, may provoke vagal inhibition and cause sudden death.

Choking as a Cause of Fatal Laryngeal Spasm

Another variation in the mode of death by choking is asphyxia due to laryngeal spasm. The cause is the entry of foreign material which, on these occasions, need not be large in size or amount; its irritant nature may be of much greater importance. This is likely if acid gastric juice, alone, suddenly enters the air passages. A man aged 20 was found dead outside his home; he was deeply cyanosed and had died from asphyxia. Some acid fluid, resembling the gastric contents, was present in the air passages, but they were not occluded by it; the cause of the asphyxia was considered to be laryngeal spasm, following the sudden entry of regurgitated acid fluid. He had returned home under the influence of drink and had vomited (Gardner, 1942).

Traumatic or Crush Asphyxia

The clinical picture of this form of asphyxia, first adequately described by Perthes (1900), is now well recognised. It is characterised by the deep red or purple discoloration of the skin of the head, neck and upper chest. On most occasions it is the result of an accident in which the body of the victim is subjected to direct compression by a heavy weight against a resisting surface.

Traumatic asphyxia is uncommon. It has occurred once in about 6000 patients or even less often, e.g. once in 18,500. Our experience has been relatively extensive, since we have seen five examples in a consecutive series of about 8500 autopsies and I had opportunity to see one non-fatal case, at the General Infirmary at Leeds in 1958 (Professor Pyrah's patient).

The degree of force required to produce traumatic asphyxia and the manner of its application is such that a fatality can only occur by accident. There is no record of suicide, homicide or even infanticide by traumatic asphyxia.

The Circumstances of Traumatic Asphyxia

The usual circumstances are those of an accident, which leads to gross compression of the chest, if not the whole of the body, by a powerful force. The first known victims, observed by Ollivier in 1834, had been crushed by mob violence. It is an accident likely to occur when panic results from an outbreak of fire in a theatre, or whenever large crowds gather in an enclosed place, e.g. a football ground. The worst example in modern times occurred during the Second World War when, in 1943, the air raid siren sounded and people sought refuge in an underground railway station. As they descended the stairs someone at the front slipped on the stairs and fell. In a matter of seconds a mass of people were heaped together. Forward progress became impossible and the incoming flow continued. In consequence, 173 persons died of traumatic asphyxia (Simpson, 1943). Another serious accident of this kind occurred at a football ground. One section was already full. Unfortunately someone unlocked the gate to this section and there was an immediate inrush of people. Very soon the crush barriers gave way and overfilling of the area led to several deaths from traumatic asphyxia.

Another of these disasters occurred in January 1971 after a football match at Ibrox Park, Glasgow. A crowd of 80,000 had watched the game and, just after its close there was a rush to the exits. A barrier collapsed. Someone stumbled and fell and soon there was a mound of casualties. Sixty-six persons were killed and several hundreds were injured. The report in the *Sunday Times* of 3 January 1971 cited the disaster in Lima in 1964. A disallowed goal at the football match started a stampede in which 350 people lost their lives.

In 1896 the mad struggle for food at public feasts during the coronation fêtes in Moscow led to 1500 deaths. Panic in a theatre in Sunderland in 1883 led to the death, from traumatic asphyxia, of 202 children attending a matinee performance. Someone raised the alarm of "fire"; when the children rushed to escape, they found the doors closed (Aitchison Robertson, 1916).

It is also a risk whenever tunnelling is done by unskilled persons who fail to construct proper support for the roof and walls. Small boys may tunnel into sandhills. On 27 July 1953 a boy lost his life at St. Annes-on-Sea when the tunnel he had made collapsed; a few days later, on 11 August, another boy was trapped in a tunnel he had made near the pier. Fortunately he was promptly rescued by his aunt. Although unconscious when extricated, he recovered after receiving artificial respiration. In the example reported below, a man lost his life when an inadequately supported shaft, driven into a slag heap, collapsed (F.M. 250). Falls of stone or earth in coal mines are illustrated by another of the examples below (F.M. 2447). It is also a risk in the demolition of buildings or the digging of deep trenches.

On other occasions the victim is pinned to the ground by some heavy weight, as by a motor vehicle or other machinery. Keith Simpson (1960) has drawn attention to the importance of recognising traumatic asphyxia in the victims of road accidents, since it indicates pinning by the vehicle. In other cases the victim has been pinned by a cow-catcher, steam shovel or an hydraulic lift. It occurred when a man was crushed by the tail section of a jet aircraft, beneath which he had been at work (Fred and Chandler, 1960). In yet other cases the victim has been crushed between the buffers of railway waggons or, as in the non-fatal case below, between tubs in a coal mine. Another victim lost his life when pinned to the ground in a coal mine by a moving coal conveyor belt [F.M. 703 (see below)].

In all of the foregoing circumstances the bodies of the victims had been subjected to severe, direct compression against a resisting surface. When known, or estimated, the degree of force responsible has been of the order of not less than 1400 lb and up to 7 tons; in one case it was estimated to have been equal to a pressure of $18^1/_2$ lb/in^2.

Rarely, traumatic asphyxia is the result of indirect compression in circumstances where the body is subjected to force in such a manner that his thighs and knees are driven against his chest, the so-called "jack-knife" position. An example (F.M. 4744) is described below; this victim was crushed by sheets of metal.

A unique case of traumatic asphyxia was the result of an attempt to reduce an umbilical hernia in an infant aged 17 hours by the exertion of great pressure on the liver (Kredel, 1970 cited Heuer, 1923).

A mild variant of traumatic asphyxia, in which there is no lasting discoloration of the skin, can occur when the abdominal and thoracic muscles are violently contracted at a time when the glottis is closed, e.g. during bouts of severe coughing or of vomiting or, perhaps, during an epileptic fit.

External Appearances

The outstanding feature of these bodies is an intense cyanosis, of deep purple or purple-red colour, of the upper parts. It involves the head and neck and upper chest, down to a level of about the third rib. Below this the skin is pale or, at most, only mildly cyanosed. The appearances are sufficiently remarkable to permit their recognition at an appreciable distance, without any knowledge of the circumstances. It can be, as in the case of Fred and

Chandler (1960), that, initially, the skin is bright red, changing within seconds to blue.

The cyanosis is general in the exposed parts, but there may be a pale band at the level of the collar or neck-band of the shirt, or around the head, if a hat was worn at the time of the accident. Clothing will also yield an irregular pale pattern which corresponds with the folds or creases in the garments; pale impressions may be made by buttons or braces. These areas of pallor are another characteristic feature of traumatic asphyxia.

If a woollen cardigan or pullover be worn, compression of the body may reproduce its pattern in the skin. A zig-zag pattern in red, due to local bleeding, on the otherwise pale skin of the lower chest, corresponded with the pattern of the inner surface of the garment (F.M. 703; 17a, b, p. 99).

In addition to these changes there are also well-developed signs of a slow asphyxia. Haemorrhages into the eyelids and beneath the conjunctivae are considerable; there is also oedema of the conjunctivae. The abnormal purple-red colour of the skin may persist for several days. It has been ascribed, by biopsy, to vaso-dilatation, without bleeding into the tissues, e.g. by Beach and Cobb (1904) and Winslow (1905), but haemorrhage into the tissues around the vessels has been reported by Bolt (1908) and Heuer (1923). In our specimens, haemorrhages were general in the corium and this is the the only satisfactory explanation of the persisting colour change in these cases.

Compression may be sufficient to fracture the ribs; in one of my cases (F.M. 703) ribs 1 to 9 on the right and 1 to 10 on the left were fractured at their convexities and several of them had also been torn away at their costo-chondral junctions; there were no other fractures. In other cases the thoracic cage remained intact. Fractures of the pelvis, spine and limb bones have also occurred, but fracture of the skull is distinctly uncommon. Intracranial haemorrhage is also uncommon for, on most occasions, the brain shows only congestion.

Symptoms. As might be expected, the patient experiences the sensation of tremendous pressure on his body. Fred and Chandler's patient then lost his vision. He felt as if his eyes were going to pop out and his head would blow up. He had a clonic seizure a minute after his rescue; he also had urinary and faecal incontinence.

Prognosis and treatment. Not a little depends, obviously, on the time during which the victim is exposed to compression. Fred and Chandler (1960) found that if the victim was alive when released and survived the accident by over an hour, recovery then occurred in 90 per cent of the cases. Thus, in a series of 143 cases, twenty-seven of the victims were dead or died within a short time of their admission to hospital. Of the 116 who survived over an hour, 104 recovered. Delayed death may be due to associated injuries or infection.

There is no specific treatment. Appropriate treatment of any injuries and "supportive" treatment will be given.

Case Reports

1. *Traumatic asphyxia due to collapse of a tunnel in a slag heap.* At a time when good coal was scarce as well as costly, it was the practice of some employees of a firm near to a slag heap, a tip for mine refuse, to forage for coal during their lunch break. They had driven a crude shaft into the heap and it was lit by candles. The heap rose to 40 ft. above the ground and they had burrowed into it at ground level for a distance of about 20 yd. No props had been used to support the tunnel. They were unaware of the risk and it had not been pointed out to them. On 26 February 1948 the deceased, aged 28, and his brother were at work in the tunnel when there was a shout "Get clear". The deceased, who was at the "coal face", was buried by about 4 tons of fine powdery slag

and his brother, who was nearer to the entrance, was buried to his waist. He was saved, but his brother died before the rescuers could extricate him. This practice had existed for some time; they had been digging in the heap during the previous winter. It was not part of their work to do this and they went there at their own risk; it was realised they ought not to have done this. But "it was really good coal which we got from the slag heap; it is better than what we bought".

The appearances of the body were characteristic of traumatic asphyxia. A pale band, about 3 cm broad, at the front of the neck coincided with the position of his collar and tie and other well-marked pale areas were beneath folds in his clothing and braces. Bleeding had occurred beneath the conjunctivae in the form of petechiae and in larger, triangular areas. Fine grit was abundant on the skin and in the conjunctival sacs. Petechial haemorrhages were plentiful, $^1/_2$ to 3 mm in diameter, in the deeper layers of the scalp and along the upper border of each temporal muscle. The skull was intact. The brain was congested, but there were no haemorrhages in it or within the skull. All structures between the trachea and the base of the tongue, i.e. larynx, thyroid gland, pharynx, tonsils and base of the tongue were engorged and of purple colour. Small haemorrhages were present in the mucosa of the larynx, especially at the base of the epiglottis. There were subcapsular haemorrhages over the lower two-thirds of each lobe of the thyroid gland. The larynx was intact. Scanty petechial haemorrhages were present beneath the visceral pleura in the interlobar sulci, and on the diaphragmatic surface of the lungs. More petechiae were present beneath the visceral pericardium. There was a deep and extensive wound of the right thigh, associated with a fracture of the femur, but the appearances were those of a post-mortem injury sustained during extrication of the body. The chest cage was intact. He had been a healthy man. Microscopical examination of the skin showed that the vessels were engorged and scattered haemorrhages of relatively small size were present in the corium (F.M. 250).

2. *Traumatic asphyxia due to a roof fall in a clay mine*. The deceased, aged 42, was a haulage corporal, engaged in the maintenance of the road in a clay mine when, on 4 February 1952, he was killed by a fall of the roof. He was found lying in one of the tubs with a rock on top of his body; the stone had to be split before it could be lifted to release him. He was then dead. Precisely what happened was not elicited. It appeared that the tub in which he lay was derailed and a girder supporting the roof had been dislodged so as to lie against the tub. The road was obstructed by a fall of the roof. At this point the tunnel was 5 ft 6 in. high and about 5 ft wide. The train was one of about twenty tubs, mechanically driven from the surface. In all probability his tub had been derailed, which caused it to strike the support and by dislodging it, it caused the fall. Something had derailed the tub immediately alongside the girder, but when the track was examined nothing abnormal was found; no repair was required. It could have been that something fell off a tub so as to cause the derailment, but there had been only one big fall, i.e. that which followed the derailment. Vibration in the tunnel sometimes caused small bits to fall. The stone which trapped the deceased measured 4 × 4 ft and was up to 1 ft thick; it was estimated to weigh "a good ton".

The appearances of the body were characteristic of traumatic asphyxia. The deep purple of the skin was interrupted by pale areas, e.g. in the region of the collar and shoulder straps of his garments. The larynx was intact, but innumerable petechiae were present in its congested mucosa. Although the muscles of the left side of his chest were severely bruised between the 2nd to 8th ribs, the chest cage was intact. Visceral petechiae were negligible; one only was observed, beneath the pleura at the back of the lower lobe of the right lung. Bleeding had occurred into the base of the tongue and each tonsillar region. Petechial haemorrhages were plentiful in the deeper layers of the scalp. The skull was intact. The brain was congested, but there was no intracranial haemorrhage. He had been a healthy man. Microscopical examination of the skin showed extensive haemorrhage into the corium (F.M. 2447).

3. *Traumatic asphyxia due to crushing by a coal conveyor belt in a mine*. The deceased was a Hindu, aged 20, who was operating the conveyor belt in a pit. The belt stopped working and when another miner went to see what had happened he found the deceased pinned by the belt to the floor of the pit and wedged against the dust plough; he lay on his right side, pinned from his shoulder to his waist. His head, although clear of the belt, was fast by the nape against a pit prop; his miner's helmet was in position and his lamp was still lit. It can only be surmised what had happened. It was his job to clean a part of the machinery at intervals and to do this he would have had to walk a distance of about 10 ft to reach it. He could have done this without crossing the belt, but it appeared he had taken a "short cut" and gone under the belt. The clearance, at best, was only about 17 in., but, at the point where his body lay, the pit bottom sloped upwards so that the clearance was there reduced to a few inches. I found it difficult to accept that it was safe to go under the belt, which travelled at 160 ft a minute, even where it was at 17 in. above the pit bottom. It was no part of his duties to crawl under the belt and he had been warned not to do so unless the belt was at rest. To do so while it was in motion entailed serious risk of being caught and crushed. A witness said, "You have to have all your wits about you to go under the belt which is travelling". It was necessary to cut the belt before he could be released; he was under it at least 15 minutes.

Despite his natural dark brown colour, it was apparent that a deep purple tint was superimposed in the skin of the face, but it was less evident in the neck and upper chest. Gross engorgement with haemorrhage was seen in the conjunctivae. The skin of the trunk was unusual in that it was covered with parallel lines of bleeding arranged vertically in a zig-zag course; these appeared as small bars of up to 5 mm long and 1 mm broad, spaced at intervals of 3 mm. It was evidently a pattern and my first impression was that it was an imprint of the weave of the conveyor belt. Inspection of the belt disproved this. He had worn a woollen fisherman's jumper and my mortuary technician, Mr. Ratcliffe, himself an accomplished knitter, identified the pattern as that of the inside of the garment. On this occasion the chest cage was severely damaged; ribs 1 to 9 on the right and 1 to 10 on the left side were broken near the spine; ribs 2 to 5 on each side were broken also at their convexities and had been disarticulated from the sternum. Bleeding into the deeper layers of the scalp was general, as was bleeding into each temporal muscle. The skull was intact, but scanty subarachnoid haemorrhages were present in relation to the occipital lobes. The fractured ribs had perforated the visceral pleura of both lungs and there was a bilateral pneumothorax. There was no engorgement of the neck structures and the larynx was intact. The liver was ruptured; a ragged tear, 10 cm. long, through the substance of the liver, separated the right and left lobes. The restricted distribution of the skin discolouration might be accounted for by death from coincident grave injuries before the complete external picture had developed (F.M. 703).

4. *Traumatic asphyxia due to crushing by steel plates; the victim was held in the "jack-knife" posture.* The deceased, aged 47, was engaged in moving some large sheets of steel which were propped against a wall. The sheets were about 8 to 10 ft long. 6 ft wide and up to $^1/_4$ in. thick. Five of these sheets had been stacked in a new position when the whole batch collapsed. One man was knocked clear, a second was partly trapped and the deceased was completely beneath the sheets. When they were cleared he was in the jack-knife position and this had kept the sheets sufficiently clear of the ground to protect his workmate from a similar fate; the latter, however, sustained a fractured femur and dislocation of the hip.

The post-mortem appearances were characteristic of traumatic asphyxia and the details are therefore omitted. The left femur and ribs 4 to 6 on the left side were fractured and there was a traumatic hernia of the diaphragm with prolapse of the stomach into the left pleural sac. The skull was intact and the only change in the brain was congestion. Microscopical examination demonstrated haemorrhages in the corium and subcutaneous tissues (F.M. 4744).

5. *Traumatic asphyxia; pinned inside a motor vehicle.* The deceased, a man aged 47, was driving a mechanical shovel. It was raised at the time and it came into contact with a low bridge. The impact forced the heavy metal counterpoise downwards so as to crush the cabin in which he was seated.

The signs of traumatic asphyxia were negligible. The 7th and 8th ribs were broken at their convexities. The skull was intact and the brain appeared healthy. The case is of interest in that it demonstrates the point made by Simpson (1960) that in some of these "pinning" cases the demonstration of traumatic asphyxia is not easy and close scrutiny is required. In the present case, the fact that death was due to pinning was established by an examination of the damaged vehicle and the evidence of those who extricated him from the crushed cabin. He was a healthy man.

It took about 3 hours to extricate his body. Death was not instantaneous; on the contrary he survived for several minutes. He was pinned laterally and thus unable to breathe, but there was no gross obstruction to his circulation and thus none of the characteristic purple discolouration (F.M. 7692A).

6. *Traumatic asphyxia due to being trapped between coal tubs and a wall. Non-fatal case.* The patient, a man aged 40, was involved in an accident on 5 November 1958 at the pit where he worked. He was trapped between two coal tubs and a wall at the pit head, for a period of about 20 minutes; the tubs were each estimated to weigh $2^1/_2$ tons. He was admitted to the local hospital, but, because he developed anuria, he was transferred to Professor Pyrah's department at the Leeds General Infirmary on 12 November.

I had an opportunity to see him on 14 November, when he still had the external appearances of traumatic asphyxia (Plate 9). The skin of his head, neck and upper chest almost to nipple level was still distinctly purple-red and there were haemorrhages beneath the conjunctivae. White streaking of the skin, reproducing the pattern of folds in his clothing at the time of the accident, was also apparent. He was then quite rational and his general condition was apparently satisfactory. Unfortunately, a few days later it deteriorated and his blood urea content began to rise. By 21 November the purple colour of his skin began to fade and he had improved. He was passing adequate amounts of urine, but the blood urea was still above normal. Unfortunately, the further history of the patient is not available, but it appears he made a complete recovery (See also p. 468).

Overlying

Overlying usually occurs when a parent or other person shares a bed with an infant. During sleep the older person rolls on to or otherwise crushes the infant and asphyxiates it. At one time this was by no means an infrequent cause of infant mortality, but now that the danger is more widely recognised, the incidence has been greatly reduced. The provision of a separate bed, even if it be in a drawer or box, for a small infant, is imperative. Poverty and, more especially, overcrowding continue to operate as potential causes. It may be that the housing shortage, which had been acute at that time, was responsible in part for a rise to 517 deaths in 1947; there was, however, a fall to 374 in 1948, notwithstanding that overcrowding was much the same. The risk is illustrated by one of my cases, in which a mother had shared her bed with three of her children. She had the baby beside her and, during the night her son, aged 18 months, who slept at the foot of the bed had crept up to the top and overlaid the baby.

It is a criminal offence, under the Children and Young Persons Act, 1933, if a person aged 16 years or over, when drunk, shares his bed with a child under the age of 3 years, and that child dies of suffocation other than the result of natural disease or the inhalation of a foreign body. The offence then committed is neglect of the child in a manner likely to cause injury to its health. Proof is required of suffocation or asphyxia, but the medical examiner is not required to prove that the child was overlaid. This must come from collateral evidence. The usual age incidence of overlying in the Leeds series, confirming the findings of Templeman (1892), is between 2 weeks and about 4 months. When an older infant is found dead in these circumstances, care is required before concluding that death was by overlying. In the Leeds series, however, there have been two instances of overlying of infants aged 7 months; there were five aged 7 months and four aged 8 months in that of Templeman. On another occasion, where it was impossible to determine whether the infant had been overlaid or smothered by deliberate compression against his father's chest, the infant was aged 11 months. This age is well outside the likely range unless, as in that case, there are changes, e.g. excess of lymphoid tissue, which may indicate undue susceptibility to stress. The father received the benefit of the doubt and was acquitted of murder (F.M. 1153).

Post-mortem Appearances

The usual findings are limited to those of asphyxia, notably the presence of petechial haemorrhages beneath the conjunctivae, the epicardium and pleurae. There may, or may not, be evidence of flattening of the nose and face. Contact flattening may indicate only that the infant was laid on its face at the time of or after death. Sometimes this may have a distinctive pattern, when, for example, the face has been pressed against a baby's dummy. On one occasion there was a circular band of pallor of the precise shape of a ring on the dummy on the infant's cheek (F.M. 110). There may be a little froth, sometimes bloodstained, at the nostrils and in the lower air passages; there may be staining of the pillow or bedding or garment. These findings, however, are not peculiar to overlying. Marks of violence, notably abrasions and bruises, are absent in overlying; if these are present, other possibilities must be at once in mind.

It is impossible to exclude, by medical examination alone, smothering of an infant by a soft agent, for example by a pillow or against the chest of an adult.

The physique of the child, as well as its age, is material. Obviously, the frail or ill child is the more liable to succumb. Moreover, such infants require little to precipitate their deaths and, in consequence, even asphyxial changes may be slight.

Death by Crucifixion

This form of punishment was introduced to the Romans by the Phoenicians and developed by the Romans into an exact science. It was an extreme form of bloodless torture. The upright of the cross was fitted with a support for the feet and one for the buttocks or perineum. In order to breathe the victim had to raise his body and throw the weight on his feet. When this became painful, he slumped to ease the foot pain. He then had to raise his body in order to breathe. When slumped his intercostal muscles were stretched and the chest cage was fixed. The alternation of rising and sitting eventually led to exhaustion, unconsciousness and death from asphyxia (De Pasquale and Burch, 1963).

Burking

This form of asphyxia is a result of a procedure used, and apparently invented, by the murderers Burke and Hare during the 1820s. A victim, preferably one without any family, was invited to their house and plied with drink. The murderer then knelt or sat on the chest and closed the nose and mouth with his hands. According to Hare, who turned King's evidence, Burke "got stridelegs on the top of the woman on the floor, and she cried out a little, and he kept in her breath. . . . He pressed down her head with his breast. . . . He put one hand under the nose and the other under her chin, under her mouth . . . " (Roughead, 1948). External injury was absent and, but for Hare, the precise mechanism of this asphyxia might not have been discovered. Burke later confessed to no less than sixteen of these murders, which were committed for gain. The bodies were sold to a school of anatomy for dissection. Christison (1829) said of one victim "The body presented the signs of death by asphyxia—vague enough in general and in this instance particularly so, because the method of the murderers left no external local marks . . . and there were no external marks about the neck or face to indicate how respiration had been obstructed." There was some bleeding into the tissues about the cervical spine but it was concluded that this injury occurred shortly after death.

Suffocation due to Subcutaneous Rupture of the Larynx and Trachea

Subcutaneous rupture of the larynx and trachea is normally associated with surgical emphysema and a number of cases have been recorded (Atlee, 1858; Bryce, 1956; Buch, 1937–8; Dalmark, 1945; Gardner, 1933; Heiberg, 1934–5; Lattemant *et al.*, 1950; Leicher, 1954; Quirico, 1950; Rieman and Goldsmith, 1937; Story, 1897; Veng-Christensen, 1958; Zeuch, 1922; and Zwergius, 1955). Complication by pneumothorax, on the other hand, is distinctly uncommon. By coincidence two cases occurred within about a fortnight, one in Denmark and the other in England. Both of the victims were boys who rapidly developed surgical emphysema and bilateral pneumothorax following a blow to the neck, without sustaining any gross external injury. The rarity of these cases prompted a report and comment on the probable mechanism of the production of the rupture of the air passages and the subsequent pneumothorax (Polson and Hornback, 1960).

Case 1. Department of Forensic Medicine, University of Leeds, F.M. 6427A.

During the afternoon of 15 March 1959, a party of boys were playing rounders, using a short wooden stump as the striker. The batsman threw down the stump and the deceased boy dived to catch it; the stump struck the front of his neck. He may have trodden on one end of it, thereby bringing the other into violent contact with his neck. Although no external sign of injury was noticed, the boy's breathing was obviously affected and a doctor was at once summoned.

The boy was sent to hospital and on arrival at 7 p.m. he had difficulty in breathing and was cyanosed; he also had surgical emphysema of the neck and front of his chest. It was decided to perform a tracheotomy forthwith. As soon as an incision had been made across the front of his neck it was apparent that there was a vertical tear in the trachea. A tracheotomy tube was inserted into the opening. Half a minute later the boy's cyanosis and respiratory distress increased and his heart stopped. At 7.30 p.m. adrenaline was injected into the heart and the left chest was opened to permit cardiac massage. Spontaneous action of the heart was restored at 7.40 p.m. and by 7.45 p.m. the pulse was good and the child's colour was again normal. During this interval a right pneumothorax was recognized and pressure in the right chest was relieved by inserting a needle of relatively wide bore. Air in the left chest following the operation was liberated by an under-water drain, passed through the surgical wound in the chest.

The boy remained unconscious until his death at 2.30 a.m. on 17 March, i.e. at about 35 hours after the accident. At 6 a.m. on 16 March there was pyrexia, 102.3°F, but surgical emphysema was less severe. At 10 a.m. he had severe convulsions. Shortly before his death his temperature rose to 107°F, pulse rate 105, and respiration rate 48, but there was a rapid fall in temperature immediately before his death.

Radiological examination in the operating theatre on 15 March confirmed the presence of gross surgical emphysema of the neck, axillae and thorax but the film did not then demonstrate a pneumothorax; there was no mediastinal shift.

The post-mortem examination was made on 18 March at 36 hours after the death. The boy was of normal size and weight for his age, i.e. about 9 years. A recent surgical incision, 3 in. long, crossed the front of the neck

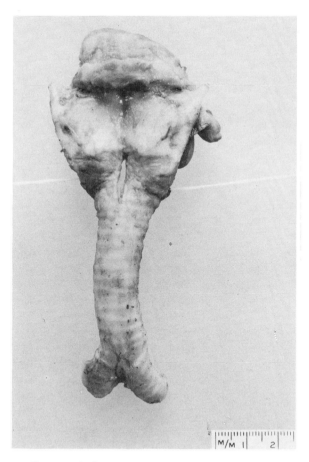

Fig. 157. Suffocation: subcutaneous rupture of the larynx and trachea (external aspect).

at the level of the lower border of the larynx. No abrasion or bruising of the skin was apparent in this area. Surgical emphysema was present; the upper part of the body, especially in the supraclavicular regions, was puffy and crepitant. A vertical fracture $^3/_4$ in. long, was present in the middle line at the front of the upper air passages (Fig. 157/158). It involved the cricoid cartilage and the upper three rings of the trachea. Internally, the fracture line was slightly irregular and oedematous in its upper part but, below, the breach was a clean break as if the tracheal rings had been cut with a knife. (No surgical wound had been made in order to insert the tracheotomy tube.) Slight bruising was present in the margins of the injured parts and there was slight bruising of the pharynx near the upper border of the larynx, where the tissues were a little oedematous. There was no bruising of the neck muscles nor of the parts in the carotid region. The trachea and bronchi contained viscid, red-green, slightly acid material (pH 6.0).

The mediastinal tissues were normal. No surgical emphysema or air blisters were seen. No tear was detected. Both lungs were collapsed and the right lung was contracted down so as to lie against the spine. The right pleural sac had been punctured to release air but it still contained air under pressure. The left pleural sac had been opened for cardiac massage.

The brain (1414 g) was somewhat bulky and slight flattening of the cerebral convolutions, but no pressure cone, was noted. Its substance was pale and oedematous. The other organs were all healthy. Death was due to respiratory and circulatory embarrassment by surgical emphysema and pneumothorax. A temporary arrest of circulation during the illness had caused cerebral anoxia. Microscopical examination of the brain by

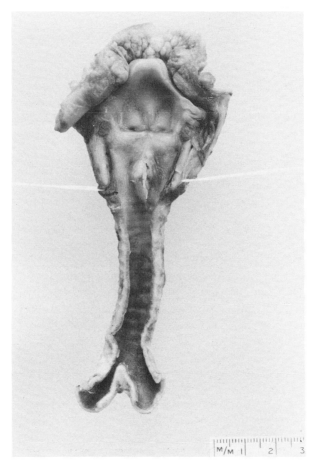

FIG. 158. Suffocation: subcutaneous rupture of the larynx
and trachea (internal aspect).

Dr. Harriman demonstrated ischaemic changes in the larger neurones of the cerebral cortex and in the Purkinje cells of the cerebellum.

Case 2. University Institute of Forensic Medicine, Copenhagen, No. F. 38/59.

On 3 April 1959, a boy aged 7 years collided with a motor cycle. The vehicle was being driven at about 6 miles per hour into a courtyard where the boy was playing marbles. He ran into the motor cycle and was struck on the neck by the handlebars. He fell but got up immediately and ran to his home nearby. On his arrival he had difficulty in breathing and was cyanosed. He was able to speak, and he complained of pains in the laryngeal region, moving his hand up to this region incessantly. A few minutes later his parents noticed that his face was swollen. They sent for an ambulance but before it arrived the boy was unconscious. When he reached the hospital, about 10 minutes after the accident, he was still unconscious. His breathing was stertorous and he was cyanosed. There was extensive subcutaneous emphysema of the face, the neck, the anterior thoracic and abdominal walls, and of the scrotum and arms. A laryngotracheal tube was introduced and oxygen was administered. This gave relief and his breathing was spontaneous and satisfactory. Subcutaneous emphysema, however, extended and his pulse became irregular and rapid. He died 8 hours after the accident and, because he did not regain consciousness, death was attributed to an intra-cranial lesion.

The post-mortem examination, at about 36 hours after death, showed the presence of a superficial abrasion 0.5 × 0.5 cm, at the front of the neck. Subcutaneous emphysema, as described, was widespread. Examination of the neck structures detected a rupture of the tissues between the thyroid and cricoid cartilages; the gap was about 1 cm broad. There was a recent bruise at the right-hand margin of the rupture. Bilateral pneumothorax was also present and both lungs were completely collapsed against the spine; there was now no visible emphysema of the mediastinal tissues. No lesion of the thoracic cage or thoracic organs was found. The skull and its contents were healthy.

Rupture of the trachea has occurred without any blow to the neck, e.g. in straining during labour, during a bout of coughing to dislodge a foreign body, or even by a sudden backward extension of the head.

This rupture may also be caused by a blow to the front of the neck and, as Zeuch (1922) has commented, the blow is often relatively trivial, as in the present two cases. This is only an apparent paradox. If, at the moment of impact, the trachea is filled with air and the glottis is closed, the tube is a relatively rigid one and, if it is suddenly compressed between the agent and the spine, the upper tracheal rings may readily rupture. Air then rapidly escapes into the subcutaneous tissues and, as is usual, in the absence of any breach of the skin, widespread subcutaneous emphysema can occur in a matter of minutes. Less often there may be a delay of several hours before this occurs. One patient described by Metson (1953) had tenderness and swelling at the front of her neck immediately after the blow but remained otherwise normal at school. It was not until the evening, 6 hours after the accident, that a bout of coughing was immediately followed by surgical emphysema.

Extension of emphysema to the mediastinum is less common but it can be of sufficient degree of itself to cause death by raising intrathoracic pressure (Jackson and Jackson, 1943). On the other hand, if treated appropriately in time, patients may recover, notwithstanding the occurrence of mediastinal emphysema (Metson, 1953, case 2).

Pneumothorax following tracheal rupture is not mentioned in any of the twenty-nine fatal cases in the series of fifty-three reports collected by Zeuch (1922). Reports have been published by Hume (1882), Goldstein (1949), two cases, and Baumann (1957). The mechanism of its production is at times, as in our two cases, obscure because, at the post-mortem examination, there may be no trace of mediastinal emphysema. The experiments of Goldberg, Mitchell and Angrist (1942) indicate the probable mechanism. Air was injected into the soft parts of the neck and was observed to reach the mediastinum, where blisters of air formed. As the injection proceeded a point was reached when no more air could be introduced unless the pressure was considerably raised. The pressure, when raised to 40 mm Hg, rapidly fell to zero and at that moment the mediastinal air blisters ruptured. More air could then be injected at a much lower pressure. Joannides and Tsoulus (1930) also produced mediastinal air blisters in dogs and noted that these were distributed principally around the roots of lungs. Emphysematous bullae were seen in the mediastinum by Goldstein (1949) but they were ruptured during the removal of the thoracic contents.

The absence of mediastinal emphysema, in the presence of bilateral pneumothorax, may be explained in some cases by rupture of the blisters during removal of the thoracic viscera. If the post-mortem has been made with care, however, these blisters will have been noted prior to removal of the viscera even if they are then burst. On other occasions failure to observe mediastinal emphysema may be due, as found by Macklin and Macklin (1944) and, as we believe, in our cases, to the escape or reabsorption of air during the period between death and post-mortem. In that event rupture of the mediastinal pleura may escape detection because the tear is small and no blister remains to mark its site. It is not beyond the bounds of possibility that the mediastinal pleura may rupture without the prior formation of an air blister. Such small tears, perhaps, could be demonstrated by the injection of fluid into the mediastinal tissues, in order to show the free communication with the pleura. It may be that the pleural sac is not the air-tight membrane it is assumed to be and that in fact there is a normal communication with the mediastinum, in the hilar regions.

(The foregoing by Polson and Hornback (1960), is reproduced by permission of the editor, Dr. Gavin Thurston, of the *Medico-Legal Journal*).

References

ATLEE, J. L., Jr (1858) *Amer. J. Med. Sci.*, **35**, 120.
BAUMANN, J. (1957) *Mémoires de l'Académie de Chir.*, **83**, 180.
BEACH, H. H. A. and COBB, F. (1904) *Ann. Surg.*, **39**, 481–94.
BOLT, R. A. (1908). *Cleveland med. J.* 7, 647.
BRYCE, D. P. (1956) *Canad. Med. Ass. J.*, **75**, 400.
BUCH, A. (1937–8) *Dansk Oto-layngologisk Selsk. Forh.*, p. 27.
BURKE and HARE (1828) *The Trial of Burke and Hare, Notable British Trials Series*, 3rd ed., 1948, W. Roughead. Edinburgh and London: Hodge.
CHRISTISON, R. (1829) *Edinb. Med. J.*, **31**, 236–50 (243).
DALMARK, G. (1945) *Nord. Med.*, **28**, 2226.
DE PASQUALE, N. P. and BURCH, G. E. (1963) *Amer. Heart J.*, **66**, 434.
DUMONT, G., PROTEAU, J., TABBARA, W. and DÉROBERT, L. (1962) Mort par asphyxie dans un sac en matière plastique au cours d'une masturbation: *Ann. Méd. lég. Criminol. Police Scient.*, **42**, 477.
FRED, H. L. and CHANDLER, F. W. (1960) *Amer. J. Med.*, **29**, 508–17.
GARDNER, E. (1942) *Med.-leg. Rev.*, **10**, 120–31.
GARDNER, H. O. (1933) *Arch. Otolaryng. (Chicago)*, **18**, 449.
GLAISTER, J. and RENTOUL, E. (1966) *Medical Jurisprudence and Toxicology*, 12th ed., Edinburgh: Livingstone.
GOLDBERG, J. D., MITCHELL, N. and ANGRIST, A. (1942) *Amer. J. Surg.*, **56**, 448.
GOLDSTEIN, P. (1949) *Amer. J. Dis. Child.*, **78**, 375.
GONZALES, T. A., VANCE, M., HELPERN, M. and UMBERGER, C. J. (1954) *Legal Medicine and Toxicology*, 2nd ed., p. 478. New York: Appleton Century.
HANDYSIDE, P. D. (1842) *Edinb. Med. J.*, **57**, 391–4.
HEIBERG, S. (1934–5). *Dansk Oto-laryngologisk Selsk. Forh.*, p. 75.
HEUER, G. J. (1923) *Surg. Gynec. Obstet.*, **36**, 686–96.
HOLZHAUSEN, G. and HUNGER, H. (1960) *Arch. Kriminol.*, **125**, 164–7.
HUME (1882) *The Lancet*, i, 987.
HUNT, A. C. and CAMPS, F. E. (1962) *Brit. Med. J.*, i, 378.
JACKSON, C. and JACKSON, C. L. (1943) *Arch. Otolaryng. (Chicago)*, **38**, 413.
JOANNIDES, M. and TSOULUS, G. D. (1930) *Arch. Surg.*, **21**, 333.

JOHNSTONE, J. M., HUNT, A. C. and WARD, E. M. (1960) *Brit. Med. J.*, **ii**, 1714–15.
KEARNEY, M. S. DAHL, L. B. and STALSBERG, H. (1982) *Brit. Med. J.*, **285**, 777 (short report: Tromsø.)
LATTEMANT, M., HENROT, H. and MERCIER, J. (1950) *Ann. Oto-laryng. (Paris)*, **67**, 196.
LEICHER, H. (1954) *Dtsch. Med. Wschr.*, **79** (i), 301.
LENNOX BROWN (1891) *J. Laryng.*, **5**, 28–30.
LITTLEJOHN, HARVEY.(1925) *Forensic Medicine*. London: Churchill.
LITTLEJOHN, H. D. (1855–6) *Edinb. Med. J.*, **1**, 551–4.
MACKLIN, M. T. and MACKLIN, C. C. (1944) *Medicine (Baltimore)*, **23**, 281.
MANN, DIXON (1908) *Forensic Medicine and Toxicology*. London: Griffin.
MARTIN, É. (1950) *Précis de Médicine Légale*, 3rd ed. Paris: Doin.
METSON, B. F. (1953) *Arch. Otolaryng. (Chicago)*, **57**, 182.
OLLIVIER (D'ANGAS) (1834) *Ann. d'Hyg.*, **18**, 485–98. (Photostat; R.S.M.)
PERTHES, G. (1900) *Dtsch. Z. Chir.*, **55**, 384–92.
POLSON, C. J. (1965) *The Essentials of Forensic Medicine*, 2nd. ed. p. 308, fig. 117; p. 347, fig. 140 and plate 8; Oxford: Pergamon Press.
POLSON, C. J. and GEE, D. J. (1972) *Z. Retsmed.-J. Leg.-med.*, **70**, 184–92.
POLSON, C. J. and HORNBACK, H. (1960) *Med.-leg. J. (Camb.)*, **28**, 88.
PUPPE, G. (1908) *Atlas u. Grundiss.* Munich: Lehmann.
QUIRICO, E. (1950) *Accad. Med.*, **65**, 129.
R. v. DONALD (1934) *The Trial of Jeannie Donald*, ed. J. G. Wilson (1953), p. 194. Edinburgh, etc.: Hodge.
RAVENEL (1891) *Abstr., J. Laryng.*, **5**, 213–14.
RENTON, J. M. (1908) *Brit. Med. J.*, **i**, 493.
RHAINEY, K. and MACGREGOR, A. R. (1948) *Arch. Dis. Childh.*, **23**, 254–8.
RIEMAN, A. P. and GOLDSMITH, A. S. (1937) *J. Amer. Med. Ass.*, **108**, 1605.
ROBERTSON, A. (1916) *Manual of Medical Jurisprudence*, 3rd ed. London: Black.
ROSSELET, E. (1927) *Ann. Méd. lég.*, **7**, 222–6.
ROUGHEAD, W. (1948) *Burke and Hare*, 3rd ed. Edinburgh, etc.: Hodge.
SANKEY, H. (1883) *Brit. Med. J.*, **i**, 88.
SCHOLLMEYER, W. (1966) *Arch. Kriminol.*, **137**, 12.
SHARMAN, S. (1937) *Lancet*, **i**, 1227–8.
SIMPSON, C. K. (1943) *Lancet*, **ii**, 309–11.
SIMPSON, C. K. (1960) *Med. Sci. Law*, **1**, 420–8 (428).
SMITH, Sir SYDNEY (1948), in a lecture in his course on Forensic Medicine, Univ. Edinburgh, 20 April.
SMITH, Sir SYDNEY and FIDDES, F. S. (1955) *Forensic Medicine*, 10th ed., p. 262. London: Churchill.
SPILSBURY, BERNARD (1934) *Med.-leg. Rev.*, **2**, 340–4.
STORY, G. B. (1897) *Med. Rec.* (N.Y.), **51**, 636.
TAYLOR, A. S. (1956) *Principles and Practice of Medical Jurisprudence*, 11th ed., vol. 1, p. 468, ed. Smith and Simpson. London: Churchill.
TEMPLEMAN (1892) *Edinb. Med. J.*, **38**, 322–9.
TIDY, C. M. (1883) *Legal Medicine*, vol. 2. London: Smith Elder.
TOLNAY, L. (1963) *Arch. Kriminol.*, **132**, 42.
VENG-CHRISTENSEN, E. (1958) *Ungeskr. Laeg.*, **120**, 189.
WEIMANN, W. (1962) *Arch. Kriminol.*, **129**, 16.
WEIMANN, W. and PROKOP, O. (1963) *Atlas der gerichtlichen Medizin*, p. 639. Berlin: Verlag Volk and Gesundheit.
WINSLOW, R. (1905) *Med. News*, **86**, 207–8.
ZEUCH, L. H. (1922) *Illinois Med. J.*, **41**, 451. (Photostat, Royal Society of Medicine.)
ZWERGIUS, E. (1955) *Ugeskr. Laeg.*, **117**, 680.

CHAPTER 13

Sexual Offences

THE law relating to sexual offences was consolidated in the Sexual Offences Act, 1956. The several crimes are grouped as follows: (a) intercourse by force, intimidation, false pretences or the administration of drugs to obtain or facilitate intercourse; (b) intercourse with girls under 16; (c) intercourse with defective (now "severely subnormal persons"); (d) incest; (e) unnatural offences, and (f) indecent assaults. Other provisions deal with abduction, prostitution, solicitation and the suppression of brothels. Certain gaps in this otherwise comprehensive statute were closed by the Indecency with Children Act, 1960. It was discovered that no crime was committed where a person, without committing an assault, invited a child to handle him or otherwise behaved indecently towards a child under 14. This is now a criminal offence with a maximum penalty of 2 years' imprisonment. The opportunity was also taken, in section 2, to increase the maximum punishment for attempted sexual intercourse with a girl under 13, or an indecent assault on a girl under that age, to 7 years' imprisonment in respect of the former and 5 years in respect of the latter offence. Attempted incest with a girl under 13 is also liable to punishment by a term of up to 7 years' imprisonment.

Sexual intercourse is defined by the Sexual Offences Act, 1956, s.44. It is not necessary to prove the completion of the intercourse by the emission of seed, but the intercourse shall be deemed complete on proof of penetration only.

An advisory group, chaired by the Hon. Mrs. Justice Heilbron, D.B.E., reported in 1975 on various aspects of the law relating to sexual offences, notably the lack of definition of rape; any evidence of the previous sexual history of the complainant; anonymity and the constitution of juries in rape cases (H.M.S.O. Cmnd. 6352).

This led to the enactment of the Sexual Offences (Amendment) Act, 1976. Rape is now defined as unlawful intercourse with a woman, who, at the time of the intercourse, did not consent to it and at that time the man knew she did not consent to intercourse or he was reckless as to whether she had consented or not. Provision is also made for restrictions on evidence of previous sexual experience and the anonymity of the complainant. The Sexual Offences (Scotland) Act, 1976 deals with a number of matters whereby the law in Scotland is now more closely in line with that of England.

Procedure at an Examination of the Victim of Rape

Consent to the examination is first obtained from the woman or, if a child, from her parent or guardian. The examination should be carried out in a well-lit room. The late

W. H. Grace, recommended that the victim be seated on the least comfortable chair; if she does not fidget, the genuineness of her complaint is suspect.

The date and time of the examination must be recorded, because the interval between the alleged incident and the examination is material. An interval of undue length will call for explanation and, more important to the doctor, will permit repair to obscure signs of rape. Negative findings at the examination of an adult are to be expected if a few days have elapsed, the more so if she is also a married woman or one otherwise accustomed to sexual intercourse.

The doctor will take opportunity to observe the gait of the victim as she enters the consulting room or by specific test. He will observe her general demeanour and bodily habit. Does walking cause pain of a kind likely to result from injury to the genitalia? Is the victim excited, distressed, or otherwise disturbed, as is consistent with the circumstances of recent rape? Is she a woman of poor or robust physique and of what kind of resistance would she be capable?

Case History

When the victim is accompanied by a parent or friend, the doctor should first obtain an account from the latter, separately from the victim; he should then hear the victim's own story and both statements should be recorded in detail.

The specific questions to be put to each of them will elicit the personal details of the victim, i.e. the name, age and status; the date, time and place of the incident; the course of events during it, with particular reference to the position of the parties; the steps taken by the victim to resist her assailant, and whether she lost consciousness at any time during the attack. It is important to determine whether the victim was menstruating at that time.

The Examination

(a) *The clothing.* When the victim has undressed, her clothing should be examined. Paul (1975) recommends that, if possible, the clothing should be removed while the subject stands on a clean sheet of paper so that any trace evidence which is dislodged can be collected and preserved. Examination with an ultra-violet light lamp may indicate areas of probable seminal staining. It should be ascertained whether the garments were those worn at the time of the attack. If so, are they soiled by mud or grass? Do they bear blood or seminal stains and are they torn, and is there any loss of buttons? The condition of the footwear may negative part of the victim's story. When a young nanny returned to her employer's house late at night, she alleged that she had been raped and left to walk several miles. A police sergeant examined her shoes; they showed no signs of wear. The police surgeon found no signs of rape; she was menstruating. Later, other circumstances indicated she was a liar and a thief.

(b) *The person.* The physique and, in the case of children, bodily development, especially of the breasts and genitalia, will be noted. Could the victim have offered resistance? Was the child older than her years to the extent that she appeared to be over 16 years old? It is here relevant to note whether cosmetics are used and also the style of dress. Youngsters of 14 or thereabouts not rarely, it seems, are prone to dress and use "make-up" in a manner beyond their years.

Injuries: General Consideration

The whole of the exterior of the body of the victim must be examined for injuries, notably abrasions and bruises. The details of any such injuries must be recorded and their probable age assessed. Do they appear in situations consistent with an injury received during a struggle and a forcible attempt at intercourse? Are they of an age which coincides with the date of the alleged attack? Special attention will be given to the arms, face, neck and the inner aspect of the thighs. Rape of young children of under 13 years may well be accomplished without the production of external injuries because these victims are unlikely to offer resistance to the assailant. Some may be willing parties to intercourse, and it appears, may even invite it! A visit to the scene may also be highly instructive (Figs. 45, p. 135 and 149, p. 419).

Bruises on the neck of oval shape may, in fact, be "love bites" occurring during consenting intercourse. Petechiae on the face or conjunctivae should be looked for as evidence of partial asphyxia caused during forcible restraint or with intent to render the victim unconscious, or to silence her.

The Genitalia and the Breasts

Breasts. One or both breasts may be bruised by rough handling. They may be bitten and the imprint of the assailant's teeth may be clear, as in the Gorringe case (see p. 69); the nipples may have been bitten off.

The opinion of a forensic odontologist should be sought before the marks are interfered with. Traces of saliva present can be identified as such and sometimes grouped by a forensic scientist. It is important, therefore, that such marks receive close and appropriate attention, before washing or post-mortem examination.

Genitalia. The normal examination is made but the vulva and hymen call for close attention.

Pubic hair. Samples are required and should be taken at a late stage of the examination because the hairs should be plucked and not cut from the part. Matting of the hairs may be caused by dried seminal fluid. Sample hairs are required to prove this and may be required also for comparison with hairs found on the clothing of the accused.

Vulva. Injury of the vulva is indicated by tenderness, swelling, redness, bruises and lacerations.

Hymen. Examination of the hymen, especially of a child, in whom it is somewhat inaccessible, is facilitated by the use of graduated glass bulbs of the kind described by Glaister and Rentoul (1966). A model, in plastic material and illuminated electrically, was prepared in our Department by R. P. Brittain.

Recent tears in the hymen (Fig. 159), associated with bleeding or swelling and inflammation, may be obvious but, when repair is advanced, care is required to distinguish between a ruptured hymen and certain forms of intact hymen.

Vagina. Undue dilatation in a child may point to intercourse but it can follow the insertion of foreign bodies like Tampax. Bruising, abrasion or laceration are at all times consistent with forcible intercourse and do not necessarily indicate rape.

This is well illustrated by the case of the vaginal rupture during lawful coitus, reported by Victor Bonney (1912). She was admitted to hospital suffering from vaginal bleeding and early peritonitis. A tear in the

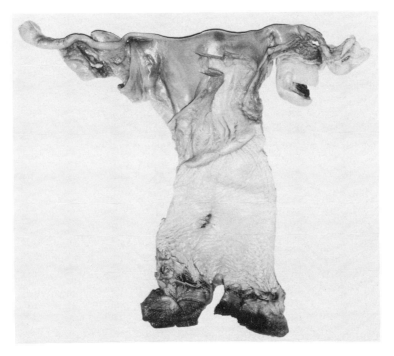

FIG. 159. Sexual interference: tearing of hymen and abrasion of vagina by digital interference (victim murdered by strangulation).

posterior fornix communicated with the peritoneum. It admitted the examiner's thumb. Bonney at first thought he was dealing with a criminal abortion, attempted with an instrument (she was a woman who had had several children). The injury, however, was not due to any criminal act. When drunk, she had accepted intercourse in the standing posture; it caused instant pain. She immediately disengaged. There was then considerable bleeding and she experienced agonising pain, which persisted until she was admitted to hospital, about 12 hours later. The tear was repaired and the peritoneum drained. Her recovery was rapid and she was discharged cured on the 24th day.

Tearing or perforation of the vagina may occur when it is thin or of frail texture. Bonney cited an instance of perforation of the vagina in the course of a vaginal examination, performed without undue force. There is also the case, originally reported by Fehling (1873–4), of the woman who perforated her own vagina in an attempt to rectify a sudden prolapse of the uterus, which occurred whilst she was carrying a pail of water. Spontaneous rupture of the vagina can also occur; Bonney also cited the case of a woman, who had had ten children, who had a sudden extroversion of the genitalia, with rupture of the vagina, whilst under strain when carrying coal. Operative cure was achieved.

There is yet another possibility, namely the infliction of injuries in order to simulate rape, when killing has been due to some other cause. The case of *R. v. Donald* (1934) concerned the murder of a girl aged 8 by throttling, but "extreme violence had been applied to the genitals". It had been the hope of the accused that this would have been deemed a sexual murder but that defence failed. The medical witnesses rejected this interpretation; Dr. Richards, for instance, did not think the injuries could have been caused by a male organ because of their size and direction. An instrument about the thickness of a middle finger or possibly two fingers used very roughly might have caused the injuries. Sir Sydney Smith also rejected rape.

It remains an open question if rape be excluded does it follow the injuries could not, none the less, have been inflicted by a man? There is such a thing as injury by digital interference by the male. Moreover, this can occur without, or prior to, sexual interference, in the course of a sexual murder (F.M. 1326A; *R.* v. *Blake*).

Samples, notably of vaginal fluid, swabs from the anus and, when appropriate, from the mouth, should be obtained in such a way as to counter subsequent allegations that the results are vitiated by contamination during sampling. Paul (1975) recommends swabs of the anal verge, perineum, vulva and introitus, first. Then the passage of a small and unlubricated vaginal speculum and proctoscope to enable samples to be taken from inside the passages without fear of contamination. Visual and digital examination can follow the taking of samples.

Vaginal fluid should be collected on swabs or preferably into a pipette and stains (see p. 489) and fresh smears prepared as described in the section on "Seminal Fluid". A swab should be reserved for bacteriological investigation, with especial reference to gonorrhoea. Vaginal discharge, e.g. leucorrhoea, of itself is not proof of sexual intercourse for it is a common manifestation wholly unrelated to venereal disease. Even when the cause be proved to be gonorrhoea, it by no means follows that it was a result of rape or unlawful carnal knowledge. A child may be infected accidentally by parents or other members of the household. The duration of the discharge should be determined; if said to have begun within 24 hours of alleged rape, infection must have occurred prior to it. Gonorrhoeal infection of these victims has significance, such as it is, only when it is proved that the victim had had no prior discharge, that it made its appearance at a time between the third to eighth day after intercourse, that it is gonorrhoeal in origin and that the accused was at the time a potential source of infection. The latter criterion in particular must be proved since otherwise, the victim may, by accident or design, accuse an innocent man.

Although it is not necessary, in rape, to prove the presence of seminal fluid in the vagina, its presence confirms that sexual intercourse had taken place. Seminal fluid on the external parts or pubic hair, or seminal stains on the clothing, are also important, the more so when the victim is a child. Fibres of cloth found on or near the genitalia must be preserved for expert examination; they may be proved to be derived from a garment worn by the accused. A blood sample, for grouping, should also be obtained.

Examination of the Accused

Consent to examine the accused must never be omitted and should be obtained by the doctor in writing and witnessed.

The examiner will note his age, size and physique. A search must be made for injuries of a kind and age consistent with an alleged struggle, e.g. scratches on his face, bite marks on the hands.

The demonstration of seminal stains on his clothing is always capable of innocent explanation. It is of greater moment to note the size of the penis and to determine whether the man is potent or impotent. An accumulation of smegma in the prepuce is inconsistent, but a torn frenum is consistent with recent copulation.

He should be examined for evidence of active venereal disease, notably gonorrhoea. A blood sample for grouping should be obtained.

His clothing should be examined for the presence of hair, blood and seminal stains.

When bloodstains are present, an attempt should be made to determine the group to which they belong. If other than that of the accused, but similar to that of the victim, it may be corroborative evidence of rape, especially when the stains belong to the rare group AB. Bloodstains on the victim may be the result of injury to the male's penis. Nail scrapings may include fibres or blood.

Summary

At times it is possible to prove that violent and probably unlawful intercourse with an adult had taken place and that the victim offered strong resistance. It may also be possible, on other occasions, to prove that a child had been the subject of an attempt at intercourse, the accomplishment of the act being precluded by the youth of the victim. There is then likely to be severe injury of the genitalia but, if the child is under 13 years, she may be uninjured elsewhere because she was unable to offer resistance; when unaware of their purpose she may have complied with the accused's advances; she may have been held down by his body.

When the victim is an adult, however, it must always be in mind that severe injuries can be consistent with violent intercourse with a consenting party. Glaister and Rentoul (1966) tell of a woman who was found in a distressed condition and who had injuries of her external genitalia; the circumstances led to a man being charged with her rape. The prisoner alleged that he had called at the house and this woman, notwithstanding that he was a stranger, invited him inside. She received his advances favourably and although she was unfamiliar with the procedure she allowed intercourse to take place. When the man was examined he was found to have a penis of exceptional size, capable of causing injury to a consenting party, especially one like the victim, who was unused to intercourse. His story was thus confirmed and he was acquitted.

Conversely, failure to demonstrate signs of intercourse or injury, local or general, does not permit an opinion that rape did not take place. If the victim be a child, however, a negative examination, made shortly after an alleged rape, indicates that, in all probability, this offence had not been committed.

Several authors have given detailed descriptions of the examination of the victim and alleged assailant in rape cases: Paul (1975, 1977) Burges (1978) McLay (1978) and Huntington (1976). Sexual offences against children have been considered by Tilelli *et al.* (1980) and Woodling and Kossoris (1981).

Sexually-orientated Homicide.

Although there is a sexual element in the majority of the murders of women, over 75 per cent of the killings occur during a domestic quarrel or are provoked by jealousy; only in 10–20 per cent is the murder prompted by the urge for sexual gratification.

Murder for sexual reasons may assume various forms. The simplest is an approach by the male, rebuff by the victim, leading to an attack and killing.

A girl was crossing some waste land on her way home when she was accosted by a youth, who, lived in the same estate. She rebuffed him. Whereupon he attacked her, strangled her and then inflicted severe head injuries with a boulder lying nearby. Autopsy showed the fatal injuries and a patterned abrasion on the cheek; the pattern was that of a zip. Search of the scene in daylight yielded a key fob and this had produced the abrasion on the cheek. It was beside a rock, which was soiled by blood and bore hairs and was thus the probable agent which caused her head injuries. The search also found nearby a set of darts which were traced to a particular youth. When examined he had a bite mark on his abdomen, inflicted by the dead girl. She had not been raped (F.M. 24,574A).

On various occasions, when a woman's body is discovered, the clothing has been displaced but there has not been sexual intercourse. This was a feature of several of the "Yorkshire Ripper's" murders. Blouses were ripped open or the jumper was raised to expose the breasts and slacks were pulled down to expose the panties. On most of these occasions the breasts were undamaged and sexual intercourse had not taken place. It seems that in some cases the element of voyeurism arises after an attack.

When murder occurs during the act of rape, or intercourse occurs immediately after the killing, the body is then likely to be found with the limbs in a position suitable for sexual intercourse; the legs wide apart, flexed at the hips and knees, with bared genitalia exposed. In such circumstances the injuries inflicted may be gross, suggesting that both the assailant and the victim may have been under the influence of drink or drugs.

A female prostitute was found spreadeagled across an old mattress in a derelict house, in a position of sexual intercourse; there were head injuries and gross damage to the neck, indicative to crushing of the larynx. The assailant proved to have been a large man with a history of violence. The death occurred shortly after both had left a public house together (F.M. 25,401A).

Gross injuries on a woman obviously prepared for intercourse, without it having taken place, may have been inflicted by an incensed client, who had been ridiculed because he had failed to achieve intercourse.

This may have been the situation when the naked body of a woman was found at the edge of a car park. She had gross head injuries, the result of several blows to the skull with a brick. The night was extremely cold. There was no evidence of sexual intercourse having taken place (F.M. 12,915). This murder was never solved. It seemed possible that the cold had rendered the man temporarily impotent, that he had been taunted and incensed to cause him to attack and inflict gross injuries.

Death may occur during sexual intercourse. This may be the result of natural disease, e.g. rupture of a cerebral aneurysm. On other occasions it could be misadventure, the result of abnormal intercourse. The victim may die of choking especially at the moment of ejaculation during oral intercourse or be choked by a plug of wool, or similar material, placed in the mouth to retain the seminal fluid. (An unsolved murder was due to asphyxia and a plug of cotton wool escaped from the throat during the autopsy; it was later found to have been contaminated by semen. (F.M. 9400B).

As stated earlier, intercourse may follow a killing. It is difficult to decide whether necrophilia was the motive or the killing was proved by sexual urge. This situation may arise when elderly ladies are murdered in the course of a burglary. An old lady, a cripple, was murdered by an intruder in her flat. Sexual intercourse had taken place, since the body was disposed as for such a purpose. There was a minor genital injury without any vital reaction. In the course of intercourse, the assailant's necktie, soiled by the woman's blood, had left a clear impression of the pattern of its fabric on the front of her nightdress (F.M. 13,074A).

Murder of children, above the age of "Battered Babies", especially of young girls is often prompted by sexual motives. Very bizarre findings may often occur. In our experience of up to 40 per cent of murders of these children are due to sexual motives. A girl, aged about 10, was way-laid when on her way home from school. She was dragged into some bushes in the front garden of a house, strangled, stripped naked and pieces of wood were thrust into her throat, and the abdomen, via the vagina. The assailant then masturbated and left seminal fluid on the front of her abdomen; it was found as a dried trace (F.M. 13,106 A).

A more recent variety of murder, with some sexual connotations, has occurred in our practice. It arises among ethnic minority groups by whom infidelity or disobedience may be punished by the infliction of severe injuries. A woman we examined, a married Asian woman, was suspected of infidelity. Her throat was cut and severe incised wounds had been inflicted on her genitalia (F.M. 9843 A). The daughter of Asian parents, who refused to marry the man chosen for her by her father, had her throat cut by him; he used the blade of a wood-plane. (F.M. 21286).

Homosexual affairs may end in violence. Our experience has been limited to murders, by stabbing, or head injuries of extreme violence. The accused's explanation was that they had reacted in disgust after homosexual advances had been made to them. Similar cases have been reported by McLay (1978) and Usher (1975).

In all such murders the circumstances and the scene of death should raise the possibility of a sexual motive. This should prompt the pathologist to be particularly careful to look for trace evidence, such as seminal fluid on the skin, as well as in the orifices; for saliva on bite marks or around nipples and for obscure bite marks themselves, etc. Any genital injuries should be preserved by dissecting out the whole female genital tract *en bloc* as in cases of suspected abortion. Great care should also be taken in the description of the distribution of the clothing, etc.

Indecent Assault

The range of acts which constitute indecent assaults is wide and proof is by other than medical evidence. For example, proof of interference with clothing is not normally determined by a medical examination, although evidence of it should be sought for at the medical examination of the victims of rape.

Doctors and dentists are open to accusations of indecent assault, arising out of professional attendance. It will be recalled that an intimate medical examination of a woman, undertaken without her consent, may result in a charge of indecent assault. Examinations of this kind, undertaken with consent, but in the absence of a disinterested third party, also expose the doctor to a false charge of indecent assault. The administration of a general anaesthetic to a woman, in the absence of others, carries the same risk; there should always be at least one other disinterested person present.

The Rape of a Male

Although the law provides grave penalties for the rape of females, the rape of a male by a female is not a specific crime. The woman may be convicted only of an indecent assault, notwithstanding she had deliberately instigated intercourse with a boy. The principal medical evidence in such circumstances is proof of the transmission of venereal disease from the woman to the victim, whose examination is unlikely to yield any other evidence of the crime.

Offences between Males

Sodomy and Paederasty

Medical evidence is restricted, in the main, to an examination of the passive agent. Examination of the active agent can yield, at most, evidence only of contamination of the penis by faecal material, lubricant or secretion from the anal glands, and, in any event, this must be determined promptly, at or near to the time of the act.

The passive agent unless accustomed to the practice, must also be examined at an early date, because reparative changes can rapidly obliterate signs of the crime. Recent tears in the anal wall are important but are unusual, since the act, as it must be, is committed with a consenting party. When the passive agent is of an age at which an emission is impossible, but only in these circumstances, seminal stains upon his clothing, especially at the back, have significance. A swab should be taken of the contents of the anal canal and examined for the presence of seminal fluid. (This is also relevant when intercourse *per anum* with a woman is alleged. This also is a serious crime, and is a species of buggery.)

Under the Sexual Offences Act, 1967, certain forms of buggery and gross indecency are no longer offences. If the parties are aged 21 or over, a homosexual act in private, with the consent of the parties, is not an offence. It is an offence if more than two persons are present or if the act takes place in a public lavatory.

Those who are accustomed to play the passive part may acquire permanent changes in the anus. It may become funnel-shaped; the anal walls are patulous and its sphincter is relaxed; a lax anus, however, is not of itself sufficient proof. Healed lacerations may produce a triangular wound, the appearances of which are characteristic of sodomy. A widely-gaping anal canal has of itself great significance. The presence of these changes, originally described in detail by Tardieu (confirmed by Brouardel (1909), with amplification), is important but their absence has no significance. In the latter event, however, the medical examiner is not entitled to assert that the offence has not been committed. Those who undertake these examinations should acquire first-hand experience under the tuition of a police surgeon.

It is important to avoid confusion with changes due to natural disease and, in the dead, with dilatation of the anal canal and prolapse of the tissues, due to putrefactive changes.

Gonorrhoeal or syphilitic infection of the anal canal, especially of boys, can be important corroborative evidence of paederasty.

The signs of sodomy were succinctly summarised by Fatteh (1962). They include not only an anal sphincter which is ready to receive the examining finger when the cheeks are separated, and dilatation of the sphincter with the appearance of a central hole as the mucosal folds separate (Gancz, 1962), but several other signs. These include: (1) spermatazoa within or around the anal canal (evidence of recent intercourse); (2) a funnel-shaped depression of the buttocks towards the anal orifice; (3) a shaved anal region but an unshaved pubic region; (4) a patulous anus with absence of radial folds and prolapse of the rectal mucosa; (5) healed coital injuries near the ano-rectal junction and, sometimes, (6) a gonorrhoeal discharge, condylomata or a chancre.

Burges (1978) detailed the examination procedure of the victim of an alleged homosexual offence.

Bestiality

Intercourse with animals is sometimes practised, especially, but not exclusively, amongst those who have charge of horses and cattle.

These offences rarely require medical evidence for their proof, since a conviction turns, as a rule, upon the evidence of an eye-witness. The forensic scientist is sometimes required to demonstrate hairs of the animal upon the underclothing of the accused; their presence on his outer garments is proof only of innocent association.

The Medico-legal Aspects of Seminal Fluid

The demonstration of seminal fluid, or the stains which it produces, may play a part in charges of rape or attempted rape, sexual murder of the female and in buggery and, possibly, bestiality.

Potency of the fluid is material in civil causes, e.g. disputed paternity or nullity when the defence is one of impotence; this may be pleaded also as a defence to a charge of rape.

It is necessary, according to the circumstances, to prove that a stain was produced by seminal fluid or this fluid is present either in the vagina or on the labia minora or in the anal canal. On other occasions it is required to demonstrate the potency of the fluid.

Proof of the presence of seminal fluid is by way of naked-eye inspection, chemical tests and microscopical study of smears; the latter must be fresh, fixed and appropriately stained to demonstrate sperms. Potency is determined by seminal analysis.

Collection of Material

It is convenient to consider seminal stains on clothing, etc., and fluid from the vagina or anal canal together, since the procedure differs only in the manner in which the specimens are obtained and prepared for examination.

In suspected rape it is necessary to look for seminal fluid in stains on the clothing, on the skin of the perineum and thighs, on the labia minora, pubic hair, in the vagina and the anal canal. It is not essential to prove that seminal fluid is present in the vagina; it is normally sufficient when it is found on the labia minora or pubic hair since penetration by the male need not be complete.

Dried or drying seminal fluid on the perineum or labia minora is best collected with a throat swab. Samples of pubic hair, which may be required also for comparison with hairs on the clothing of the accused, should be plucked carefully and transferred to a small glass container. Hairs which are cut will not include the roots and are therefore unsatisfactory.

Fluid from the vagina is collected with a pipette or throat swab inserted with or without the aid of a speculum. Since sperms may disintegrate rapidly, it is important to make one or more smears on glass slides immediately and to send them with the corresponding specimens for investigation. Similarly, smears of anal swabs should also be made forthwith.

A search for seminal stains on clothing is facilitated by its examination under filtered ultraviolet light. Fluorescent areas are suitably marked to permit subsequent identification and a portion of fabric in each is cut out and preserved for laboratory investigation. Fluorescence is not proof that the stain is seminal because this property is common also to pus, urine and milk, which may be present. It is necessary to submit the selected specimens to further tests which are described later in this chapter.

This search is normally the duty of the forensic scientist, but the doctor should himself make his own examination of the clothing for tears, blood or seminal stains, since their presence and distribution may play a part in the interpretation of the medical findings.

Seminal Fluid

Seminal fluid is gelatinous and of yellow-white colour and is ejaculated in amounts of from 2 to 5 ml; the volume is excessive if it be 6 ml or over, but it can be as much as 13.5 ml (Glaister and Rentoul, 1966). The fluid normally contains some 60 million sperms per millilitre of which 90 per cent are motile at the time of ejaculation. When the fluid is allowed to stand at room temperature for about $^1/_2$ hour it becomes watery and there is a progressive reduction in the number of motile sperms. The fluid is alkaline and has a pH of 7.4.

Seminal Analysis

The determination of potency takes several factors into account, namely, the volume and viscosity of the specimen, its cell content and the motility and morphology of the sperms.

The volume, normally about 2 to 5 ml must be adequate, first, to neutralise the acid vaginal secretion and, second, to enable the sperms to reach the cervix. Viscosity should be within normal limits since motility and vigour of the sperms are reduced by excessive viscosity of the fluid.

A potent fluid should normally contain not less than 60 million sperms per millilitre but counts within a wide range are consistent with potency. Conception has occurred when the seminal fluid contained as few as 15 to 20 million sperms. On the other hand, counts much in excess of 100 millions are frequent (Baird, 1950). Complete absence of sperms, azoospermia or aspermia, must not be assumed unless confirmed by an examination of at least three ejaculates. The cause of azoospermia is either a failure in their production by the testis or an obstruction of the ducts which convey the sperms to the urethra. The distinction will rest on a biopsy of the testis.

Motility of the sperms enables them to gain the uterine cavity. The proportion of motile sperms is determined by an examination of a fresh ejaculate, collected from the male. Specimens from the vagina are unsatisfactory, if not valueless, because contact with the vaginal secretion, the acidity of which approximates to N/10 HCl, rapidly destroys motility of the sperms; motility in the vagina may cease within $^1/_2$ hour and is invariably absent by the end of 2 hours. It is unlikely, therefore, that vaginal specimens obtained from the victims of rape will include motile sperms. When an ejaculate from the male is kept at room temperature full motility persists for about 3 hours; by the end of 8 hours only half of the sperms are motile but 10 per cent may remain motile for 24 hours (Baird, 1950). Motility persists for several hours if the specimen is kept at 98.4° F, i.e. body temperature.

Specimens obtained from the uterine cavity where the secretion is alkaline may include living sperms even at the end of a fortnight after insemination.

Opinions regarding the length of time that seminal fluid may be detectable in the genital tract after intercourse vary. Summers (1969) says that spermatozoa may be found in the rectum some days after the offence, and in the vagina up to 8 days after coitus. Rupp (1969) finds that within 8 hours there is an equal chance of finding motile or non-motile sperm in vaginal aspirates. Non-motile sperm were found for periods up to 14 hours. Positive acid phosphatase reactions were found for periods in excess of 24 hours.

Willmott (1975) reviewed the literature and reported that sperm had been found in the vagina up to 9 days and 12 days in the cervix after intercourse. Davies and Wilson (1974) found that the longest time sperm could be found after intercourse was 6 days. Apparently complete sperm do not persist as long as the heads alone; complete sperm are said to be found only up to 72 hours after intercourse. Soules *et al.* (1978) reported that sperm were present in nearly 50 per cent of the vaginal samples taken at 72 hours after intercourse. After death semen can persist much longer; they were found at up to 3 to 4 months in the bodies of the victims of murder (Nicholls, 1956).

A summary of the length of time semen can be detected in the various body orifices has been given by Williams (1978). He indicated that semen would be found in the vagina at up to 24 hours after intercourse; are likely to be found at up to 72 hours and may be found at up to 6 days. In the anus they have been found at up to 2 days and in the mouth at up to 9 hours after intercourse.

The Demonstration of Seminal Stains

A search for seminal stains should always be under satisfactory lighting and, preferably, under filtered ultraviolet light.

Stains on absorbent fabrics, especially those of light colour, have a grey or yellow-grey colour and an irregular shape, map-like in outline; the colour is deeper in a narrow zone at the periphery of the stain. The fluid penetrates the fabric, which, when dried, is stiffened as if starched. Under filtered ultraviolet light the stain fluoresces but, as already stated, other substances, notably pus and urine, are also fluorescent.

Stains on smooth, impervious surfaces, when dried, are seen as slightly yellow, brittle scales, which yield the characteristic odour of seminal fluid when warmed. They should be gently scraped off with the point of a knife into a watch-glass or other suitable glass container.

Fabric bearing a suspected stain is thoroughly soaked in a watchglass in Ungar's solution, i.e. HCl or acetic acid in a concentration of 0.8 per cent; enough is used to soak the fabric and no more. The time required for soaking may be only a few minutes or it may be several hours; the process *must not be hurried* because this is likely to break up the sperms. When the stain has been softened, the fabric is drained and applied to a series of clean glass slides. The films are then submitted to histo-chemical tests and microscopical examination.

In the modification described by Ellis (1960) the stain is agitated in saline and the eluate is then filtered under pressure. Suitable filter discs are stained with Weigert's iron haematoxylin-eosin. The filtrate is used for phosphatase analysis.

HISTO-CHEMICAL TESTS FOR SEMINAL FLUID

Two preliminary tests, namely the Florence (Beeman, 1942) and Barberio tests are used in the search for semen. Moist smears of the stain-extract are required for the test.

The Florence Test

The moist smear is covered with a cover glass and a few drops of the reagent are placed at its edge; capillary attraction draws the reagent under the cover-glass.

The reagent is an aqueous solution of iodine and potassium iodide prepared by adding to 30 cm^3 of distilled water, 2.54 g of iodine and 1.65 g of potassium iodide.

A positive result is indicated by prompt precipitation at the junction of the reagent and the extract under test. Microscopical examination will then show rhombic crystals, which resemble haemin but are larger, arranged in clusters, rosettes, crosses, etc. They are a product of choline.

The test is not proof of seminal fluid but only of the presence of some vegetable or animal substance. A positive result in these circumstances, however, is presumptive evidence of seminal fluid; a negative result means that the stain is in all probability other than that of seminal fluid. (See reviews by Beeman (1942) and Pollak (1963).)

Barberio's Test

The procedure already described is followed but with another reagent, i.e. a saturated aqueous solution of picric acid.

A positive result is obtained when a bright yellow precipitate forms. It contains rhombic crystals of spermine picrate; once they form they increase in size rapidly.

Although it is a less sensitive test than the Florence test, a positive result raises a strong presumption that the stain is that of seminal fluid.

These two tests narrow down the search and indicate which of the stained areas are the best to choose for microscopical examination.

The Acid Phosphatase Content of Seminal Stains

It was found by Gutman and Gutman (1941) that the human ejaculate is rich in acid phosphatase; the amount was from 540 to 4000 units per ml in ejaculates obtained from sixteen healthy young males. The amount was much higher in samples obtained by prostatic massage, namely 3300 to 23,200 units per ml (Hansen, 1946). Many vegetable substances were tested and none was found to yield results of this order. The maximum content in vegetable matter was only 48 units, yielded by the juice of beech leaves. Top yeast in a little water was the nearest to seminal fluid, but it contained only about 130 units per ml. Of animals, monkeys alone yielded results which approximate to those obtained from man; in other tests, with rats, for example, fluid from the preputial glands contained only from 27 to 104 units per ml.

Stains on fabric are suitable for this test since the kind and colour of the fabric does not vitiate the results. Riisfeldt (1946) obtained positive results with stains on seventy-six fabrics of different kinds. Interference occurred only when the fabrics were impregnated with sodium arsenate or phenylmercuric acetate but this is a remote possibility in circumstances which ordinarily call for the demonstration of seminal fluid.

The concentration of acid phosphatase is slowly reduced when the stain is left at room temperature and exposed to light. Heating of the specimen to 60°C or over destroys acid phosphatase within 5 minutes but stains kept in a refrigerator will retain acid phosphatase, unimpaired, indefinitely.

Several methods for the demonstration of acid phosphatase have been devised. The value of the test was first suggested by Lundquist (1945) and the first method was described by Rasmussen (1945). Other methods and modifications were subsequently published by Hansen (1946), Riisfeldt (1946), Kaye (1947) and Faulds (1951).

The demonstration of an acid phosphatase concentration of 300 units per ml in a stain raises a presumption that it is seminal. It is unlikely to be anything else if values of 500 or over are obtained. The technique is more elaborate than that of the Florence and Barberio Tests but, where the facilities are available, it should be a routine step in the investigation of seminal stains. It cannot, however, displace the microscopical demonstration of sperms as proof of seminal fluid.

The test was the subject of a review by Kind (1964) which should be consulted.

Estimation of time since intercourse from acid phosphatase/U.V.270 absorbence ratios has been described by Rutter *et al.* (1980).

Acid phosphatase is only detectable for up to 2 days after intercourse (Davies and Wilson, 1974).

Another substance which has been advocated as a test for semen is sperm-specific lactate dehydrogenase isoenzyme (Mokashi and Maniwale (1976).

The modern trend for sterilisation vasectomy renders these males aspermic. However, the emission of prostatic fluid, containing acid phosphatase, will still occur. Acid phosphatase also occurs in vaginal secretion but the two kinds of phosphatase can be distinguished by the technique of iso-electric focusing (Toates, 1979).

The Morphology of Spermatozoa

Microscopical examination of fresh, unstained smears and those which have been fixed and stained is the principal test for seminal fluid.

Films dried in the air without heat are fixed for 1 minute in methyl alcohol and then stained. I have found that staining with haemalum, 2 to 5 minutes and eosin, 2 to 5 minutes is satisfactory. Alternatively, staining by methyl blue-acid fuchsin (Baeechi's method) may be preferred. This is a mixture, freshly prepared, of three stock solutions, namely methyl blue 1 per cent, one part, acid fuchsin (aqueous solution) 1 per cent, one part, and HCl 1 per cent, 40 parts. With this stain the heads of the sperms are red and their collars and tails are blue or sky-blue.

Sperms are unique structures which, once seen, create no difficulty in recognition thereafter. The head is a thin oval structure, which is from 4.5 to 5.2 microns long and 2.9 to 3.6 microns broad; a narrow collar or neck joins the head and tail of filament, which is from 50 to 55 microns long.

A positive result is obtained, and is proof of seminal fluid, when one unbroken sperm is found. Although this gives sufficient evidence, it is desirable to demonstrate two or more sperms to support a charge of rape; it is insufficient to find only broken sperms.

A negative result does not exclude seminal fluid as the source of the stain. The fabric may have been washed or the sperms may have been filtered to leave only the fluid fraction on the fabric, or, again, the male concerned may have had aspermia.

Washing the fabric does not necessarily preclude proof; although the substances in the fluid which yield positive chemical tests may be dissolved and removed, sperms, which are not destroyed by soap of alkalis, may remain.

Old stains, even when several years old, may yield positive results, but, the older they are the less is the chance of finding intact sperms.

Grouping of Seminal Fluid

Under suitable conditions it is possible to determine the group of seminal fluid or a seminal stain by the procedure normally adopted for the determination of blood groups. Seminal fluid from the anal canal may be sufficiently contaminated by faecal matter to render the grouping test valueless.

Grouping of seminal fluid by the ABO and GM systems has been described by Willmott (1975) and Williams (1978) but difficulties have been indicated by Pereira and Martin (1976).

Faecal Stains

The possibility of identifying the origin of faecal stains by comparison with faecal material of known origin, e.g. from the body of the victim, and a method of examination, was reported by Giertsen (1961).

Other methods

Methods for analysis of seminal stains include gel diffusion precipitate reactions (Coombs, *et al.* 1963), immuno-diffusion (Thornton and Dillon, 1968), iso-electric focusing (Sutton 1975).

References

BAIRD, D. (1950) *Combined Textbook of obstetrics and Gynaecology*, 5th ed., p. 83. Edinburgh: Livingstone.
BARNES, J. (1967) *Brit. Med. J.*, **1**, 293.
BEEMAN, J. (1942) *Arch. Path.*, **34**, 932–3: Florence test; a review.
BONNEY, V. (1912) *Arch. Middlesex Hosp.*, **28**, 57–60.
BROUARDEL, P. (1909) *Les Attentats aux moeurs*. Paris: Baillière.
BURGES, S. H. (1978) in *The New Police Surgeon*. London. Hutchinson.
COOMBS, R. R. A., RICHARDS, C. B. and DODD, B. (1963) *Med. Sci. Law*, **3**, 65.
COSGROVE, M. ST. J. (1962) *J. Forens. Sci. Soc.*, **3**, 94.
DAVIES, A. and Wilson, E. (1974) *Forensic Sci.*, **3**, 45–55.
ELLIS, H. D. (1960) *Amer. J. Clin. Path.*, **34**, 95–98; *Techn. Bull. Regist. med. Technol.*, **30**, 111–14.
FATTEH, A. (1962) *Brit. Med. J.*, **i**, 486.
FAULDS, J. S. (1951) *Edinb. Med. J.*, **58**, 94–98.
GANCZ, E. (1962) *Brit. Med. J.*, **i**, 263.
GIERTSEN, J. CHR. (1961) *J. Forens. Med.*, **8**, 99–109.
GLAISTER, J. and RENTOUL, E. (1966) *Medical Jurisprudence and Toxicology*, 12th ed. Edinburgh: Livingstone.
GUTMAN, A. B., and GUTMAN, E. B. (1941) *Endocrinology*, **28**, 115–18.
HANSEN, P. F. (1946) *Acta path. microbiol. scand.*, **23**, 187–214.

HUNTINGTON, K. (1976) *Practitioner*, **216**, 519–28.

KAYE, S. (1947) *J. Crim. Law and Criminol.*, **38**, 79–83.

KIND, S. S. (1964) Methods of Forensic science, *Interscience*, **3**, 267.

LUNDQUIST, F. (1945) *Nord. Med.*, **28**, 2131–2.

McLay, W. D. S. (1978) in *The Pathology of Violent Injury*. Ed. Mason, J. K. London. Ed. Arnold.

MOKASHI, R. H. and MANIWALE, M. S. (1976) *Forensic Sci.*, **8**, 269–75.

NICHOLLS, L. C. (1956) *The Scientific Investigation of Crime*. Butterworths.

PAUL, D. M. (1975) *Med. Sci. Law*, **15**, 154–162.

PAUL, D. M. (1977) *Leg. Med. Annu.* Ed. Wecht, C. H. New York. Appleton-Century-Crofts.

PEREIRA, M. and MARTIN, P. D. (1976) *J. Forensic Sci. Soc.*, **16**, 151–154.

POLLAK, O. J. (1943) *Arch. Path.*, **35**, 140–96 (review of methods).

R. v. DONALD (1934) *Trial of Jeannie Donald, Notable British Trials Series*, ed. J. G. Wilson, vol. 79, 1953. Edinburgh, etc.: Hodge.

RASMUSSEN, P. S. (1945) *Nord. Med.*, **28**, 2523–5.

RIISFELDT, O. (1946) *Acta path. microbiol. scand.*, Supplement 58.

RUPP, J. C. (1969) *J. Forens. Sci.*, **14**, 177.

RUTTER, E. R., KIND, S. S., and SMALLDON, K. W. (1980) *J. Forensic Sci. Soc.*, **20**, 271.

SOULES, M. R., POLLARD, A. A., BROWN, K. M., and VERMA, M. (1978) *Am. J. obstet. Gynek.*, **130**, 142–147.

SUMMERS, R. D. (1969) *The Practical Police Surgeon*, chap. 17, p. 157. London: Sweet & Maxwell.

SUTTON, J. *et al* (1975) *Forensic Sci. Soc.*, **6**, 109–14.

THORNTON, J. I. and DILLON, D. J. (1968) *J. Forens. Sci.*, **13**, 262.

TOATES, P. (1979) *Forensic Sci. Int.* **14**, 191–214.

USHER, A. (1975) *Forensic Sci. Int.*, **5**, 245–253.

WILLIAMS, R. L. (1978) in *The New Police Surgeon*. London. Hutchinson.

WILLMOTT, G. M. (1975) *J. Forensic Sci. Soc.* **15**, 269–76.

STATUTES

Indecency with Children Act, 1960; 8 & 9 Eliz. 2, Ch. 33.

Sexual Offences Act, 1956; 4 & 5 Eliz. 2, Ch. 69.

Sexual Offences Act, 1967; Eliz. 2, Ch. 24.

Sexual Offences (amendment) Act, 1976; Eliz. 2, Ch.

Sexual Offences (Scotland) Act, 1976; Eliz. 2, Ch.

CHAPTER 14

Criminal Abortion

ABORTION is defined as the untimely birth of offspring or the procuring of premature delivery so as to destroy offspring. "Miscarriage", the statutory term, is usually deemed synonymous with "abortion" (*O.E.D.*). The present chapter is concerned with the illegal procuring of abortion, i.e. in circumstances other than those permitted by the Abortion Act, 1967.

The Offences against the Person Act, 1861, section 58, enacts that "Every woman being with child who, with intent to procure her own miscarriage, shall unlawfully administer to herself any poison or other noxious thing, or shall unlawfully use any instrument or other means whatsoever with the like intent, and whosoever, with intent to procure the miscarriage of any woman, whether she be or be not with child, shall unlawfully administer to her or cause to be taken by her any poison or other noxious thing, or shall unlawfully use any instrument or other means whatsoever with the like intent, shall be guilty of felony", and it is further enacted, in section 59, that "Whosoever shall unlawfully supply or procure any poison or other noxious thing, or any instrument or thing whatsoever, knowing that the same is intended to be unlawfully used or employed with intent to procure the miscarriage of any woman, whether she be or be not with child, shall be guilty of a misdemeanour . . .".

In the Pharmacy and Medicines Act, 1941, under section 9, it is unlawful to advertise goods in terms calculated to lead to their use in the procurement of an abortion. It is provided, however, that such advertisements are lawful in a publication of a technical character intended for circulation in professional circles, e.g. to doctors, nurses and registered pharmacists.

The law prohibits the administration of poison or any noxious thing or the use of an instrument to procure an abortion. In the case of the woman herself, it must be shown that she was pregnant at the time if the attempt at abortion was made by herself. It is unlawful to supply poisons or instruments for the purpose of procuring an illegal abortion and it is unlawful to advertise goods in terms calculated to lead to their use in the procurement of such an abortion. It is lawful, however, to buy a Higginson's syringe and, indeed, a fitment which can be used to increase the length of such a syringe. It is also lawful to purchase soap, Lysol and Dettol, without restriction.

The Incidence of Criminal Abortion

There is no doubt that a considerable number of abortions are still procured by unqualified persons, and occasionally by qualified persons, in criminal circumstances. In 1939 the Interdepartmental Committee on Abortion estimated that the annual incidence of abortion in England and Wales was between 110,000 and 150,000 cases and there was reason to believe that about 40 per cent were the result of criminal interference. The situation regarding the incidence of criminal abortions since the coming into operation of the Abortion Act, 1967, is not clear, but opinion suggests that there are still a substantial number of illegal operations (*Lancet*, 9 Aug. 1969).

McDaniel and Krotki (1979), using special survey methods, studied the incidence of illegal abortion in Edmonton, Alberta. They estimated that in 1973 one conception in five ended in an illegal abortion. Francome (1977) tried to estimate the occurrence of illegal abortions after the Abortion Act 1967. On the basis that before the Act the number of abortions was 100,000, he estimated that the number of illegal abortions in 1973 in England and Wales was 8,000 and that this figure since then was likely to have decreased. Kahan *et al.* (1975) have shown that the effects in America of providing legal abortion had a corresponding fall in the number of illegal abortions.

When Davis (1950) reviewed a series of 2665 abortions, a consecutive series of patients under his personal care, his opinion was that only about 10 per cent were cases of spontaneous natural abortion. The choice of mode by the majority for self-induction was vaginal douching under pressure.

Teare (1951) reviewed a series of 89 deaths from abortion; 51 of these were unlawful.

Beric *et al.* (1973) in a review of morbidity due to legal and "other" abortions, showed that the mortality rate for "other" abortions in Yugoslavia was more than 100 times greater than for legal abortions. Therefore the likelihood of a doctor encountering death or illness after illegal abortion must still be anticipated.

Our experience is that since the Abortion Act, 1967 a death following abortion is a rare event. However such cases still occur and, therefore, the present account is deemed necessary information for the doctor, who has to deal with a sudden death in a woman of child-bearing age.

The Cause of Death following Criminal Abortion

Simpson (1949a) divided his series of 100 fatal cases into "immediate" deaths, "delayed" deaths and "remote" deaths. The major group, one of sixty-two cases, was that of "delayed" deaths and all of these were the result of infection, including eleven cases of infection by *Clostridium Welchii* and one by tetanus. There was no instance of fatal haemorrhage in this group.

The group of "immediate" deaths, which totalled thirty-four cases, included twenty-one due to air embolism and eleven due to vagal inhibition; there were two instances of fatal haemorrhage. Simpson (1949b) again drew attention to the then frequency of vagal inhibition due to criminal abortion.

Vagal inhibition is a hazard of criminal abortion, when carried out, as it almost always is, without anaesthesia and in circumstances of stress and haste. It can result from instrumental interference or the sudden injection of fluid, which is either too hot or too cold.

Immediate death following abortion is to be dreaded by victim and abortionist alike. If self-inflicted, the scene is often self-explanatory. The abortionist may conceal the apparatus and alter the scene but it is still necessary to explain the presence on the premises of a dead pregnant woman, whose body bears evidence of abortion, or attempted abortion. The possibility that the abortion had been self-induced elsewhere and the person went to the house to seek advice was raised in one case of death from air embolism. It was then a question as to whether the victim could have walked for a mile, after attempting to procure abortion in her own home. In view of the reports of delayed air embolism, although few (not then available) this possibility must be considered on future occasions.

Death following abortion in this area occurred in the following circumstances: air embolism, following syringing, four cases; perforation of the uterus and heavy infection, three cases, of which only one was within the last 10 years; shock due to syringing; shock and inhalation of gastric contents following syringing; shock due to digital dilatation of the cervix by the woman's husband; *Clostridium Welchii* infection; and uraemia, complicating septic abortion.

Although abortion other than therapeutic abortion is probably the result of criminal interference, it should not be forgotten that about 10 per cent are spontaneous, natural abortions. Moreover, there is the possibility that the death of a pregnant woman in circumstances which are distinctly suspicious can have been the result of an accident. Vaginal douching is not rarely practised for hygienic reasons and Forbes (1944) and Teare (1951) have each recorded a case in which this practice resulted in the entry of fluid and air into the uterus, to cause air embolism. Where douching is practised under pressure, as with a Higginson's syringe, about 40 ml of fluid at each squeeze of the bulb can be introduced under a pressure of as much as 28 cm of mercury or the eqʻivalent of 3 atmospheres. When the ball-valve end of the syringe be raised into froth, about 25 ml of air may be introduced into the uterus at each squeeze of the bulb (Teare, 1944).

The Methods used in Procuring Illegal Abortions

Although many methods have been devised to bring about abortion they fall into one of two principal groups, namely the application of violence, which may be general or local, or the administration of drugs. A proportion of abortions are the result of a combination of these methods. The inexperienced may first resort to drugs and, when these fail, some instrumental method is used.

General Violence

It is a popular belief that abortion is readily precipitated by violence and the pregnant woman must not be exposed to any undue exercise. No doubt abortion can be traced to some minor accident, for example, a trip over a rug, but in all probability it is merely a coincidence. It is certain that violence of severe degree can fail to disturb a pregnancy. The mother can be the victim of a motor accident and sustain multiple fractures and yet be delivered at term. One woman had the misfortune to sustain a fracture-dislocation of her neck. Despite this and the arduous treatment she had to undergo, she was successfully delivered at term. The case described by Wagner (cited Ogston, 1878) is yet another illustration. After applying a stout leather strap, a man then knelt on the woman's abdomen and compressed it with all his strength. He then trampled on her as she lay on her back. In spite of this she did not abort and recourse was had to local violence, with a pair of scissors. Although there was perforation of the uterus, with pain and haemorrhage, the woman not only survived this brutality but, it is alleged, the child was born at term.

The victim of poliomyelitis confined to an "iron lung" may yet be delivered at term of a healthy child, during a brief release from the apparatus.

Some of the past attempts by general violence, almost unbelievable because of their brutality, failed to cause abortion. Women have suffered serious bodily injuries, for example by falling headlong down a flight of stairs, without achieving their object. Tight lacing or violent kneading of the abdomen have also failed. It may still be the practice to indulge in severe exercise for example, horse riding or cycling, in the belief that it will induce abortion. All these attempts, however, are unlikely to be effective. The occasions on which abortion appears to result from accidents are often those of a trivial kind and the women are usually anxious to bear children. On the other hand, compensation or damages have been paid when an abortion followed a motor accident, although it was not clear whether traumatic or psychic shock caused the abortion (Hertig and Sheldon, 1943).

Injury to the child *in utero*, produced by general violence, is rarely described. We have experience of a case in which a pregnant girl's repeated attempts to dislodge a pregnancy by blows and falls on her abdomen was followed ultimately by the still-birth of the child, which at autopsy was found to have healing fractured ribs and brain damage (Seymour-Shove *et al.*, 1968).

Local Violence

The choice of method and its results will depend upon the skill of the operator. If used by a person possessed of medical knowledge and equipment, the method will approximate to therapeutic procedure. Its detection is then difficult because there may be no trace of interference and no septic or other complications. Unskilled attempts, however, may result in perforation of the vagina or uterus, in grave haemorrhage, sepsis or, it may be, sudden death, either from shock or air embolism.

It is true, as a general proposition, that women can and do procure their own abortions by local violence. The practicability of such self-abortion, however, depends upon the circumstances. The multipara, especially if she has some knowledge of her anatomy, can readily succeed and may do so without inflicting any injury upon herself. The primipara, if a young person, ignorant of both anatomy and procedure, will have great difficulty and is almost certain to injure herself, within the vagina alone or, if she passes the instrument into her womb, it is likely to cause injury also to the cervix and body of the womb. She may also injure her urethra and bladder. If the damage be limited to the body of the womb alone, when there is no injury to the vagina, cervix or bladder then, in my opinion, someone else, with anatomical knowledge, had assisted her (F.M. 3758A). It is regretted that Taylor (1948) did not give more details of the young girl who pushed the handle of a paint brush into her womb and succeeded in procuring her own abortion.

The well informed can introduce an instrument without causing any injury and succeed in procuring their own abortion. A well-educated woman, the mother of three children, procured her own abortion at about the 7th or 8th week by passing a sound into her uterus. When she informed her doctor, he expressed disbelief. She then produced a No. 16 sound and passed it, while under his observation. She had successfully procured her own abortion on another occasion, 3 years previously. She had been taught the method by a midwife (Anon., 1894).

On all occasions, however skilled the operator and adequate his facilities, criminal abortion is inevitably fraught with danger. The need of secrecy and haste and the criminal nature of the operation are bound to create an emotional disturbance in the mind of the victim which predisposes to shock. There are, it appears, certain operators who conduct their trade in circumstances which conform closely with surgical standards but most are compelled to interfere without the aid of anaesthesia or aseptic technique. No doubt their skill may then avert disaster, especially sudden death, but many of their victims are subsequently compelled to seek treatment, usually in hospital, either for haemorrhage or sepsis.

The medically trained abortionists are likely to use methods which ensure immediate and complete evacuation of the uterus, whereas the lay operator will use methods which aim only at rupture of the membranes and an inevitable abortion, which takes place, elsewhere, several hours later. Not rarely the victims may seek medical aid for the relief of bleeding, without disclosing the cause. If a sound is introduced, abortion is likely to occur whether the membranes are ruptured or not; when the membranes are ruptured abortion is inevitable. The interval at which abortion then takes place may range from minutes to days but it is usually at about 55 to 60 hours.

Instruments Used in Abortion

Many instruments have been used in attempts to procure abortion. A nursing sister had on more than one occasion successfully procured her own abortion by inserting her finger into the uterine cervix. The abortionist who has medical knowledge is likely to use the same instruments, for example, sounds, bougies or flushing curettes, as are used for therapeutic evacuation of a gravid uterus. Hat pins, paint brushes, knitting needles and even pokers, have been used by the lay operator who, however, was more likely to choose slippery elm bark.

Slippery elm bark was a favourite household remedy, where it was used as a demulcent drink. It can be purchased, without restriction, by members of the public, either in powder or in strips of the bark. The latter are sheets of about $9 \times 5 \times {}^1/_{10}$ in., and the soft wood is easily shaped with a penknife or table-knife into an instrument for abortion. When brought into contact with moisture a mucilage is formed; within a few minutes each side of the bark may bear a jelly-like layer as thick as the bark itself. This property makes the bark a self-lubricating instrument because the mucilage forms when in contact with the vaginal secretions, and the cervical canal is dilated when the bark is inserted. The disadvantages are that when sharply pointed it may be forced through the vaginal or uterine walls; it is not sterilised for use and therefore it may infect the uterus. Occasionally, either by accident or because of imperfect knowledge of the anatomy, the bark may be passed into the urethra and be lost in the bladder, whence it is retrieved some weeks or months later as an encrusted foreign body. Three examples, in one of which the foreign body measured $6 \times {}^1/_2$ in. were reported by Dodds and Mayeur (1939); a fourth, unpublished, was examined by Polson in 1933.

Instrumental methods may cause sudden death from cardiac inhibition as a result of vagal shock. Rough instrumental manipulation of the cervix of a person who is in an emotional state and not anaesthetised, is always attended by this risk. Septic endometritis and profuse haemorrhage are common complications. Occasionally, there is perforation of the vagina or uterus, followed by peritonitis, but, if the instrument is sterile, perforation of the uterus may not have any untoward result; this is not unknown in surgical practice.

Abortion by digital interference: shock due to dilatation of the cervix

Case Report:

A woman aged 23 died when alone with her husband. He admitted that 3 weeks earlier she had allowed him to attempt to procedure her abortion. She had bought some ether and he administered it to her on cotton wool. She lay on the bathroom floor and when she was "off" her husband swayed on her abdomen with one hand and put three fingers of his left hand into her vagina. Nothing happened, so he stopped. She regained consciousness, asked for a drink and was sick. She was then quite well. Three weeks later he agreed to try again. His wife undressed and lay on the bathroom floor on two pillows. Again he administered ether and he repeated his manipulation as before. She started to moan and gasp for breath. A small amount of blood escaped from the vagina, and she passed faeces. She went blue and then went limp, and ceased to breathe.

There were no external signs of asphyxia, nor any visible injury of the external genitalia. A little blood escaped from the vagina. She was pregnant at about the 24th week; a male foetus, weight 550 g. crown-heel length $11^3/_4$ in. was in the uterus. Recent bruising of the tissues of the left broad ligament and beside the cervix had occurred. The cervical canal was open and an index finger could be inserted for a distance of $^3/_4$ in. but beyond the canal only admitted the tip of the little finger. The cervix was $1^1/_2$ in. long and firm. She was a parous woman. The mucus plug had been displaced, the membranes had ruptured and the amniotic fluid had escaped. A single oval placenta, $4^1/_2 \times 3 \times 1$ in. was situated in the right half of the back of the uterus; its lower border had been detached for a distance of about 2 in. The appearances were those of recent interference. There were no signs of infection. A shallow scratch, $1^3/_4$ in. long by $^1/_5$ in., was present in the mucosa of the posterior vaginal fornix.

The lungs were collapsed and the lower lobes were congested, but there was no visible disease.

There was no evidence of syringing or the use of slippery elm. No perforation or laceration had occurred; the vaginal scratch could have been caused by a fingernail.

The opinion given was that there had been digital interference, but that the changes found were inconsistent with self-induction of abortion. The possibility of amniotic embolism was considered, but an examination of thirty-six samples of lung was entirely negative. Death was presumed due to shock (F.M. 4176A; *R.* v. *Scarr*, 1955).

Syringing Methods

The enema syringe has been used frequently in the past as an instrument of abortion. The standard Higginson's syringe may be used or its nozzle may be exchanged for one which is long and slender, to facilitate entry of the uterus. Abortion can be produced by injection of sterile water, since the method depends essentially on a mechanical separation of the membranes and placenta by a fluid wedge driven between them and the uterine wall (Figs. 160, 161). In practice, however, soapy solution is often used, possibly as a lubricant or irritant; other operators favour solutions of Lysol, pearl ash or Dettol, presumably to disinfect the parts.

There is no doubt that a high proportion of successful abortions result from syringing. The morbidity rate is high but the mortality rate, despite the dangers of the method, is low, possibly because, when self-applied, the fluid only enters the vagina and does not reach the uterus.

Two major risks attach to this method. Rough insertion of the syringe into the cervix, or rapid injection of cold or unduly hot fluid, may cause sudden death from vagal inhibition. This may also follow rapid separation of the placenta, which is likely to cause severe pain (F.M. 6951A Polson).

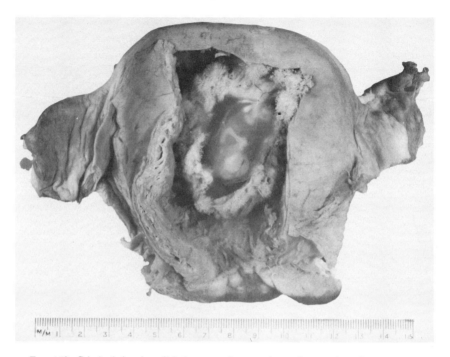

FIG. 160. Criminal abortion: dislodgement of mucus plug and separation of the choriori frondosum (death from air embolism: syringing).

The other risk, probably a common cause of sudden death in these circumstances, is air embolism (F.M. 892 and 2739). So long as the syringe is completely filled with fluid during use this will not arise but, in the haste which attends these operations, it is easy for the bulb to be filled with a mixture of air and fluid. The distal end of the syringe may be lifted into the foam of a soapy solution or completely leave the container. It then requires only a few squeezes of the bulb to drive a lethal quantity of air into the uterus. If, as is likely, the edge of the placenta has already been stripped, even by an inch, the venous spaces are opened and the air passes forthwith into the circulation. The danger is appreciably greater later in the pregnancy, i.e. at 24 weeks or later, when the vessels may be as much as $^1/_5$ in. in diameter. Collapse, in about 2 minutes, and death, by the end of about 10 minutes follow the entry of air. It is said delay in the onset of symptoms can occur. This is possible only if the victim be at rest and the air is temporarily locked in the uterus. As soon as the woman begins to move about, transfer of the air to the heart takes only a matter of seconds. If the amount of air is sufficient to kill, a matter of about 100 cm^3, the heart beats it into a foam, which effectively and promptly obstructs the pulmonary circulation. Deaths from cerebral or coronary embolism in these circumstances are rare and the victims are likely to have a defect in the auricular or ventricular septa.

The danger of perforation during syringing is remote so long as the ordinary nozzle of an enema (Higginson's) syringe is used. It is otherwise if a special nozzle or an adaptor is used since this increases the normal length from just over 2 in. ($2^1/_{10}$ in. to $2^1/_5$ in. from the mouth to the base of the collar) to one of about $4^1/_2$ in. Adaptors could be bought by the public whereby the syringe is thus lengthened for vaginal douching.

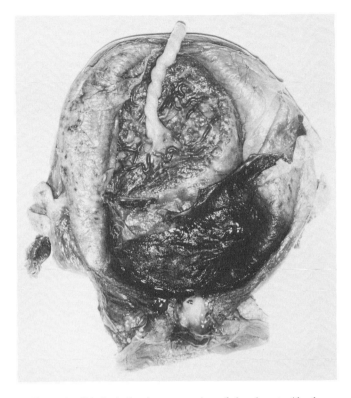

FIG. 161. Criminal abortion: separation of the placenta (death
from air embolism: syringing).

It is not necessary for the nozzle to have a less blunt end than that of the normal model. It was found that when the normal nozzle was held by the index finger and thumb it was possible to push it into the wall of a pregnant uterus by using only firm pressure. Counter-pressure with the other hand outside the uterus greatly facilitated perforation with the nozzle (Fig. 162).

If, therefore, a normal nozzle be inserted into the cervical canal until its collar is flush with the cervix, it is possible for this agent to perforate the back of the womb, the more so if the operator's other hand presses upon the abdomen to provide counter-pressure on the uterus (F.M. 3758A Polson).

Perforation of the vagina is more likely; Dodds and Mayeur (1939) recorded a case in which the nozzle was pushed through the vaginal fornix. This accident is normally avoided by the abortionist by passing his index finger into the vagina and then sliding the nozzle beside his finger, into the external os. He may hold the nozzle between his index and second fingers with the end of the nozzle just beyond his finger tips, as demonstrated by an abortionist in the witness box (F.M. 3758A).

Mobility of the Victim of Air Embolism; Delayed Air Embolism

The accident of air embolism during attempted abortion normally causes immediate collapse and rapid death, i.e. within minutes. Sufficient time may elapse for the woman to

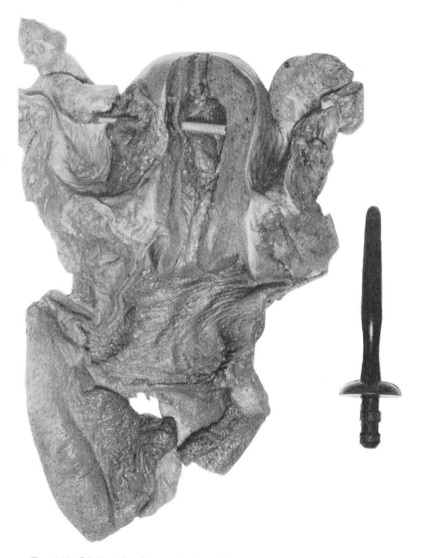

FIG. 162. Criminal abortion: perforation of the uterus by nozzle of a Higginson's
syringe (a probe is inserted through the track). Death from peritonitis.

take a few paces or to replace the syringe on a hook or, possibly, throw it on the fire.

It is now beyond doubt that *delayed death from air embolism* in criminal abortion has occurred. Simpson (1958) has recorded the case of a woman aged 35 who collapsed and died in a toilet. Her death was due to air embolism following syringing. She had been under direct observation for at least 2 hours prior to her death, because she was working as a cook in the company of several other persons, in circumstances which precluded privacy. It is probable that the interval between instrumentation was even longer and that had occurred during the previous night or earlier on the morning of the day of her death, which occurred at about 3 p.m. Gormsen (1960) has had four cases of abortion with a symptom-free interval of several hours between syringing and death. The circumstantial evidence of at least one left no doubt that no additional interference could have occurred during the interval between the syringing and the death. Another example was recorded by Shapiro (1965).

Simonin (1955) recognised three clinical forms of fatal air embolism: (a) sudden death, in the course of a few minutes; (b) slow death, at any time between 12 and 24 hours: loss of consciousness and the commencement of symptoms—convulsions and paralysis—occur immediately, but persist for some time; (c) delayed embolism, produced in two stages, separated by a clear interval: the air does not reach the heart until some time—sometimes several hours—after the injection.

Delayed air embolism does occur, but its mechanism has yet to be explained. The air is held in some fashion in the uterus until such time that placental separation opens vessels to allow it to pass into the circulation. The mucus plug could possibly prevent escape via the cervix.

A dogmatic opinion which denies the possibility of the occurrence of delayed embolism, like most, if not all, dogmatic opinions, is dangerous. (In the case of *R.* v. *King* (1952) (Polson) I expressed the view that there was no delay; in the circumstances of that case I believe I was right.) On all occasions where delayed air embolism is alleged, it requires the support of strong, if not unequivocal, circumstantial evidence. Otherwise an abortionist may be left free to ply his or her nefarious trade, to the danger of other women.

Although a fatal issue is the normal result of air embolism, it is not invariable. Not a little depends on the amount of air introduced. The victim may suffer no ill-effects when the amount is small or, with larger, sublethal amounts, there may be a temporary respiratory crisis, with or without convulsions, and then recovery.

The Lethal Dose of Air

The volume of air required to kill was considered by Forbes (1944). There is no doubt that normally it must be appreciable, approximating to the capacity of the right heart or at least that of the pulmonary trunk. In that event, it is of the order of at least 100 ml, as noted by Dible *et al.* (1938) in reports of fatal cases. A volume of 480 ml, as estimated from animal experiments, or one as little as 10 ml are extreme limits. The actual amount which kills is modified by the general condition of the victim and more so by the rate at which the air is introduced. Whatever the volume, the amount which reaches and collects in the circulation must be sufficient to cause a substantial air lock in the heart, the pulmonary trunk or both pulmonary arteries. Except in an enfeebled or gravely ill subject, it is unlikely that obstruction of one pulmonary artery is enough to kill. Slow but continued embolism, if it results in cumulative cerebral embolism, is another variant, but in the absence of a patent foramen ovale, cerebral air embolism is rarely the cause, or even a factor, in death from air embolism.

A simple but effective apparatus was designed in Copenhagen for the measurement of the volume of air in the heart and the collection of a sample for analysis (Gormsen, 1960).

Examples

Abortion by Syringing: Death from Air Embolism

The deceased, a woman of 28, collapsed and died at the house of a known abortionist. There were no external injuries, nor was there any injury to the vagina. The cervix was that of a parous woman and the canal was widened, so that a tip of the finger could be inserted in the lower part and scissors were then readily passed onwards into the uterus. The mucous plug had been displaced, but there were remains of it at the upper end of the canal, acting as a ball valve to prevent the escape of fluid from the uterus. The uterine cavity contained about 4 oz of red-brown, watery fluid in which there were scanty bubbles. The placenta was attached to the anterior wall of the uterus and there had been separation of its lower border by about 1 in. The membranes were intact and contained a male foetus, 1050 g, i.e. at about the 6th to 7th month of pregnancy. No bubbles of gas were seen in the pelvic veins, but when the right heart, which was dilated, was opened dark frothy blood was present, and a similar condition was noted in the blood in the pulmonary trunk and both pulmonary arteries. Bubbles of air were also seen in the veins of the neck.

The defence suggested that this woman had syringed herself in her own home and had walked to the house of the abortionist for advice. The distance travelled, when checked by a healthy policewoman, took 15 minutes. It was my opinion that the deceased could not have walked this distance after syringing herself, so as to cause air embolism.

Since 1952, as was mentioned earlier, a few instances of unequivocal delayed air embolism have been recorded and, on the face of it, my opinion might have been wrong. Reflecting on the case, however I think it would have been impossible for this woman to have covered the distance and yet retain in her uterus the quantity of fluid which was found there. The ball valve action of the mucus plug could well have retained it if the woman was at rest, i.e. had she collapsed and died at the abortionist's house immediately after syringing, but it would have been insufficient to retain the fluid in an erect woman walking a distance of about a mile.

The accused was found to be guilty and sentenced to 4 years' imprisonment.

(F.M. 2739 Polson; Fig. 160; *R. v. King*, Leeds Assizes 1952.)

Attempted Abortion by Syringing: Death from Shock

This was a woman aged 20, who collapsed and died suddenly after abortion had been attempted by syringing. There was a little bloodstained material on the skin around the anus and genitalia, but no local bleeding point, other than a mildly varicosed anal vein, was found to account for it. There was no escape of blood from the vagina, nor was there any injury of the external genitalia. The woman's face was slightly dusky and one or two small petechial haemorrhages were observed in the eyelids of the right eye; there were none on the left side or face.

The peritoneum was healthy. The uterus was also healthy externally. The fundus was at a hand's breadth above the pelvis. The uterine cervix was scarred by a former pregnancy, but showed no recent injury. A little tag of opaque elastic material projected from the external os. The cervix was $1^1/_2$ in. long and $^1/_4$ in. thick and the canal was $^1/_3$ in. in diameter. It was closed by a plug of tenacious, jelly-like material, slightly yellow in colour. No displacement was apparent, nor was there now any evidence of the track of the passage of the nozzle of the syringe. The membranes were intact and contained a female foetus, 327 g, $9^1/_8$ in. crown-heel length, representing one at about the 12th week of gestation. There was no evidence of infection. The placenta was attached to the right and posterior walls of the uterus and the lower border of it had been separated for a distance of about $1^1/_2$ in. In the space between the placenta and the uterus there was a little red-brown fluid, of which only about $^1/_2$ g was available for examination. There was no evidence of blood from this region between it and the cervix. A single healthy placenta, $4^3/_4$ in. diameter, was present.

Proof of attempted abortion in this case rested primarily upon the scientific investigation. Dr. A. S. Curry was able to recover soap from the small sample of blood obtained from within the uterus and to demonstrate that it was the same kind of soap as that found in a pan and elsewhere at the house of the deceased, and in a bag, the property of the accused. His keen sense of smell was able to identify the fact that the fluid in the uterus still retained the smell of this soap.

A woman was found guilty of attempted abortion and her son was found guilty of aiding and abetting this attempted abortion. They received, respectively, sentences of $4^1/_2$ years and 18 months. (F.M. 6951A Polson; *R. v. Buck and Buck*, Leeds Assizes, March 1960.)

[The medico-legal demonstration of soap abortion and soap intoxication was discussed at length, supported by a comprehensive bibliography, by Schwerd (1959).]

Abortion by Syringing: Perforation of the Uterus and Death from Septicaemia

This girl, aged 17, had first attempted abortion with "female" pills and had then sought the assistance of an abortionist. She was admitted to hospital complaining of generalised abdominal pain of 48 hours' duration; her bowels had not been open for 3 days; she had been sick and had passed very little urine. Examination detected generalised abdominal tenderness and tenderness in the Pouch of Douglas. She received vigorous antibiotic treatment, but deteriorated. Her blood urea rose from 106 mg to 256 mg per cent. The pus from the vagina contained *bacillus coli* and *staphylococcus albus*. The patient was incoherent throughout and could not make a dying declaration.

Post-mortem examination demonstrated peritonitis and septicaemia due to perforation of the uterus (Fig. 162). The uterus was now empty and contracted, so as to be $3^1/_4$ in. from fundus to cervix. There was inflammatory exudate on its surface and a ragged opening, 1 in. in diameter, was present on the left side of the back of the uterus, centred 1 in. below the fundus and 1 in. internal to the left cornu. It was a circular hole covered by chocolate-brown inflammatory material. Probe examination demonstrated free communication with the interior of the uterus. The appearances were those of a perforation by an instrument, enlarged by inflammation and necrosis of tissue. The uterus still contained brown-coloured fragments of necrotic products of conception. The cervical canal was $^1/_4$ in. in diameter, and there was no injury to the cervix or the vagina. It was estimated that peritonitis had existed for about 7 days.

An incidental finding was ante-mortem digestion of the oesophagus.

The appearances were consistent with an abortion having procured at about the 3rd month and with a rod-like instrument by an unskilled operator. It could have been the nozzle of a Higginson's syringe, the more so if that had been lengthened by an adaptor. It was believed that this injury was unlikely to have been self-induced in the circumstances. Had she used a knitting needle, it was more likely that she would have perforated the vagina.

The accused admitted in the witness box that he had attempted her abortion with a Higginson's syringe and demonstrated the manner in which he inserted the nozzle into the cervix. It seems probable that by excessive pressure from below, accompanied by pressure on the abdomen, he had caused the nozzle to perforate the uterus. Since it was suggested by the defence that she had said she would use a knitting needle and that this injury was due to a rod-like instrument, sufficient doubt was thrown upon the matter to acquit the accused of the charge of her manslaughter. He was found guilty of attempted abortion (F.M. 3758A Polson).

Abortion Pastes

Abortion is sometimes procured by the injection of a prepared paste into the uterus. Interruptin which contains iodine and thymol is an example. The use of this paste is not without risk, because it may lead to death from fat or air embolism or poisoning.

Another paste, recommended for medical use, is a soap medicated with iodine, potassium iodide and thymol. It is supplied in a collapsible tube with a uterine applicator and a turn-key, to empty the tube during injection. It is an effective local method of induction of labour at full term and is also used when evacuation is deemed necessary to save the life of a nephritic or tuberculous patient. The dose ranges from 10 to 30 cm³, according to the stage of gestation; the tube is marked to show the amount expelled. The injection is usually uneventful. The patient should experience little change during the ensuing 12 hours but abortion, preceded by moderate pain and bleeding, takes place in from 20 to 36 hours. It is claimed by the makers that no complications occur "in the great majority of cases", but some patients may subsequently require curettage. There is no fat or air in the paste and the manufacturers state that there is no danger of embolism from its use. The amount of iodine not exceeding 2 per cent, precludes poisoning. It is, however, made clear that care and skill must be exercised. The injection should be slow, at a rate not exceeding 2 cm³ per minute. These claims are substantially confirmed by a colleague, who has had occasion to subject the paste to clinical trial. Some regard the method as unsuitable for clinical use.

Abortion by Drugs

Many substances have been used to procure abortion, but evidence of their value is scanty and unsatisfactory. The essence of the matter is that successful use of drugs for this purpose is likely only when they are taken in quantities which are dangerous to life.

The drugs belong either to the group of emmenagogues, i.e. those alleged to hasten the menstrual flow, or they are ecbolics, i.e. drugs which increase the power of uterine contraction. Emmenagogues are further subdivided into those which act directly upon the uterine muscle and those which have an indirect action, for example, reflexly, by causing pelvic and intestinal congestion.

David (1974) examined several different preparations which were on sale as abortifacients. Most contained the traditional substances, such as apiol and tansy. Several women had used a synthetic vasopressive nasal spray.

Emmenagogues Having a Direct Action on the Uterus

This is the largest and least effective group. It includes a number of vegetable poisons, many of ancient repute as abortifacients—Savin from the *Juniperus sabina*, Tansy, Penny Royal, Rue, Broom, Laburnum, Hellebore, *Anemone pulsatilla* and so on. Saffron, an established abortifacient in Germany, was responsible for several deaths (Fasal and Wachner, 1933). To those interested in gardening the list is reminiscent of a nurseryman's catalogue.

Cantharides has also been used but it is likely to be effective only when taken in highly dangerous doses. Apiol, an extract of parsley, is reputed to have been successful in no less than sixteen of twenty attempted abortions. There is a difference of opinion concerning its effectiveness, whether with or without the production also of toxic symptoms (Schifferli, 1938) but fatalities are rare (Trillat *et al.*, 1931).

Emmenagogues Having an Indirect Action on the Uterus

These drugs are purgatives which, when taken in excessive doses, may induce abortion. Aloes and colocynth take pride of place. Hiera picra (Holy bitter) is a mixture of aloes (4 parts), and canella bark (1 part); the latter is an aromatic added to minimise the disagreeably bitter taste of the aloes. Pill Cochia is a mixture of aloes, $1^1/_3$, and colocynth, $^2/_3$, Castor oil, epsom salts; even croton oil have been used. Indian brandy, also in this group, is a mixture, without any brandy, of rhubarb and spirit of nitrous ether. It was used in Leeds and one inevitable abortion is known to the author as a possible result of its use.

A subsidiary group of indirect emmenagogues includes so-called tonics, notably iron. "Widow Welch's" pills, for example, which are popular in some quarters, are one-half (52.5 per cent) composed of iron sulphate, one-quarter excipient and with about 5 per cent each of elecampane, a substitute for digitalis, curcuma, an aromatic root used in curry powders, liquorice and sulphur. Other remedies are "Dr. Reed's" extra strong female pills or his female mixture, marketed by a firm in London.

Potassium permanganate, in the form of pills, was once favoured. This substance returned to popularity in recent years, and was apparently widely used abroad, as a local abortifacient. A tablet of potassium permanganate was inserted into the vagina and, in due course, bleeding occured. The patient then visited her doctor, who was led to believe she was threatened with abortion. On occasion this diagnosis has been accepted or confirmed without any satisfactory investigation, and the uterus evacuated. It would have been found, however, that bleeding was due to ulceration of the vaginal fornix or the cervix; the changes may be such that they resemble a chancre or a carcinoma of the cervix.

Recognition of the cause is important because adequate local treatment of the ulcer is alone required; the pregnancy is to be left to take its normal course. Evacuation of the uterus is not the correct treatment.

This practice was not recorded in England until 1951 when Miller (1951) said he had seen about ten cases in Croydon.

Ecbolics

It may be that some of the indirect emmenagogues are also ecbolics. Savin, lead and mercury are said to have this property. Despite the fact that diachylon is no longer readily available to the public, those who propose to use lead can purchase machine-spread plasters of lead oleate and make pills of material scraped from the plaster.

This group includes the three most effective abortifacients, namely ergot which is a true ecbolic, pituitrin, which has a specific action on the gravid uterus, and quinine. A doctor was alleged to have supplied a noxious thing, namely ergometrine, to a patient to enable her to procure her abortion. His successful defence, apparently, was that there was a possibility she might unexpectedly have a haemorrhage and he might not be able to attend her promptly. As a safeguard, therefore, he had prescribed ergometrine (*R. v. P... W.*, Leeds Assizes, 1959).

Therapeutic abortion was sometimes practised by the administration of quinine, castor oil and pituitrin. The treatment began with a dose of 2 fluid ounces of castor oil followed, 6 hours later, by quinine hydrochloride. The latter was repeated at the end of another seven and again at the end of 9 hours. Next morning the course concluded with an injection of piturin, 0.5 ml. The results were disappointing, especially early in pregnancy.

Abortion and the Medical Practitioner

(a) *The General Practitioner* Women intent upon abortion may go to some trouble to mislead a practitioner in the hope that he will make an examination which they believe might result in abortion. They may complain of displacement of the womb and hope an instrument will be passed to rectify it. More often it is likely they have received attention from an abortionist and consult their doctor for uterine bleeding, in the expectation he will treat the threatened or incomplete abortion by emptying the uterus. No doubt this may have to be done but no practitioner should attempt it in his surgery. There might be a disaster, as once happened; two doctors later found themselves charged with manslaughter. It also opens the door to the possibility of blackmail. The moment a doctor suspects that an abortion is impending or is complete, the patient should be advised to undergo treatment at the hands of a specialist in a hospital or nursing home.

(b) *Medical Practitioners in Hospital* Although the situation may arise in. general practice, it is more probable that the problem of disclosure of criminal abortion will confront a member of a hospital staff. The Royal College of Physicians (1916) published resolutions for the guidance of medical practitioners. This document has no legal sanction and is not the law, but practitioners will bear the recommendations in mind. The College took the view that the practitioner has a moral obligation to respect the confidence of his patient and, therefore, disclosure of the fact that she had been the subject of a criminal abortion is permissible only with her consent; notwithstanding that any act or omission on his part which conceals a felony is a misdemeanour. On all occasions, before reporting the matter to the police, a practitioner, especially one who is as yet inexperienced, should obtain a second opinion, preferably from his defence society.

If the patient is about to die, the practitioner should ask her if she wishes to make a statement. Its importance should be pointed out to her, but if she refuses, the doctor should not press for one. If taken, the rules which apply to dying declarations must be observed.

If the patient dies the doctor must report the death to the coroner or the police because he cannot certify it as due to natural causes.

Post-mortem Evidence of Criminal Abortion

A pathologist carrying out an autopsy in a case of suspected criminal abortion must, of course, bear in mind the special requirements of an autopsy on any pregnant woman's body; not least because he may find himself at a later stage subjected to stringent cross-examination in Court. Rushton and Dawson (1982) detail the procedure at these autopsies and their review should be consulted.

Abortion by Drugs

Toxicological analysis may detect the drug and determine the probable quantity, if recently taken. Bodily changes may be consistent with poisoning by an abortifacient; most of these substances are gastro-intestinal irritants.

Instrumental Abortion

Proof must rest upon signs of tearing or perforation of a part of the genital tract. A perforation of the posterior vaginal fornix or the posterior or a lateral wall of the uterus, followed by death from peritonitis or severe local inflammation, points to interference by an unskilled operator. Rupture due to disease must be excluded by microscopy. The introduction of penicillin has reduced the fatalities from this cause and they are now uncommon.

Abortion by Syringing

When abortion by syringing is self-induced, the victim may be found dead in a posture consistent with recent use of a syringe. The instrument and a bowl of fluid may be near the body; occasionally, the deceased woman had had time to put these things away before she collapsed nearby.

When induced by another person, steps may be taken to make the death appear to have been due to natural causes. It is possible, however, that in her haste or panic, the abortionist may fail to remove the articles of her trade. On other occasions, a relative or friend, having found the victim dead of self-induced abortion, may interfere with the scene; for example, the syringe may be destroyed in the fire.

Circumstances which point to self-induced abortion do not exclude the possibility of an accident occurring during hygienic douching, and undue haste to presume criminality is therefore to be avoided (Teare, 1951).

Syringing is demonstrated by the following changes. The mucous plug in the cervix is usually displaced or disintegrated. The cervical canal may be dilated and injured. Fluid, which may be foamy, lies in a space between the uterine wall and the foetal membranes. Partial detachment of the edge of the placenta, with separation by an inch or more, is also common. Bubbles of gas may be traced in the venous system, from the sides of the uterus up to the right heart, which, with the pulmonary trunk and pulmonary arteries may contain foamy blood. More bubbles may be found in the branches of the pulmonary artery within the lung. Some air may have been carried to the cerebral vessels at the surface of the brain; there may be air also in the coronary arteries. In general, however, unless there is a septal defect in the heart e.g. a patent foramen ovale, air does not reach the systemic circulation or, if it does so, the amount in it is negligible. The air lock which causes these sudden deaths is essentially and unequivocally that which forms in the main pulmonary vessels and heart; these deaths are rarely due to cerebral or coronary embolism. It is easy to demonstrate bubbles in the vessels on the surface of most brains, after the calvarium has been removed; this is a common artifact which is difficult to prevent.

The fluid in the uterus is likely to be red or dark red, rather like dark red ink. Examination may detect the presence of soap or a cresol, together with blood. The right heart blood, as Teare (1951) has pointed out, may contain approximately twice the normal amount of cresols, but the value of this investigation has yet to be established. Teare also considered the examination of the blood in order to determine its content of fibrinolysin, which, if unduly high, may confirm the fact of sudden death. This point has value when it is contended that the abortion was induced at a place distant from that at which the victim died.

Syringing may occasionally be complicated by perforation of the uterus; the late Dr. Grace once examined a victim in whom the syringe had been pushed through the uterine fundus and I have had a case in which the normal nozzle of a Higginson's syringe was pushed through the back of the uterus (F.M. 3758A, Fig. 162).

The histological and other features of the detection of soap abortions were reviewed by Schwerd (1965).

Septic Abortion of Criminal Origin

When death is due to, or accelerated by, septic abortion, the death is likely to take place several days after the abortion was induced. If there was no gross interference at the time, all trace of it will have cleared, or will be obscured by the subsequent inflammation. In such circumstances it is obvious that criminality rests solely on suspicion, which does not permit the institution of criminal proceedings. If a charge is preferred, proof by medical evidence is unlikely or difficult (Warrack, 1963).

Amniocentesis

Papers (Cameron and Dayan, 1966 and Dayan *et al.*, 1967) report cases of infarction of the brain in the hippocampal region and mid-line of the brain-stem, of patients who had undergone attempted therapeutic abortion by the amniotic fluid replacement technique. The cause of the damage is thought to be cerebral oedema and systemic anoxia.

Fabricated Abortion

On rare occasions the victim of an assault may endeavour to exaggerate the offence by alleging that it caused her to abort. Some ingenuity may be shown. One woman acquired the foetus of a dog, chopped off the tail and legs, and presented it as a human foetus of about the 3rd month of gestation. The legend has it that the unsuspecting doctor, in attendance, waited an hour for the delivery of the placenta. On another occasion a woman borrowed two human foetuses, possibly in the belief that truth is reinforced by plenty. Her plan failed, however, because a difference in age was at once apparent in the alleged twins; the two foetuses were, respectively, at about the 3rd and 5th months of gestation. There are obvious difficulties in the way of success in these attempts.

Extra-uterine Pregnancy: Simulation of Criminal Abortion

The symptoms and signs of extra-uterine pregnancy may give rise to the suspicion of criminal interference. In the case reported below it so happened that the patient had been under medical observation and, at the time of the disaster, she was in hospital. Had she been elsewhere, there is a probability that, until the autopsy, strong suspicion of attempted abortion might have arisen.

The patient was a woman aged 21. She first came under observation on 31 August, 1943 when she complained of abdominal pain. Her periods had been irregular for a year. The initial diagnosis was one of twisted ovarian cyst. She appeared to be in no serious danger and a pre-operative enema at 5 a.m. yielded a satisfactory result. Three-quarters of an

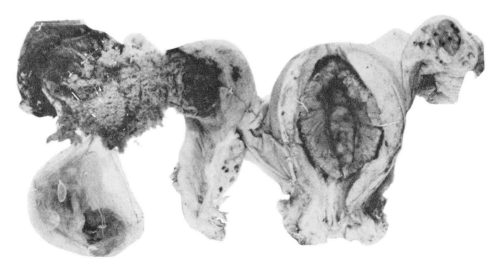

FIG. 163. Ectopic pregnancy in rudimentary horn of a bicornuate uterus. Rupture of the horn. Death from intraperitoneal haemorrhage.

hour later she called for a bed pan. While using it she became faint and collapsed. Half an hour later she was restless and complained of abdominal pain. She was then cold, pale and pulseless. Free fluid was detected in her abdomen. Her condition deteriorated rapidly and she died at 6.45 a.m. on 3 September.

The post-mortem examination demonstrated massive intraperitoneal haemorrhage due to rupture of an ectopic gestation, which had occurred in a rudimentary horn of a bicornuate uterus (P.M. 4362; Polson Fig. 163).

References

ANON (1894) *Med. Record*, **45**, 776.
ARNOLD, M. E. (1951) *Brit. Med. J.*, **i**, 760.
BERIC, B. KUPRESANIN, M. and KAPOR-STANULOVIC, N. (1973) *Amer. J. Obstet. Gynec.* **116**, 813–821.
CAMERON, J. M. and DAYAN, A. D. (1966) *Brit. Med. J.*, **1**, 1010.
DAVID, T. J. (1974) *Med. Sci. Law*, **14**, 120–123.
DAVIS, A. (1950) *Brit. Med. J.*, **ii**, 123–30.
DAYAN, A. D., CAMERON, J. M. and PHILLIPP, E. (1967) *Med. Sci. Law*, **7**, 70.
DIBLE, J. H., HEWER, T. F., ROSS, A. O. F. and WALSH, C. H. (1938) *Lancet*, **i**, 313.
DODDS, R. L. and MAYEUR, M. H. (1939) *Brit. Med. J.*, **i**, 921–2.
FORBES, G. (1944) *Brit. Med. J.*, **ii**, 529–31.
FRANCOME, C. (1977) *J. Biosoc. Sci.*, **9**(4), 467–479.
GORMSEN, H. (1960) 2nd Internat. Meeting on Forensic Path. and Med.; *Program and Abstracts*, p. 42.
HERTIG, A. T. and SHELDON, W. H. (1943) *Ann. Sug.*, **117**, 596–606; also *Abstr. Med.-leg. Rev.*, **11**, 153.
KAHAN, R. S. *et al.*, (1975) *Amer. J. Obstet. Gynec.*, **121**(1).
LANCET, Leading Article (1969) *Lancet*, **ii** (Aug.), 89.
MCDANIEL, S. A. and KROTKI, K. J. (1979) *Can. J. Public Health*, **70**(6), 393–398.
MILLER, J. C. (1951) *Brit. Med. J.*, **i**, 526.
OGSTON, F. (1878) Lectures on Medical Jurisprudence, ed. F. Ogston, Jr. London: Churchill.
ROYAL COLLEGE OF PHYSICIANS (1916) *Brit. Med. J.*, **i**, 207.
RUSHTON, D. I. and DAWSON, I. M. P. (1982) *J. Clin. Path.* **35**, 909–921.
SCHIFFERLI, E. (1938) *Dtsch. Z. ges. gerichtl. Med.*, **30**, 55–58.
SCHWERD, W. (1959) *Dtsch. Z. ges. gerichtl. Med.*, **48**, 202–46.
SCHWERD, W. (1965) in *Methods of Forensic Science*, **4**, 249, ed. A. S. Curry London: Interscience.
SEYMOUR-SHOVE, R., GEE, D. J. and CROSS, A. P. (1968) *Brit. Med. J.*, **1**, 686.
SHAPIRO, H. A. (1965) *J. Forens. Med.*, **2**, 3.
SIMONIN, C. (1955) *Medicine Legale Judiciaire*, 3rd ed., p. 425. Paris: Maloine.
SIMPSON, C. K. (1949a) *Lancet*, **i**, 47.
SIMPSON, C. K. (1949b) *Lancet*, 558.
SIMPSON, C. K. (1958) *Med.-leg. J.* (Camb.), **26**, 132–4.
TAYLOR, A. S. (1948) Principles and Practice of Medical Jurisprudence, 10th ed. vol, ii, p. 114. Sydney Smith. London: Churchill.
TEARE, R. D. (1944) *Lancet*, **ii**, 242.
TEARE, R. D. (1951) *Med.-leg. J.* (Camb.), **19**, 81–88.
TEARE, R. D. (1964) *Med. Sci. Law*, **4**, 177.
TRILLAT, P., MICHON, L., and THIERS, H. (1931) *Bull. Soc. belge Gynec. Obstet.*, **20**, 615.
WARRACK, A. J. N. (1963) *Med. Sci. Law*, **3**, 207.
WATKINS, R. E. (1933) *Amer. J. Obstet. Gynec.*, **26**, 161–72.

CHAPTER 15

Infanticide and Child Destruction

UNTIL 1922 the unlawful killing of a newly-born infant was (in any circumstances) murder. This made no allowance for the fact that the effects of delivery may temporarily disturb the balance of the mother's mind and she would not then be responsible if, at that time, her act or omission led to the destruction of her child. The Infanticide Act, 1922, which created the crime of infanticide, made provision for this possibility but failed to define "newly-born" nor did it take into account the further possibility that lactation may also cause temporary mental unbalance. The Act was repealed and re-enacted, with amendments, in 1938. There is no such Act in Scotland but provision was made in Scots law to take into account the mental state of the offender, long before English law considered this aspect (Mason, 1978).

The Infanticide Act, 1938, section 1, enacts that "Where a woman by any wilful act or omission causes the death of her child being a child under the age of 12 months, but at the time of the act or omission the balance of her mind was disturbed by reason of her not having fully recovered from the effect of giving birth to the child or by reason of the effect of lactation consequent upon the birth of the child, then, notwithstanding that the circumstances were such that but for this Act the offence would have amounted to murder . . ." she is guilty of the felony of infanticide and may be dealt with and punished as if she had committed manslaughter. Provision is also made whereby, if she be indicted for murder, the alternative verdicts of manslaughter, guilty but insane or concealment of birth are within the power of the jury.

The charge of infanticide, in practice, is likely to succeed only on the clearest evidence of deliberate killing. The law, moreover, presumes the child to have been still-born until the contrary be proved. The mother is given the full benefit of any doubt and, in consequence, many of those who are charged with infanticide are convicted only of concealment of birth.

Infanticide is most likely to be committed by a young unmarried woman, although there may be a motive for infanticide by married women. Allowance is made for inexperience of the mother and the circumstances of the birth, which is likely to take place in secret; this prejudices the survival of the infant because of the lack of adequate care and attention. A mother who finds herself alone in labour, might experience panic and inadvertently destroy the child; on the other hand, it is possible for a woman to give birth at noon and be on night-duty the same day. The factors of drink, drugs, or natural illness causing a fainting attack or a fit have also to be taken into account. Eclampsia or puerperal mania must be excluded.

Asch and Rubin (1974) described the psychological basis of infanticide and child battering as one of several different forms of postpartum psychological reaction. d'Orban (1979) reviewed the cases of 89 women admitted to a prison over a six-period, having killed or attempted to kill their natural children. Eleven of the women had killed their children within 24 hours of the birth. They were found to be the least likely to have social or psychiatric disturbances and were younger than the other women. d'Orban drew attention to the fact that although these women are the most likely to be dealt with under the Infanticide Act, they are not suffering from mental disorder as defined by the Mental Health Act, 1959.

Kukull *et al.* (1977) studied the hypothesis that a majority of S.I.D.S. cases were actually homicides but found no evidence to support this view. They base their opinion on the finding that the rate of increase of known numbers of infant homicides showed no alteration after the condition of S.I.D.S. was recognised in 1963.

Although secret disposal of the remains may strengthen the evidence of infanticide, it is likely that it will serve only to establish a charge of concealment of birth.

Proof of a separate existence, an essential ingredient of infanticide, is notoriously difficult and for this reason alone the charge is likely to fail.

It is material to know the mode of birth, because an abnormal presentation adds to the natural risks run by the infant. If, however, the mother alleges the birth to have been a breech delivery and the infant's lungs are fully expanded, the probability is that it not only was a live-birth but also it was not a breech delivery.

In the absence of a history, breech delivery may be inferred from the external examination of the infant's body. In one such case a child's body was found in a plastic bag on waste land. There was a ragged wound of the mouth. Further examination revealed an area of intense congestion of the buttock, and rupture of the mandibular symphysis. There was no evidence of separate existence. It was concluded that the congested buttock was the presenting part, and the facial injury was due to unskilled traction on the aftercoming head (F.M. 15,753B).

Viability of the infant is not an ingredient of infanticide but, where it can be shown the child was premature, there is a strong presumption of still-birth or death from prematurity, shortly after live-birth.

Still-birth is relatively common and its incidence is estimated to be one in eighteen of all legitimate births; it is appreciably higher in illegitimacy. Labour complications, particularly intra-cranial damage and especially tearing of the tentorium, are not rare.

Injuries suggestive of infanticide vary. The infant may be struck over the head or wounded with a knife or scissors, but some form of mechanical asphyxia, other than drowning, is the common mode. Attention is to be paid therefore to the face and neck for signs of nail-marks, scratches or bruising consistent with smothering or strangulation; in the latter event a ligature may be left *in situ*. Although infanticide without leaving external traces is practicable, undue force is generally used and its marks are then evident.

The umbilical cord requires close attention. Is it torn or cut across? Does it show signs of rough handling, likely to result from its use as a ligature? What is the length of the cord? Could the infant have fallen on its head in the course of precipitate labour and sustained a fracture? Fractures in these circumstances must be a rare event because, in view of the distance fallen, which, even when the mother is erect, can only be a short one, there would have to be forcible propulsion towards the ground. This is not normally the manner of delivery because a child is not expelled like a missile.

Conversely, signs of prolonged labour, i.e. oedema and bleeding into the scalp, a caput succedaneum, and severe moulding of the head, point to the possibility of still-birth or death from natural causes shortly after birth. Prolonged labour is the common mode of a first delivery and women charged with infanticide are nearly always primipara.

Although statements by the mother may be inconsistent or even demonstrably false, the principal evidence to support a charge of infanticide is that of the medical witness. If the charge is to succeed he must be able to prove not only that the child had had a separate existence but that its death was due to violence which has to be distinguished from injuries incidental to the birth. Secondary matters on which his opinion may be required include the viability of the child, and probable duration of life, when the child was live-born. It may also be necessary to prove that the mother was recently delivered and that the date of delivery coincides with the probable duration of the life of the infant. It may be necessary to prove that the accused was in fact the mother of the child.

The defence will test, as is thought necessary, the evidence of separate existence and ensure, when this is established, that the possible influences of maternal disease, the complications of labour, and neonatal disease are adequately excluded. The probability of still-birth, especially when the infant is illegitimate, will also be considered.

If the death of the child is ascribed to asphyxia and there is no clear evidence of criminal interference as the cause, due weight will be given to natural disease as the explanation. It has been found that asphyxia due to natural factors was responsible for over a third (37 per cent) of foetal deaths and nearly a fifth (17.8 per cent) of neonatal deaths, i.e. those which occur within the 1st week after delivery.

It will be apparent from the foregoing that the task of the medical examiner is one of considerable difficulty.

These considerations in no way permit the attitude that, because proof of infanticide is difficult, there is no need to search diligently for evidence of it. On all occasions the medical examination should be pressed to the limits of the examiner's resources.

The autopsy of a newly-born child requires techniques which differ in many respects from those of the adult's examination. The pathologist examining a suspected case of infanticide must follow an accepted technique, though it may be modified to suit the particular case where necessary. Details of such procedures were reviewed by Pryse-Davies (1981), Langley (1971) and Barson (1982).

Viability

The courts sometimes require to know whether the infant had attained the 28th week of gestation at the date on which the pregnancy terminated. Proof of this is relatively simple, since most of the victims of infanticide and child destruction are mature, i.e. have attained the 36th week of gestation. There are several criteria which can be applied to assess viability. Although an opinion based on only one criterion is of doubtful value, the demonstration of all of them permits a confident and reliable opinion.

The general condition of the body of the infant, its plumpness and absence of apparent disease or malformation, is not to be ignored; closer attention, however, is given to the weight, the crown-heel length of the child and the distribution of centres of ossification in its skeleton.

It has been established that there is a reasonably close relationship between the age and *weight* of a foetus. At 28 weeks the average weight is between $2^1/_2$ lb (1.1 kg) and 3 lb (1.3 kg); although when the weight is under 3 lb (1.3 kg) opinion should be guarded. At 32 weeks the expected weight is from $3^1/_2$ lb (1.6 kg) to 4 lb (1.8 kg); at 36 weeks, i.e. maturity, it is about 5 lb (2.2 kg) and at 40 weeks it is from 6 lb (2.7 kg) to 7 lb (3.2 kg). The corresponding crown-heel lengths are: 14 in. (35 cm), 16 in. (40 cm), 18 in. (45 cm) and 20 in. (50 cm).

When the birth is *multiple*, the weight of each of the infants is appreciably less than that of a single birth at the same stage of gestation. Due allowance must also be made for difference in sex since the female foetus is about 3 oz (100 g) lighter than a male at the same stage of gestation. The weight of an infant is easy to ascertain and, therefore, this criterion has value.

The crown–heel length is probably the best criterion. The length of a foetus up to the 5th month (20th week) of gestation represents the square of its age in months. Thus, a length of 16 cm is that of a foetus at about the 4th month. This is the rule of Haase (1895).

Beyond the 5th month, the length of the foetus measured in centimetres, on division by five, represents the age in months; if the length be measured in inches, division is by two, e.g. a length of 25 cm, i.e. 10 in., is that of a foetus at about the 5th month (Morison, 1964). Although length is a better criterion than weight, accurate measurement calls for skill (Dunham, 1948).

In the past considerable reliance was placed upon the distribution of *centres of ossification*. It is now more widely appreciated that the time of their appearance is distinctly variable. This, however, does not preclude use of them as an index of age. There are usually centres of ossification in the heel and ankle bones, i.e. the os calcis and astragalus, at the 28th week. By the time the child is mature, i.e. the 36th week, other centres usually will be found in the lower end of the thigh bone, in the cuboid and cunate (capitate) bones and, sometimes, in the upper end of the tibia. The centre in the lower end of the thigh bone is the most important because it is exceptional for it to be absent in a mature infant. Conversely, its absence does not exclude maturity. Glaister and Rentoul (1966) had noted its absence in two apparently mature infants.

The researches of Christie showed that of ten centres of ossification, only three, namely those in the proximal end of the tibia, the cunate or capitate and cuboid centres, were reliable as a means of distinguishing between infants in the weight groups of 2000 g or less and those whose weights were from 2000 to 2499 g. In his experience, the centre in the proximal end of the tibia was the most, and that of the cunate the least, reliable; the cuboid centre had an intermediate value (Dunham, 1948).

These centres may be sought for by radiological examination or, as is more usual and convenient, by direct inspection of the bones. The lower end of the thigh bone and upper end of the tibia are sliced across (coronally) until the centre is found or until the cuts have passed well beyond its usual site. The centre in the cuboid bone is best demonstrated by an incision which runs back from the cleft between the third and fourth toes towards the centre of the heel.

Another method of assessing maturity of the foetus is a study of the development of the teeth. (see page 66).

Separate Existence: Live Birth

These two terms are not infrequently deemed synonymous. Although they are not, this misuse does not normally lead to misunderstanding or error. The fact is, however, that the principal requirement of legal birth is that the child had had, or was capable of having, a separate existence, independent of its mother.

In respect of the crime of child destruction, it is required to be proved that the child was capable of being born alive. The pregnancy must have reached the twenty-eight week or over, i.e. the child was viable, and, further, it must be proved that a wilful act caused its death before it had an existence independent of its mother. Viability is the crux of this matter.

Infanticide, on the other hand, requires proof that the child had had a separate existence; that it had lived after the complete extrusion of its body from that of its mother. Viability need not be proved, but when there is doubt about this, it is improbable that the child had had a separate existence. In consequence, a charge of infanticide is then unlikely to be preferred or the mother, if charged with infanticide, has a strong defence.

A separate existence requires complete extrusion from the body of the mother, but not severance of the cord. A child can have a separate existence when its body has been completely delivered, but it is still attached to the placenta within the uterus of the mother.

The complete extrusion of the child is also relevant to still-birth. This is defined by the Births and Deaths Registration Act, 1953, s.41 as "a child which has issued forth from its mother after the twenty-eighth week of pregnancy and which did not at any time after being completely expelled from its mother breathe or show any other signs of life . . .". When in doubt, as stated earlier, still-birth is to be presumed.

External Signs of a Separate Existence

The external signs of a separate existence are few. They are limited, in fact, to changes in the umbilical cord and the presence of injuries which cannot be ascribed to labour and delivery.

On the other hand, external examination may reveal signs which prove that the child could not have achieved a separate existence. For instance, the body may show evidence of maceration, indicating intra-uterine death; the head may be enveloped in the amniotic membranes, the "caul", preventing the establishment of respiration; or there may be some gross congenital abnormality, incompatible with life (Plate 8).

The umbilical cord is cast off within the 1st week of life. During the first 12 to 24 hours the cord becomes a dry, shrivelled structure but this appearance is also seen in the body of a still-born infant. At 36 hours, or thereabouts, a zone of reddening of the skin appears around the attachment of the cord. Separation is well advanced at 4 to 5 days and is completed in from 6 to 7 days; the scar at the site of the cord remains active for up to about 12 days. None of these changes, which constitute a "vital reaction", can be found in a still-born child and, since they do not appear until the end of about 36 hours, their presence is proof of a separate existence.

The mode of severance of the umbilical cord is also important. The mother may allege that it was torn when the child fell on its head following precipitate labour. It can be shown that the cord has been cut across and not torn. When accidentally torn, the break is usually close to one of its attachments, either near the placenta or the navel of the infant; in the latter event haemorrhage is not excessive and is unlikely to be sufficient to cause the infant's death.

Morris and Hunt (1966) have found that the cord is relatively easily broken by hand. They describe the appearances of the cord ends produced by different modes of severance.

The ends of the cord should be examined by placing the two portions in water or on a board and their ends are then gently spread out; they should be examined also under low magnification. Gross irregularity is consistent with tearing whereas a linear break with regular margins is indicative of separation by cutting. An opinion, however, must take into account the possibility that a blunt instrument may have been used, producing a ragged line of separation and also the fact that it is possible for a tear superficially to resemble a clean-cut division of the cord. In any event, the occurrence of post-mortem change or severe drying usually precludes any opinion on the mode of severance of the cord.

Internal examination may provide strong, if not unequivocal evidence of a separate existence. It can be shown that extraneous material, which could enter only after complete extrusion of the infant, is present in the air passages or the digestive tract. Extraneous material can enter the air passages for a limited distance after death but its entry into the intrapulmonary bronchi is resisted by the air in the lungs. If, therefore, extraneous material be demonstrated in the secondary bronchi and beyond, it must have been inhaled. This, however, is capable of proof only in circumstances which preclude contamination and "milking" of the material downwards from the trachea and major bronchi by compression of the infant's body. The examination, therefore, must avoid these artifacts. The thoracic viscera must be removed with delicate "no touch" technique and placed on a clean slab or dish before any attempt is made to obtain samples of the bronchial contents and, of course, the pipette or syringe used must be clean. The specimen obtained must be accompanied by a sample of the probable source of extraneous material, e.g. soil or sand, in order that a comparison may be made and, as may be, proof obtained that the two samples are identical.

Extraneous material may enter the gullet, stomach and pass beyond, even into the small intestine, during life, but is unlikely to reach even as far as the stomach after death. A sample taken in a manner which precludes contamination is preserved for examination, together with a sample of material from its probable source.

The demonstration of food, e.g. milk, in the infant's stomach is of first importance since the possibility of its ingestion prior to complete extrusion is, to say the least, remote.

For the rest, the demonstration of a separate existence enters a field of investigation in which a definitive assessment of the value of its criteria has yet to be made.

In the past particular attention was paid to *the respiratory system*, always bearing in mind that proof of breathing is not proof of live-birth. It is sufficiently established to say, without adducing further evidence—of which there is an abundance in the books—that breathing can occur before complete extrusion of the infant. Breathing is by no means rare while the head of the child still remains in the vagina and there are authentic examples of its occurrence while the child is still in the womb (e.g. Clouston, 1933). It would appear there have been over 130 cases recorded, of which 122 were authentic; the earliest is ascribed to Vincelius, who had two cases. The record of Lebarius's case (1596) alleges that the child's cry could be heard from quite a distance. Ryder (1943) reviewed the literature and gives a comprehensive bibliography of vagitus uterinus.

It is still important to pay attention, even closer attention than in the past, to the respiratory system. The mode of approach, however, has radically altered.

The main test in the past, that known as the *hydrostatic test*, consisted in the determination of the buoyancy of the lungs. If they sank in water they were those of a still-born; if they floated freely this was taken to indicate live-birth. The test was suspect even in 1900 and requires no detailed discussion, because it is now known to have no value. The lungs of the live-born, even those who have been known to live for days, may sink (Dilworth, 1900; Randolph, 1901), and those which float are not necessarily those of live-born infants. They may have breathed before complete extrusion or their lungs may have been insufflated after delivery when still-born; the putrefied lung will also float. When the thoracic contents as a whole are sufficiently buoyant to float high in the water and putrefaction is absent it is probable that the infant was live-born. This degree of aeration is apparent to the eye; it is therefore pointless to apply the hydrostatic test which, moreover, will impair the material for other and more important investigations.

Aeration of the lungs increases their weight because, when the pulmonary circulation is established, the vessels fill with blood. An increase in the lung-weight of from one-seventieth to one-thirty-fifth of the total body-weight is then usual. This, however, is a test of minor importance and, since it also may interfere with the histological investigation, it can be omitted without detriment to the final opinion.

Naked-eye inspection of the lungs has importance. When they are generally distended, soft and crepitant, they have been aerated but, as Osborn (1953) has emphasised, the size of the lungs is no criterion of still-birth. He has disproved the former belief that small solid lungs indicate still-birth. Whether the child is born alive or not, it is his experience that the lungs fill the thorax in at least three-quarters of all cases. He has demonstrated that failure to expand may be due, for example, to bilateral pneumothorax with surgical emphysema, a result of artificial respiration. The presence of Tardieu's spots of asphyxia and evidence of broncho-pneumonia are not signs of live-birth, since they may be seen in the still-born. Occasionally sub-pleural interstitial emphysema may be seen and may represent attempted resuscitation by mouth-to-mouth respiration after birth.

Preparation of the Lungs for Microscopical Examination

Before attempting to draw practical conclusions from the researches of Osborn (1953), which should be consulted, it is necessary to mention his technique. He stresses the importance of the "no touch" technique, which aims at the elimination of artifacts produced by careless manipulation. The thoracic contents should be removed intact by cuts with a scalpel, the parts being controlled by holding the tongue or larynx with forceps. After fixation for 48 hours, samples for microscopy are taken of the whole lung in cross-section. In any case where there is doubt about the naked-eye interpretation or when criminal proceedings might arise, this procedure must be followed. The coroner and police will no doubt demur at the delay but they should then be informed of its advantages and of the disadvantages of hasty, inadequate treatment of the material.

Once the thoracic viscera are preserved and a complete examination has been made of the rest of the body, the coroner can safely permit its disposal. The police, also, may be glad of an interval in order to complete their inquiries before deciding to prefer a charge.

Microscopical Changes in the Lungs

In the past, microscopical examination of the lungs was a secondary line of investigation and was confined almost exclusively to one feature, namely, the condition of the lining of the air sacs. If these retained a gland-like appearance it was concluded that the child had not breathed and, therefore, it was a still-born. It is now realised that change in the kind of cell which lines the air sacs is not abrupt nor is it coincident with the onset of breathing, and, moreover, it has been proved that gland-like air sacs may be present in the lungs of live-born infants. The current interpretation is that persistence of this appearance is probably indicative only of prematurity, or of some disease state in the mature foetus which prevents normal differentiation, e.g. hydrops foetalis.

Microscopical examination of the lungs of these infants is now the dominant investigation and, indeed, is the only reliable means of solving many of the problems which arise. Some infants, it is true, are clearly still-born because, on naked-eye inspection alone, it is obvious the body is macerated. This appearance, however, is uncommon and unless the body is seen soon after delivery, interpretation may be made difficult by the onset of putrefaction. There are other children, representing at least a third of the cases in Osborn's series, where the appearances of the lungs were obviously those of infants which had breathed; some also showed signs of obstructive emphysema. The real difficulty arises over those infants who have succumbed to "the struggle to breathe". The recognition of this condition is of first importance and much is due to Osborn for his description of the changes indicative of it.

The victims of the "struggle to breathe" may be still-born or they die shortly after delivery. The gross changes are similar in both groups. The condition is a progressive one but it may terminate at any stage.

At the outset there is haemo-concentration, which is followed by cyanosis. It is important to note that the lungs are usually well expanded which, Osborn found, may be due to inhalation of liquor amnii or vomit, or to obstructive emphysema, or to oedema, with or without inhalation of air or liquor amnii.

Tardieu's spots are another feature but, it must be repeated, these can be seen in still- and live-born infants alike and are now discounted as evidence of asphyxia.

Osborn also emphasised the importance of distension of the large bowel with meconium. This may be extruded into the liquor and later inhaled, a point of importance in the recognition of still-birth because phagocytosis of meconium may then be demonstrated in the lungs.

The development of oedema of the lungs is a late change and is not always seen. Osborn found that not all new-born infants are prone to oedema. It can arise with remarkable speed, and, in Osborn's experience, it can cause death within as little as a minute or two. It is not, he emphasises, a "terminal" event; its development is incompatible with life. Acute neonatal oedema is a probable valid primary cause of death.

The recognition of oedema, however, may be difficult when the fluid has drained from the air sacs during the preparation of microscopical sections and especially when its cellular content is negligible. The air sacs then appear as if they had been aerated, although their distension was, in fact, due to the accumulation of fluid.

Another change found in these lungs may be recognised in sections specifically stained to demonstrate fat. It may be then seen that the alveolar ducts, i.e. the passages which lead to the air sacs, are lined by a membrane which is made prominent by the stain. The precise nature of the membrane has yet to be ascertained; it may be fatty material derived from the vernix (Ahlström, 1942) or it may not.

Osborn called it "alveolar duct membrane". It is now well-known as "hyaline membrane disease", which is usually associated with the respiratory distress syndrome (Pryse-Davies, 1981).

Gross oedema was common in Osborn's series and present in live-births in the proportion of 17:1 still-births. There was some oedema in five out of seven, and gross oedema in just under half of the lungs of the live-born. Absence of oedema in the still-born is to be expected since a rise of blood pressure, which normally follows delivery and favours the production of oedema, does not then occur. The haemorrhagic variant of oedema represents the last stage in its development and occurs when increased capillary permeability permits the escape of red cells into the fluid in the air sacs.

Desquamation of bronchial epithelium is noteworthy, providing, as Osborn warns, the specimen has been obtained by the "no touch" technique and the lungs are thoroughly fixed prior to sampling. Its occurrence is then a probable indication of early "maceration" of the lungs and, therefore, an indication of death *in utero* and thus of still-birth.

Bronchopneumonia, even when unequivocal, is not proof of live-birth, because Osborn found this change in the lungs of one in eight of the still-born examined by him.

Phagocytosis of meconium by the cells which line the air sacs, providing artifact be excluded, is important evidence of inhalation of liquor amnii and thus of still-birth. Osborn demonstrated this phagocytosis in eleven of thirty-one still-born infants.

The History of the Case

The value of the *history of the case* is also stressed by Osborn. When the circumstances do not give rise to the possibility of criticism of any person or create the possibility of criminal proceedings, it is permissible to reach conclusions on the basis of a reliable history and the naked-eye appearances of the infant's body. It is otherwise when there is no history, or that which is available is unreliable or incomplete; a full investigation is then necessary.

The presence of *contusion of the lungs* is important. This subpleural bleeding is readily distinguished from Tardieu's spots, because it has the pattern of "rib markings" and is more extensive. If, however, contusion be gross, Osborn found it resembled the severe phase of oedema of the lung, i.e. the haemorrhagic phase. He points out, also, that contusion must be distinguished from changes which are a part of the syndrome of haemorrhagic disease of the new-born. Pulmonary contusions, in Osborn's view, are the result of unduly vigorous artificial respiration. He found them in the proportion of 1:14 live-births but in none of the still-births. Although prepared to find their occurrence very good evidence of live-birth, he has deferred a definitive opinion until he has stronger proof of this. (The article on neonatal pulmonary disease by Aherne (1964) should be consulted.)

Summary

From the foregoing it appears that a diagnosis of *still-birth* is permissible in the presence of the following changes.

1. Maceration of the infant, preferably in the absence of coincident putrefaction.
2. Flooding of the lungs with liquor amnii and, more especially, evidence of phagocytosis of meconium by the cells lining the air sacs.
3. Desquamation of bronchial epithelium, providing technique which avoids artifact has been used.
4. The large bowel is distended with meconium, this being a sign of the struggle to breathe.

Still-birth is not necessarily indicated by small solid lungs of uniformly dark colour. Gross oedema makes still-birth doubtful and probably excludes it.

Live-birth is a probable event when:

1. The lungs are fully expanded in all lobes, with or without obstructive emphysema.
2. There is oedema, especially gross oedema, of the lungs.
3. An alveolar duct membrane is present and has widespread distribution in the lungs.
4. Pulmonary atelectasis, due to obstruction by an alveolar duct membrane, is present.
5. There are pulmonary contusions, and haemorrhagic disease of the new-born has been excluded.

A gland-like appearance of the alveoli does not exclude live-birth but indicates only prematurity. Tardieu's spots, although indicative of the struggle to breathe, may be present in live- and still-born alike; this is true also of broncho-pneumonia. Osborn believes the latter to be an important cause of abortion. He requires evidence of changes which must have occurred before birth, e.g. a fibrinous pleurisy, as proof of its congenital origin since other pneumonic changes can develop within a few hours of the birth; he does not accept the 6-hour limit sometimes regarded as the criterion (Osborn, 1954).

Osborn was able to diagnose live-birth correctly on eight or nine occasions out of ten by a study of the history, whereas diagnosis by an examination of the lungs alone is not easy, even when the preparations are good. Unfortunately it is unusual to obtain reliable case histories, except from obstetricians. Osborn (1954) told me of a baby which had gross bruising of its lungs and a ruptured liver and yet the nurse was positive that artificial respiration had not been performed, ". . . There never has been when it is the main cause of death . . . it has to be a very strong baby to stand artificial respiration."

Other Tests of a Separate Existence

(a) *Saliva in the stomach* Diniz (1932) maintained that saliva was always present in the stomach of any new-born infant who had survived a few hours after birth. No saliva was found in the stomachs of still-born infants.

(b) *Air in the gastro-intestinal tract* Hajkis (1934) believed the radiological demonstration of air in the stomach and intestine to be a confirmatory sign of respiration. If air had reached the duodenum he considered this strong evidence of a separate existence. Air was not shown in the stomach and intestine of the still-born.

Jobba (1970) has drawn attention to the need for reservation in evaluating such tests, because of the possibility of the application, at birth, of artificial respiration.

On occasion an infant's remains will be presented for examination, which have been concealed for such a long period of time that no soft tissue remains. In such cases it is sometimes worth submitting the jaws, containing the unerupted teeth, for skilled dental examination, since demonstration of an unequivocal neonatal line in the enamel will indicate that the infant achieved a separate existence (Gustafson, 1966). Gravimetric observations may also indicate the maturity of the infant (Stack, 1960).

On one occasion a trunk which had been abandoned in a left luggage office was opened prior to being disposed of at the end of a year. It contained the partially mummified and skeletonalised remains of two infants, some paper tissues and a knitting needle. An attempt, unsuccessful, was made to ascertain evidence of post-natal growth but a clear neonatal line could not be demonstrated. The owner of the trunk, a young girl, was traced. Although the presence of a knitting needle was viewed with considerable suspicion, no connection between it and the babies's deaths could be demonstrated. In consequence, the girl was charged only with concealment of birth (F.M. 13,965 A: Gee).

Prematurity

A birth is premature when delivery occurs prior to the full period of pregnancy, but precisely what that period is has yet to be fixed. The courts, loath to bastardise a child born in wedlock, are liberal in their interpretation of the possible limits of pregnancy. Legitimacy has been established when the period of pregnancy was no less than 349 days (*Hadlum* v. *Hadlum* [1949] P. 197). On the other hand, periods of 338 and 340 days were held to have precluded legitimacy. The average period of pregnancy is one of about 250 days.

The obstetrician will regard an infant premature where the birth weight is under $5^1/_2$ lb (2500 g). Viability in law is acquired at the 28th week or over, i.e. at a time when the foetus weighs as little as $2^1/_2$ lb (1000 g). Some remarkable cases of survival of premature infants have been recorded. One which weighed only 735 g (26 oz) at birth survived (Hoffman *et al.*, 1938). Another, which weighed 15 oz at birth, having been born at the beginning of the 7th month of pregnancy, was alive and well 6 weeks later, when it then weighed $32^3/_4$ oz (Hubbard, 1928). Shackleton (1928) also recorded the birth of a child on 27 February 1927, when it weighed only 17 oz; 10 months later it weighed $22^1/_2$ lb.

The Modes of Infanticide

Although it is proper, whenever practicable, not only to demonstrate the fact of still-birth but also to explain its cause, the essential finding is that the infant was still-born because in that event there cannot be a charge of infanticide.

When it is probable that the infant was live-born, it is important, whenever practicable, to ascertain the cause of death. For present purposes, however, niceties of precise diagnosis, which may depend upon minute structural changes, have minor importance. The first step is to determine whether death was by violence; it is next imperative to distinguish between injuries due to labour, or those which may rarely occur during gestation, and those which are the result of a criminal act. Unequivocal evidence of the latter is necessary to support a charge of infanticide; the signs are described in the chapters on wounds, head injuries and asphyxia.

No attempt is here made to detail the many ways in which natural disease can cause foetal or neonatal death. This is adequately treated by others, notably by Morison (1970) in his monograph, and complications of labour are adequately described in textbooks of midwifery, which should also be consulted. See also Berry (1982).

The present concern is to consider the possible modes of infanticide or murder and to indicate where caution is necessary before ascribing the findings to a criminal act.

Smothering is a simple and convenient mode and one which, as is described elsewhere (see p. 460), can leave no trace, but the application of more force than is necessary, the usual event, will leave marks of violence.

Strangulation is another common mode. If it is effected by a ligature, which may be left round the neck, it must be shown that this was applied before death. It may be alleged that the ligature was applied by the mother to assist self-delivery. Another possible explanation is that the infant was strangled accidentally by the umbilical cord. The length of the cord is here material. Considerable variation occurs; the normal length is about 20 in. but it may be up to 57 in. (Bandlocque, cited by Smith (1850) who recorded one of $59^{1}/_{2}$ in. in length). Examination of the cord, however, may show that it had been roughly handled, e.g. there is displacement of Wharton's jelly, which would exclude accidental strangulation and point to the use of the cord by the mother (or another person) as a ligature. In that event, also, there are likely to be marks of violence on the neck of the infant.

Manual strangulation, or throttling, is likely to produce only relatively insignificant bruises or scratches on the skin of the neck, though there is likely to be considerable internal bruising of the neck structures. Widespread bruises and scratches on the neck, sometimes extending on to the face and chest, are more likely to have been caused in a panic by an inexperienced mother attempting forceful self-delivery.

The infant may be choked. Littlejohn (1855–6) demonstrated a mass of dough or paste blocking the pharynx, and he was of the opinion that the use of a plug was then a common mode of infanticide. Difficulty arises if the agent is a plug of cloth, removed shortly after death. There may then be no trace other than pallor of the parts to indicate their compression by a plug. Mud, as in Easton's case, or newspaper, have also been used; in a French case the police were able to prove that the plug was part of a newspaper found in the woman's room (Littlejohn, 1855–6).

Infanticide by dashing the infant's head against a wall or the floor is infrequent. This is liable to produce a comminuted fracture with laceration of the scalp and it may be possible, also, to show marks which indicate that the infant's limbs were held during the crime. It may be suggested that the fracture occurred as the result of precipitate labour while the mother was erect. Labour, however, does not result in a forcible and rapid expulsion of the infant and, moreover, the normal length of the cord, namely 20 in., is likely to check a violent fall; the length of the cord, of course, is distinctly variable, i.e. within limits of from about 6 in. to 5 ft. Even if the infant did fall on the ground, the force is insufficient to cause a fracture; none occurred in 183 precipitate labours in Klein's experience. The experiments of Chaussier (also cited by Taylor, 1957) did not properly reproduce the circumstances of precipitate labour and, therefore, the relatively high incidence of his experimental fractures is not representative of the probable results of precipitate labour. When a caput succedaneum and moulding are apparent, the labour was not precipitate and this will throw doubt upon the mother's story.

A newly-born child's body was discovered in a compost heap, apparently dead. While awaiting an ambulance to take the body to the mortuary, the infant began to show signs of life and was taken to hospital. The only external sign of injury was a tiny abrasion on the forehead. The child died 12 hours later. Autopsy disclosed a massive fracture of the frontal bone, with laceration of the dura and brain. The mother admitted that she had thrown the child down a flight of steps on to a concrete floor (F.M. 11,216A).

Fractures of the skull which occur during and as a result of labour have certain characteristics. They are not associated with laceration of the scalp. They usually involve the parietal bones and run downwards at right angles to the saggital suture for an inch or so; they are fissured fractures; less often, these fractures may run from the anterior fontanelle to the frontal eminence. Fractures produced by forceps may be accompanied by laceration of the scalp; the fractures lie at points normally gripped by the instrument and are usually "gutter" or "pond" fractures. The person who applied forceps, also, should be available to give evidence concerning the injuries.

Infanticide by drowning is unusual. A woman was charged in 1940 with murder of her infant aged 16 days by drowning. She was thought to have recovered from the effects of giving birth, but, when the prison medical officer examined her 6 weeks later he found she was still bleeding and in his opinion the balance of her mind was probably disturbed at the time of the crime; she was acquitted of murder but convicted of infanticide and placed on probation. It is more usual for the mother to attempt to dispose of the body by submersion after infanticide than by some other means.

We once saw a dead, apparently still-born, child recovered from a river, still attached by its umbilical cord to the placenta where there was a second umbilical cord. The twin's body was recovered, further down the river, several days later.

Submersion may, of course, be the mode of disposal of a still-born. The mother may put the body in a closet and allege she gave birth while using it, or, as is not rare, where a bucket serves, she may allege the infant was delivered into the bucket. The investigation will then be directed to the possibility of precipitate labour, unusual in a primipara, and the demonstration of fluid, resembling the contents of the bucket, in the air passages and digestive tract of the infant.

A woman gave birth when in bed in the middle of the night. She alleged the child was still-born because it did not cry. She placed the body in a chamber utensil and next morning transferred it to a closet, where the body was found by the police. A medical examination showed that the infant was probably live-born and had died of asphyxia. The learned judge properly drew the attention of the jury to the importance of proof of a separate existence, of which the evidence was inadequate. The woman was acquitted of infanticide but found guilty of concealment of birth (*Brit. Med. J.*, 1940, **ii,** 652). Drowning was the mode in *R. v. Kemp*, 1950, Leeds Assizes, 13 August (F.M. 1565).

Infanticide by burning is rare though, again, like submersion, burning is often a mode of disposal of the victim of infanticide or of a still-born infant. Radtke (1933) found that the usual tests of death by burning were not generally applicable, but he emphasised the importance of the presence of foreign bodies, something more than carbon particles, in the burnt lungs of the infant. Presumably the demonstration of a high saturation by carbon monoxide is proof of death by burning in these circumstances, as it is in others. Calcined remains may be found in the firegrate but obviously it is then impossible to prove infanticide; a conviction of concealment of birth may be recorded.

One child's body we examined was found submerged in the cistern of a toilet in a ladies lavatory in a Polytechnic. One side of the body was badly burnt, with a well-marked red band of vital reaction bordering the burnt area. It appeared that there had been an attempt to dispose of the body by fire before death had occurred. The mother was never discovered, she may not have known the child was still alive when exposed to fire (F.M. 15,673 A).

Infanticide by wounding, e.g. by cut-throat, is uncommon. This mode is indicative of intent to kill. It may be alleged, however, that the injury resulted from an accident when cutting the cord. The kind of instrument used is then important because, although not impossible, it is highly improbable that wounds caused by an open razor or a penknife are accidental; it is otherwise if scissors were used. In any event, it is further necessary to determine whether the particular kind of injuries on the infant's body could have been accidental. An extensive, incised wound of the throat almost certainly excludes an accident; the possibility of frenzy or panic at the time of delivery, however, might lead a woman to perform acts for which she is wholly irresponsible, yet they might appear to indicate a determined attack. Infanticide by decapitation, followed by dismemberment, was described by Amoroso (1935). In his opinion the child was alive at the time of the crime since he found signs of vital reaction in the tissues. Six cases of infanticide by cut-throat were described by Busatto (1935). A newly-born female was found dead with a cut-throat on 4 August 1954. The wound extended from below the right ear, across the front of the neck to just below the left ear. Its margins were clean-cut and were without bruising. On the left side of the neck there was notching of the skin, indicating that there had been three separate cuts. The main incision had severed the right internal and external carotid arteries and the trachea; there was also a deep incision into the vertebral column. Bleeding had occurred into the tissues of the neck and blood had been inhaled to give each lung a notable red mottling. Bruising of the child was also apparent over the left temple on the left side of the neck and over the front of the chest. Although the former bruises could have occurred in the course of self-delivery, it was highly improbable that bruising of the chest had occurred except after complete extrusion. The lungs were well expanded. The mother was an unmarried woman aged 18, who pleaded guilty to infanticide and was bound over for 3 years (F.M. 3744 A; *R.* v. *Larkin*, Leeds Assizes, Nov. 1954).

Cutting the umbilical cord so as to cause exsanguination of the infant could be a mode of infanticide. A child's body was found in a bus-shelter, wrapped in newspapers drenched with blood. The umbilical cord had been cut flush with the abdominal wall. This could have been due to the mother's ignorance or it was a deliberate act. This was not determined (F.M. 15,769 A).

Punctured wounds are also uncommon; they may be alleged to have been accidental. The point of a scissor blade could enter the child's body during the cutting of the cord, e.g. its body might slip on to the blade. The position and nature of the wound, however, may be wholly inconsistent with accidental injury; frenzy or panic might then be pleaded as the explanation. Instruments which are not of a kind normally used to sever the cord, e.g. a needle, a hatpin or a knife with a fine blade, tend to exclude accidents. These may be inserted with skill through a fontanelle, inner canthus of the eye, temple, or into the spine; in such circumstances neither accident nor panic can be readily accepted as an explanation of the injuries. It appears to be a mode used in India today but it is not new because cases were cited by Ogston (1878).

We have examined a newly-born infant who was found to have suffered two penetrating wounds of the neck, produced by a pair of nail scissors; in one wound the agent had completely transfixed the neck, from before backwards, but the blades had been closed, and no vital structures had been injured. This child also had healed fractured ribs, and an old area of brain damage, apparently produced during attempted self-abortion in the early stages of pregnancy, the mechanism being repeated impacts inflicted on the abdomen by the mother throwing herself against tables, downstairs, etc. (Seymour-Shove *et al.*, 1968) (F.M. 12,118 B).

Infanticide by withholding food or by undue exposure is rare. It is consistent with a planned crime and inconsistent with temporary mental unbalance. The usual experience is that the mother who "abandons" her infant leaves it well clad and in a place where it will soon be found and cared for by others; in all probability she will stay nearby until she knows that the infant is in safe hands.

The demonstration of starvation and exposure by medical examination is distinctly difficult; the absence of food in the stomach may be of some importance. Proof of infanticide on these occasions must be, in the main, by collateral evidence. The mother, for example, must have left the nude or ill-clad infant at the roadside, where it remained for several hours.

Poisoning is now a rare mode of infanticide. In the past, tincture of opium, arsenic, antimony, concentrated sulphuric acid and yellow phosphorus, obtained from matches, or an overdose of a purgative have been used. The possibilities of the present abundance of barbiturates do not yet appear to have been exploited. It is a premeditated crime to which a defence of accident or mental unbalance may be weak.

Burial alive is an uncommon mode of infanticide. Instances are reported from time to time and the case of Berardinelli (1935) is an example. An unmarried woman aged 23 was found by her father shortly after she had given birth. The child appeared to be dead and the man buried the body in the backyard. A doctor was summoned and he asked to see the body. When it was exhumed, $^3/_4$ hour after burial, it moved and cried feebly. No charge was preferred because it was accepted that the father really thought it dead when he buried it. The author cited other instances of live burial of infants. In her opinion the common modes of infanticide were, first, smothering, second, violence, especially to the head, then strangulation; next in frequency were drowning and exposure. Burial alive was commoner on the continent than elsewhere.

It is believed that, subject to rare exceptions, infanticide is the result only of some act which is unpremeditated and which is effected by means immediately to hand, by a person who for the time being is irresponsible. The maternal instinct is strong and usually prevents planned infanticide. (see d'Orban, 1979)

Child Destruction

The crime of abortion was defined by the Offences against the Person Act, 1861, and that of infanticide by the Infanticide Act, 1922, but it was still no offence to kill the child during labour before it had a separate existence. This defect in the law was remedied by the Infant Life (Preservation) Act, 1929, which created and defined the crime of child destruction. "Any person who, with intent to destroy the life of a child capable of being born alive, by any wilful act causes a child to die before it has an existence independent of its mother, shall be guilty of felony, to wit of child destruction and shall be liable on conviction thereof on indictment to penal servitude (now imprisonment) for life." It is, however, a statutory defence to this charge that the act which caused the death of the child was done in good faith for the purpose only of preserving the life of the mother.

It will be noted that viability requires proof. It was enacted by section 1 (2), that, for the purpose of this Act, evidence that a woman had at any material time been pregnant for a period of 28 weeks or more shall be *prima facie* proof that she was at that time pregnant of a child capable of being born alive.

The offence may be committed almost by coincidence, as in one case (F.M. 12,641 A) where a man stabbed a pregnant woman. The wound was in the abdomen and the knife penetrated the uterus. The mother survived but the child was born dead, with a stab-wound in the left side of the trunk with transfixion of the heart.

Concealment of Birth

It is an offence, in England, to conceal a birth; in Scotland it is an offence to conceal pregnancy. The Offences against the Person Act, 1861, s.60, provides that "if any woman shall be delivered of a child, every person who shall, by any secret disposition of the dead body . . . whether such child died before, at, or after its birth, endeavour to conceal the birth thereof, shall be guilty of a misdemeanour . . .".

A verdict of concealment of birth is an alternative to that of infanticide and, in view of the difficulties of proving the major charge, the prisoner is usually convicted of concealment of birth.

It will be noted that there is no need to prove live-birth. It is sufficient that there has been a birth and that the child was dead at the time of concealment; there is no need to produce the body. It does not appear to be necessary to prove the child had been viable. All parties to the concealment stand as principals.

A conviction will result when there is evidence of concealment, essentially a legal matter; medical evidence on these occasions is of minor importance. It has been held that placing the dead body between a bed and the mattress, or under a bolster on which the prisoner laid her head, was concealment. On the other hand, it was not concealment when the body was placed in a box within another box, neither of which was locked, when kept in a room much resorted to by other persons in the house, and it occupied a position likely to attract attention. It is not concealment to leave the body exposed in a public street.

Medical evidence will relate to proof of still-birth or the death of the child and its identification as the child of the prisoner, e.g. that she was recently delivered and at a time consistent with the date of birth of the dead infant.

On occasion medical examination of the concealed body may provide evidence by which the mother may be traced. A newly-born coloured child's body was found, wrapped in a sheet, on the bank of a river. It had been skilfully layed-out; the orifices packed with cotton-wool, and the head covered by a piece of adhesive plaster of the type usually only found in hospital. It was clear that the person responsible was likely to have medical knowledge, and she was soon traced and found to be a nurse in training (F.M. 11,722 A).

Viability may also be relevant but convictions have been recorded when the child was "a foetus, not bigger than a man's finger, but having the shape of a child".

Although the mother is the person usually convicted of concealment of birth, all who may be concerned, as stated, stand as principals.

In 1940 a doctor was charged with the murder of the newly-born child of a young woman with whom he had been intimate. Death was due to asphyxia, alleged to have been caused by the forcible insertion of cotton wool plugs into its mouth. The successful defence was that at the time of the delivery the mother had a severe haemorrhage, which required all the doctor's attention. The infant died in spite of attempts at resuscitation. Its body was later wrapped in cotton wool and placed in the doctor's bag, which he took about with him in his car for 2 days. Evidence was also led to show that asphyxia could have been caused by congenital heart disease, there being a patent ductus arteriosus. The cotton wool could have entered the mouth after death, and, except for a bruise on the infant's tongue, all the other signs could have been accounted for by circulatory defect. The doctor was acquitted of murder but convicted of concealment of birth. A nominal sentence of 3 day's imprisonment was imposed, due allowance being made for the fact that the prisoner had stood his trial for murder and that he would also have to face another tribunal.

References

AHERNE, W. (1964) in *Recent Advances in Clinical Pathology*, Series iv, pp. 284–305, ed. Dyke, S.C. London: J. & A. Churchill.

AHLSTROM, C. G. (1942) *Dtsch. Z. ges. gerichtl. Med.*, **36**, 63–74.

AMOROSO, M. (1935) Abstr., *Med.-leg. Rev.*, **3**, 234–5.

AREY, L. B. (1947) *Amer. J. Obstet. Gynec.*, **54**, 872–3.

ASCH, S. S. and RUBIN, L. J. (1974) *Amer. J. psychiatry*, **131**, 870–874.

BARSON, A. J. (1982) *Fetal & Neonatal Pathology*; Praeger, New York.

BERARDINELLI, C. C. (1935) *Amer. J. Surg.*, **29**, 455–6.

BERRY, C. L. (1982) edit. *Paediatric Pathology*; Springer-Verlag. Berlin.

BUSATTO, S. (1935) Abstr., *Med.-leg. Rev.*, **3**, 321–2.

CLOUARON, E. C. T. (1933) *Brit. Med. J.*, **i**, 200–1.

D'ORBAN, P. T. (1979) *Br. J. psychiatry*, **134**, 560–571.

DILWORTH, T. (1900) *Brit. Med. J.*, **ii**, 1567.

DINIZ, S. (1932) *Ann. Med.-leg.*, **5**, 60–62; also abstr. *Med.-leg. Rev.* (1934) **2**, 384.

DUNHAM, E. C. (1948) Premature Infants, Children's Bureau Publication, No. 325, Washington: U.S. Govt. Pub. Office.

GLAISTER, J. and RENTOUL, E. (1966) *Medical Jurisprudence and Toxicology*, 12th ed., p. 393. Edinburgh: Livingstone.

GUSTAFSON, G. (1966) *Forensic Odontology*. London: Staples Press.

HAASE, – (1895) *Charite-Annalen*, **ii**, 668–96, cited Arey (1947).

HAJKIS, M. (1934) *Lancet*, **ii**, 134–5.

HOFFMAN, S. J., GREENHILL, J. P. and LUNDEEN, E. C. (1938) *J. Amer. Med. Ass.*, **90**, 283–5.

HUBBARD, W. L. (1928) *Brit. Med. J.*, **ii**, 878: ibid., p. 1076.

JOBBA, G. (1970) *Ztschr. f. Rechtsmed.-J. Leg. Med.*, **67**, 119; ibid., p. 364.

LANGLEY, F. A. (1971) *J. Clin Pathol.* **24**, 159–169.

LITTLEJOHN, H. D. (1855–56) *Edinb. Med. J.*, **1**, 521–2.

MASON, J. K. (1978) *Forensic Medicine for Lawyers*. Bristol. J. Wright and Sons.

MORISON, J. E. (1970) *Foetal and Neonatal Pathology*, 3rd ed., London: Butterworth.

MORRIS, J. F. and HUNT, A. C. (1966) *J. Forens. Sci.*, **11**, 43.

OGSTON, F. (1878) *Lectures on Medical Jurisprudence*, ed. F. Ogston, Jr. London: Churchill.

OSBORN, G. R. (1943) *Lancet*, **ii**, 277–84.

OSBORN, G. R. (1953) in *Modern Trends in Forensic Medicine M*. 33–52; ed. K. Simpson. London: Butterworth.

OSBORN, G. R. (1954) Personal communication.

PRYSE-DAVIES, J. (1981) in *Recent Advances in Histopathology*. No. 11. Ed. Anthony P. P. & MacSweeny R. V. London Churchill-Livingstone.

RADKE, W. (1933) *Dtsch. Z. ges. gerichtl. Med.*, **20**, 267–77; abstr. *Med.-leg. Rev.*, **i**, 255.

RANDOLPH, C. (1901) *Brit. Med. J.*, **i**, 146.

RYDER, G. H. (1943) *Amer. J. Obstet. Gynec.*, **46**, 867–72.

SEYMOUR-SHOVE, R., GEE, D. J. and CROSS, A. P. (1968) *Brit. Med. J.*, **1**, 686.

SHACKLETON, H. (1928) *Brit. Med. J.*, **ii**, 1076.

SMITH, T. (1850) *Lancet*, **i**, 95.

STACK, M. V. (1960) *J. Forens. Sci. Soc.*, **1**, 49.

TAYLOR, A. S. (1957) Principles and Practice of Medical Jurisprudence, 11th ed., Sydney Smith and K. Simpson, vol. 2. p. 190. London: Churchill.

STATUTES

Births and Deaths Registration Act, 1953; 1 & 2, Eliz. 2, Ch. 20.
Infanticide Act, 1922; 12 & 13 Geo. 5, Ch. 18.
Infanticide Act, 1938; 1 & 2 Geo. 6, Ch. 36.
Infant Life (Preservation) Act, 1929; 19 & 20 Geo. 5 Ch. 34.
Offences against the Person Act, 1861; 24 & 25 Vict., Ch. 100.

CHAPTER 16

Cruelty to Children: the "Battered Baby" (Non-Accidental Injury)

Introduction

Cruelty to children is not recent nor has it escaped the notice of Parliament but there has been public indifference, even callous indifference, to its existence. In 1946 attention was focused on one of its worst aspects when Caffey, a radiologist, published his observations on the occurrence of "Multiple fractures of the long bones of infants suffering from chronic sub-dural haematoma". These results of deliberate injury to children, and other ill-effects due to the same cause, came to be known as the "Battered Baby Syndrome", a term introduced by Kempe *et al.* (1962). The term "non-accidental injury" is now more generally accepted. Since 1946 there has been a spate of publications, including a journal (*Child Abuse and Neglect* Ed. Kempe, C.H.) devoted to this subject.

Cruelty to children in any form, but more especially physical cruelty, is mean and despicable. It arouses indignation but the pathologist must view the ill-effects without allowing this natural reaction to influence his interpretation of his findings, since they play an important part in the distinction between injuries which are accidental and those which are the result of a deliberate assault. It is in these circumstances that this distinction is specially difficult to make. The examination must be thorough and complete and should be undertaken only by those with special experience of these cases.

THE EXAMINATION OF AN ALLEGED BATTERED CHILD

(a) *The History of the Case* It is important that the pathologist is given a satisfactory history of the case before he begins his examination. Unfortunately that is not the rule. It is material for him to know about the environment of the dead child. It is usually one from a lower-income group but it must be remembered that cruelty to children occurs at all levels of the social scale and it has been said that intelligent people, under the guise of strict discipline, can be "efficient torturers" (Halton, 1964). (These, however, are more likely to inflict mental cruelty, which leaves no tell-tale injuries.)

The alleged culprit is usually a parent or guardian. It could be a child minder or a foster parent but those who occupy these positions, for payment, are under the supervision of the social services department of the local authority; applicants, moreover, have to be approved. There are times when the child has been injured by an older brother or sister.

Kaplin and Reich (1976) studied 12 cases of child homicide in New York. The victims were more often males, of whom two-thirds were born out of wedlock and the most frequent assailant was the mother. Densen-Gerber (1978) drew attention to the frequency in New York with which children dying as the result of cruelty had parents who were drug abusers or alcoholics. She reports cases of children injected with heroin or morphine, or given these substances orally, to quieten them. (It was an ancient custom to let infants suck a finger dipped in Tr. Opii.)

The child is often the first born and may be either illegitimate or unwanted; it may be one suffering from severe subnormality. The majority are infants aged less than 2 years and almost all are under school age; the mean age of the series studied by Cameron *et al.* (1966) was 14.3 months. There is a preponderance of males, which Camps and Cameron (1971) found to be in the ratio of 30:11 in the living and 24.5:12 in the dead.

There may be a history that the child was "accident-prone"; if so, it is a clear warning to scrutinise the body for old as well as recent injuries. In several of these children it is clear that the fatal injuries were the last of a series of assaults upon the child.

d'Orban (1979) comments on the frequency with which children who are battered to death are suffering from some illness at the time of their assault. Many battering mothers had multiple social and psychiatric problems with a chaotic and violent home background.

It is important to know what steps the parent took when the child was injured. If accidental it is to be expected that the parent is prompt to seek medical aid and other assistance. But it must be appreciated that this does not exclude the possibility of deliberate violence as the cause of the child's injuries. They may have been inflicted by the father, and the mother, anxious to know how much damage has been done, may take the child forthwith to hospital or infant clinic. Injured children brought to hospital during the night should excite suspicion and undue delay in seeking medical aid is certainly a warning that the injuries may not have been accidental. Any attempt to resuscitate the child and the mode employed can be important information.

Any explanation given by the parent should be recorded. It is true that several "stock" explanations are now well known. "He was always tumbling and bumping his head (against furniture: against a flower pot, against the wainscotting, etc.). "She fell downstairs (and hit her head on the metal base of a lamp standard)".

"He often threw himself on to the floor in a fit of temper." "The child would not stop crying so I threw a pillow at him (the new pillow had burst open!). These have been termed frivolous (Turner, 1964) and, indeed, they often are blatant lies but it is within our experience that some were in fact true. Obviously, in the presence of grave injuries these explanations must be received with considerable circumspection and suspicion. The police should persist in their inquiries and if these elicit fresh explanations none of which are adequate, further persistence may at last yield the truth. Dr. George Manning (1965) told of the mother whose initial explanation failed to satisfy him and, in the end, the mother admitted that she had bashed the child's head against furniture. It is otherwise when the explanation offered is feasible; on these occasions the inquiries must be conducted with considerable tact. Serious harm can be done by blundering inquiry which imputes blame where none exists.

A British Medical Journal Editorial (1981) suggested that the tendency might have moved too far towards immediate suspicion of the parents and warned of the dangers of too hasty a diagnosis of child abuse.

On the other hand a recent paper, Oliver, (1983) puts the opposite point of view. Oliver studied 147 families in one county where child neglect or abuse was known to have occurred over two generations. In these families 560 children were born during 21 years. Of these 513 were known to have been neglected or assaulted, and 41 died. Only three of the deaths resulted in criminal convictions. However, confidential information indicated that parental behaviour had often caused or contributed to the other deaths.

In the event that the parent adheres rigidly to his explanation, even if unsatisfactory, a court may be obliged to accept it. On many of these occasions, since the parent is almost always alone with the child, the course of events is purely conjectural. The one occasion in our series when battery was witnessed by the boy's elder sister, aged 8 years, enabled her to give the police a clear account of it. Her evidence, however, was immediately excluded, when in answer to the first question put to her in the witness box she truthfully said she had discussed the case with her mother. (Other evidence led to the conviction of her father of manslaughter and the judge imposed a long sentence of imprisonment.)

It is sometimes suggested that child abuse is a problem peculiar to the Anglo-Saxon countries. Not so, however. Several publications have drawn attention to its occurrence elsewhere, e.g. Nigeria (Nwako, 1979) and Hong Kong (Law, 1979).

(b) *External Appearances of the Body* As already indicated it is more likely to be that of a male than a female and the age will be somewhere between 3 and 15 months; but it may be female and either sex may be over that age. That it is dirty and verminous, and the clothing of poor quality and amount and in poor repair, should be noted but undue importance should not be attached to these details since they are common to many circumstances. The body weight and nutrition may or may not be relevant; this should be determined and recorded. Some are well below normal weight for age but this may be due to natural disease.

Emery (1978) described the problem faced by the pathologist when examining a dead wasted child and trying to decide whether this was due to natural or unnatural cause. He described a situation in which the mother fails to develop normal rapport with the infant; the result is the child is quiet and does not stimulate her to give food and this establishes a vicious circle. Characteristic findings are: extreme wasting of fat pannicles in the skin and viscera and a terminal respiratory infection producing a "retention lung". The pancreas shows shrinkage of endocrine cells. Differentiation from coeliac disease is difficult. Full body measurements must be taken and, possibly, blood and skin for chromosome studies.

Bruising

The report should include a detailed account of all bruises present, with special reference to size, position and probable age.

Multiplicity of bruising, and more especially when the bruises are of differing ages, has significance. Bruising of the forehead can occur because the child was often bumping his head. Bruising of the arms can result from a firm grip applied in the course of legitimate restraint or in an attempt to prevent a fall. Bruising of the ankles may be due to gripping. It is important to remember that children bruise more readily than adults. Bruising of the buttocks may be due to a fall (but at under a year the child is likely to be well protected by a napkin) or it may be due to legitimate chastisement; it could be due to a kick.

Patterned bruising is unusual but on one occasion the presence of groups of small circular bruises matched the distribution of small metal cones on a leather belt and the mother was obliged to admit that she had thrashed the child with the belt. (She differed with the pathologist in regard to the age of the bruises; in her view they had been inflicted several hours before the child died.) (Fig. 18a, p. 100).

It is usually initially suggested that bruises and other superficial injuries are the result of accidents. (Pascoe *et al* (1979) compared the patterns of soft tissue injuries in the victims of child abuse and those due to accidents. The abused children had significantly more soft tissue injuries over cheeks, trunk, genitals and upper legs. Lacerations were commoner as the result of accidents. Ellerstein (1979) lists cutaneous manifestations of child abuse, including injuries, traumatic alopecia, dermatoses, animal bites etc. But even quite dramatic injuries are not necessarily evidence of cruelty. Anderson and Hudson (1976) described a battered child whose bite marks on the arms were shown to have been self-inflicted. A child who died of abdominal injuries inflicted by the father had its body covered with rounded, back scabs which were at first thought to have been cigarette burns. Closer examination showed that they were the residual scabs of chicken pox infection (F.M. 13,341A).

Wilson (1977) summarised current views of the determination of the age of bruises in cases of alleged child abuse.

Burns and Scalds

All too often toddlers sustain burns or scalds by accident. The presence of these injuries or their scars calls for satisfactory explanation. Now and again the burn may have distinctive pattern, e.g. the blade of a heated knife or the top of a stove. The practice of applying a lighted cigarette is likely to produce small circular, pitted burns. In the presence of other grave injuries, a father's explanation that the burn of the child's foot occurred while the child was sat on his knee and he was unaware that the foot was too close to a fire was not accepted. Lenoski and Hunter (1977) described specific patterns of burns in child abuse and consider that the position of the body at the time of burning can be determined by analysis of the position and depth of the burns. We have found this approach of value in alleged accidental scalding. Running water produces characteristic trickle marks. Their study made it possible to show the direction of the flow of water down the body from the back of the head. The original story was one of accidental scalding in a bath. The truth was that the mother had poured a kettleful of boiling water over the child (F.M. 8634A). Keen *et al.* (1975) reported the deliberate infliction of burns and scalds, involving 16 children. They described typical "dip scalds" on the hands and feet. Ayoub and Pfeifer (1979) also describe burns as a manifestation of child abuse.

Lacerations, Incised and Stab Wounds

These injuries are infrequent; the most likely injury is laceration of the scalp, which could, of course, be due to an accidental fall. The occurrence of laceration of the inner side of the upper lip, especially when associated with laceration of the frenum, is important and Camps and Cameron (1971) consider it diagnostic of battery.

Fractures

The usual sites are the skull, chest cage and long bones. In their series of 100 cases, Camps and Cameron (1971) found fracture of the skull in forty-three, fracture of the chest cage in twenty-seven and of the long bones in twelve of those recently injured. As might be expected, old skull fractures were the least common of old fractures since skull fractures are usually associated with recent subdural haemorrhage and death. Rib fractures were the commonest of the old fractures, twenty-two cases, although old fractures of long bones were almost as common, seventeen cases; there were only seven old fractures of the skull.

Akbarnia *et al.* (1974) reviewed 231 cases of child abuse with reference to orthopaedic findings. The commonest sites of fracture were ribs, humerus, femur and tibia. The epiphyses were almost never involved. Characteristic lesions were metaphyseal impaction fractures and symmetrical periosteal new bone formation, secondary to sub-periosteal haemorrhage. Multiple fractures at various stages of healing were deemed pathognomonic of the syndrome.

It is good practice to make a radiological examination of the skeleton as a routine procedure but, if this be impracticable, the finding of a single fracture merits this step. Although, ideally, radiological examination should precede the autopsy, on occasion it may be easier to postpone this until the dissection is completed. We have not found this impracticable. Although it means the radiological examination of the skull and spine is no longer practicable. Keeling (1981) states that whenever the pathologist has the slightest suspicion of child abuse an X-ray examination should precede the autopsy. She also recommends the fixation and histological examination of the eyes. An X-ray examination may disclose a congenital malformation which may have a bearing on the interpretation of the course of death.

Fractures of the skull may be simple fissures, local depressed fractures or comminuted fractures. Camps and Cameron (1971) drew attention to the possibility that a skull injury can result from a blow with the side of the hand (a karaté blow) when cuffing the child without intent to injure it.

Fractures of differing ages are significant and there is general agreement that this is a special feature of battery. Only three of twenty-nine subjects were without fractures in the series examined by Cameron *et al.* (1966).

Fractures of the long bones are likely in the femur or humerus. The injury may be recent or healing. Akbarnia *et al.* (1974) did not find damage of the epiphyses. We agree with them that the sub periosteal calcification, unaccompanied by fracture, of the long bones is a feature. These bony envelopes are the end result of periosteal bleeding of traumatic origin. This may have been by a blow or the result of a twisting or shearing strain of the limb. We have seen it involve all of the long bones of the limbs. At the outset the parents ascribed the injuries to a single fall from a pram. (F.M. 13,941A). It is often that at the outset the parents attempt to explain the injuries as a result of an accidental fall. The pathologist is then asked to give his views. In many cases the injuries are far too gross to have been the result of a single fall; on other occasions, when the injuries are less severe, it is then difficult to interpret their cause. Helfer *et al.* (1977) studied 246 children, aged 5 years or less, who had fallen out of bed, either at home or in hospital. None had any serious injury as a result. Only 3 had an identifiable skull fracture on subsequent X-ray examination and none had resultant C.N.S. damage. Levin (1972) studied 100 infants who had fallen. None had serious injuries. His view was that fatal injuries could be expected only if the child had fallen at least 10 feet, or had been abused. (Edit. *Can. med. ass. J.* 1973).

The spine may be injured. Cullen (1975), Dickson and Leatherman (1978), Gosnold and Sivaloganathan (1980) describe such cases. Kerley (1978) found healing fractures of the spines of murdered children at an examination of their bodies after burial; they were members of the same family.

Injuries can be produced either by lifting the child by its extended arm, whereby the whole of the body weight is thrown on the shoulder region (a practice one observes all too often in entirely innocent but stupid circumstances) or the child may have been held by one or both ankles and swung against furniture or dragged along. (The ankles should be inspected as a routine for evidence of bruising consistent with gripping.)

Fractures of the Chest Cage

Fracture of one or several ribs, on one or both sides of the chest cage, is a common finding in the living as well as the dead, battered child. The usual sites of these fractures are the convexity of the rib or at a point an inch or so nearer the spine (The appearances are well illustrated in one of our cases, which was published by Fairburn and Hunt, 1964.) When these fractures are of differing ages they are probably the result of battery but if they are all of the same age it is essential to exclude external cardiac massage as the cause; this form of resuscitation, even in skilled hands, can fracture ribs and rupture the liver or heart. (The police should ask, as a routine question, what steps were taken by the parent or others to attempt to resuscitate the child.)

On various occasions we have found in the body of an infant, 3 or 4 weeks of age, that there are one or two healed fractures of ribs, at the back of the chest, close to the spine, with prominent bony callus formation. There seems to be no reason to think this is a manifestation of child abuse; it is probable that at the time of birth the fractures were the result of handling the trunk during delivery.

Sub-dural Haemorrhage

Sub-dural haemorrhage is the commonest immediate cause of death of battered children. It may be associated with bruising of the scalp and fracture of the skull. Bruising is usually present, if not fracture of the skull, but both forms of injury may be absent. Sub-dural haemorrhage alone may be caused by severe shaking (Guthkeltch, 1971). Incidentally a good shaking is sometimes a form of chastisement and some, it appears, regard it as a proper form of resuscitation.

A baby admitted moribund to hospital was diagnosed as having meningitis. Autopsy disclosed a fresh sub-dural haemorrhage. Suspicion fell upon the father. He explained that the child had collapsed and stopped breathing; he had shaken it to revive it. This explanation was supported by the bacteriological and histological examinations, which confirmed the presence of *E. coli* meningitis and the absence of other injuries.

Caffey (1974) described the effects of shaking a child as a major cause of sub-dural haematoma and intra-ocular bleeding in battered babies: the "infantile whip-lash syndrome". Such children have no external signs of trauma to the head or fractures of the skull but there may be traction lesions of the periosteum of the long bones, without fracture. Habitual, prolonged shakings can produce permanent brain damage. Oliver (1975) described microcephally and permanent brain damage in three victims of child abuse.

On most occasions the bleeding is fresh but evidence of prior bleeding should be sought for, e.g. golden-brown staining of the dura mater. Histological examination of the dura should be a routine procedure since this may disclose iron-containing deposits of haemosiderin, which is derived from the disintegration of haemoglobin and is evidence of prior bleeding and thus of trauma.

It should be remembered that sub-dural haemorrhage can result from slight trauma (Russell, 1965).

Abdominal Injuries

The majority of abdominal injuries are the result of force applied to the centre of the upper abdomen. In consequence the liver is the organ most often injured; this occurred in 10 per cent of the cases examined by Camps and Cameron (1971). Injury to the mesentery and the duodeno-jejunal junction was also seen; it results from crushing force compressing the structures against the spine. Injury to the kidneys or bladder was also seen in 3 per cent of cases.

Boysen (1975) described a case of chylous ascites due to abdominal trauma during a battering. Green (1980) described chylothorax due to the same cause. Rees *et al.* (1975) reported traumatic V.S.D. due to child abuse of a girl aged 5 years.

Other Varieties of Child Abuse

Deliberate poisoning, often repeated, and sometimes administered during the child's stay in hospital, has been described by several authors, who include: Rogers *et al.* (1976), Derschwitz *et al.* (1979), Watson *et al.* (1979), Meadow (1977), Lorber *et al.* (1980) and Schnaps *et al.* (1981).

Needles inserted into a child's body is a form of abuse reported by Ramu (1977) and Bhaskaran (1978). Abuse, murder, by drowning was reported by Nixon and Peam (1977), Berger (1979) and Minford (1981) reported deliberate, partial suffocation, presenting as "near-miss" cases of "sudden infant death" syndrome. Kempe and Kempe (1978) drew attention to the problem of sexual abuse as another aspect of child abuse.

Kempe (1975) listed as uncommon manifestations of the battered child syndrome: isolated retinal haemorrhages; sub-galeal haemotomas, caused by pulling the hair; hand print bruises; human bite marks; genital injuries, especially biting or tying the penis; tear of the floor of the mouth due to forced feeding; intra-mural haematoma of the bowel; traumatic cysts of the pancreas; hypernatraemic dehydration; repeated poisonings and uncommonly jittery babies with neurological signs which resolve, for no apparent cause, in hospital.

It is as well to bear in mind, although not within the province of the pathologist, that grave mental damage can be inflected.

Natural Disease

It is, of course, imperative to exclude natural disease as the cause of, or as a contributary factor, in the death.

Haemorrhage may be the result of, or may be exaggerated by, haemophilia. The rare possibility of scurvy required consideration in one of our cases.

Toxic epidermal necrolysis may simulate injury by burns or scalds. As mentioned earlier, "burns" may prove to be the scars of chicken pox.

Diseases of bone, e.g. fragilitas ossium, usually associated with blue sclera, or infantile cortical hyperostosis must be excluded. The latter may simulate a fracture undergoing repair. Histological examination of the affected portion of the bone is essential and it may be necessary to obtain expert opinion from one familiar with the appearances of rare bone disorders. Congenital malformation of the spine may have played a significant part in the death.

Sub-dural haemorrhage may be the final complication of death from otitis media associated with thrombosis of venous sinuses.

Records

At all stages it is extremely important that good records are kept by those in medical charge of the child. Note in particular the nature, position, age, etc, of any injuries. (This concerns health visitors just as much as doctors). Solomons (1980) drew attention to the difficulties which arise in any subsequent medico-legal procedures if the initial medical records are inadequate. It is wise to supplement these, when appropriate, by clinical photographs, preferably in colour.

SUMMARY

The pathological diagnosis of a "battered baby" may be made if all, or most of, the following features are observed:

1. The subject is a child under the age of 5 and, especially, if aged between 3 and 15 months; it is more likely to be a male than a female, and an unwanted or illegitimate child.
2. There are multiple bruises and, especially, when they are of differing ages.
3. There is laceration of the upper lip, with laceration of its frenum.
4. There are multiple fractures, again more especially when these are of differing ages; this fact is more accurately ascertainable than the age of bruising. The fractures are of the skull, chest cage or long bones.
5. There is sub-dural haemorrhage. This sign is enhanced if there be evidence of prior haemorrhage.
6. Natural disease and poisoning have been excluded.
7. There is no satisfactory explanation of the injuries; the explanation is either palpably false or unreasonable.

THE LIVING BATTERED BABY

Medical practitioners should be alert to recognise the possibility that a child in their care is being subjected to cruel treatment. The practitioner himself is not the best person to pursue inquiries in this matter since he has neither the time nor the necessary training; his relationship to the family also places him at a disadvantage to handle the matter to best advantage. His health visitor, if one is attached to the practice, can make tactful inquiries. (Although she has a statutory duty to visit the new-born, the parents can deny her entry.) Alternatively, the Medical Defence Union (1966) have indicated that the doctor can send a confidential report to the local Medical Officer of Health, to an officer of the local Department of Social Services (formerly the Children's Department) or to an officer of the National Society for the Prevention of Cruelty to Children. These persons are well qualified to undertake the necessary inquiries.

If the child be ill, arrangements should be made for its admission to hospital; this may be a wise step, even when the child is not seriously ill but is in danger of further ill-treatment.

If the child dies, its death must be reported to the coroner. A current medical certificate of cause of death should not be issued.

Illustrative Case Reports

The following case reports illustrate the text and are self-explanatory. They illustrate unequivocal battery and also illustrate the need for caution in arriving at this diagnosis.

The first two reports are examples of battery and the third, although in all probability another, could not be proved and therefore the mother was properly acquitted. The fourth was in all probability an accident. The fifth occurred in circumstances of neglect but there was no proof of battery. The sixth is an example of battery by another child in the family. The seventh was an unusual accident.

Case 1. A boy aged 3 years died of internal bleeding due to rupture of the liver and left kidney; there was fresh blood, about 6 oz, in the peritoneal cavity and a considerable quantity, at least $1/2$ pint, of blood behind the peritoneum on the left side. The liver had been ruptured between the right and left lobes, through the thickness of the organ, and the left kidney was completely divided between the upper two and lower thirds; there were subsidiary tears. Externally, bruising of relatively recent date was widely distributed over the trunk, limbs and face, with a substantial bruise in the right parietal region. Only six bruises, four at the front of the chest, exceeded $1/4$ in. in diameter and none was directly related either to the liver or left kidney. There was no bodily disease; the child was somewhat underweight (23 lb 2 oz), but of normal stature ($38^1/_2$ in.). It was conceded that some of the bruises were probably accidental, as by falls, tumbles or bumps, but the number and distribution could not be satisfactorily explained in this way. The internal injury was believed to be due to blunt force of at least moderate severity and by two blows rather than by one alone. Both had occurred within 24 hours of the death and the agent could have been a fist or an unshod foot. While another child could have produced the skin bruises, it was believed that only an adult (or teenage) person could have caused the internal injuries. It so happened that the culprit had been seen by a child aged 8 years, the boy's sister, to maltreat the boy, but she was properly prevented from giving evidence when she admitted that she had discussed the case with her mother. The child, however, had made a detailed statement long beforehand, in which she said the accused had thrown the boy towards the ceiling of their living room and allowed him to fall violently to the ground. She had seen him kick the boy. The accused endeavoured to shift the blame to the boy's mother, alleging that she had hit him with a shoe fitted with a stiletto heel. The bruises and the complete absence of any abrasions in relation to them were inconsistent with such treatment; nor could it have ruptured the liver and kidney. When first questioned the accused had admitted that he had punched the boy a few times. "I killed him. I want to hang." The mother had seen him hit the boy and likened the blows to those normally given to a grown-up person. The jury rejected his story; he was acquitted of murder but convicted of manslaughter.

Mr. Justice Streatfield imposed a sentence of 12 years imprisonment (F.M. 8143B; *R*. v. *Wilson*, Leeds Assizes, 27 Mar. 1962).

Case 2. The victim was a boy aged 3 years, who was poorly nourished but not emaciated (wt. 17 lb; ht. 32 in.). His death was due to bilateral pneumothorax following fracture dislocation of the lumbar spine (L. 1-2) and rupture of the diaphragm. He too had numerous recent bruises, widely distributed, on the face and limbs. Some of the bruises were fading; others were recent. There was no natural disease to account for this death, but it was alleged he had had diarrhoea a few days before this death; the intestinal contents were scanty and fluid or only slightly inspissated; no pathogenic bacteria were present in them.

In view of the nature of the principal injury, the Crown was advised also to call an orthopaedic surgeon as a witness. He examined the spine and confirmed the occurrence of a fracture dislocation between L. 1-2; there was partial separation of each vertebral body and no signs of repair. The spinal cord was visible in the depths of the fracture line; the anterior spinal ligament was completely torn across. The psoas minor muscles and the attachments of the diaphragm were torn. It was a recent injury. Deep bruising of the muscles beside the spine at the level of the fracture dislocation was seen in three places, lying in the same horizontal line. This fracture was produced by hyperextension and not by flexion nor by rotation. There was no disease. Mr. Fitton, F.R.C.S., had not seen such a fracture before and it is one of some rarity. In adults it is produced only by great violence, e.g. falls from a height or crushing by a roof-fall in a coal mine. The accused, the boy's mother, admitted injuring the child, but did not disclose what had happened. The fracture dislocation certainly did not occur, as suggested by the defence, by falling from the sideboard on to the arm of a well-upholstered armchair. We believe the child had stood beside her, inside the arm of a fireside chair, and she had bent the child's spine forcibly over the wooden arm. It was noted, later, that the room contained such a chair with a broken arm. She was acquitted of murder because there was no intent to do serious injury, but she was convicted of manslaughter. There was a strong recommendation to mercy and she was placed on probation for 3 years (*R*. v. *Barker*, Leeds Assizes, 2 May 1961; F.M. 7492).

Case 3. This boy, aged 2 years, died of compression of the brain by bilateral subdural haemorrhage. There were numerous bruises on his body, including nine on the forehead. At the back of each knee joint and on the outer side of the right thigh there were patterned bruises in the form of circles, each $^1/_4$ in. in diameter, arranged in equilateral triangles, the sides of which were $^1/_2$ in. long (Fig. 18a, b, p. 100). The left lower incisors had recently been lost and there was accompanying laceration of the adjacent gum and of the mucosa of the upper lip. These changes were without any sign of vital reaction or repair (Fig. 25a, p. 110). Although due to blunt injury, probably a blow, this occurred so close to the moment of death that it was impossible to say whether the child still lived at the time; his injury was therefore deemed to have been sustained after death. (In consequence, the judge at once excluded it from the medical evidence.)

The mother was charged with murder. It was alleged that she had beaten the child and pushed it violently so that it sustained a head injury, causing the sub-dural haemorrhage. It was also alleged that for some time she had ill-treated this child in a manner sufficient at least to cause grievous bodily harm. The evidence concerning the last day of the child's life was conflicting. The family lived in one room in a house in which several families resided and there were other young children in the house. A child was heard screaming, but was it the deceased boy? A leather belt about $1^1/_2$ in. wide, bearing brass cones arranged in equilateral triangles, was present in the room and she admitted she had chastised the child with it, but not later than the morning of the day on which he died. She admitted she had felt impelled to chastise this child on other occasions, e.g. when her husband had chastised an elder child. In a statement she made, she was alleged to have said, "I had to hit David (the deceased) because I could not see Paul being scolded. I seemed to have taken every opportunity of punishing David. I have not a clue why I have done this, nor why I hated him so."

In my opinion, the bruising, although widely distributed and, as to some of it, clearly due to chastisement with a belt of the kind produced, did not cause this death. It was due to sub-dural haemorrhage, but it was impossible to say which of the several bruises on the head was related to the injury which caused the internal bleeding. Such haemorrhages, nearly always due to injury, could result from a fall or blow, if a fall, it would be more probably accelerated by running or a push. The accused said that a few days prior to his death he had fallen and hit his head on an open drawer which contained his toys. He then became unconscious, but recovered after her husband had applied artificial respiration. The defence suggested that the child, confined to this room for hours in wet weather, had developed a habit of walking round and round the settee clockwise and had banged his head on the settee. It had hard, relatively sharp edges and the child could have slipped and bumped his head on one of them. The accused admitted having pushed the child about 15 minutes before he died, but sub-dural haemorrhage does not normally kill quickly; the shortest time is about 4 hours. I was unable to say whether the sub-dural haemorrhage was due to a blow or a fall. The dislodgement of the teeth and injury to the gum was left unexplained, but, in my opinion, this could not have occurred during the transport of the body to the mortuary or at the mortuary. It is now recognised (1971) as a hallmark of battery; but even so, in this case it could not be proved to have been inflicted during life. Exactly what occurred during that evening will never be known, since the accused was alone with the child.

On the medical evidence alone, the jury was bound to acquit the accused of murder and manslaughter. She was discharged (*R. v. C.*, Leeds Assizes, 29 and 30 April 1960).

Case 4. A female infant, aged 5 months, had a few superficial bruises of different ages, of from $^1/_4$ to $^1/_2$ in. in diameter over both knees, on the outer side of an ankle, the left cheek, and one or two on the arms. She was a well nourished, clean child. There was no external injury of the scalp but a small circular bruise was found in the deeper layers, over the right parietal bone. There was no fracture of the skull but she had a recent sub-dural haemorrhage with soft red clot of up to $^3/_8$ in. in thickness on both sides; the brain was not damaged. A few petechial haemorrhages were present beneath the conjunctivae. The upper air passages contained a small quantity of creamy material which had an acid reaction. There was a scoliosis, with deviation to the right, near D. 7. Two thin areas of bright red blood between the pleura and the upper ribs on the left side marked the sites of recent fractures of ribs 3, 4, 7 and 8. The skin of the back was normal and extensive cuts into the muscles showed no definite bruising. A healing fracture of the eighth rib was present on the right side. There were no fractures of the long bones.

The body was subjected to radiological examination which disclosed a remarkable degree of skeletal malformation. In addition to scoliosis, there was an extensive cervical spina bifida, hemivertebra in the mid-dorsal region and fusion of the spinal ends of ribs on both sides in the upper part of the chest. The radiologist (Dr. Michael Winn) was of the opinion that the ribs were abnormally thin (Fig. 164).

The police were satisfied that the home conditions were satisfactory; there was no evidence of neglect. The parents were young, in their twenties, not over-intelligent, who gave no grounds for suspicion. The child was their only child, legitimised by wedlock. On the day the child died she was alone with her father; she then appeared to be in normal health. He had fed the child with a bottle of milk and supported her on a cushion against the arm of the settee. This was close to a slightly raised, tiled hearth. (The distance from the seat of the settee to the hearth was 14 in.) He sat near the child to watch television. When the set needed adjustment he got up and crossed the room to do this. As he turned he saw the child topple on to the hearth; the right side of her head hit the edge. He immediately picked the child up and noticed she had difficulty in breathing. He attempted mouth-to-mouth artificial respiration and shook her, without success. An ambulance was summoned and the attendant attempted resuscitation and, it appeared, performed external cardiac massage. This was unsuccessful. The impression given by the father was that he was undoubtedly telling the truth.

The interpretation of the findings was that the immediate cause of death was asphyxia due to inhaling stomach contents. This could have been precipitated by, or resulted from, the fall. The fall produced the bruising of the scalp and the sub-dural haemorrhage, the principal cause of death. The rib fractures, so recent that they could have occurred shortly after death, were a result of attempted resuscitation, either by the father or the ambulance attendant. The malformation of the skeleton was such that slight force could have broken these ribs. By the same token, some minor injury on an earlier occasion could have broken the rib on the right side. In the circumstances, a verdict of accidental death was a proper one. An open verdict in this case would have been unjust to the parents (Polson, 1966A).

Case 5. A female infant aged 3 years was brought by her mother into a police station during the early hours of 7 January. The mother was distracted and begged the police to save her child. It is not surprising that the initial impression gained by the police was that the child had been ill-treated. She was wasted, bore numerous bruises, and appeared to have a laceration at the back of her head—she was, in fact, dead. The child had been normal and well until about 3 weeks before when she "caught cold" and refused all solid food; she was fed on baby foods. During the day prior to her death she had felt sick and was retching. Her mother gave her some salt and water. Shortly before she died she was sick and then "became quiet". The child had been liable to tantrums during which she would bang her head on the bed or a chair. No doctor had attended the child nor had she been seen by a health visitor during the 3 weeks prior to her death. The deceased was one of four children and her mother, aged 33 years, was expecting a fifth. The mother was separated from her husband and depended solely on National Assistance. The home conditions were deplorable. The body weighed 14 lb and was 29 in. in length; wasting was obvious but it was not emaciated; it was moderately clean and not verminous. (Although severely underweight, due account was taken of the fact that she was small for her age.)

Many bruises were present; details of twenty-six were recorded. The majority were less than $^1/_2$ in. in diameter; they were all superficial, bruising being limited in most to the skin and immediately adjacent subcutaneous tissues. They had been sustained on different occasions; a few were recent but some could have been several days old. They were distributed in areas which could have been the sites of accidental injury, for example, the forehead and face, and the arms and legs. There was a fresh abraded bruise at the back of the head 1 in. in diameter but no laceration of the scalp. There was no fracture of skull, spine, ribs or long bones, nor any intra-cranial abnormality. The nasopharynx was flooded with stomach contents but there was no sign of asphyxia. Her large bowel, from caecum to anus, was filled with masses of firm faecal material of up to $1^1/_2 \times ^1/_2$ in. in diameter. The stomach still contained about 8 oz. of an ochre-coloured, digesting meal. (No poison was detected by toxicological analysis).

The interpretation was that the child had been sick; flooding of the nasopharynx had caused abrupt cardiac arrest (she had suddenly "become quiet"). Sickness was ascribed to delayed emptying of the stomach (her last

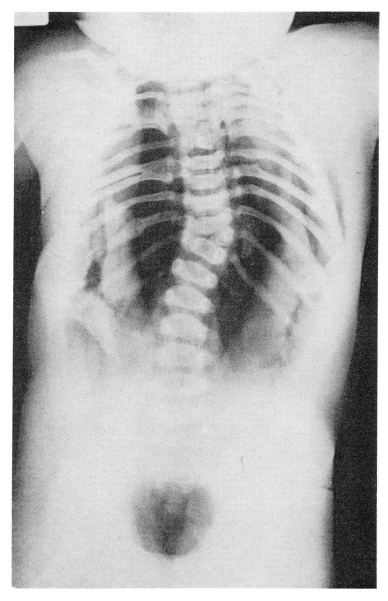

FIG. 164. Spinal deformity—alleged battered baby.

meal had been taken several hours before death) and grave constipation. This could have begun 3 weeks earlier when the child was first off-colour.

The bruising of her body was not the cause of death, nor was it deemed sufficient to cause ill-health. It was not of sufficient gravity to suggest criminal violence. It could have occurred during tantrums or from accidental bumps; some of the bruises could have been sustained during play with the other children.

The dead child had all the superficial appearance of a "battered baby" but as the investigation proceeded, and more information concerning her background was available, it was clearly unsafe, if not quite wrong, to allege ill-treatment.

The only criticism of the mother was on the question of neglect. Why had she not taken the child to her doctor? The mother, however, may not have realised that the child was really ill until it "became quiet". The mother, in the last stages of pregnancy, and with four children to care for, in deplorable home conditions and stringent financial circumstances, may have been doing her best.

The circumstances may well have been those of lack of care but, again, having regard to the circumstances, how far did this mother, in late pregnancy, fall short of what she could have been expected to do? (F.M. 11,121A; H. M. Coroner, Craven District, S. E. Brown Esq., I.I. M.) (Polson, 1966B).

Case 6. An unusual accident: death from crush asphyxia. A coloured child, aged 15 months, when found dead had suspicious marks on its body. The investigation of the circumstances established that the child had climbed out of its cot and proceeded to explore the interior of a large console radiogram, which was in the room. The gramophone compartment had a hinged front. He had succeeded in opening this compartment and had leant on the flap in order to reach the gramophone. It was shown, by test, that his weight on the flap would have been sufficient to cause the radiogram to topple over. When this happened his body was trapped between it and the flap of the gramophone compartment and he died of crush asphyxia (F.M. 14,011A).

Case 7. A male child, aged 6 months, lived with its mother, aged 22 years, in a fourth floor flat. At the time of the incident, in January, her husband, who was unemployed, was away from home. It was said to have been the first time that she had been alone with the child at night. It would not stop crying so she put him in his carry cot on an outside window ledge. She then went to sleep and did not wake up until 10 a.m. When she retrieved the baby, he was dead. The over-night air temperature was just above freezing.

An X-ray photograph, taken prior to the autopsy, revealed a fresh fracture of the right femur. There was no other evidence of recent or old bony injury. The autopsy findings were consistent with acute hypothermia; there was also some pulmonary fat embolism, some bruising of the scalp and a congenital abnormality of the skull; with premature closure of the frontal suture and anterior fontanelle.

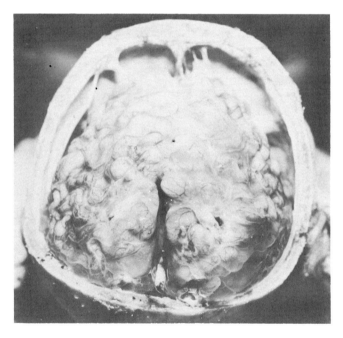

FIG. 165, Cerebral atrophy in child dying 1 year after severe battering (F.M. 15467A).

Subsequently the mother told the police that she had thrown the baby on to the floor and had slapped his head. She was convicted of manslaughter, (F.M. 23,630A).

Case 8. A male child, aged 8 months, died of strangulation and obstruction of the air passages by a disposable table napkin. There multiple abrasions and bruises of the face and neck. There were large quantities of white fibrous material adhering to the face and clothing. There was also extensive bruising of the muscles of the neck; a piece of cellulose wadding from a nappy was wedged in the pharynx and extended down, over the epiglottis, to reach the vocal cords.

At the trial the father was stated to have married the mother when she was pregnant by him. The child was delivered by Caesarian section and was not presented to his mother until a day or two later. This caused her to reject the child as not having been born naturally. Neither parent cared greatly for the child, although it was well fed and tended. On the night of the child's death the parents had been watching the film *Psycho* and during the night the father had become depressed. He decided that it was best that the child should die because he was not happy. The father strangled the baby in its carry cot. The father pleaded guilty to murder (F.M. 25,832A: Dr. Michael Green)

Case 9. Twins died as the result of sub-dural haemorrhage, caused by shaking. One of the babies was found dead at home. There were no external injuries nor bruising of the scalp but death was due to a fresh sub-dural haemorrhage and extra-dural haemorrhage, surrounding the spinal cord, from the 4th. cervical down to the thoracic vertebrae. No other internal injury was present.

The other twin died a week later, in hospital, from necrosis of the brain due to sub-dural haemorrhage, which had been operated upon. There was bleeding around both kidneys and the pancreas: chylous ascities was apparently due to rupture of the thoracic duct. These internal injuries were consistent with firm gripping of the child's abdomen during the shaking.

It was stated that the babies had been shaken during a row between the parents, who were not married. Both were convicted of manslaughter. (F.M. 28,535A and 28,569A: Dr. Michael Green).

References

ANDERSON, W. R. and HUDSON, R. P. (1976) *Forensic Sci.*, **7** (1), 71–74.
AKBARNIA, B., TORG, J. S., KIRKPATRICK, J. and SUSSMAN, S. (1974) *J. Bone Joint Surg.*, (Am) **56**-A (6) 1159–1166.
AYOUB, C. and PFEIFER, D. (1979) *Am. J. Dis. Child.*, **133** (9), 910–914.
BERGER, D. (1979) *J. Pediatrics*, **95** (4), 554–556.
BHASKARAN, C. K. (1978) *Arch. Dis. Child.*, **53** (12), 968.
BOYSEN, B. E. (1975) *Am. J. Dis. Child.* **129** (11), 1338–1339.
CAFFEY, J. (1946) *Am. J. Roentgenol*, **56**, 163–173.
CAFFEY, J. (1974) *J. Pediatrics*, **54** (4), 376–403.
CAMERON, J. M. JOHNSON, H. R. M. and CAMPS, F. E. (1966) *Med. Sci. Law*, 6–21.
CAMPS, F. E. and CAMERON, J. M. (1971) *Practical Forensic Medicine*. 2nd ed. London. Hutchinson Medical Publications.
CULLEN, J. C. (1975) *J. Bone Joint Surg.* (Br) **57** (3), 364–366.
DENSEN-GERBER, J. (1978) *Med. Leg. Ann.,* 135–147.
D'ORBAN, P. T. (1979) *Brit. J. Psychiat,* **134**, 560–571.
DICKSON, R. A. and LEATHERMAN, K.D. (1978) *J. Trauma* **18** (12), 811–812.
DERSCHWITZ, R. VESTAL, B. MACLAREN, N. K. and CORNBLATH, M. (1976) *Am. J. Dis. Child*, **130** (9), 998–999.
EDITORIAL (1981) *Brit. Med. J.,* **283**, 170.
ELLERSTEIN, H. S. (1979) *Am. J. Dis. Child.,* **133**, 906–909.
EMERY, J. L. (1978) *Med. Sci. Law,* **18** (2), 138–142.
FAIRBURN, A. D. and HUNT, A. C. (1964) *Med. Sci. Law,* **4**, 123–126.
GOSNOLD, J. K. and SIVALOGANATHAN, S. (1980) *Med. Sci. Law,* **20** (1), 54–57.
GREEN, H. G. (1980) *Pediatrics,* **66** (4), 620–621.
GUTHKELCH, A. N. (1971) *Brit. Med. J.* **ii**, 430–431.
HALTON, K. (1964) *Sunday Times Magazine,* 29 August.
HELFER, R. E., SLOVIS, T. L. and BLACK, M. (1977) *Pediatrics,* **60** (4), 533–5.
KAPLUN, D. and REICH, R. (1976) *Am. J. Psychiat.,* **133** (7), 809–813.
KEELING, J. W. (1981) in *Pediatric Pathology*. Ed. Berry, C. L. Berlin. Springer-Verlag.
KEEN, J. H., LENDROM, J. and WOLMAN, B. (1975) *Brit. Med. J.,* **4**, 268–269.
KEMPE, C. H. (1975) *Am. J. Dis. Child,* **29** (11), 1265.
KEMPE, C. H., SILVERMAN, F. M., STEELE, B. F., DROEGEMUELLER, W. and SILVER, H. K. (1962) *J. Am. Med. Ass.,* **181**, 17–24.
KEMPE, R. S. and KEMPE, C. H. (1978) *Child Abuse.* London. Fontana. Open Books.
KERLEY, E. R. (1978) *J. forensic sci.,* **23** (1), 163–168.
LAW, S. K. (1979) *Med. Sci. Law.,* **19** (1), 55–60.
EDITORIAL (1973) *Can. med. ass. J.,* **108**, 130–131.
LEVIN, S. (1972) *S. Afr. Med. J.* **46**, 586–588.
LENOSKI, E. F. and HUNTER (1977) *J. Trauma,* **17** (11), 842–846.

LORBER, J. RECKLESS, J. P. D. and WATSON, J. B. G. (1980) *Arch. Dis. Child.*, **55** (8), 643–647.
MANNING, G. B. (1964) Personal communication.
MEADOW, R. (1977) *Lancet*, **ii**, 343–345.
Medical Defence Union (1966) Annual Report. London. M. D. U.
MINFORD, A. M. B. (1981) *Brit. Med. J.*, **282**, 521.
NIXON, J. and PEARN, J. (1977) *Brit. Med. J.*, **1**, 271–272.
NWAKO, F. A. (1979) *Med. Sci. Law*, **19** (2), 130–133.
OLIVER, J. F. (1977) *Brit. Med. J.*, **2**, 262–264.
OLIVER, J. E. (1983) *Brit. Med. J.*, **1**, 115–117.
PASCOE, J. M., HILDEBRANDT, H. M., TARRIER, A. and MURPHY, M. (1979) *Pediatrics*, **64** (2), 245–247.
POLSON, C. J. (1966A) *Med. Sci. Law*, **6**, 163.
POLSON, C. J. (1966B) in "Medical Progress", *Brit. Encyc. Med. Pract.* Ed-in-Chief: Lord Cohen of Birkenhead.
    London Butterworth, page 152.
RAMU, M. (1977) *Med. Sci. Law*, **17** (4), 259–260.
REES, A., SYMONS, J., JOSEPH, M., and CINCOLN, C. (1975) *Brit. Med. J.*, **i**, 20–21.
ROGERS, D., TRIPP, J., BENTOVIM, A., ROBINSON, A., BERRY, D. and GOULDING, R. (1976) *Brit. Med. J.*, **i**,
    793–
RUSSELL, P. A. (1965) *Brit. Med. J.*, **ii**, 446–448.
SCHNAPS, Y., FRAND, M., ROTEM, Y., and TIVOS, L. M. (1981) *Pediatrics*, 68 (1), 110–121.
SOLOMONS, G. (1980) *Am. J. Dis. Child*, **134**, (5) 503–505.
TURNER, E. A. (1964) *Brit Med. J.*, **i**, 308.
WATSON, J. B., DAVIES, J. M. and HUNTER, J. L. P. (1979) *Arch. Dis. Child.*, **54** (2), 143–144.
WILSON, E. F. (1977) *Pediatrics*, **60** (5), 750–752.

GENERAL REFERENCES

CAMERON, J. M. (1974) *Leg. Med. Annu.*, 123–34.
PALMER, C. H. and WESTON, J. T. (1976) *J. Forensic Sci.*, **21**, 851–5.
SCOTT, P. D. (1977). *Brit. J. Psychiatry*, **131**, 366–80.
HORAN, F. T. and BEIGHTON, P. H. (1980) *J. Bone Joint Surg.*, **62**-B, 243–7.
ZUMWALT, R. E. and HIRSCH, C. S. (1980) *Hum. Pathol.*, **11**, 167–74.
WECHT, C. H. and LARKIN, G. M. (1980) *Leg. Med.*, 31–55.
O'DOHERTY, N. (1982) *The Battered Child*, London, Bailliere Tindall.

CHAPTER 17

Sudden Natural Death

Introduction

Of the cases of sudden death investigated by the forensic pathologist, after adequate examination, about 75 per cent of the total number will be found to be deaths from natural causes.

Many unnatural causes of death produce few, and slight changes which can be recognised with the naked eye at post-mortem examination. Therefore, unless the pathologist is thoroughly familiar with the features of the various natural causes of death, he will not appreciate when there is insufficient natural disease to account for death; moreover, unless he is acquainted with the uncommon varieties of natural death, he may incorrectly attribute a death to unnatural causes, such as poisoning, when it was a natural death.

The major potential cause of mistakes is the approach to a post-mortem examination with a preconceived idea of the cause of death. It is easy to recommend caution, but difficult to avoid forming an opinion from the medical history of the case, or other information received, for instance, from the Coroner's officer. Of course, it is essential to have such information, lest appropriate tests for certain less obvious conditions, such as diabetes, may not be carried out until it is too late and suitable specimens have been destroyed.

Nevertheless, there is a risk, especially in a busy practice, sooner or later to assume, for instance, "this man has had pains in the chest, the cause must be, obviously, 'coronary occlusion'", and open the chest as the first step, in order to examine the heart as quickly as possible, thereby missing the evidence of spontaneous pneumothorax.

Functional causes of death, such as hyper- or hypoglycaemic coma, epilepsy, asthma, etc., are especially liable to be overlooked.

Also, when the history suggests death due to poisoning, the pathologist may not take material for histological examination and later may find that the analysis has not detected any poison; he will then be unable to determine the cause of death.

Histological examination of selected material should be an integral part of any of these post-mortems.

Moreover, a danger is to ignore the coincidence of non-fatal natural disease, for example osteo-arthritis, in the presence of an overdose of poison. Later, when it is too late to make a further examination, natural disease may assume a considerable importance as a factor leading to taking an overdose, and a reason for the treatment received by the deceased before death.

Therefore it follows that a complete autopsy is imperative on all occasions when investigating a case for the Coroner. The omission to open the skull and examine the brain is inexcusable. The case which seems the simplest and most obvious at the time is the one which may cause the greatest trouble later on.

It is essential that in any medico-legal autopsy, even when there is no suspicion of an unnatural cause of death, or any possible dispute over factors not related to the cause of death, always to make a thorough external and internal examination of the body.

The spinal cord should be examined if there appears to be any possible disease or injury of the spine or nervous system. In children the middle ear, in elderly persons the femora, and the bone marrow where there seems a likelihood of a blood disorder, must receive attention.

Incidence of Natural Disease

The table gives an indication of the distribution of the different causes of death in a year, as found in the Department of Forensic Medicine at Leeds. The area served by the Department is a typical industrial urban area. Areas with other geographical characteristics such as a major sea-port, or a predominantly rural district, might be expected to show differences in the proportions of different categories of disease.

NATURAL DEATHS,

	1981	1970		1981	1970
Cardiovascular system			*Respiratory system*		
Haemopericardium	44	35	Pulmonary embolism	33	31
Coronary thrombosis	161	129	Broncho-pneumonia (secondary)	54	47
Coronary atheroma	422	325	Lobar pneumonia	10	24
Aortic/mitral valve	20	27	Virus pneumonia	—	1
Hypertension	37	21	Acute/chronic bronchitis	38 + 1	14
Ruptured aneurysm	48	19	Asthma	8	7
Senility	—	2	Cot death	5	39
Atrial myxoma	—	2	Pneumoconiosis		1
Myocarditis	3	5	Bronchiectasis		1
Fatty heart	—	1	Ca. of bronchus	10	10
Ball thrombus	—	1	Hamman Rich		1
Amyloid	—	1	TB		1
			Broncho pneumonia (primary)	24	—
Central nervous system			*Others*		
Cerebral haemorrhage	25	18	Haemorrhage-ulcer	9	3
Sub-arachnoid haemorrhage	16	10	Intestinal obstruction	3	8
Cerebral thrombosis	5	2	Peritonitis	13	6
Epilepsy	3	4	Gastro-enteritis		1
Brain abscess	—	1	Mesenteric thrombosis	1	2
			Pyloric stenosis	—	1
Genito-urinary system			Carcinoma/pancreas	—	1
			Carcinoma/colon	1	3
Pyelonephritis	4	3	Carcinoma/stomach	2	3
Carcinoma/bladder	1	2	Hepatitis	1	2
Carcinoma/kidney	1	1	Fat embolism	—	1
			Thyrotoxicosis	—	1
			Liver cirrhosis	4	—

UNNATURAL DEATHS,

	1981	1970		1981	1970
Poisoning by analgesics	15	—	Falls	16	4
Poisoning/CO	1111	15	Burns/fires	10	3
Poisoning/barbiturates	3	36	Electrocution	1	5
Poisoning/other	15	10	Self-strangulation	1	2
Hanging	13	6	Intoxication	—	2
Drowning	7	11	Cut-throat	2	4
Vehicle road accidents	44	39	Gunshot	2	1
Exposure	5	2	Stabbing	—	2
Plastic bag/suffocation	1	2	Anoxia	—	2

HOMICIDE,

	1981	1970		1981	1970
Stabbing	10	4	Shooting	3	2
Head injuries	8	8	Incised wounds	1	1
Strangulation/ligature	3	4	Smothering	—	2
Strangulation/manual	4	2	Duod. haematoma	—	1
Cut-throat	1	—	Abortion	—	1

Almost any disease capable of causing death may be disclosed at a Coroner's autopsy, since many of these subjects have not died suddenly. They were persons known to have had chronic disease but the patient's practitioner, not having seen the patient for some time found himself unable to issue a certificate of cause of death. The present account, however, restricts attention of disease capable of causing sudden or undiagnosed cause of death.

DISEASES OF THE CARDIO-VASCULAR SYSTEM

Coronary Artery Disease

This group represents the commonest cause of sudden natural death at this time, in this country. Narrowing or occlusion of the coronary arteries by atheroma is the commonest condition to be found; coronary thrombosis, although figuring frequently on certificates of cause of death, given without autopsy, only accounts for about a quarter of the total number of deaths from coronary artery disease; embolism of the coronary arteries, aneurysms, both mycotic and dissecting, and arteritis are comparatively rare.

The aetiology of atheroma in general, especially that affecting the coronary arteries, remains in doubt, despite a vast amount of research. The older idea of simple accumulation of lipids within the vessel walls has been superseded by the concept of recurrent mural fibrin thrombi becoming incorporated into the vessel walls.

For reviews of the current concepts of pathogenesis of coronary atheroma the reader should refer to Crawford (1977). The sites of atheroma may be determined by hydrodynamic factors. The distribution of the disease is distinctly irregular. In younger age groups it tends to occur primarily in the left coronary artery, mainly in the descending branch; usually in the form of plaques of soft yellow-white material which reduce the lumen of the vessel (at their site) to an eccentric slit-like form. In older persons the thickening of the vessel walls is concentric and the dimensions of the lumen are progressively reduced until of pin-hole size. Davies and Popple (1979) consider that 85 per cent stenosis is the minimum reasonably associated with sudden death.

Patches of calcification may affect the vessel walls in some areas, often the descending branch of the left artery, and on occasion render considerable lengths of the vessels too hard to cut. Although it may be possible to sever these vessels by using a knife with a serrated edge, this often causes disruption; the crushed vessel can give little indication of its condition in life. On these occasions decalcification of the intact artery, as recommended by Osborn, or perfusion by radio-opaque solutions and radiography of the heart (Crawford *et al.*, 1961) is necessary.

In elderly persons, calcification of the vessel walls is likely to occur, converting them into quite rigid tubes, but with little atheromatous disease, and no encroachment on the lumen of the vessel, so that palpation and attempts to section the vessels may give a false impression of their state of patency.

The soft central constituents of an atheromatous plaque are liable to burst through the overlying intima, into the lumen of the vessel. Sometimes this appearance may be artificially produced during the section of the vessel by the knife. However, microscopical examination will usually demonstrate when the rupture is an artifact. If it occurred before death, the extruded contents of the plaque may often become incorporated in a thrombus within the lumen of the vessel. Alternatively there may be bleeding into the intima of the side of the rupture, with some fibrin formation, and serial sections may reveal small areas of dissection of the wall above the level of the rupture. Details of the examination of coronary arteries are described by Osborn (1967).

AGE DISTRIBUTION OF CASES SHOWING CORONARY OCCLUSION BY ATHEROMA	
Age	%
Up to 40 years	1.7
40 to 50 years	7
50 to 60 years	18
Over 60 years	72

The extent of atheromatous disease of the vessels increases with age, but on occasions gross disease is found in the vessels of young persons in the second or third decades. In such cases it is well to consider the possibility of some biochemical disorder, often familial such as hypercholesterolaemic atheromatosis, e.g. a man of 40 who had visible coronary occlusion due to a lesion of an unusual greenish hue. A sample of his blood, on standing, sedimented rapidly producing a layer of serum which had a pronounced milky-white appearance. Post-mortem biochemical tests (Dr. Payne) demonstrated:

N.E.F.A. Plasma . . .	0.98 m Eq/litre
T.E.F.A. 1440	m/100 ml
Electrophoresis . . . Plasma	Massive pre-beta
Lipo-protein Band:	Present
Plasma Cholesterol	444 mg/100 ml.

Coronary thrombosis, in our experience, is found in the same age distribution as coronary atheroma.

Age	%
AGE DISTRIBUTION OF CASES SHOWING CORONARY THROMBOSIS	
Up to 40 years	2.4
40 to 50 years	9.8
50 to 60 years	14.7
Over 60 years	73.7

It is only found in about one-quarter of deaths from coronary artery disease, though other authors (Crawford, 1969) have reported it as occurring much more frequently in their series.

Thromboses occur most frequently in the descending branch of the left coronary artery, next in the right coronary artery and then the left circumflex, and least frequently in the left main artery. Fresh thrombi are dark red-brown and attached to the vessel walls. Occasional thrombi, which are mainly composed of platelets, are pale pink-red in colour.

Although they frequently occur in vessels which are narrowed by atheroma, they are not infrequently found in vessels, especially the right main coronary artery, which have an otherwise patent lumen. Such thrombi have been seen in the Department recently in several young married women who had taken contraceptive pills. This association was noted by Radford and Oliver (1973).

With the passage of time, for coronary thrombosis is not always immediately fatal, the thrombus becomes organised, by ingrowth of connective tissue from the vessel walls, and ultimately there may be some re-canalisation. Old coronary thromboses, which were survived, may often be seen in persons, dead of a subsequent heart attack, as homogeneous yellowish or grey firm plugs blocking the vessels.

Sub-intimal haemorrhage is another common lesion of the coronary arteries, which may be associated with sudden death. Sometimes these appear as narrow crescentic bands of dark-red bleeding into the middle of the vessel wall, but often they present as a mass of soft pasty atheromatous debris in a large plaque in the wall, associated with bleeding into the mass. This is more often detected by microscopic examination of the occluded portion of the vessel.

It is suggested that much of the progressive atheromatous disease of the vessel walls is due to sub-intimal haemorrhages, with organisation and endothelial proliferation, due to poorly supported and nourished arteries in the vessel walls, subjected to sheering strains (Morgan, 1956).

Other lesions of the coronary arteries are rare. Embolism may be due to impacted atheromatous debris from ulcerated plaques further up the vessel, to fragments of thrombus or tumour in the atria or vegetations from heart valves in bacterial endocarditis, or any other embolic substances, such as fat.

Dissecting aneurysms of the coronary arteries have been described especially in young women in the post-mortem period (Burton and Zawadzki, 1962). Saccular aneurysms are especially rare. Only one has been seen in the Department in recent years. Arteritis, apparently polyarteritis nodosa, is also rare.

With any of these lesions of the arteries, but especially with occlusion of the vessels by atheroma, death may occur without any detectable injury of the myocardium, though there may be patches of fibrosis or larger fibrous scars indicating the sites of previous infarcts. The mode of death is presumably sudden fibrillation, due to a localised area of ischaemia in the heart muscle.

Where occlusion by a thrombus and death has been postponed for several hours after the occlusion damage to the heart muscle may be detectable. On naked-eye examination this may be seen first as a slightly congested, roughened area of the muscle, or a zone of pallor with waxy appearance of the muscle. The characteristic yellow area of established myocardial infarction, usually with a red peripheral zone, is not apparent for about 24 hours after the establishment of the occlusion. In the succeeding few days patches of the centre of this infarct may become softened, translucent and even rather cystic. Fibrosis of the tissue is apparent to the naked eye after about 2 weeks, progressing ultimately to a fully established dense white fibrous scar. However, it is not uncommon to see an area of heart muscle showing a mixture of changes, e.g. small white fibrous scars set in a zone of yellow infarcted muscle. Presumably this represents a progressively widening zone of ischaemia in the area of distribution of a particular artery. At about 12 hours or more after the commencement of the infarction microscopical evidence of damaged muscle fibres will appear slightly hazy, and will show increased staining with eosin, in haematoxylin eosin preparations. Nuclei become square and pyknotic. Sections stained by phosphotungstic acid haematoxylin, which shows up the cross striation of the muscle, will demonstrate heaping up of these regular bands and an alteration in colour of staining from the normal blue-black to a reddish brown. With periodic acid–Schiffe stains, infarcted areas assume a purple-blue compared to the pale-lilac colour of normal muscle tissue. Such changes in isolated individual muscle fibres scattered throughout a section are not uncommonly seen associated with any form of anoxia, but in cardiac infarction the change may be expected to be seen in large groups of fibres. Congestion, with diapedesis and polymorph infiltration of areas of infarcted muscle is seen at about 12 hours.

Connor (1970) has described the use of a stain containing cresyl violet and acid fuchsin, which he has found valuable in the early demonstration of myocardial infarction.

Hudson (1965) cites a study by Lodge-Patch as giving a calendar of events, macro- and microscopical, in the development of myocardial infarcts. Thus neutrophil polymorphs appear by 6 hours, and are prominent at the edge of the area by 48 hours. Mononuclear cells commence to appear by the 4th day, and contain golden-brown pigment during the 3rd week. Fibroblasts and ingrowing capillaries begin to appear at the 4th day. (For full details the original articles must be consulted.)

For the histochemical demonstration of myocardial infarction, using macroscopic and microscopic techniques, the reader is referred to the articles by Knight (1965) in *Medicine, Science and the Law*, and in *Gradwohl's Legal Medicine*, and by Sahai and Knight (1976) and by Crawford (1969; 1977) the latter described the chronological order of microscopical changes.

Death may occur within the first few hours or days after infarction, and the immediate cause is ventricular fibrillation. Another cause of sudden death soon after the onset of infarction is rupture of the ventricular wall in the infarcted area, and death from cardiac tamponade. The quantity of fluid and clotted blood within the pericardial sac at autopsy usually amounts to about 10–15 oz. Such ruptures may occur in the centre of an infarcted area, appearing as a small linear tear in the epicardium, approximately $^1/_2-1$ in. long, and a haemorrhagic tract can be demonstrated through the infarcted muscle. Death in such cases occurs in 2 or 3 days after the onset of the infarction, and is apparently due to rupture of the softened necrotic centre of the infarct.

In many cases rupture of the heart and death occurs much sooner after the onset of infarction. It is then possible to demonstrate an occlusion of the artery supplying the area by atheroma or thrombus, but no definite zone of infarction of the muscle surrounding the site of rupture; the myocardium may have a faint pallor in that region.

In our experience ruptures leading to haemopericardium are only found in the wall of the left ventricle.

Rare complications of myocardial infarction which may cause sudden death are ruptures of an infarcted papillary muscle with sudden failure of function of the mitral valve with or without rupture of the interventricular septum, creating an interventricular septal defect. The infarcted muscle is not contractile and usually a layer of thrombus forms on the endocardium overlying the area of infarction, with small nodules of thrombus between the columnae carnae. Fragments may become detached and cause embolism of the coronary arteries or remote organs such as the brain.

Occasionally when an infarction is survived for a long time the fibrous scar at the site of the infarct may become distended and a cardiac aneurysm may form which contains layers of mural thrombus from which emboli may be derived. The sac can exceed the size of a normal left ventricle (Polson, 1941).

Many hearts, by the time that death occurs, show a mixture of lesions, widely scattered through the myocardium. Frequently there is extensive fibrosis, scars representing old areas of infarction, or there may be a diffuse fibrosis of the ventricular wall, which is sometimes associated with a thin yellow layer of fresh infarction of the sub-endocardial tissues, appearing extensive in the area of the inner surface of the ventricle affected, but only forming a thin layer of the muscle wall.

Cardiac infarction, when well developed, may be associated with a fibrinous pericarditis and opaque pericardial effusion. Resolution of this may result in the formation of localised adhesions between the pericardial sac and the epicardium, or complete obliteration of the pericardial sac by fine fibrous adhesions, which do not, however, cause constriction of the heart. There may be calcification of the organised tissue.

Deaths from coronary occlusion or thrombosis are invariably associated with pulmonary oedema, due to acute left ventricular failure; whereas long-standing failure produces severe oedema, greatest in amount in the lower parts of the lungs, in acute coronary deaths with sudden collapse it is usual to find oedema much more prominent in the upper lobes.

Hypertensive Heart Disease

Cardiac hypertrophy beyond the recognised weights for the deceased's age, especially above 400 g, are a frequent finding in sudden deaths from heart disease. Such hypertrophy is usually associated with severe coronary artery disease and death appears to be principally due to the ischaemia of the muscle resulting from this. It is uncommon to find cases in which there is evidence of left ventricular failure, with pulmonary oedema, with uncomplicated cardiac hypertrophy.

A cause for the hypertension can rarely be found. Occasionally renal disease, for example hydronephrosis, ureteric obstruction by calculi or renal artery stenosis can be demonstrated. Very rarely a phaeochromocytoma is revealed.

Valvular Heart Disease

Valve lesions may be found not infrequently in cases of sudden death and appear in many cases to be tolerated well until relatively late in life (Hargreaves, 1961).

A specific valve lesion occurring in the older age groups is calcific aortic stenosis (annular sclerosis), which is apparently due to atheromatous degeneration of the valve cusps and ring, and not a legacy from rheumatic heart disease in earlier years. Such rigid stenosed valves frequently appear to be bicuspid due to contraction of the cusp margins (may give the erroneous impression of a congenitally abnormal valve). They may be associated with considerable degrees of left ventricular hypertrophy. Aortic stenosis is uncommon, probably related to the decreased incidence of tertiary syphilis. Mitral stenosis in milder degree may be found in middle-aged persons, and may be associated with a ball-valve thrombus in the left auricle or signs of atrial fibrillation, thrombus in the left auricular appendage and evidence of previous embolic episodes in spleen, kidney or brain.

A degenerative change of the cusps of the mitral valve, recently recognised, which may be associated with sudden death is the "floppy-valve syndrome". The affected cusp is much larger than the other, white, and, microscopically, shows mucoid degeneration (Pomerance, 1975). This may be the sole finding at autopsy. For example: an elderly woman was imprisoned in a cupboard by a burglar. She was released unharmed but died a few minutes later. The sole pathological finding was a "floppy" mitral valve (F.M. 24,161).

Bacterial endocarditis is now rarely a cause of sudden death since almost all cases, especially of sub-acute bacterial endocarditis, are diagnosed and treated in life, but fulminating bacterial endocarditis sometimes occurs (F.M. 9439).

Cardiomyopathies

These represent an uncommon group of causes of sudden death, many of which do not advertise their presence by visible changes in heart muscle. In any autopsy where the cause of death is not apparent the whole heart, or at least representative blocks from it, should be taken for histological examination. These should include a block from each of the lateral walls of the right and left ventricles, and from the interventricular septum.

Lesions may be scattered and infrequent and may be absent from a single block of tissue. Isolated myocarditis as a cause of sudden death was recorded by Corby (1960).

Asymmetrical cardiomyopathy, or cardiac hypertrophy, was first described by Teare (1958) and cases occurring in Northern Ireland were described by Marshall (1970).

This condition can affect persons in any age group and in our experience their ages ranged from 13 to 60 years. It is usually undiagnosed or diagnosed as sub-aortic stenosis in the living. More often it is the cause of sudden, unexpected collapse and death.

Externally the heart appears normal, or slightly hypertrophied, but when opened in the usual manner, the characteristic feature is a swelling of the right side of the inter-ventricular septum. The columnae carnae over the septum are considerably enlarged by as much as three or four times normal size; they are pallid and yellow-brown in colour. These abnormal columnae are in striking contrast to the adjacent normal muscle bundles over the inner surface of the ventricle. The appearance is equally striking on the left side of the septum, but, because the columnae are normally larger on that side, there is less contrast between the normal and abnormal muscles. The septum is thickened and the muscle on the cut surface is pallid, coarse, and sometimes flecked with areas of white fibrosis. The enlarged septum protrudes into the cavities of the ventricles, especially the left, and makes a pronounced ridge of tissue below the aortic valve.

On microscopic examination the abnormal tissue consists of hypertrophied muscle fibres arranged in a wholly irregular fashion, and associated with interstitial fibrosis.

The aetiology of the condition is unknown. The cause of sudden death due to this abnormality is also unknown, but it could be that the hyperplastic muscle acts as an ectopic focus of abnormal rhythms, and, presumably, may initiate ventricular fibrillation.

The other variety of cardiomyopathy which occurs in normal forensic practice from time to time is amyloid infiltration of the heart of the elderly, often aged over 80 years (McKeown, 1965). The heart muscle has a waxy, translucent appearance. Microscopical examination reveals widespread infiltration by strands of pink, amorphous material between the muscle fibres and some of the muscle fibres are atrophic and have been replaced by amyloid material. This condition is easy to overlook but, if in mind when examining the bodies of the elderly, it is not uncommon. It is distinct from the condition of primary amyloidism of younger persons, affecting the heart, tongue, etc.

Arterial Diseases

As causes of sudden death the only diseases of the arteries which are of any importance are those giving rise to aneurysms which are likely to rupture. Of these, the commonest today is an atheromatous aneurysm of the abdominal aorta, in persons usually male and over the age of 50. It is usually fusiform, situated between the origin of the renal arteries and the aortic bifurcation, and it is sometimes associated with aneurysmal dilatation of the common iliac arteries. As the walls of the aorta dilate they become coated with multiple layers of soft yellow-brown blood clot. Ultimately, it would seem, blood tracks through a defect in this layer of thrombus to reach, and rupture, the outer wall of the vessel, can lead to a massive retroperitoneal haemorrhage, mainly beneath the root of the mesentery and in the para-colic gutters; the amount of blood then extravasated may amount to $^1/_2-1$ litre. (It is not a true "sudden death"; it can take hours, and the lesion has been diagnosed in life.) Atheromatous aneurysms, except of the cerebral arteries and aorta, are rare.

Dissecting aneurysms of the aorta, though less common than the abdominal atheromatous aneurysm, usually occur in the thoracic portion of the aorta. They originate in rupture of the intima of the vessel at a weakened point overlying a plaque of atheroma or at a point of stress. This seems particularly liable to occur in the arch of the aorta, and the dissection between the intima and adventitia of the vessel usually extends proximally, leading to rupture of the adventitia near to the aortic valve into the pericardium causing death from cardiac tamponade. The total length of dissection is only a few centimetres. Less commonly the dissection may extend downwards, even to the level of the common iliac arteries. There may sometimes be re-entry into the lumen of the vessel at this lower level, a condition which the patient may survive for months or years, when the aneurysm is an incidental finding at autopsy.

In younger persons the rupture of the vessel wall leading to the dissection is more likely to be associated with the condition of cystic medial necrosis, which in turn may be one of the abnormalities associated with Marfan's Syndrome. Microscopic sections from blocks of intact aortic wall taken away from the region of the dissection, if a suitable area can be found, should be stained for elastic tissue (Voerhoff–Van Geison), and mucopolysaccharides (Alcian Blue), in order to demonstrate that these cystic spaces are related to destruction of the elastic laminae and contain muco-polysaccharides.

Occasionally the wall of the ascending aorta appears to become weakened, dilated, and thinned, just above the aortic valve, and may rupture into the pericardial sac, with no dissection of the layers of the wall or thrombus formation. Such rupture is a not infrequent cause of haemopericardium, and must be sought whenever a ruptured myocardial infarct cannot be found. The site of rupture of the aortic wall may be difficult to demonstrate, as it may be situated at the back of the aorta or in the wall abutting the pulmonary artery. Microscopic examination of the adjacent aortic wall demonstrates moderate atheromatous disease alone. The incidence of these aneurysms was reviewed by Fothergill *et al.* (1979).

Aneurysms due to tertiary syphilis are rarely encountered nowadays. Other diseases affecting the arterial walls, such as giant-cell arteritis, temporal arteritis, aortic arch syndrome, Takayashu's disease, etc., are extremely rare associated with sudden death.

In the venous system, although disease of the vessels, notably in the form of varicose veins in the legs, is common, this rarely is associated with sudden death. However, on occasion a trivial injury to the leg may cause rupture of a varicosity, with profuse haemorrhage, which in an elderly person, especially if left on their own, is liable to cause fatal exsanguination.

The quantity of blood at the scene of death, and the fact that bloodstaining of the body is usually confined to the hands and legs, is of itself suggestive of the diagnosis, but the actual hole in the skin communicating with the varicosity is usually very small—of the order of $^1/_8$ in. or so in diameter—and readily overlooked in the mass of dried blood and blood clot adhering to the leg (F.M. 11,896ᴀ).

Varicose veins are also one of the factors predisposing to venous thrombosis, which may in turn lead to sudden death from pulmonary embolism. Air embolism due to unusual sexual activity (Aronson and Campbell, 1960); self-induced air embolism (Cooke, 1961), following vacuum injury to the penis (Fox and Barret, 1960) and Hendry (1964) are examples of unusual sudden death and of air embolism.

Amniotic fluid embolism

Amniotic fluid embolism is, fortunately, a rare cause of sudden death in pregnancy; it appears that there are less than a hundred case reports. Its recognition is important since, as in one of our cases, it may give rise to an unwarranted suspicion of criminal interference.

This accident usually presents as a sudden attack of respiratory failure during an otherwise uneventful labour in a healthy woman. In one of our cases, however, although in the 8th. month of pregnancy, she was not in labour. During the evening of her death, while in bed, she had a sudden attack of severe abdominal pain; she lost consciousness and died within a few minutes. The autopsy demonstrated a tear 15 cm long in the amniotic sac but no signs of any interference. The cause of death was established by the history and the demonstration of fatty material in the pulmonary blood vessels. In the second case, the cause of death was not established until frozen sections of lung, stained for fat, were available. (Dennis, R. G., Goldie, W. and Polson, C. J. (1954) *J. Obstet. Gynaec. Brit. Emp.*, **61.** 620). Two subsequent case reports were by Hunt, A. C. (1960) *J. Forens. Med.*, **7**, 74, and by Nichols, G. P. and Raney, E. H. (1966) *Archs. intern. Med.*, **117,** 807.

Cardiac Conducting Tissue

The conducting tissue of the heart may be overlooked when seeking the obscure cause of sudden death. Technique for its examination is described by Davies (1971) and the pathological changes were discussed by Ferris (1974), Davies and Anderson (1975) and Voigt (1977).

Ageing changes, such as fibrosis or fatty infiltration, are not uncommon and cannot be used to indicate a cause of death. On the other hand, localised patches of myocarditis may be found (see page 181). We have found small areas of haemorrhage into the bundle or its branches, and, on occasion, associated with infection. On one occasion the haemorrhages were associated with hyperpyrexia, following poisoning by amphetamine. We usually adopt the simple technique of Lumb and Shackett (1960). We are of the opinion that the examination of the conducting tissue is essential whenever a sudden death is not readily explained by obvious macroscopic changes.

Respiratory System

Relatively few diseases of the respiratory system cause sudden and unexpected death, although many cases seen by the forensic pathologist, especially in winter, include acute bronchitis or broncho-pneumonia, superimposed upon an existing disease complex of chronic bronchitis, pulmonary fibrosis, and emphysema, the existence of which is well-known to the patient's medical practitioner, who is, however, unable to issue a death certificate due to the fact that he has not seen the patient during the 14 days before death.

However, such acute infections may occur rapidly and cause death after only a short period of illness, possibly 1 or 2 days, before the patient has received any attention. This is particularly so in cases of lobar pneumonia. Such an infection has reached the stage of grey hepatisation when seen at autopsy, and pneumococci can be cultured quite easily from swabs from the lung surface or from muco-pus in the smaller bronchi. Staphylococcal broncho-pneumonia may also kill very rapidly, especially when associated with fulminating tracheo-bronchitis. One such recent case seen in the Department caused sudden death within 36 hours of the onset of mild symptoms, which had not been deemed sufficiently severe to require medical treatment.

The appearances of inhalation pneumonia, which are distinct from those due to infection, were described by Macgregor (1939) and Rhainey and Macgregor (1948).

Influenzal pneumonia in the virulent and widespread form which caused the pandemic of the 1920s, with violaceous cyanosis and death within a few hours, has not since recurred. Nevertheless, sporadic cases of acute virus pneumonia occur; they are associated with an acute tracheo-bronchitis of haemorrhagic type; the lungs are intensely congested and contain scattered areas of haemorrhagic consolidation. Microscopical examination reveals severe bronchitis and bronchiolitis, characterised by intense congestion and oedema, and, in addition, round-celled infiltration of the bronchial walls associated with necrosis and desquamation of the epithelium; the alveolar walls are indistinct and hazy. It is sometimes possible to isolate a virus from portions of the lung tissue or from strips of the tracheal wall. The material must be delivered without delay to the virologist, or kept deep frozen or placed in some suitable transport medium, e.g. Dubos media. By the time the case comes to autopsy extensive secondary bacterial infection makes isolation of the virus difficult if not impossible. These virus infections are sometimes associated with neurological symptoms, such as coma, which may give rise to an initial suspicion of poisoning as the cause of death. The correct interpretation is made by the presence of naked-eye signs of slight patchy sub-arachnoid bleeding and the microscopic picture of haemorrhagic leuco-encephalopathy.

Apart from infections the principal cause of sudden death from disease of the respiratory system is pulmonary embolism by thrombus, derived from the peripheral venous system. This, of course, is well recognised as a complication of recumbancy following trauma, especially fractures and surgical operations (Sevitt and Gallagher, 1959), or prolonged bed rest in medical cases. However, it occurs quite frequently as a cause of sudden death unassociated with such unnatural conditions (Knight, 1966). Predisposing causes may be anything which diminishes the rate of circulation, such as thrombophlebitis, congestive heart failure or obesity, or any local disease of the vessels, e.g. varicose veins of the legs, dilatation and varicosity of the vessels in the prostatic plexus.

A less frequent finding is an unsuspected carcinoma of the lung, which, by eroding a blood vessel, gives rise to a massive haemoptysis.

On occasions, when blood becomes widely distributed at the scene of death and no other person was present at the time to describe the circumstances, the initial presumption of those first discovering the body is likely to be that the deceased has been murdered. Rupture of an emphysematous bulla, with production of sudden spontaneous pneumo-thorax, is a rare cause of sudden death.

Although bronchial asthma is not usually considered to be a fatal illness, deaths due to it occur in twos and threes a year in most forensic practices. Such deaths are usually of well-established young or middle-aged asthmatics, who collapse during a severe attack, and who at post-mortem show considerable over-distension of their lungs which are bulky, pale, overlay the pericardial sac anteriorly, feel rubbery, and pit easily on pressure. On the cut surfaces of the lungs the bronchi are prominent with congested thickened walls and contain obvious plugs of sticky, almost creamy, grey opaque mucus, which can be expressed with difficulty from the bronchi as threads. Elsewhere the tissue is rather pallid and well aerated. Microscopically the walls of the bronchi show hypertrophied layers of smooth muscle and are extensively infiltrated by eosinophils, and the lumena contain masses, often rather whorled in outline, of eosinophilic amorphus mucoid debris containing clumps of eosinophils. Often the smaller blood vessels within the lung will also contain large numbers of eosinophils. The mechanism of death in such cases is presumably acute right ventricular failure and respiratory failure due to persistent over-distension of the lungs.

In the past some victims died during an acute asthmatic attack, following an overdose of iso-prenaline, taken by means of an inhaler (Greenberg and Pines, 1967; Price, 1967). The use of such inhalers has been almost totally discontinued and the chance of a pathologist dealing with one of these deaths is now remote. However, he must always be on the look-out for some other form of drug-induced attack. A middle-aged man, who had a vague history of a previous wheezy chest, took the first dose, a single tablet, of a beta-blocking drug, prescribed for hypertension. He died in intense broncho-spasm, within half an hour of taking the tablet. The risks of such drugs with chronic asthmatics are well-documented (F.M. 29,867).

A rare cause of sudden death from affection of the respiratory system is acute epiglottitis (Leading Article *Brit. Med. J.*, Aug. 1969). Though more frequently occurring in children (see p. 480), it may also cause sudden death in adults. Bacterial examination in reported cases has usually revealed infection by Haemophilis influenzae type B. Occasionally a meningitis is also discovered.

Severe pulmonary oedema, in the absence of an obvious cardiac or cerebral cause, raises the possibility of poisoning. Acute barbiturate poisoning and other sedative and narcotic drugs, if all the drug has been absorbed from the stomach, may produce severe pulmonary oedema as the sole autopsy finding. Much rarer, and correspondingly easily overlooked, is some inhaled poison, e.g. cadmium fume (Winston, 1971), or phosgene (Polson and Tattersall, 1971). Finally, sudden death can occur from acute obstruction of the air passages by inhaled foreign material; this, of course, means that death results from choking (see p. 461).

Central Nervous System

Unexpected and relatively rapid death from disease of the central nervous system is the result of haemorrhage. Numerically these are roughly equally divided between intra-cerebral haemorrhage associated with hypertension, or sub-arachnoid haemorrhage due to rupture of an aneurysm of one of the vessels comprising the Circle of Willis at the base of the brain. Much more rarely a sudden haemorrhage into necrotic tumour tissue within the brain may cause a rapid fatal rise in intra-cranial pressure. In our experience sudden death from intra-cerebral haemorrhage is more common in females than males—ratio 3:2 and at average age 66 years. Normally there is found to be a large cavity within the centre of a cerebral hemisphere, filled by blood clot, with extension of haemorrhage into the ventricular system and swelling of the brain with flattening of the convolutions. Occasionally the haemorrhage has burst through the overlying cerebral cortex at one point, often through the lateral surface of the frontal or temporal lobe into the sub-dural space. This has to be distinguished from sub-dural haemorrhage of traumatic origin. If natural, there is usually evidence of hypertension, e.g. hypertrophy of the left ventricle of the heart; there may also be a history of hypertension. The vessels of the brain may not appear grossly atheromatous on naked eye examination. There are no signs of injury or if so these are mild and consistent with collapse.

A rather less frequent form of intra-cranial haemorrhage is pontine haemorrhage. This also is frequently associated with hypertension and occurs at average age 69 years, twice as often in women as in men. There is usually found to be a large central cavity in the pons filled by fresh blood clot, but on a transverse slice of the pons there are often apparent small subsidiary haemorrhages in the tissues around the margins of the major haemorrhages, apparently due to blood tracking between the bundles of nerve fibres.

It is usually fairly obvious that such haemorrhages are spontaneous, since there is no evidence or history of injury, but on occasion the onset of haemorrhage may be associated with a fall or a vehicle accident, resulting in injury to the head such as bruising or laceration of the scalp or fracture of the skull. It may then be difficult to decide whether the injuries were the cause or the consequence of the haemorrhage, but in the latter case the injuries are usually in a different region of the head from the haemorrhage and there is no bruising of the cortex overlying the site of haemorrhage. Traumatic cerebral haemorrhages are considered in greater detail in Chapter 4, p. 148 *et. seq.*

Spontaneous sub-arachnoid haemorrhage is almost always due to rupture of a cerebral aneurysm, though on occasion this may be difficult to detect, if the actual rupture and consequent haemorrhage has destroyed the greater part of a small aneurysm. Although the accepted view of the aetiology of such "berry" aneurysms, on the vessels of the Circle of Willis at the base of the brain, is that they arise in sites of weakness of the vessel wall, due to absence of the muscle layer at the points of division of the vessels and so are congenital abnormalities causing sub-arachnoid haemorrhages in young adults, yet as a cause of sudden death they are usually found in older persons. In our present series the average age at death from this condition is 60 years and it occurs in females about twice as frequently as in males. In an early series the age was appreciably lower, 30–50 years. The atheromatous aneurysm of the elderly is more often an incidental finding.

A few of the aneurysms show evidence of a previous leak, with brownish staining by altered blood of the pia-arachnoid and brain surface around the aneurysm. Some also show histological evidence of a dissection of the wall of the aneurysm, with leucocytic reaction, apparently occurring hours or even days before the fatal haemorrhage. Occasionally the haemorrhage presents initially with the appearance of an intra-cerebral haemorrhage, because the aneurysm has been in close contact with the brain surface, and evidently once rupture of the aspect of the aneurysm has occurred, the escaping jet of blood has ploughed a track into the underlying brain tissue and produced an intra-cerebral haematoma.

As in the case of intra-cerebral haemorrhages, the spontaneous nature of the sub-arachnoid haemorrhage is usually obvious. There may often, however, be no evidence of hypertension in the form of cardiac hypertrophy. Evidently degeneration, usually from atheroma of the wall of the aneurysm, is sufficient to cause the final rupture. However, it must be appreciated that an exertion or emotion, which causes a rise in blood pressure, may cause the aneurysm to burst, so that such an event sometimes occurs during a heated altercation in which no blows, or very trivial blows, are struck. Alternatively a minor jolt to the head, several hours or days earlier may cause a partial dissection or splitting of the wall of the aneurysm, and so predispose to the final rupture.

Although the dangers of many kinds of drug interaction are now fully understood, and such drugs as the mono-amine oxidase inhibitors are so much less frequently prescribed, it may be advisable when finding a cerebral haemorrhage in a case of sudden death to ascertain whether the patient could have developed a hypertensive crisis from the combined effects, for instance, of a mono-amine oxidase inhibitor drug and a tyramine-containing food such as cheese or Marmite.

The other forms of natural disease of the central nervous system are much less frequently responsible for sudden death. Although cerebral thrombosis is a not infrequent diagnosis before autopsy, such occlusion of the vessels are scarcely ever demonstrable at post-mortem, and although old cystic areas of softening of the brain are not uncommon, fresh red areas of cerebral infarction are rare. The more frequent site of obstruction of blood vessels supplying the brain is in the carotid arteries in the neck, where the lumen may be considerably encroached upon by atheromatous plaques in the vessel walls at, or just above, the bifurcation of the common carotid artery, and the remaining lumen may be completely occluded by thrombus.

Such arterial obstruction may be responsible for episodes of cerebral ischaemia, but frank infarction is rarely seen, and the more common finding in the brain is the presence of multiple tiny cystic spaces, about $^7/_{16}$ in. or less in diameter, grouped principally in the sub-cortical matter.

Various methods are described for the macroscopic demonstration of early cerebral infarction. An alteration in the pH of the infarcted tissue may be demonstrated by pouring liquid Universal Indicator over a thin slice of brain. The infarcted tissue should then assume a pink colour, in contrast to the greeny-yellow hue of normal tissue. Alternatively macro-enzyme techniques similar to those described for detection of early myocardial infarction may be employed (Knight, 1968).

Infections of the nervous system rarely cause unexpected death. However, an encephalitis may be associated with a sudden convulsion and death and is one of the conditions which should always be sought if the autopsy fails to reveal an obvious explanation for death. In the same way de-myelinating conditions will usually have been diagnosed long before death, but should be considered if the autopsy fails to disclose naked-eye evidence of cause of death. An area of acute degeneration in the brain-stem could cause sudden respiratory failure or cardiac failure.

Undiagnosed cerebral tumours are not infrequent discoveries during medico-legal autopsies, but usually are incidental to the cause of death. Such tumours are usually either meningiomas or pituitary fossa tumours, in our experience. However, an astrocytoma in a cerebral hemisphere may be the seat of a sudden haemorrhage into necrotic tissue, causing death, and tumours of the lining of the ventricular system may obstruct the flow of cerebro-spinal fluid suddenly, and by this means cause death.

Epilepsy as a cause of sudden death is often very difficult to diagnose. It may be suspected if there is a known history of epilepsy, or the victim was witnessed to be having a fit at the time of death. However, if death should occur during the first, or one of the earlier fits, as for instance in a child, then it may be virtually impossible to make the diagnosis at post-mortem.

Death may occur from asphyxia or heart failure during a prolonged fit or status epilepticus, or the victim may sustain some accident during the fit, such as becoming smothered by bedclothes, or from turning face down into a mattress, or from falls, burns, drowning, etc. The possibility of such an event should always cross the pathologist's mind when examining, for instance, a person who has drowned in a domestic bath. Even so, proof is likely to be very difficult in the absence of a well-established history of epilepsy, as in the case of a 10-year-old girl who was found drowned in her bath, with no explanation other than a story of mild gastro-enteritis earlier in the day, which was not substantiated by bacteriological examination. A vague story of the girl having had one or two fits earlier in childhood could not be confirmed and there were no morbid anatomical features to suggest the cause of drowning. However, while waiting to give evidence at the inquest, the child's mother, who was not known to have epilepsy, collapsed in the waiting room and had a fit. This may have been due to hysteria, but it seems likely that the child had a similar convulsion while in the bath (F.M. 15,486A).

Apart from the history, evidence which one may obtain from the post-mortem examination, which will indicate the cause of death, is slender. Apart from non-specific signs of asphyxia or acute heart failure, the tongue may be bitten and the bladder empty. A full bladder suggests death in coma rather than in a convulsion. The occurrence of many previous fits may be indicated by old scars of previous injuries, cuts, or burns of the limbs, scarring of the tongue, or of the inner surface of the lips due to the lips being pressed against the teeth, and a feeling on palpation of the cut surface of the brain of unusual firmness, suggesting fibrosis of the region of Ammon's horn, or the hippocampal gyrus, compared to the surrounding brain. Microscopical examination of this region will reveal neuron loss in Sommer's sector of the hippocampal gyrus, sometimes associated with tiny areas of softening due to infarction of the tissue, or minute areas of haemorrhage. In death after several hours in status epilepticus, as has been shown by Norman (1964), staining of large sections of the brain by Nissl's method (toluidine blue) will reveal patchy areas of pallor of the cortex, between the normally blue-staining tissue.

Some years ago we recorded a case of sudden death from haemorrhage into a neuro-fibroma, in a patient suffering from von Recklinghausen's disease. This man, aged 36, was in good health until 6 March 1933. That evening he complained of pain in his right shoulder, where there was a "birthmark". This began to swell in an alarming fashion and he felt ill. Soon after, he collapsed and was admitted at 11 p.m. The swelling on his shoulder had then reached the size of a football and he had the signs and symptoms of internal haemorrhage. He died next morning at 6.50 a.m. There was a swelling over his right shoulder which measured $9 \times 6 \times 6$ in.; its wall was $1\frac{1}{2}$ in. thick and contained neurofibromatous tissue; it formed the sac of a haemorrhage; clotted and fluid blood representing about 1500 ml was collected from it. The precise bleeding point or points were not identified but it was established that the larger blood vessels were intact. Several other neurofibromata were present, e.g. at the back of the neck, inner aspect of the left arm and on the front of the abdomen. Two gliomata were found in the brain (P.M. 908; St. James's Hospital, Leeds; Polson, 1934).

Alimentary System

As in the case of the nervous system, the usual cause of sudden death is from haemorrhage. In this case the cause of such massive haematemesis, or melaena, is almost always erosion of a large blood vessel in the floor of a gastric or duodenal ulcer, usually a large chronic ulcer. The eroded vessel can usually be seen projecting in the floor of the ulcer and bearing a plug of thrombus.

Much less common causes are rupture of oesophageal varices associated with cirrhosis of the liver, or bleeding from gastric tumours, either large ulcerating carcinomas, or occasionally from erosion of the apex of a large lieomyoma of the stomach wall. As in the case of haemoptysis, a massive haematemesis may cause so much blood to be apparent at the scene of death, that initially the victim may be thought to have been murdered (Polson, 1936). Spontaneous rupture of the stomach was recorded by Davis *et al.* (1963).

The other major complication of ulcers, i.e. perforation, is less often found as a cause of sudden death. However, an acute peritonitis may cause death within a few hours before medical advice has been sought by the patient or the relatives. Another occasional cause of acute peritonitis, in the older age group, is perforation of a diverticulum of the colon.

A ruptured appendix is very rarely found, presumably because in the younger age group medical treatment is sought and an early diagnosis made.

Another cause of peritonitis, with relatively early death especially in older persons, is acute intestinal obstruction, either from strangulation of a hernia or from a carcinoma of the colon. In such cases the immediate cause of death is often acute inhalation pneumonia due to regurgitation of intestinal contents.

Very occasionally one may come across an example of peritonitis due to intestinal infarction due to thrombosis of the mesenteric vessels, usually the artery. This may be associated with atheromatous disease of the aorta and mesenteric artery, or with a carcinoma at some distant site, but it may occur in young people with no apparent predisposing cause. In the elderly it is a condition which is prone to be overlooked in life, but at autopsy the distended, plum-coloured coils of bowel are very striking.

Disease of the individual abdominal organs does not usually lead to sudden death. One exception is acute haemorrhagic pancreatitis, which may, on occasion, cause such severe shock as to precipitate sudden death. The commoner variety of pancreatitis in forensic practice is the firm white pancreas of elderly people, associated with some fat necrosis on the surface of the gland, but no haemorrhage, and usually found in association with some disease which of itself would cause hypotension and death, such as ischaemic heart disease.

Of the diseases of the pancreas, apart from acute haemorrhagic pancreatitis, the only one likely to be associated with sudden or apparently unexplained death is diabetes mellitus. Hypoglycaemic coma, due to an overdose of insulin, or rarely a functioning Islet-cell adenoma, may cause abrupt unconsciousness, and soon produce irreversible cerebral damage. According to Courville (1963), this will be associated with acute congestion of the brain, and if the acute episode is survived for some time, by focal and laminar necrosis.

Hyperglycaemic coma will usually take many hours to kill, by biochemical disturbance, but rarely death occurs abruptly in the early stages, especially in children. Disturbance of the potassium levels in the plasma are, of course, particularly liable to cause abrupt cardiac arrest. The morbid anatomical evidence of diabetes is likely to be scanty or non-existent. The pancreas usually appears normal, though rarely it may be small, and show gross fatty infiltration. On microscopical examination the Islets are also usually normal, but may show hyaline changes or fibrosis, and in the unlikely event of really fresh tissue being available, histo-chemical stains may demonstrate deficiency of the insulin-producing beta cells. Otherwise the post-mortem diagnosis of diabetic coma may be extremely difficult, especially if the diagnosis is not entertained initially. Provided urine samples are kept in all such obscure cases, it should be possible to demonstrate the presence of sugar and ketone bodies in the sample, unless the cases is one of the rare non-glycosuric types of diabetic coma. Blood sugar determinations are unlikely to be of much value unless the blood is taken fairly soon after death, and from the left side of the heart, not the right, since the blood sugar level rises precipitately in the right heart within a few hours of death, due to breakdown of liver glycogen. If the sample cannot be analysed at once it should be preserved by the addition of sodium fluoride.

Another useful sample is the vitreous fluid. Normal amounts of glucose disappear rapidly after death so that within a few hours none is usually found in this fluid. However, in hyperglycaemic coma high levels of glucose will have accumulated in the fluid and, even many hours after death, substantial amounts may still be detectable in it .

Very rarely the forensic pathologist may come across sudden collapse and rapid death associated with disease of some other organ, e.g. the liver. Fulminating liver necrosis, due to viral infection, might cause such a sequence and the possibility would then have to be considered of liver damage from poisoning.

Sudden death has been described in association with severe fatty change in the liver, (Randall, 1980). The authors have only seen one such case in which it would appear that the fatty change in the liver was probably due to an early unsuspected diabetes mellitus.

Rapid death may also occur in association with severe fatty change in the liver, where the deceased is an alcoholic. The liver then shows signs of acute alcoholic hepatitis, and after a spell of heavy drinking the victim becomes hypoglycaemic and may die if treatment for the lowered blood sugar is not rapidly available.

Haemopoietic System

Diseases of the spleen are only likely to cause sudden death if they cause the organ to rupture. This can occur with relatively slight trauma in diseases such as malaria or Leishmaniasis, and of course, by tradition constitute a simple method of committing murder in oriental countries by striking the victim a slight, and subsequently undetectable, blow over the left flank.

In this country glandular fever has been incriminated in causing spontaneous rupture of the spleen in a few patients and such spontaneous ruptures have, rarely, occurred in otherwise healthy pregnant women.

Diseases of the blood and bone marrow will very rarely cause sudden death, except by producing unsuspected myocardial degeneration due to anaemia, in which case the "thrush-breast" appearance of the heart may be seen. In non-Europeans, however, other blood disorders may sometimes cause sudden death. Such a fatality, due to an acute episode of sickling in a West Indian male, with sickle-cell anaemia, has been described (Mant, 1967).

Genito-urinary System

It is most uncommon for diseases of the renal or genital tracts of cause sudden or unexpected death, although pathological conditions coincident to the death are frequently found in forensic autopsies. Abrupt onset of renal colic due to a stone caused collapse and death from drowning in a bath (Simpson, 1965). However, in persons living alone and not being seen for a day or two before death, autopsy may reveal death due to toxaemia from acute pyelonephritis, and occasionally, examination of the kidneys may demonstrate acute renal papillary necrosis, usually associated with diabetes, sometimes with obstruction of the urinary tract by tumour or stone. Uraemia, and its underlying cause, is usually diagnosed in life, but occasionally may be unsuspected and in that event will usually present with fibrinous pericarditis, showing little reaction either to naked-eye examination or on histological examination, and also often pulmonary oedema with uraemic pneumonitis, with slight round-celled reaction but many hyaline membranes and patchy haemorrhage. The body cavities tend to have an odour reminiscent of shoe polish.

Endocrine System

Although very rare, diseases of any of the endocrine glands can produce unexpected death, usually by their remote effects on other organs or systems. Both thyrotoxicosis (Goodbody, 1963) and myxoedema have been described as rarely causing sudden death from effects on the heart. In neither case is the heart likely to appear remarkable to naked-eye examination, except possibly for some dilatation. Thyroid disease may also sometimes cause sudden death if a haemorrhage into a thyroid nodule causes rapid compression of the trachea.

The adrenal gland at the medico-legal autopsy is more likely to show pathological changes associated with other diseases than to be the primary cause of death. A phaeochromocytoma, arising from the adrenal medulla, might conceivably, by producing paroxysmal hypertension, precipitate sudden heart failure. Atrophy of the cortex may very rarely be found in otherwise unexplained sudden death. It is more likely to be associated with death in an asthmatic who has been on steroid therapy. Voigt (1966) has made an extensive survey of adrenal pathology in medico-legal autopsies.

Post-mortem Biochemistry

The use of biochemical measurements, although having distinct possibilities as an aid to the diagnosis of the cause of death, is commonly neglected. In the past it was generally assumed that the usual parameters used with the living altered after death in a way so variable that the results could never be relied upon to indicate the state of the deceased at the time of death. Research during the past few years has shown that this attitude was not necessarily true. Biochemical tests can be used to a much greater extent than formerly. The use of samples other than or in addition to, blood, notably the vitreous fluid, has provided wider possibilities for diagnosis.

The substance first studied in any detail was glucose. Hill (1941), by experiments with dogs, found a dramatic post-mortem rise in the amount of glucose in the blood in the right side of the heart and that its source was the liver. This and other changes were reviewed by Evans (1963) in his *The Chemistry of Death*.

Sanders (1923) studied nitrogenous compounds, notably urea, Naumann (1956), cholesterol and lipids; Enticknap (1960) enzymes, and Schorup (1950) the cerebrospinal fluid. Jetter (1959) studied a wide range of substances. Coe (1976) has covered the widest field in recent years and his original publications should be consulted.

His findings may be summarised as follows: glucose in the blood usually falls rapidly after death; urea is relatively stable; cholesterol and lipids are stable; bilirubin shows a very slight increase after death but not enough to interfere with the diagnosis of liver dysfunction; proteins remain stable as also calcium. On the other hand, most enzyme levels rise after death; adrenalin and insulin also rise; and, of the electrolytes, potassium shows a rapid rise, while sodium and chloride fall, but more slowly.

We have studied parameters similar to those studied by Coe and have obtained similar results (Lythgoe, 1981). We also found that the site of sampling the blood makes a considerable difference in the result. Thus the enzyme L.D.H. was found to have risen in all samples but its concentration was up to 15 times higher in blood from the right side of the heart than in blood samples from the limbs. This was found to have been due to leakage of the enzyme from the liver. Similar results were obtained with alkaline phosphatase (Lythgoe, 1980, 1981).

Intra-cellular enzymes from red cells, such as glutathione reductase, declined slowly after death and the amount did not vary according to the site of the sample. Other tests, examining the stability of the red cell membrane and glucose metabolism in cells, indicated different metabolism of cells after death according to site; the metabolism lasted longer and electrolyte levels remained normal for a longer period in peripheral sites than in the heart (Tsunenari *et al.*, 1981).

Uraemia and associated renal disorders can easily be detected by biochemical measurements after death. So also can dehydration, due to some inter-current disease. A woman aged 84, whose death was due to coronary thrombosis and acute enterocolitis, was found to have a vitreous content of urea of 286 mg./100 ml. and a sodium content of 145 mMol/100 ml (F.M. 25,713). Similarly diabetic hyperglycaemia may show obvious results. A diabetic male, aged 24, insulin dependent, who was found dead at home, had a vitreous glucose content of 60 mMol/litre (1081 mg./100 ml.). The vitreous sodium level was 140 mMol/litre and ketones were present (F.M. 23,871).

On the other hand, it is rarely possible to demonstrate the existence of hypoglycaemic coma, but it may be possible to exclude it. A female, aged 64, collapsed and died soon after an injection of insulin, administered by the district nurse. Hypoglycaemia was mooted but the blood level of glucose was 175 mg./100 ml. and the vitreous glucose level was 150 mg./100 ml. whereby hypoglycaemia was excluded (F.M. 22,618). It is unlikely that enzyme estimations will help much towards confirming a diagnosis of disease but in some recent instances of suspected hypothermia in our practice the level of amylase in the vitreous was very high and appeared to support this diagnosis.

It is apparent that when the cause of death is obscure, and the interval between death and the post-mortem examination does not exceed 48 hours, there is room to undertake biochemical analysis as an adjunct to morbid anatomical diagnosis. It is a possible aid in the diagnosis of metabolic diseases and such unnatural conditions as hypothermia and drowning (see page 432). It is important to indicate the site of the sample of blood and where practicable, to take several samples, preferably from a peripheral site, to take urine when available and, by no means least important, of the vitreous fluid.

Poisons and Sudden Death

Details of the appearances at autopsy of the effects of various poisons are available in textbooks of toxicology (e.g. Polson and Tattersall, 1971). However, unless the pathologist is forewarned, from the history of the case, of the possibility of poison, he may easily overlook its presence, especially if the autopsy demonstrates a considerable degree of natural disease, and the following are only intended as examples of the hazards.

The more dramatic, and nowadays rarer, poisons may make their presence very obvious, even in the absence of a history to suggest them. Thus, the corrosive and irritant substances, such as the mineral acids, sodium and potassium hydroxide, ammonia, and the phenolic substances, will advertise themselves by acute inflammation or corrosion of the stomach, and by a characteristic smell in the case of ammonia or phenol. Cyanide in large amount will also have a characteristic smell, or the stomach may smell of ammonia in cases of poisoning with old and deteriorated alkaline cyanide substances, and the stomach will appear acutely congested. Oxalates, fluorides, and oxidising substances such as permanganates and chlorates are also likely to cause sufficient chemical damage to make their presence obvious.

Poisons damaging the liver, such as phosphorus, by producing acute fatty change, necrosis, and haemorrhages in the tissues, may initially resemble liver disease from natural causes, such as acute infective hepatitis. Similarly the mono-amine oxidase inhibitor drugs and the phenothiazines may produce hepatitis or acute hepatic necrosis, apparently resembling viral hepatitis. Histological examination and toxicology is usually necessary to attempt a definite diagnosis, which even then may be difficult. Alcoholism may also produce a fatty liver, which, at periods of heavy drinking, may present the histological picture of a superimposed acute hepatitis, usually characterised by the presence of Mallory's hyaline material. Probably the commonest cause of acute liver necrosis due to poisoning nowadays is an overdose of paracetamol.

Inflammation of the kidneys, or urinary tract, may be caused by metallic salts such as mercuric compounds, associated with inflammation of the bowel, especially the colon, but this is unlikely to be confused with naturally occurring pyelitis. Rare cases of cantharides poisons may produce haemorrhages into the renal pelves and haematuria, and can be mimicked by blood diseases, e.g. leukaemia. More subtle in occurrence is chronic nephritis and renal fibrosis, associated either with the long-continued over-use of analgesics such as phenacetin, or chronic lead poisoning.

With the increasing frequency of drug abuse in this country the pathologist has to keep in mind the possibility that a sudden or suspicious death may be due to this cause. Often the features at the scene of death draw attention to the possibility, as when death is due to the inhalation of a volatile substance contained in a plastic bag, which may be over the deceased's head, or on the ground nearby. However the evidence may be less obtrusive. Thus a young girl was found dead, lying on her bed. At autopsy a strange odour of the brain was noticed when the skull was opened; analysis showed this to be due to carbon tetrachloride. Further enquiries revealed that she had said she enjoyed sniffing cleaning fluid. A corked bottle of such fluid was present in her room. She must have spilt some on the bedclothes, recorked the bottle, and then succumbed from the fumes arising from the bedclothes.

Drugs taken by injection usually reveal their presence by injection marks on the limbs, but these may be very small and inconspicuous, especially when, as is often the case, the deceased's arms are heavily tattooed. Scrutiny with a hand lens may then be necessary to detect them. The internal evidence of drug abuse, apart from at the injection site, may be slight. However the presence of chronic hepatitis, or of severe pulmonary oedema, in a young person, should suggest this possibility (Froede, 1975; Tomashefski and Hirsh, 1980; Kamm, 1975; Whayne and Spitz, 1978; Rajs and Falconer, 1979; Gerlach, 1980).

Unexpected Death in Childhood

Death occurring unexpectedly, or as is usual, suddenly, from natural causes is obviously far less common in childhood than later in adult life. The most likely causes are fulminating infections, especially of the respiratory and nervous systems.

Thus, acute epiglottitis, laryngitis, tracheo-bronchitis, and broncho-pneumonia can all kill within hours, especially when associated with one of the acute exanthemata such as measles. Similarly meningitis, especially acute meningococcal septicaemia, with its characteristic purpuric rash, viral encephalitis, and encephalo-myelitis, may produce collapse and death within hours. Acute infections, of many kinds, by often producing convulsions in their early stages, may cause sudden death from asphyxia, e.g. by inhalation of vomit during a fit. Similarly, acute intestinal obstruction, causing vomiting, may lead to the inhalation of vomit.

Unsuspected congenital abnormalities of the heart, such as endocardial fibro-elastosis, or the cardio-myopathies, such as asymmetrical hypertrophy, predispose to sudden death. The youngest person in our series of deaths due to asymmetrical hypertrophy was 13 years old, but it has been reported in younger children.

The acute metabolic disorders, diabetic coma, acute acidosis, etc., may be responsible for sudden deaths, as may such conditions as congenital adrenal hyperplasia.

Other causes of sudden death in infancy and childhood which have been reported are internal haemorrhages, pulmonary thrombosis etc.

The Sudden Infant Death Syndrome—"Cot or Crib Deaths"

Though cot deaths have been recognised for many centuries—the first reported case being in the *Old Testament* (I Kings, Ch. 3 v. 19)—only in the last two decades has any intensive research been applied to the problem.

The Sudden Infant Death Syndrome (now internationally known as S.I.D.S.) has profound pathological, epidemiological, sociological and psychological aspects, as it not only encompasses the actual death of the infant, but the family and legal consequences.

The incidence of S.I.D.S. in Europe, North America and Australasia makes it the prime cause of death in infants after the perinatal period of up to one week. In some series, it exceeds all other causes of infant death combined, at its peak incidence of about 3–4 months of age.

Incidence

This varies in different series, but about one of every 500 live births ends in a cot death. As many as 4 per thousand have been reported and in special groups, such as families of the Armed Services, even higher rates occur.

The 1 in 500 rate is for singleton babies, as twinning markedly increases the risk, up to four-fold in some investigations.

At least half-a-dozen tragedies have been reported where both members of a twin pair have suffered a cot death on the same day. There appears to be no variation in risk between uniovular and biovular twins, suggesting that environment is more important than heredity; most twins are premature and of low birth-weight, both of which are known to be predisposing factors.

Age

Sudden infant death does not afflict babies in the perinatal period and is uncommon under 1 month of age. The accepted age range is from 2 weeks to 2 years, though most occur between 6 to 30 weeks, with a peak at 3–4 months. There is a typical distribution curve for age incidence and undoubtedly cases do occur at the extremes of the curve, though rarely after 1 year.

Seasonal Variation

In the northern hemisphere, there is a strikingly significant excess of cot deaths between October and April, the colder, wetter months when respiratory infections are common. In Australasia, this seasonal peak occurs between May and September. There is considerable controversy over the role of climatic factors in the aetiology of S.I.D.S., especially in relation to temperature. A number of investigations point to an excess of deaths in colder weather, yet one series implicated domestic hyperthermia as a factor.

Social Class Incidence

There is a marked excess of deaths in the less advantaged social classes, whether measured by paternal occupation or housing standards. Though S.I.D.S. can occur in children of professional parents, it is far more common in the lower and middle social groups. This may not be related directly to financial status, but also to family size, housing and readiness to utilise medical and social services.

Sex Incidence

There is a slight but definite trend to an excess of cot deaths amongst male infants. The variation seems to be of the order of three males to two females, though it must be remembered that the male is more vulnerable to many disease states throughout life.

The Typical History

A child within the usual age range is either quite well on the day preceding death or has apparently minimal symptoms, usually of an upper respiratory infection or minor gastro-intestinal disturbance. The condition is not sufficient to give rise to parental anxiety in most cases and if a doctor is called, he has no reason to consider the babe to be seriously ill.

The child is put to bed and is either found dead in its sleeping place in the early morning or is found to be dead some hours after its early feed. Most deaths occur before noon.

Post-mortem Appearances

As S.I.D.S. are sudden and unexpected deaths, most are the subject of a coroner's or other medico-legal investigation and an autopsy is almost always performed. There are no specific findings in cot death, either naked eye or on microscopic examination. In about 15 per cent of babies dying with a typical history, some overt pathological condition may be found, such as frank pneumonia, congenital heart disease, Down's syndrome or a true tracheobronchitis. However, whether these are actually the cause of death or a concomitant finding is hard to decide. Histologically, opinions differ as to the threshold of minimal findings, such as a bronchiolitis, which can be accepted as a cause of death.

Several spurious findings may be present, the significance of which is either nil or in doubt. Petechial haemorrhages on the visceral pleura, epicardium and thymus are agonal in nature, perhaps from terminal respiratory efforts against a closed glottis. Unfortunately, in former years they reinforced the baseless claims that S.I.D.S. was due to mechanical asphyxia.

The finding of gastric contents in the air passages is also unhelpful and can be misleading, if used as a sole cause of death. Such contents can be found in up to 25 per cent of an autopsy series, both adult and infant and is either agonal or actually post-mortem. Unless aspiration of regurgitated stomach contents is witnessed during life, it cannot be claimed to be a vital phenomenon purely on post-mortem examination.

Theories of Causation of S.I.D.S.

In former years, much social and psychological damage was caused by unsubstantiated theories about the causation of cot deaths. For centuries, they were attributed to "overlying", that is, the mechanical suffocation of an infant in the maternal bed, due to an adult smothering it during sleep. When babies began to be placed in separate cots, S.I.D.S. continued unabated, so disproving the overlaying theory – though in fact the Children and Young Persons Acts, still in force, include "overlaying" by a drunken adult as an offence, an example of legislation for what was probably a non-existent condition.

Partly because of the lack of any specific autopsy signs of disease and partly because of the frequent finding of intra-thoracic petechiae, the mechanical asphyxia theory persisted, but was now blamed upon "heavy bedclothes", "soft pillows", etc. It has now been shown that normal bed clothes can admit sufficient air to sustain infant respiration and a significant proportion of undoubted S.I.D.S. victims are found dead on their back with no obstruction whatsoever to their external respiratory passages.

More recently, it was postulated that there was a single cause for S.I.D.S., such as a specific virus or an allergy to cow's milk protein. At least forty hypotheses have been advanced, but now it seems clear that there is no single cause of cot death, but that there is a common final fatal pathway which is reached by the confluence of several factors. There may well be different permutations of this "multi-factorial situation" in different cot deaths, but several factors seem to be common. It is rather difficult to make some of these postulated factors compatible with the epidemiology of S.I.D.S., but respiratory infection and sleep apnoea are now widely accepted as playing an important role.

There would appear to be predisposing factors which are developmental and environmental, rather than hereditary. Prematurity and low birth-weight definitely increase the risks and because of this and the obvious tendency for infants to "grow out" of the risk zone in the second half of the first year, it would seem that immaturity, probably of respiratory drive and control, is a potent factor.

The literature of S.I.D.S. is now voluminous and much modern research is in the field of respiratory patho-physiology.

The currently favoured hypothesis suggests that some infants have prolonged sleep apnoea which renders them susceptible to hypoxia. Additional factors which potentiate this state will favour a descending spiral of *hypoxia→respiratory depression→hypoxia* which eventually leads to bradycardia and cardiac arrest.

Foremost amongst such accelerating factors is a respiratory infection; this may produce a viraemia which itself adds to the sleep depression of the respiratory centres. Nasal oedema and mucus secretion may further narrow the small upper respiratory passages (many small babies are obligatory nose-breathers) and in some hypotonic babies, a flaccid pharynx and even neck posture may further reduce the air-way. One hypothesis also suggests that there may be an element of laryngeal spasm.

There may therefore be both central and obstructive apnoea, leading to silent cardio-respiratory failure during sleep. Pathological evidence of chronic hypoxia is claimed by some workers, which includes thickened pulmonary vessels, increased brown fat and fine gliosis in the brain stem.

One interesting feature is the relatively recent recognition of "near miss" cot death, where an infant is detected whilst in a still reversible stage of apnoea-hypoxia. Clinical examination of these babies and sometimes their siblings may reveal abnormal cardio-respiratory function, especially E.C.G. changes.

Because of the fear which parents of a cot death have in regard to subsequent births, efforts have been made to monitor "at risk" infants by means of respiratory alarms, which are set to give an audible signal after a certain period of apnoea. There is considerable controversy over the efficacy of these devices, but whatever their physiological value, they appear to provide welcome support to apprehensive parents.

The social and psychological aspects of cot death are profound, revolving mainly about the guilt feelings of the mother, which may lead to acute anxiety states and even suicide. Counselling is vital in many cases and a number of supporting organisations have been established in Britain and the United States.

The pathologist should be willing to participate in this task, by explaining the autopsy findings to those parents who desire it, emphasising that the death was due to natural causes and not to some act of commission or omission on their part. This function of the pathologist has been recommended in leading articles in both the *Journal of the American Medical Association* and in the *British Medical Journal*.

REFERENCES AND RECOMMENDED READING (S.I.D.S)

Bergman, A. B., Beckwith, J. B. and Ray, C. G. (eds), (1970) *Sudden infant death syndrome* (Proceedings of the Second International Conference on SIDS, Seattle, 1969), Univ. of Washington Press.

Bergman, A. B., Beckwith, J. B. and Ray, C. G. (1975) The Apnoea Monitor Business, *Pediatrics*, **56**, 1.

Camos, F. E. and Carpenter, R. J. (eds) (1972) *Sudden and Unexpected Deaths in Infancy (Cot Deaths)* (Proceedings of the Cambridge Symposium) John Wright, Bristol.

Knight, B. (1983) *Sudden Infant Death Syndrome* Faber & Faber, London.

Leading article (Adelson), 1977, *J.A.M.A.* **237**, 1585.

Leading article (Knight), 1977, *Brit. Med. J.*, **2**, 6080, 148.

Robinson, R (ed) (1975) *SIDS 1974* (Proceedings of the Toronto Symposium, 1974), Canadian Foundation for the Study of Infant Deaths.

Valdes-Daepena, M. (1981) Sudden infant death syndrome; a review of the medical literature 1974–79. *Pediatrics*, **66**, 597.

Valdes-Dapena, M. (1977) Sudden unexplained infant deaths, 1970 through 1975; an evolution in understanding. *Pathology Annual*, **12**, 177.

Wedgwood, R. J. and Benditt, E. P. (eds) (1964) *Sudden Death in Infancy* (Proceedings of the Conference in Seattle, 1963), US Dept of Health, Education and Welfare, Bethesda, Maryland.

ORGANISATIONS PROVIDING COUNSELLING

The Foundation for the Study of Infant Deaths,
5th Floor, 4 Grosvenor Place, London SW1X 7HD; tel 01-235 1721

National Sudden Infant Death Syndrome Foundation
2 Metro Plaza, Suite 205, 8240 Professional Place
Landover, Maryland 20785, USA.

References

ARONSON, M. E. and CAMPBELL J. E. (1960) *2nd Internat meeting on Forensic Pathology and Medicine*, N. Y., Program and Abstracts, p. 43.
British Medical Journal (Leading Article) (1969) **3**, 487.
British Medical Journal (Leading Article) (1971) **4**, 25.
BURTON, J. F. and ZAWADZKI, E. S. (1962) *J. Forens. Sci.* **7**, 486.
COE, J. I. (1976) *Leg. Med. Ann.* Edit. Wecht, Appleton-Century-Crofts.
COE, J. I. and PETERSON, R. D. A. (1963) *J. Lab. Clin. Med.*, **62**, 477.
CONNOR, R. C. R. (1970) *J. Path.*, **101**, 71.
COOKE, R. T. (1961) *Brit. Med. J.*, **2**, 1197.
CORBY, C. (1960) *Med. Sci. Law*, **1**, 23 (Excellent illustrations).
COURVILLE, C. B. (1963) *J. Forens. Sci.*, **8**, 392.
CRAWFORD, T. (1969) *Trends in Clinical Pathology*, p. 63. London: B.M.A.
CRAWFORD, T., DEXTER, D. and TEARE, R. D. (1961) *Lancet* i, 181.
CRAWFORD, SIR T. (1977) *The Pathology of Ischaemic Heart Disease*. London. Butterworths.
DAVIES, M. J. (1971) *The Pathology of Conducting Tissue of the Heart*. London. Butterworths.
DAVIES, M. J. and ANDERSON, R. H. (1975) in *The Pathology of the Heart*. Ed. Pomerance, A. and Davies, M. J. Oxford. Blackwell.
DAVIES, M. J. and POPPLE, A. (1979) *Histopathology*, **3**, 255–277.
DAVIS *et. al.* (1963) *Arch. Surg. Chicago*, **86**, 170.
ELLIS, H. A. and KNIGHT, B. (1969) *Pediatrics*, **44**, 225.
EMERY, J. L. (1964) *Med. Sci. Law*, **4**, 39.
EMERY, J. L. and MACDONALD, M. S. (1960) *Amer. J. Path.*, **36**, 713.
ENGLANDER, O. (1971) *Brit. Med. J.*, **4**, 625.
ENTICKNAP, J. B. (1960) *J. Forensic Med.*, **7**, 135–146.
EVANS, W. E. D. (1963) *The Chemistry of Death*. Springfield. Thomas.
FERRIS, J. A. J. (1974) *Med. Sci. Law*, **14**, 36–39.
FOTHERGILL, D. F. BOWEN, D. A. L. and MASON, J. K. (1979) *Med. Sci. Law* **19**, 253–260.
FROEDE, R. C. (1975) *Leg. Med. Annu.*, pp 1–15.
FOX, M. and BARRET, E. L. (1960) *Brit. Med. J.*, **1**, 1942.
FRASER, G. R. and FROGGATT, P. (1966) *Lancet*, ii, 56.
FROGGATT, P., LYNAS, M. A. and MARSHALL, T. K. (1968) *Amer. J. Cardiol.*, **22**, 457.
FROGGATT, P. (1970) in *Proc. 2nd Int. Conf. on Causes of Sudden Death in Infants*, p. 32, ed. A. B. Bergman, J. B. Beckwith and C. G. Ray, Seattle: University of Washington Press.
FROGGATT, P., LYNAS, M. A. and MACKENZIE, G. (1971) *Brit. J. Prev. Soc. Med.* **25**, 119.
GEERTINGER, P. (1967) *Pediatrics*, **39**, 43.
GERLACH, D. (1980) *For. Sci. Internat.*, **15**, 31–39.
GOODBODY, R. A. (1963) *Med. Sci. Law*, **3**, 214.
Gradwohl's Legal Medicine, (1968) 2nd ed. Francis E. Camps, p. 257. Bristol: John Wright & Sons Ltd.
GRAHAM, R. L. (1944) *Bull. Johns Hopkins Hosp.*, **74**, 16.
GREENBERG, M. J. and PINES, A. (1967) *Brit. Med. J.*, **2**, 441.
HARGREAVES, T. (1961) *Brit. Med. J.*, **2**, 342.
HENDRY, W. T. (1964) *Med. Sci. Law*, **4**, 179.
HILL, E. V. (1941) *Arch. Path.*, **32**, 452.
HUDSON, R. E. B. (1965) *Cardiovascular Pathology*. London: Edward Arnold.
JAMES, T. N. (1970) in *Proc. 2nd Int. Conf. on Causes of Sudden Death in Infants*, p. 118, ed. by A. B. Bergman, J. B. Beckwith and C. G. Ray, Seattle: University of Washington Press.
JETTER, W. W. (1959) *J. Forens. Sci.*, **4**, 335.
KAMM, R. C. (1975) *For. Sci.*, **5**, 91–93.
KNIGHT, B. H. (1965) *Med. Sci. Law*, **5**, 31.
KNIGHT, B. H. (1966) *Med. Sci. Law*, **6**, 150, and personal communication.
KNIGHT, B. H. (1968) *The Criminologist*, No. 9, p. 29.
LUMB, G. and SHAKLETT, R. S. (1960) *Amer. J. Pathol.*, **36**, 411–422.
LYTHGOE, A. S. (1980) *Med. Sci. Law* **20**, 48–53.
LYTHGOE, A. S. (1981) Ph.D. Thesis. Univ. Leeds.

LYTHGOE, A. S. (1981) *J. Forensic Sci. Soc.*, **21**. 337–340.

MACGREGOR, A. R. (1939) *Arch. Dis. Childh.* **14**, 323.

MCKEOWN, F. (1965) *Pathology of the Aged.* London: Butterworths.

MANT, A. K. (1967) *Med. Sci. Law*, **7**, 135.

MARSHALL, T. K. (1970) *Med. Sci. Law*, **10**, 3.

MINISTRY OF HEALTH (1965) *Enquiry into Sudden Death in Infancy*, Ref. No. 113, London; H.M.S.O.

MORGAN, A. D. (1956) *The Pathogenesis of Coronary Occlusion*, p. 97, Oxford: Blackwell.

NAUMANN, H. N. (1956) *Amer. J. Clin. Pathol.*, **26**, 495–505.

NEAME, P. B. and JOUBERT, S. M. (1961) *Lancet*, **ii**, 893.

NORMAN, R. M. (1964) *Med. Sci. Law*, **4**, 46.

OSBORN, G. R. (1967) in *Modern Trends in Forensic Medicine*, Chap. 10, pp. 233–80, ed. C. K. Simpson. London: Butterworths.

PETERSON, R. D. A. and GOOD, R. A. (1963) *Pediatrics*, **31**, 209.

POLSON, C. J. (1934) *Queen. Med. Mag. (Bir.)* **31**, 102.

POLSON, C. J. (1936) *J. Path. Bact.* **42**, 317.

POLSON, C. J. (1941) *Univ. Leeds Med. Mag.*, **11**, 51.

POLSON, C. J. FREEN M. A. and LEE, M. R. (1983) Clinical Toxicology, London: Pitman.

POLSON, C. J. and TATTERSALL, R. N. (1971) *Clinical Toxicology*. Reprint of 2nd ed. London: Pitmans Medical Publications.

POMERANCE, A. (1975) *The Pathology of the Heart*. Ed. Pomerance, A. and Davies, M. J. Oxford. Blackwell.

PRICE, D. E. (1967) *Med. Sci. Law*, **7**, 215.

RADFORD, D. J. and OLIVER, M. R. (1973) *Brit. Med. J.*, **3**, 428–430.

RANDALL, B. (1980) *Hum. Path.*, **11**, 147–153.

RAJS, J. and FALCONER, B. (1979) *For. Sci. Internat.*, **13**, 193–209.

RHAINEY, K. and MACGREGOR, A. R. (1948) *Arch. Dis. Childh.*, **23**, 254.

SAHAI, V. B. and KNIGHT, B. (1976) *Med. Sci. Law*, **16**, 17–20.

SANDERS, F. W. (1923) *J. Biol. Chem.*, **58**, 1–15.

SCHORUP, K. Dodstidsbestemmelse, Copenhagen. Dansk Videnskabs Forlag.

SEVITT, S. and GALLAGHER, N. G. (1959) *Lancet*, **ii**, 981.

SIMPSON, C. K. (1965) in *Taylor's Principles and Practice of Medical Jurisprudence*, 12th ed., **1**, p. 374, London: J. & A. Churchill.

SPRINGATE, C. S. and ADELSON, L. (1966) *Med. Sci. Law*, **6**, 215.

TEARE, R. D. (1958) *Brit. Heart J.*, **20**, 1.

TOMASHEFSKI, J. F. and HIRSCH, C. S. (1980) *Hum. Path.*, **11**, 133–145.

TSUNENARI, S., LYTHGOE, A. S. and GEE, D. J. (1981) *J. Forens. Sci. Sco.*, **21**, 333–336.

VALDES-DAPENA, M. (1970) in *Proc. 2nd Int. Conf. on Causes of Sudden Death in Infants*, p. 3, ed. A. B. Bergman, J. B. Beckwith and C. G. Ray, Seattle: University of Washington Press.

VOIGT, J. (1966) *J. Forens. Med.*, **13**, 3.

VOIGT, J. A. (1977) *Leg. Med. Annu*, pp 83–95.

WERNE, J. (1953) *Amer. J. Path.*, **29**, 633: *ibid.*, pp. 817, 833.

WERNE, J. and GARROW, J. (1947) *Amer. J. Publ. Hlth.*, **37**, 675.

WHAYNE, N. G. and SPITZ, W. U. (1978) *Z. Rechtsmed.*, **81**, 147–149.

WINSTON, R. M. (1971) *Brit. Med. J.*, **2**, 401.

CHAPTER 18

Scenes of Crime

DURING the course of the practice of forensic medicine a pathologist will be called upon many times to attend the scene of a suspicious death, and view the body *in situ*. Some may doubt the value of such an exercise, considering that the examination of the locus of a crime is the duty of the police, and that the pathologist can contribute little or nothing in such circumstances. However, such is not the view of the authors. In our experience such an examination is of considerable value often in assisting the police investigations, and always in enabling the pathologist to formulate conclusions based on his autopsy findings.

Thus if a body is viewed for the first time by the pathologist in the post-mortem room, he may form quite erroneous opinions about the origin of various injuries. However, seeing the body *in situ*, with the various surrounding objects, goes a long way towards avoiding such mistakes. Even viewing the scene of death for the first time after completing the autopsy may be of considerable value; this course may be obligatory if the victim has been found alive, and removed to hospital before death has occurred.

Examination of the scene of death may be especially valuable if the body bears a patterned injury, the origin of which is in doubt.

On one such occasion I was called to the scene of death of an elderly woman in a house. Suspicion had been aroused because smoke had been seen coming from the house, and when the fire was extinguished, in the bedroom, five other separate seats of fire had been found, all of which had obviously died-out of their own accord, and the dead body of the woman, who lived alone, was found in the kitchen, well away from the fire, lying on the floor near to the kitchen window. On examination at the scene her body bore no evidence of burns, or presence of carboxyhaemoglobin; it showed various superficial injuries— notably a bruise of a peculiar pattern on the skin of her left temple. None of the surrounding articles of kitchen furniture matched it, and it was possible to assure the police that it had not been caused by impact with any of the objects in the kitchen, as by a fall. The autopsy revealed a broken neck and ribs. When a youth was subsequently accused of her murder, he alleged that he accidentally knocked the woman down and had trodden on her while trying to make his escape through the broken window. However scrutiny of his clothing revealed a belt buckle which exactly matched the pattern of the bruise, and indicated that his story could not be true, and that he must have held the woman's head, possibly against his waist. He was convicted of her murder. (F.M. 25,947 A)

However, there are occasions when preservation of the scene so that the pathologist can view the body *in situ* is a waste of police and pathologist's time. In particular this is the case where death is due to a fight, and stabbing in the street. The most that is likely to be visible then is a pool of blood around the body, or a trail of bloodspots along the pavement, and these can be perfectly well recorded by photography, and if necessary viewed by the pathologist after the autopsy examination.

There is no doubt that for the maximum value to be derived from the examination of a scene, the close co-ordination of a team of experts working together is necessary, especially if they are accustomed to working together. Then, the activities of the pathologist, the forensic scientist, the fingerprint expert, the scenes of crime officer, and the police photographer are likely to be complementary, and their combined experience of great value to the investigating police officer. Nevertheless it often happens that, for instance, the pathologist alone is called to the scene, on the grounds that if his examination and autopsy indicate that death was due to homicide, then further examination of the scene can be carried out by other experts later. The danger of this course is that when the body is removed to enable the pathologist to carry out his autopsy with the inevitable attendant disturbance of the scene, evidence may be destroyed which could only have been detected by an expert in a different discipline. The most obvious example of this is the improbability of finding reliable evidence of fibre transfer subsequently.

At the early stages of the investigation of a suspicious death the duty of preserving the scene falls on the police. It is vitally important that this is done as thoroughly as possible and any inevitable disturbance recorded. Thus, it may obviously be essential for a doctor certifying the fact of death, in the very early stages of the investigation, to approach, and sometimes move the body to a slight extent. Providing that the nature of the movement is known, and slight, no significant harm will be done to the subsequent investigation. However, if the fact that the body or its surroundings have been disturbed is not made clear, then false conclusions may be drawn subsequently.

In the usual uncertain weather conditions of the British Isles, retaining a dead body *in situ* out of doors, until it can undergo expert examination, may be difficult, especially on windy days, or where rain or snow is falling, or expected. It may then be necessary to erect some form of temporary covering over the body; this should never be a blanket or sheet layed directly on the body. Obviously such covering will gravely interfere with the possible recovery of contact trace evidence from the surface of the body. Some form of tent is best, so long as it can be erected easily, without the necessity of many men trampling over the adjacent parts of the scene. Various tents of this type have been devised by different police forces, for instance one illustrated in the *Police Research Bulletin* (1982). Another simple shelter can be the kind used by cemetery workers when digging a grave in inclement weather. On occasions it is wisest to remove the body as soon as it has undergone a brief preliminary inspection *in situ*. In one such case the body was found (F.M. 20,891) lying in a narrow alleyway between derelict buildings, but a strong wind and intermittent showers of rain meant that a detailed examination with displacement of clothing, and movement of the body would have been very likely to dislodge any trace evidence which in this case was of far greater potential importance than was an early diagnosis of the nature of the injuries, or the recording of body temperatures. Therefore the body was lifted straight on to a plastic sheet, wrapped up and transferred to the mortuary, where the detailed examination was carried out under more reasonable conditions.

On another occasion (F.M. 24,574 A) the body of a young girl was found at night, by a neighbour, on rough ground and moved a short distance by him and covered by a blanket before help was summoned. In view of this, and the difficulty in carrying out an adequate search of the area in the dark, with the danger of destroying evidence if an incomplete preliminary search were made, the body was removed at once and the whole area sealed off until daylight. The autopsy carried out during the night revealed severe head injuries and manual strangulation, and an area of patterned abrasion was found on the girl's cheek, of small interlocking lines. Search of the scene in daylight revealed a large rock bearing traces of blood and hair, evidently the agent responsible for the head injuries. Also on the adjacent grass there was a key ring with zipped cover; the teeth of the zip precisely matched the patterned abrasion on the cheek. Most important of all, close-by, lay a set of darts which could have dropped from the pocket of an assailant crouching over the girl's body. These subsequently proved to belong to a youth who was suspected causing her death. All these items could easily have been displaced or lost, during a casual search in the dark.

Of course the mode of preservation of the scene, and examination, may be made easier, or more difficult by its location. Thus bodies out of doors suffer from the effects of the weather, while those lying in rooms of houses are well protected and securing the site from outside interference is easier. However more bizarre scenes have their own attendant difficulties, and the authors at various times have been called to view bodies in chimneys, in sewers, in manholes, in caves and down mineshafts, underwater, in the underdrawings of floors, embedded in concrete, in the foundations of roadways, in sand-heaps, haystacks, cowsheds, etc., and of course most experienced forensic pathologists can recount experiences in similar or even more bizarre and unusual situations. In each of such situations, the examination has to be modified to suit the exigencies of the situation.

However there are certain basic precepts which are applicable to the examination of most scenes. In the first place, if a scene is to be visited, then obviously it is important for the pathologist to go to it as quickly as possible, whether that means in the middle of the night, or whenever it occurs. Delay wastes police time, considerably decreases the value of any evidence to be derived from recording the temperature of the body, and makes the loss of surface trace evidence more probable. Ideally all those involved in the examination, scientists, photographer, fingerprint expert, pathologist etc., should congregate at a convenient nearby location, such as the police station and then approach the scene together, after initial briefing.

On arrival, approach to the body should be by a single predetermined and marked route, which if at all possible should not be the route used by the murderer. Lack of this precaution may destroy valuable evidence. On one occasion (F.M. 18,812 A) a man's body was seen lying a short way down a steep wooded slope at the side of the road which was bordered by a rough stone wall. The police took care to ensure that everyone entered the wood over the wall some distance further down the road, and approached the body along the slope. Subsequent detailed examination of the wall just above the position of the body by the forensic scientist revealed the presence of a few red dog hairs and green woollen fibres adhering to the rough stone surface. Later, when a man was arrested for the crime, the hairs were proved to match those of his red setter dog, and the green fibres a carpet in his van in which he had brought the dead body to the scene and dumped it.

Often it is sufficient to approach the body simply by walking along a predetermined path. However on occasion, if a fingertip search of the surroundings is later to be made by police officers, it may be better to arrange a line of duckboards leading up to the body.

Another suggestion might be a strip of thick plastic of the type used to protect carpets of showhouses on new housing estates.

Examination of the Body

On arrival of the body the pathologist's initial duty is one of observation. The old policeman's practice of standing still, with the hands in the pockets to prevent contamination and looking at everything for some minutes before doing anything else, has much to recommend it. Too hasty progression to handling the body may mean that some valuable observation is missed, and so destroyed. At this stage we have always found it valuable to make a simple sketch of the position of the body in its surroundings, with the location of any obvious bloodstains, or trickles, etc. The addition of *measured* distances between the body and articles of furniture or adjacent objects is also valuable. This should, of course be supplemented by photographs taken by police photographers and also perhaps by the pathologist himself. Good photography is an integral part of the investigation of crime, but even the best can unintentionally present an inaccurate view of the scene, since the distances between the body and adjacent objects may be foreshortened or apparently unduly widened, according to the angle at which the camera was sited. There are occasions, therefore, when *a sketch, even a rough sketch*, which embodies the record of distances precisely ascertained, e.g. between a body and a doorway or a fireplace, or objects, e.g. a chair or table, can be of *inestimable value* in the interpretation of the circumstances of a death. Moreover the sketch forms part of the pathologist's original notes, and so can be used to refresh his memory later in Court, and we find that the action of drawing helps to fix the attention and ensure the observation of details which might otherwise go unnoticed. Lack of artistic skill, even if to be regretted, need not affect the value of this operation. The use of two or three pens of different colours can make the recording of details much easier, for instance the position of bloodstains.

The value of this initial period of scrutiny and recording may only be appreciated much later. In one case (F.M. 18,771) the victim lay on the floor at the back of the room behind a table covered by heaps of old newspapers. Close scrutiny revealed a piece of twine around the neck, partly concealed by clothing. The man who purported to have first found the woman's dead body, and raised the alarm, told the police on subsequent questioning that she had a piece of twine round the neck which he had seen from the doorway of the room, although he had not entered the room or gone up to the body. Reconsideration of the records of the scene made at the time of the initial examination showed that this was impossible.

One important observation to be made at this stage, before the body is touched, is the direction of any bloodstains or trickle marks on the body, in relation to the wounds from which they originate. This may indicate any mobility of the deceased after receiving the wounds or indeed, movement of the body after death, and also sometimes indicate the order of infliction of the injuries.

Thus, in one case (F.M. 20,577) the body lay on its back with the clothing torn open and disarranged except for the panties which were in normal position. There were many stab wounds in the abdomen from which trickles of dried blood ran downwards towards the ground by the most direct routes as the body lay. One trickle ran down to the top of the panties and then along the upper margin towards the ground. There were also severe head injuries with a depressed fracture of the back of the skull, and several lacerations of the scalp. It was clear, therefore, from the initial inspection of the body, that the stab wounds had been inflicted while the girl lay in the position in which she was subsequently found, that the head injuries must therefore have been inflicted before the stab wounds, and that the panties had not been displaced during or after the attack, although the other clothes had, excluding rape as a motive for the attack.

On another occasion (F.M. 17,778 A) a man's body was viewed *in situ*, lying on its back in a farmyard. There were severe head injuries. The defendant later claimed that he had inflicted the injuries in self-defence during a struggle. The initial inspection of the body however had demonstrated that the dead man's hands were in the pockets of his overalls and had been recorded as such, thereby refuting the defendant's suggestions.

The initial inspection should obviously include objects adjacent to the body. On one occasion a woman's semi-naked body lay at the foot of some stairs, she had been stabbed and strangled. A small quantity of fluid on the floor between her legs was assumed to be urine, voided at the moment of death. Subsequently it became evident that it was seminal fluid ejaculated by the murderer.

Cases of suspicious death which later are found to be due to poisoning are often revealed as such by the presence of a tablet or capsule near the body. One man was thought to have been murdered, together with his wife. A single Tuinal capsule, lying on the carpetted floor of the toilet in which his body was found, was almost overlooked against the brightly-coloured carpet pattern; the death turned out to be due to an overdose of Tuinal (F.M. 16,917 A).

Blood at the Scene

The features to note include an estimation of the amount of blood shed. If a large amount, it should be remembered that a head injury or cut-throat can be followed by an appreciable blood loss after death from an open dural sinus or jugular vein. The distribution of the blood is important. Was it confined to a large pool near the body or was there a trail of small splashes or drops? Had it spurted from the victim or flowed in a slow stream, or had fallen in drops? The shape of splashes, drops or smears should be noted and, in the event of skin ridge impressions in smears, these will be the concern also of the fingerprint experts.

The relation of the blood to the body is to be noted: it may have accumulated in a pool beside or beneath it, indicating lack of mobility after the injury. On other occasions there may be a trail of blood extending from the body to some distant place. Blood at the scene may be on a wall, ceiling or on objects, at the scene or in a neighbouring place.

A trail of blood stains may indicate that the victim received his wound or wounds at some distance from the place at which the body is found. This does not of itself distinguish the circumstances of the wounding. It can happen in the course of a running attack or in circumstances of suicide. A man who first attempted suicide by cutting his wrists with a razor blade in his house, was found in his garage dead of self-inflicted stab wounds in his chest. A trail of blood led from the house to the garage (F.M. 633/48).

Smaller amounts of blood may be distributed in spurts, against a wall or on furniture, suggesting bleeding from a small or medium-sized artery, e.g. the radial artery at the wrist. Venous bleeding, on the other hand, is a slow steady flow, which will produce a pool, if the victim is at rest, and separate drops, more widely spaced than those of arterial spurts, if he was ambulant.

Spurts of blood on to a flat vertical surface, e.g. a wall, can produce a series of linear streaks which are widened, club-like, at their lower end, accompanied by separate drops which have the appearance of exclamation marks.

Single drops, as from a vein, differ in appearance according to the angle at which the drop falls on to a flat surface. When the direction is vertical the stain is circular. It is possible, moreover to assess approximately the distance through which the drop fell. At short distances the stain is likely to be almost a perfect circle without any irregularity of its periphery. At greater distances the periphery becomes more irregular and eventually radiating short projections appear. However it must also be borne in mind that the nature of the surface on which the drop falls will modify the shape as well as the distance through which it has travelled.

Drops of blood which fall at an angle other than vertically produce stains which have been most appropriately likened to exclamation marks. The "dot" of the mark points to the direction of the path of the drop of blood. If projected on to a wall by an upward sweep of an injured hand, the "dots" point upwards, or, if by a downward sweep, downwards. In similar fashion, if the long axis of the stains lie horizontally, it is possible to tell whether the drops fell in a forward or backward direction. Although a minor point, perhaps, these observations may be relevant to a reconstruction of the movements of a victim or assailant at the time of attack.

Smears of blood should also be noted. They trail off in the direction of the smear. Smears may be of first importance when they preserve the impressions of fingers or palms and may thus lead to the identification of an assailant.

Up to this point, relying only upon naked eye examination, the stains can only be presumed to be blood. It is true that fresh blood in quantity has a familiar red colour but in conditions of poor lighting, a pool of red paint may appear to be blood. Smaller stains, drops for example, can readily give rise to error since paint, dyes, jam, fruit stains, etc., may resemble fresh blood. Rust or tar stains are not easily distinguished from blood and always call for expert examination. The texture of the material also plays a part in making the detection of bloodstains by the naked-eye difficult, for example, bloodstains on dark fabrics, especially thick woollen garments. Drying, washing, or the application of chemicals can also modify the appearances of the stain.

Attempts by criminals to remove bloodstains at the scene of crime, from their clothing, or, as in *R. v. Whiteway* (1953), their footwear, are, fortunately, rarely completely successful. Even when effective measures are known, imperfect knowledge of the technique or lack of time may cause traces, capable of expert detection, to remain. It is true that washing weakens the colour and increases the difficulty in recognition. Drying, especially rapid drying, for example when the body is exposed to fire, darkens the colour of the stains. Their colour is also modified by chemicals. Soap or solutions of a chlorine bleach are likely to turn blood a greenish-brown. Chemicals added to soften or dissolve stains include alum; in practice these are likely to be less effective than water, especially with old stains. Cold water in sufficient amounts may remove all superficial stains, although this may take time; a solution of borax or normal saline may hasten the extraction of the stain. Although soaking of garments may remove external signs of blood, it is calculated to drive dissolved blood into the stuff of the garment or its lining and complete removal of blood from outer garments is usually beyond the resources of the criminal. Examination of the lining, at any rate, may yield results when traces are absent elsewhere, but well-washed stains are unlikely to admit of proof.

A photograph of bloodstains at the scene of a crime is always valuable but it is important to bear in mind the limitations of black and white prints, especially when they lack detail, because it is then difficult to distinguish bloodstains from other marks. This is calculated to exaggerate the severity of the victim's injuries. The police now have facilities for colour.

ILLUSTRATIVE EXAMPLES

Case 1: Death from Natural Causes: Suspected Homicide

The scene was one in which a doctor had died in distinctly suspicious circumstances. His body was found lying face down, beside his bed; an eiderdown covered the body and the room was in disorder. There was a pool of blood beneath his face, but he had not sustained any obvious injury. With Sir Sydney's case in mind, I suggested that he had collapsed on to his nose as a result of an accident or some natural cause. Later he was shown to have died of cerebral haemorrhage. It appeared while he had been accompanied by a woman friend, during the previous night, he was suddenly taken ill and had collapsed on to the floor. She covered him with the eiderdown and then, realising her embarrassing position, she ran away. Next day she telephoned the police to ask if Dr. "X" was "all right". The mysterious nature of her message resulted in a call at his house by a police officer. It was locked and he got no response to knocking. A panel in the back door had recently been broken and the officer thought there might have been a "breaking and entering". (It was later established that the doctor, when returning home drunk, unable to find his key, had broken the door in order to enter.) The discovery of his body in an unusual posture, beneath an eiderdown, not unnaturally aroused suspicion (F.M. 3042A).

This case resembled that of the late Sir Sydney Smith (see p. 483).

Case 2

An old woman had been battered to death with a shovel but there was no lead to the identity of her assailant. The fact that the shovel had been swung in an arc to strike the vertex of the victim was confirmed by an arc of blood spots on an adjacent wall. Amongst those questioned was a woman who had been to the local cinema that evening. When seen by the police surgeon (Dr. Alistair Sinton) he noticed that her finger nails appeared to be bloodstained. Scrapings were taken and the groupings tallied with that of the victim and not that of the subject. The latter was later convicted of the murder (R.v. Lloyd, 1955; F.M. 4067A).

Case 3

The collection of a pool of blood near the body during life indicates that the deceased fell unconscious and remained immobile after he had sustained the injury which caused bleeding. A girl who had been murdered by throat-cut was found lying on her back and the only blood at the scene was a large pool directly beneath the head and neck; downward streaking by blood was apparent on the skin of the right side of her neck; there was no blood on the front of her clothing nor on her hands and arms. It was inferred that she was unconscious and on her back at the time of her wounding and had made no movement thereafter. She had been raped and partially asphyxiated prior to this fatal injury (F.M. 1516).

Case 4

An elderly woman was found dead in a room where there were extensive blood stains and there was a quantity of blood in a bowl on the floor. Those who were first at the scene could find no obvious wound but believed that the bleeding had been due to a wound or haematemesis, without soiling the mouth. The information furnished by the police by telephone indicated that the soiling of the body by blood was restricted to one leg. The pathologist then suggested that a varicose vein had ruptured and this was confirmed by him at the autopsy; the perforation in the skin over the vein was only one-eighth of an inch in diameter (F.M. 11,596A).

Case 5

A farmer was found dead in his barn; he had an extensive shotgun injury of his head. Suspicion was aroused because the gun was not beside the body; it was at the top of some steps to the loft in the barn, about 15 feet away from the body. A trail of blood spots, most numerous on the front of the steps and on the pillars of the barn, indicated that he had sustained his injury at the top of the steps, had fallen forwards and had then somersaulted, so as to land on the floor of the barn at a distance from the steps (F.M. 9959B).

Case 6

When a middle-aged couple were found murdered in their bedroom, there were numerous bloodstains in the room and trails of wet sand across the bedroom ceiling, apparently from a sandbag used as a bludgeon which had burst, and some bloodstains on the window sill of an adjacent bedroom, accessible from the back of the house. The initial appearances suggested murder by an intruder from outside the house. However, a very few tiny bloodstains in the son's bedroom, together with traces of blood and sand in the bathroom, and especially in the bath, directed attention to the son, who ultimately was convicted of the murder. It is always wise to refrain from using sinks, etc., at a scene, until these have been examined for such traces (F.M. 12,329A and B).

Case 7

A single, middle-aged, Middle-European man, was found dead lying on the floor of his bed-sitting room. Suspicion was aroused initially by the presence of a large amount of blood on the floor and on the partially clothed body of the deceased. Examination revealed blood in large separate splashes on the floor, extending from the side of the bed to the position of the body near the door of the room. There was blood in a bucket near the feet of the deceased, blood spots on his legs and feet and extensive bloodstaining of the face around the nose and mouth. The appearances suggested some natural internal source for the haemorrhage, and the presence of marked finger-clubbing indicated a probably pulmonary source, confirmed at autopsy by the discovery of a carcinoma of the bronchus which had eroded a branch of the pulmonary artery. Evidently bleeding had commenced while the deceased was in bed, had continued as he staggered across the room and coughed blood into the bucket, and the final bleeding oozed out of nose and mouth as he lay collapsed on the floor, during his attempt to reach the door (F.M. 13,265A).

Case 8

An alcoholic, whose wife had died recently, was found in the bedroom of his house after not having been seen for several days, in a moderate state of putrefaction. A kitchen knife protruded from and transfixed his neck, from left to right. The deceased lay across the bed, feet towards a dressing table and, in addition to blood around the neck and beneath the body on the bed, there were spots of blood on the floor, between his feet and the dressing table, and on the top and front of the dressing table. No blood was apparent elsewhere in the house. Apart from the transfixion of the neck the only other wound on the body was a shallow cut extending from below the left ear, along the lower border of the lower jaw towards the chin, which appeared to be a misdirected tentative stab (F.M. 14,067A).

Cause of Death

The initial determination of the cause of death at the scene, in many cases is unlikely to be rewarding. Most often the cause is such as to be obvious even to a cursory glance by a layman, as when there are multiple stab or incised wounds, or strangulation with a ligature still in place. On such occasions the most that the pathologist is doing, though even this is not valueless, is to confirm the senior investigating police officer's suspicions. However the suspicious signs of death may be slight, and require specialist examination for their detection, as for instance in manual strangulation. Thus (F.M. 14,199A) an elderly woman's body was found lying on the floor of her sitting room. The principal grounds for suspicion were that a crash had been heard shortly before a scream which had prompted neighbours to see if she was all right. Although some broken plates were found beside the body which could have been damaged if she had accidentally fallen, yet there was also a recently broken window at the back of the house, raising the possibility of illegal entry. Inspection of the body, even in poor light, revealed tell-tale small crescentic abrasions on the neck, and subsequent autopsy confirmed the initial suspicion of manual strangulation.

On occasion the general features of the scene, especially if they have been encountered before, will alert the pathologist to the likely cause of death. This is particularly so in cases of carbon monoxide poisoning.

Two middle-aged people were found dead in the living room of their house, in wintertime, after having last been seen alive 4 days previously (F.M. 14,725 A & B). Both bodies showed advanced putrefaction, due to the fact that a gasfire was alight in the room. The dead body of the family cat also lay in the room. These features suggested the possibility of carbon-monoxide poisoning, which was further indicated by a pinkish hue of the residual hypostasis in the lesser decomposed body. It was confirmed by blood tests after the subsequent autopsy, and the source as suspected, was blockage of the flue of the gas fire by debris.

On other occasions bizarre features of the scene may enable the pathologist, at a very early stage, to relieve the suspicions of the police and indicate that the circumstances of the death were other than murder. This is particularly the case where death is due to sexual asphyxia. (See Chapter 9). Then, such things as the wearing of female apparel by a male, the presence of pornographic literature, and bizarre modes of bondage may all point to the true circumstances.

The strange features of preternatural combustion (see Chapter 7), may also raise suspicion of homicide in police minds when the scene is first viewed. It is often thought that a murder has been committed and attempts then made to conceal the fact by arson. However, the position of the body, close to a source of ignition, the wholly disproportionate damage to the body compared to the very slightly affected surroundings, and the absence of any signs of a struggle or other features of a homicidal attack enable the pathologist at the scene, to indicate the true circumstances.

Time of Death

Apart from the cause, and the circumstances of death, the other factor which the pathologist may be able to assess at the scene is the approximate time of death. The details of the methods available and their attendant problems, are fully dealt with in Chapter 18. However time can be saved if the air temperature at the scene is being measured while the initial inspection and recording are proceeding; then the sooner the body temperature is taken the better, especially if it is going to prove necessary to record several temperatures as the body cools over a period of an hour or two. Often this is considered unnecessary, as an approximate time of death is already known from other sources. In this case a single record of the body temperature will allow a very rough indication of the time of death, and if this is in agreement with the time as estimated from other sources, then the investigating police officer may well be satisfied with this, and will be anxious to have the body moved and the autopsy commenced as soon as possible. However the pathologist would do well to bear in mind that although at the time of the initial examination everyone may well be quite satisfied that they know the time of death, or that it is unimportant, yet some days, or weeks, later the situation may well have changed considerably, and he may then find himself being pressed to express a firm opinion as to the time of death. Therefore he needs either to make a very detailed examination at the scene, in spite of the views of its irrelevance expressed by others, or else agree to make a cursory examination on the clear understanding that he will not be able to give reliable evidence on this point. He should certainly avoid being trapped into expressing a dogmatic view later on insufficient data.

Apart from body temperature, an assessment of such additional features as rigor mortis and hypostasis, although notoriously uncertain, should nevertheless be made carefully. They may prove to be valuable later. Thus (F.M. 27,073) an elderly man's body was found in the pantry of his house, with severe head injuries, bearing an unusual and distinctive toothed pattern. The body temperature had reached that of the surroundings, rigor mortis was present, but very early putrefaction in the form of slight green discoloration of the abdominal wall was apparent. My view was that death had occurred some 2 to 3 days beforehand, based on the stage of rigor and putrefaction. A few days later police enquiries discovered that the next door neighbours stated that they had seen the deceased, at a bus stop, less than 24 hours before his body was found. My opinion given with some trepidation to the police, was that this was impossible. At this the neighbours came under suspicion, were questioned extensively, and eventually confessed to having committed the murder themselves. They disclosed that they had thrown the murder weapon in a local lake from whence it was recovered, and found to be part of the machinery of a washing machine; it had a shape which exactly matched the pattern of the injuries. It is of course, always necessary to remember to take an anal swab, for examination for seminal fluid, before inserting a rectal thermometer or probe into the rectum, lest there be subsequent allegations of contamination from the thermometer. Even if the clothing is in normal position, subsequent allegations may be made that an assault occurred after homosexual practices had taken place. Moreover, it is advisable in the case of a woman to take vaginal as well as anal swabs at this stage, before the body is moved since later it may be alleged that a positive anal or vaginal reaction for semen is due to fluid trickling or being transferred from the other orifice during removal of the body. For the sake of completeness an oral swab could be taken at this stage as well, subject in the case of all the investigations, to the completion of the forensic science examination of the clothing, face, etc., for trace evidence. While taking swabs it is worth considering the possibility that a bloodstain or drop of blood in an odd place, not in keeping with the other features of the wounds, may be in fact derived from the assailant rather than the deceased; so a moistened swab rubbed on to the stain will recover sufficient to enable it to be grouped if necessary.

Removal of the Body

At the completion of his examination the remaining duty of the pathologist is to superintend the preservation of the body for the recovery of any further contact evidence, and to prevent any extraneous contamination. The easiest way to do this is to lift the body on to a large polythene sheet, which can then wrap up the body completely, being secured by sellotape or string. At the post-mortem room the body can be left on it until clothing etc. has been removed and the sheet can then be carefully folded up, to preserve any material which has fallen on to it, and handed to the forensic scientists.

Alternatively plastic bags can be secured over the deceased's head, hands and feet. However in our experience this is less satisfactory than using an entire sheet. Where there are head wounds a bag leads to smearing blood more widely over the face, thus confusing subsequent examination. The pathologist should then superintend the removal of the body from the scene, so that he can be satisfied that no additional injuries have been inflicted to the body in transit.

It is obviously extremely important that the pathologist takes the utmost care to avoid damaging any evidence which may be vital to other experts in the team.

Thus on one occasion (F.M. 14,249 A) a child's body was found in a wood close to the route she would have taken from her school to her home which was in a remote farmhouse. She had been strangled with the belt of her gaberdine raincoat. Fortunately the body was removed from the scene with adequate care because subsequent examination of the belt by the forensic scientist revealed fibres which were later shown to match fibres from the rug in the car of a young man suspected of causing her death.

On another occasion (F.M. 18,977 A) an old man's body was found in his flat, with severe head injuries, and heavily bloodsoiled, with considerable bloodsoiling of the surrounding parts of the room. At the mortuary, in better light, one bloodstain on the deceased's thigh was recognised by the fingerprint expert as being a palmprint in blood, later shown to be identical with that of a suspect. I would never have recognised the print for what it was, if it had not been pointed out to me by the expert, and so, in his absence, it would easily have been destroyed. (Swann, 1976)

Indeed shaped bloodstains on the surface of a body, unless they are recognised and recorded with photographs *in situ*, are in great danger of being destroyed during the removal of the body by becoming smeared or overlain with fresh blood. On several occasions the authors have seen shaped blood smears on the bodies of victims of stabbing, caused by the knife having been wiped on the skin of the deceased. Such marks can, when recognised, give useful information about the blade of the weapon causing the injuries.

Before leaving the scene finally, the pathologist would be well advised to look around other areas away from the situation of the body. It may be possible to see clear drag marks, or trails of blood, indicating that the body has been moved or the victim had staggered to the situation where the body lies. On other occasions the absence of such a trail may be of special significance. Thus (F.M. 19,171 A) a man's body with severe facial injuries, was found, on a wet day in a yard at the back of a house at the end of an alleyway. The possibility was suggested that the deceased, a known alcoholic, had fallen elsewhere, in the street, and had sustained his injuries, then staggered to the situation where he had collapsed and died. However, the alleyway leading to the yard was roofed over, and the ground bore no traces of bloodspots such as would have been found to fall from his injuries. Although in the street, or the open yard, these could have been washed away by the rain, there was no possibility of this happening in the protected alleyway, and so it was clear that the deceased must have sustained his injuries at the place where his body was found.

Concealed Bodies

In certain circumstances, particularly where the body is partly hidden, the technique for examination of the scene has to be modified. When a body is partially concealed, it is usually discovered by accident, by a chance observation of some passer-by. A young child (F.M. 28,346 A) was missing. Near her home was a housing site in process of construction. Shortly before the concrete for a new roadway was to be poured on to the foundations of rough-cast, a workman noticed some strands of hair protruding from beneath a piece of stone in the centre of the roadway. The body of the child, who had been strangled, had been concealed in a shallow grave in amongst the stones.

In such cases it is important to expose the body slowly, a layer at a time, with photographic record of each stage. If necessary, where for instance large rocks or concrete slabs are laid on top of the body, these can be marked by a paper label, or a chalked number for photography before being removed. The position of such rocks may well be important later in relation to any injuries on the body, or any trace evidence.

Since partial concealment implies haste on the part of the murderer, some articles may fall out of his pockets, or be dropped beside the body. In the case of the young girl mentioned above, a cylindrical cigarette lighter was found between the girl's legs. At first it was thought that genital injuries were due to its insertion. However later it became apparent that the injuries were due to rape and the lighter had been accidentally dropped during the murderer's haste to conceal the body and leave the scene.

Bodies which are buried, however, pose yet different problems. In the first instance, there is the matter of the location of the body itself. Most often, in our experience, this has come about from information given to the police, while on other occasions it has occurred through reconstruction of the events by the police from other clues.

Thus one woman's body (F.M. 15,124 A) was buried in a sunbathing area within a large wild garden, by her husband. Her disappearance was noted by neighbours, and after some months had passed the alarm was raised. Only prolonged interrogation by the police caused him to reveal the situation of his wife's body. The grave by this time was wholly concealed by long grass. In the case of the two children's bodies in the "Moors Murder" case, the first, Downey, was found by police searching the area, being partly exposed in a peaty bank on moorland. However, the other, Kilbride, was found because police discovered a photograph of one of the suspects, Hindley, staring at the ground on a patch of moorland which one of the investigating police officers identified from the photograph.

Location by means of general search has always posed great problems. Often this has meant a line of policemen crossing a suspect area, and probing the ground with long sticks, to see if this reveals any telltale odours. Such a technique obviously has considerable limitations. Attempts have been made to devise more precise methods, based on the results of scientific research. Of these, infra-red photography has proved the most useful, but depends on the body being buried in an area which is fairly uniform and amenable for aerial photography. Other similar techniques which had been attempted include aerial photography of the spectral reflectance of vegetation. However such a technique is even more dependent on uniform background. It is of course well known that vegetation of certain types will be more verdant over areas containing human detritus. Thus elderberry bushes flourish on old sites of human habitation and so do nettles. The reader will probably recall seeing such plants inside iron age hill fort sites. However their value in detecting bodies buried in more recent times is clearly very limited. On one occasion police searching for a suspected missing woman in a garden used a thermal heat intensifier in an endeavour to detect human tissue buried underground. It has been suggested that a dowser or water diviner might be able to detect a buried body in the same way that pipes can be discovered around buildings. However the authors have no personal experience of the use of this method of detection, although there are recorded instances of its use.

Probably the most successful technique is the use of animals presumably because of their ability to detect odours. It is obvious that bodies which have been buried are often disturbed by animals, such as foxes or dogs. Attempts are now being made in various police forces to train certain dogs to detect buried human bodies, but the technique has yet to be tried out in practice, so far as we know. If as seems probable, the animal relies on olfactory sense to detect the body, then it would seem to be also possible to devise some chemical testing device along the lines of a gas chromatograph, also capable of selecting such odours. Research so far has indicated that the only gas generated in quantity during decomposition is ammonia. However various other substances, such as certain amines, must be produced to cause the characteristic odour of decomposition. The subject is worthy of further research.

Once a buried body has been located the correct procedure lies in slow and careful exposure of the body with photographic recording at all stages, and preservation of samples of soil and other material from above and beside the body. As in the partially buried body objects may have been accidentally dropped into the grave while the body was being covered.

Once the body has been exposed, careful cleaning of soil from the body surface is necessary to expose the clothing and detect any abnormalities which can be recorded at this stage lest they be altered during removal of the body. Thus it is often the case that where the death of a person whose body has been buried was by strangulation by a ligature, the ligature is left in position around the neck when the burial takes place. This fact has been used by the defence in a case to suggest that the victim had died accidentally, the defendant had only placed the ligature in position to ensure that the victim did not recover consciousness once buried.

More readily overlooked is the presence of foreign material in the mouth. In several of our cases, in addition to the ligature round the neck, the victim's mouth has been stuffed with cloth or handkerchiefs, or, on one occasion the horsehair stuffing of an old sofa. Unless this is detected and recorded at this stage, it may be displaced on removal of the body, or else it could be alleged that the material accidentally entered the mouth during this procedure.

Soil samples from beneath the body and at a distance from it are advisable in case any toxicological analysis becomes necessary later. The actual removal of the body may pose problems. If decomposition is not too far advanced, then it may be possible simply to lift the body on to a plastic sheet. However, if adipocerous change or skeletonisation is advanced, then it may prove necessary to dig down beside and then beneath the body so that some firm material, such as a sheet of hardboard may gradually be inserted under the body which can then be lifted and transported on it. In more formal exhumations of bodies buried in conventional circumstances in burial grounds the main problem is the avoidance of publicity. Apart from simple removal of the body to another site for administrative reasons where faculty is obtained from the ecclesiastical authorities, such exhumations where a crime has been alleged will be on the authority either of the local coroner or the Home Office. Full details of the administrative procedures may be found elsewhere (see Chapter 24).

As regards the actual procedure of exhumation, this is usually done in the early morning, to avoid publicity which usually means that it attracts even more. The site is screened off and the position of the grave, when exposed, and identity of the coffin, is established by some competent official, such as a funeral director or superintendent of the burial ground. Soil samples from above, beside, and beneath the coffin, and any water leaking from coffin, shall be collected at this stage. Further examination should be carried out in a fully-equipped modern mortuary. The days of working on trestles in a hut at the edge of the cemetery have passed.

Certain situations produce scenes which have their own peculiar difficulties. Thus, in cases of fire, where a body or bodies have been found in a burning building, they are often removed, naturally enough, by the firemen in case any chance remains of resuscitation. Where they remain *in situ* the attendant danger to the surroundings makes examination very difficult. However the possibility must always be borne in mind at the outset, that this may be a case of death due to homicide, with subsequent attempted concealment by arson. Therefore inspection for injury, ligatures, etc. and examination of the hypostasis for an initial assessment of the probable quantity of carboxyhaemoglobin is necessary. Estimation of time of death is rendered much more difficult. Confait Case; ref. Fisher report. One major problem may concern identification. In one of our cases (F.M. 12,678 A) a child's grossly incinerated body was found in the remains of a burnt haystack. Identification was achieved by a scrap of shirt collar preserved at the back of the neck, which bore a laundry mark, and a spectacle lens, the prescription for which could be established.

Where large numbers of bodies are found in a burnt building, as in some mass disasters involving hotel fires or dance halls, then a full scale mass disaster scheme must be adopted to secure the identification of all the victims.

In bodies recovered from water there is rarely anything of value to be learnt from the scene by a pathologist, though police officers may find footprints etc. Obviously the place where the body is found, if in a river, is unlikely to be the one where it also entered the water (see Chapter 11).

In cases of death from shooting the presence of a ballistics expert at the scene, though often not possible, is a great advantage, as trajectory, likely weapon, and associated circumstances can be most easily worked out by the ballistics expert and the pathologist working together at the scene.

Deaths from poisoning rarely require an initial visit to the scene, unless the death in some other way is suspicious, as in cases of unsuspected carbon-monoxide poisoning (Page 582 above).

Retrospective Visit to the Scene

Finally there may be considerable value, even if a pathologist does not see the body *in situ*, in a retrospective visit to the scene. At its least, the value resides in enabling the pathologist, at any subsequent discussion of the case, in court or elsewhere, to have a true appreciation of the nature of the surroundings. These are often found to differ markedly from the impression gained from other people's descriptions. Photographs of the scene often provide an acceptable alternative, but in any case of uncertainty it is better to visit the scene personally.

In some situations this is particularly valuable. In the case of alleged battered babies it may enable injuries to be matched with objects in the room. Similarly in road and rail accidents it may be possible to relate injuries to particular parts of the railway track, or even the locomotive.

Finally it may serve to indicate that a death being viewed as a possible accident, must in fact be the result of a homicidal attack. On one occasion in our experience (F.M. 24,396) a tramp was admitted to hospital unconscious suffering from head injuries. These took the form of three roughly parallel linear lacerations of the scalp. Suggestions were made that these could have been caused by a fall down some stairs at a derelict factory site where he was found. However a visit to the scene, and inspection of the staircase in the place where the body was found showed this to be impossible. The pathologist's view was that the injuries were the result of several blows with a rod-like instrument. This view was reinforced at the subsequent autopsy. Later another tramp confessed to having assaulted this man using a wooden club as a weapon.

References

Police Research Bulletin (1982) **38,** 75.
SWANN, P. M. (1976) *Police Journal*, **XLIX,** 158–164.
Confait Case. Report of an Inquiry by the Hon. Sir Henry Fisher into the circumstances leading to the trial of three persons on charges arising out of the death of Maxwell Confait and the fire at 27, Doggett Road, London SE 6. H.M.S.O. 13, Dec. 1977.

CHAPTER 19

Anaesthetic Deaths

IT IS preferable and more accurate to consider these as "deaths occurring during anaesthesia", since the chapter heading is calculated to imply that the main, if not the sole, cause of death, was the anaesthetic or technicalities of its administration. Investigation, however, not infrequently discloses that the anaesthetic and the anaesthetist played no part in the death.

These investigations are complex. Regardless of the fact that the majority occur in hospitals—it must not be forgotten that a few occur in dental surgeries—although the hospital pathologist is competent to perform his part, the autopsy should be, and normally is, referred to a pathologist from outside the hospital, who can be seen to be independent of the hospital administration and staff. The pathologist of the hospital concerned is thus spared much possible embarrassment. A forensic pathologist, with experience of such examinations, is ideally placed to perform such a role.

It must be realised that the pathologist's findings, although an integral part of the investigation, are often an insufficient explanation of the death. The cause may have been due to factors, the nature of which places them beyond the scope of his examination (Polson, 1955).

Not rarely the post-mortem examination yields negative findings, and the pathologist is not then in a position to express an opinion as to whether the anaesthetic, or its administration, was a factor in the death; this was confirmed by the experience of Hunt (1958) and Harrison (1968a). They took the view that the role of the pathologist was restricted, in the main, to the detection of natural disease, overt signs of damage by anaesthetic procedure or errors in surgical procedure. In the absence of positive findings the pathologist has been compelled to accept the formula "there was nothing to show that the anaesthetic was not skilfully given".

The present position, however, has been appreciably improved by access to toxicological analysis, and therefore when the autopsy findings are negative, the pathologist should collect material for this purpose, and, as may be necessary, obtain advice from the toxicologist concerned, in order to ensure that the appropriate material, in adequate amount and condition, is sent for examination (Blanke, 1960; Campbell *et al.*, 1961; Rieders, 1969).

Where it is left to the pathologist to be the sole witness to the medical findings it is imperative that he should have had the opportunity to discuss the circumstances of the case with the anaesthetist and clinician concerned. The Coroner may well wisely decide to hear their evidence in addition to that of the pathologist, if he is to reach a correct interpretation of the cause of death. He should also have information of any relevant toxicological findings.

Scepticism has been expressed by various authors about the value of an inquest or procurator-fiscal's enquiry into such deaths. It has been suggested that these enquiries are rarely in possession of the full facts, or consider the opinion of anaesthetists, in reaching a decision (Bourne, 1973a). It has also been suggested that post-mortem examinations ordered by Crown authorities in such cases may be largely unrewarding and mostly unnecessary (Gillies *et al.*, 1979).

Attention was drawn to the incidence of unexplained deaths in other spheres of medical activity and it was suggested that the assumption of fault on the part of the anaesthetist prevents adequate investigation of these deaths (Keats, 1979).

Classification of Deaths Associated with Anaesthesia

Several classifications have been published, e.g. by Schapira *et al.* (1960) and Harrison (1968b). We offer a simple grading as follows:
(a) Deaths due to the anaesthetic and/or the mode of its administration.
(b) Deaths due to surgical mishaps during anaesthesia.
(c) Deaths due to natural disease, either that for which the treatment was given, or intercurrent disease.

The hazards of anaesthesia are considered in detail by several authors, including Keating (1966). Surveys of series of cases from centres in various countries have been published by Marx, Mateo and Orkin (1973), Bodlander (1975) Harrison (1978) and Hovi-Viander (1980).

Surveys of anaesthetic morbidity and mortality have been made in Britain by the Association of Anaesthetists and the results were reported in 1956 and 1964. The most recent report is by Lunn and Mushin (1982); see also the Leading Article, *Brit. Med. J.*, 1982).

ANAESTHETICS

The report on mortality associated with anaesthesia (Lunn and Mushin, 1982), should be consulted in the original for detail. The authors make the point that autopsy reports alone are of limited value in explaining deaths associated with anaesthesia. Even so, in a table in which they list a series of events, quoted by anaesthetic assessors as occurring in deaths which are considered to be wholly due to anaesthesia, nearly half showed factors which should have been detectable at autopsy, e.g. inhaled vomit, overload of fluids, ischaemic heart disease, embolus, etc.

The most recent figures (Lunn and Mushin, 1982) give an estimated anaesthetic mortality of one patient in 10,000 or 0.001 per cent. By comparison deaths from other causes within 6 days of operation are reported as being one patient for every 1,000 operations or 0.6 per cent. Thus the numbers of deaths attributable to anaesthesia are very small. However, the list of causes remains fairly constant; inadequate management of fluid balance, respiratory insufficiency, cardio-vascular collapse, technical errors, failed intubation, inadequate supervision, respiratory failure due to drugs and inhalation of vomit.

Surveys have also been conducted into maternal death due to anaesthesia during obstetric procedures. Reports are often based on the Confidential Enquiries into Maternal Deaths in England and Wales, e.g., Crawford (1974), Scott (1974) and Moir (1980). Morgan (1980) reported on a survey conducted at Queen Charlotte's Hospital over 20 years. His findings were that anaesthesia was the greatest single cause of maternal death during the period 1958–78. The reports based on the Confidential Enquiries indicate that the proportion of deaths due to anaesthesia was of the order of 13–14 per cent, with avoidable factors in almost all cases.

The cause of death from anaesthesia is in many cases of such a nature that it cannot be detected by dissection alone. However, a knowledge of possible causes, as reported in the various surveys, coupled with the autopsy findings and, ideally, following discussion with the anaesthetist, may allow a probable cause to be assigned with some confidence.

(a) DEATHS DUE TO ANAESTHESIA AND/OR ITS MODE OF ADMINISTRATION

It should be emphasised that anaesthetic deaths are uncommon; the published reports say that the incidence of death during or shortly after an operation ranges from 0.2 to 0.6 per cent of operations and that deaths attributable to anaesthesia are of the order of only 0.03–0.1 per cent of all anaesthetics given. Of deaths occurring during or soon after operation, the reported incidence due to the anaesthetic vary from 5 to 50 per cent (Campbell, 1960). Several authors have listed the causes of death due to anaesthesia, e.g. Edwards *et al.* (1956), Campbell (1960), Schapira *et al.* (1960), Dinnick (1964), Love (1968), Harrison (1968b). (The reports by Edwards *et al.* (1956) and Dinnick (1964) were based on a series of investigations conducted by the Association of Anaesthetists.)

(i) *Inexperience* Morton and Wylie (1951) were of the opinion that the majority of deaths during anaesthesia were due to inexperience and failure to adopt precautions when clearly indicated. This may still be true. These include mishaps due to intubation (e.g. aspiration of vomit, kinked tubes, etc.) and bronchoscopy. Each may cause vagal inhibition if the depth of the anaesthesia be inadequate. Post-operative respiratory obstructions by tubing or swabs may also occur.

Attention has been drawn to the risks of inexperienced anaesthetists in obstetric anaesthesia (Moir, 1980), who quotes the view of the Obstetric Anaesthetists Association that obstetric anaesthesia should not be given by unsupervised anaesthetists, of less than one year's experience. The risks of inadequate training in anaesthetics have been described by Scott (1982) and the dangers of excessively long working hours of juniors by Heggs (1982).

A study of human factors involved in preventable anaesthetic mishaps was published by Cooper *et al.* (1978). They described interviews with anaesthetists in an urban hospital which identified 359 preventable incidents. Human error was responsible for 82 per cent of the deaths, e.g., breathing circuit disconnections. Equipment failure occurred in only 14 per cent; other factors included inadequate communication between staff, haste and distraction.

(ii) *Drugs* Drugs used in modern anaesthesia may play an important part in these incidents, for example, overdosage of intravenous barbiturate, or collapse after the administration of this drug with relaxant drugs.

Harrison (1978) drew attention to the risks of respiratory inadequacy following the use of drugs to produce myo-neural blockade. He also commented on deaths caused by circulatory collapse, produced in elderly and arteriosclerotic patients with ischaemic heart disease, by the use of such drugs as thiopentone. Moir (1980) refers to fatal bradycardia caused by suxamethonium given without atropine.

Abnormal or anaphylactic reactions to drugs may prove fatal. Hovi-Viander (1980) refers to anaphylaxis induced by dextran. A young mother was about to receive cosmetic surgery of her breast. Althesin was used as one of the anaesthetic agents. It caused immediate, violent bronchospasm during induction, resulting in fatal pulmonary rupture and tension pneumothorax.

Heart failure has been associated with trichloroethylene. Intravenous administration of urea has caused hypertension. The safety of halothane has been the subject of several reports and there is evidence that this drug can cause liver necrosis and, more recently, it has been deemed to cause malignant hyperpyrexia. Tygstrup (1963) found a clear connection between halothane and liver necrosis, but the experience of Mushin *et al.* (1964) showed that hepatitis after halothane was no more likely to occur than after any other anaesthetic. Sharpstone *et al.* (1971) have little doubt that halothane can cause hepatitis, usually after multiple exposures to this anaesthetic. Thus six of the eleven patients in their series died in from 8 to 28 days after halothane anaesthesia and the post-mortem examination disclosed massive liver necrosis and other features of acute hepatitis. Halothane alone or with suxamethonium is now recognised as the probable cause of an alarming complication of anaesthesia known as malignant hyperpyrexia.

This is characterized not only by the abrupt onset of rise in temperature to dangerous levels, even to 110°F, but also tachycardia, hyperpnoea, cyanosis and stiffening of the muscles (Barlow and Isaacs, 1970). This condition is likely to result in death in the majority of patients. It was at first thought to have been a reaction to suxamethonium but the condition has since been observed following the administration of halothane alone (Harrison, 1968a; Drury and Gilbertson, 1970). It is apparently genetically determined and likely to occur in families who have evidence of sub-clinical myopathy and an abnormally high level of serum creatinine phosphokinase (Isaacs and Barlow, 1970).

Experiments with pigs given suxamethonium showed that they developed hyperpyrexia and so an association with abnormal muscle metabolism was suspected. Later halothane was also incriminated when used as an anaesthetic agent. It was found that surviving human victims had abnormal levels of creatinine phosphokinase and aldolase enzymes in their circulation as did many of their relatives, indicating a form of genetically determined myopathy.

Techniques, such as muscle biopsy, to screen for persons at risk were described by Ellis (1972). More recently the value of such estimations has been doubted (Macrae 1979, Ellis, 1980). Doctors in America have been sued for malpractice by patients who have suffered this condition. (Mazzia and Sinion, 1978).

Nitrous oxide anaesthesia is rarely fatal and these deaths are probably due to inexperience or inefficient administration. An example is that of death during single-handed anaesthesia and surgical treatment for avulsion of a toe-nail (Polson, 1955).

The death of a girl, who had been a dentist's receptionist, occurred in circumstances which suggested fatal overdosage, following addiction to the inhalation of nitrous oxide (Enticknap, 1961).

In 1966 outbreaks of poisoning by nitrous oxide created considerable alarm and on the first occasion the outbreak was traced to the fact that there had been faulty labelling of the medical gas points. In consequence, patients who required oxygen inhaled nitrous oxide (*Brit. Med. J.*, 1966).

Later that year the deaths of two patients were ostensibly due to inhalation of nitrous oxide. Investigation disclosed that the particular supply of nitrous oxide had been contaminated by nitric oxide. This was the result of unprecedented breakdown in the elaborate safety precautions used in the manufacture of nitrous oxide. When the nitrous oxide cylinders were recalled, over 40,000 were tested; sixty-five were found to be contaminated by nitric oxide (*Lancet*, 1966a, 1966b; *Brit. Med. J.*, 1966; *Brit. J. Anaesthesia*, 1967).

Atropine used in pre-medication has been alleged to cause hypoxia, especially in the presence of respiratory and cardiac disease (Conway and Payne, 1964). See *Lancet*, 1964, vol. 1, pp. 109, 165, 220, 273. See also "Malignant Hyperpyrexia", pp. 332–3.

Atropine may cause hyperpyrexia through interference with the heat-regulating mechanism (Tattersall, 1953; Pask, 1964). Examples were reported by Harris and Hutton (1956).

Adrenaline and cocaine: Mackintosh (1948–9) drew attention to the hazards of adrenaline and cocaine. The administration of adrenaline in error for cocaine caused two sudden deaths. He also considered its addition to cocaine for local anaesthesia an unnecessary step in the production of vaso-constriction and their combination increased the toxicity of both drugs. He also drew attention to the need to distinguish between 2 per cent cocaine *in* adrenaline and 2 per cent cocaine *with* adrenaline. He doubted the existence of sensitivity to cocaine; in his experience these accidents were due either to overdosage, or the combination with adrenaline.

Berger *et al.* (1974) described two deaths of women undergoing paracervical block anaesthesia for termination of pregnancy. The drug used was lignocaine hydrochloride. Within minutes of injection generalized convulsions developed and death occurred soon after. It was possible that an overdose of the drug was administered intravenously.

(iii) *Clinical Factors* These include under-ventilation, low blood volume, and inadequate transfusion and anoxia. The latter is not infrequently due to unidentified cause; this hazard causes cerebral damage (Courville, 1960; Brierley and Miller, 1966). On one exceptional occasion in 1959 anoxia causing gross cerebral damage was the cause of the death of a child. On that occasion the death was due to inefficient administration by the anaesthetist, who was himself at that time under the influence of anaesthetic.

Inadvertent hypothermia, hyperpyrexia, sensitivity reactions and the inhalation of regurgitated material, especially during the post-operative period, are other possible hazards.

Skilled nursing during the post-operative period with the patient in a safe position is an important protection, and there should be direct observation of the patient until he recovers consciousness. Even if left alone for a few minutes fatal inhalation of vomit may occur (Mackintosh, 1948–9).

More recently the importance of adequate supervision in recovery rooms has been stressed by Boulton (1982).

(iv) *Technical Mishaps* The administration of incompatible blood today is a rare event. Abnormal abduction of the arm during transfusion can lead to brachial paralysis, though it is normally only temporary. This accident was the grounds of a civil court action in 1953 (*Crawford* v. *Charing Cross Hospital Board*). The infusion of the wrong fluid is also a rare event. A patient died when she received sodium citrate in error for normal saline. This error was largely due to the fact that both colourless solutions were contained in similar bottles with almost similar labels, in the same store cupboard. In circumstances of urgency it would, however, be easy for this mistake to occur. The two solutions should be kept in separate cupboards and bear distinctive labels. Mistakes have occurred through failure to check the label, for instance an anaesthetic of greater strength than was intended was administered, or ether has been injected in error for a local anaesthetic. The anaesthetist should personally check the label on the bottle and also check the odour of the fluid.

Gauze or other swabs used may be overlooked and inadvertently inhaled. They should be of the right design and controlled by tapes or instruments (*Garner* v. *Morrell*, 1955: *Urray and Urray* v. *Bierer*, 1955). In the past there have been rare occasions of explosion in the operating theatre during anaesthesia.

DENTAL ANAESTHESIA

The risks of dental general anaesthesia are much the same as those in the surgical theatre. There are the additional specific hazards of inhalation of blood, teeth, or mouth packs, peri-odontal lignococaine and hypotension due to fainting in a sitting posture. The injection of local anaesthetic directly into the blood stream, an accident which may happen during injection of the inferior dental nerve, may cause sudden collapse. These matters are considered in the pamphlet *Emergencies in Dental Practice* (1972) which contains criteria for safety in dental anaesthesia, but also draws attention to dental hazards created by the medical profession. [Although the Minister declined to introduce regulations implementing the recommendations in this report he hoped that it would be studied and the recommendations would be voluntarily adopted (*Brit. Med. J.*, 29 Dec. 1971)].

The hazards of dental operations on patients in sitting positions in dental chairs and of single-handed operator-anaesthetists has been increasingly a matter of concern during the past decade. Several deaths occurred and were the subject of inquests during 1973 and 1974 (Mehta, 1974: Bourne, 1973a: 1973b and Medico-legal report, *Brit. Med. J.* 1973). Authors have pointed out the difficulty of detecting that a patient has fainted while anaesthetised and hence the importance of operating with the patient in a reclining position. The importance of adequate facilities for resuscitation is also stressed. In some of the reported cases oxygen equipment was exhausted too quickly. The dangers of the administration of intravenous barbiturate anaesthesia by unskilled dental assistants was recorded (*Brit. Med. J.*, Medico-legal reports 1974; 1975 and in Correspondence, 1974: and

1975). Some have expressed reservations about the horizontal posture (*Brit. Med. J.*, 1976). A definitive view of the situation was expressed by Mr. Rodney Swiss in his presidential address to the General Dental Council: "A practitioner who regularly administers general anaesthetics single-handed for conservation work is, in my view, acting inexcusably".

The finding of a swab in a bronchus at autopsy calls for care in interpretation. It may have been impacted during life or pushed into the bronchus by inexpert post-mortem technique.

Robertson (1961) reported the presence of a swab in the main bronchus of a patient who had had a tracheotomy following a road accident. It was alleged that the swab contributed to the patient's death, and that it had been introduced into the air passages during tracheal toilet. There was, however, no evidence of collapse in the lung beyond the obstruction.

Robertson demonstrated by experiment that simulated artificial respiration did not displace a swab into the bronchus. He showed, however, that the normal practice of removing the lungs *en bloc* with traction on the trachea followed by opening of the air passages through their posterior wall with scissors, could dislodge a swab which had been inserted into a tracheotomy after death, and force it into the bronchus. He therefore recommended the opening of the air passages *in situ* in medico-legal cases, but this is practical only on those occasions when there is reason to suspect a foreign body in them.

We were asked to investigate a similar problem. This patient died of pneumonia following bronchitis and emphysema; he had required a tracheotomy. When the first pathologist removed the lungs *en bloc*, in the usual manner, he found a cotton-wool swab in the right main bronchus. There was partial collapse of the lung beyond the obstruction and the appearances were consistent with the inhalation of the swab.

A second opinion was obtained because following autopsy it was alleged that the swab had been introduced into the trachea by a nurse when sealing the tracheotomy opening with a wool plug, and strapping after death.

The pathologist's report did not indicate that the swab had been seen immediately on opening the air passages but it might have been displaced by his scissors during his examination. However, in tests which we conducted on other autopsies, pieces of cotton wool, introduced through artificial tracheotomy openings before the body was opened, were only dislodged into a bronchus, and then not firmly, if the air passages were opened by scissors equipped with sharp points. Blunt or ball-ended scissors always slipped past the swab in the trachea without displacing it.

We found that the foreign body consisted of two separate rolls of cotton wool similar in appearance to those used in the ward for tracheal toilet. They were not of the kind used to plug a tracheotomy after death.

Histological examination of the bronchus at the site of the swab and of the corresponding segment of the bronchus as a control showed that the bronchial wall around the swab was encircled by an inflammatory reaction, whereas inflammation of the wall of the control bronchus was restricted to its dependent surface.

Experiments showed that where swabs were introduced into inflamed bronchi after death they removed most of the signs of inflammation, by the compression and emptying of the dilated blood vessels in the bronchial walls.

As a result of our examination and experiments we concluded that in the specimen submitted to us the swabs must have been inhaled during life, following tracheal toilet. We were unable to say how long the swab had been impacted (F.M. 14,582 A).

(b) DEATHS DUE TO SURGICAL MISHAPS

Deaths coming within this category are usually readily detectable at autopsy, and do not require detailed discussion here. They are considered in reviews of deaths associated with anaesthesia, such as that of Harrison (1968a) and monographs on the subject are available, such as those of Beecher and Todd (1954) and Boba (1965). In the experience of one forensic pathologist (Mant, 1958) the principal findings are massive haemorrhage, as from slipped ligatures, uncontrollable oozing, etc., accidental perforation of a viscus such as the bladder, air embolism—for instance in operations in the region of the axilla—and gross surgical errors. Most well-recognised complications of surgical treatment, such as post-gastrectomy acute pancreatitis, are likely to occur outside the period of the operation or a few hours after it, and so do not come within the scope of this discussion. In the case of deaths during this period, a careful dissection of the operation site will reveal any surgical disasters.

As ever more complicated surgical procedures are developed, they carry their own peculiar risks and the pathologist has no alternative to a review of the recent literature when carrying out the investigation of such a case, e.g., open-heart surgery has hazards peculiar to its site and operative techniques.

Special difficulties may arise when a surgical mishap occurs during an operation necessitated by a criminal act (F.M. 24957B). A youth suffered a single stab wound of his chest in a fracas. This had punctured a lung and the surgeons suspected the onset of a tension pneumothorax. A pleural drain was inserted through a surgical "stab" incision. The patient died some hours later.

The autopsy disclosed that in addition to the wound caused during a fight there was a second identical stab wound beneath the surgical drain. The two wounds were indistinguishable in size and gravity. In consequence the original charge of murder was reduced to one of manslaughter.

(c) DEATHS FROM DISEASE

In the majority of cases of death associated with anaesthesia, the cause of death is disease. This is often the disease for which the surgical treatment was being given, and in a gravely ill patient the death was often obviously inevitable, as, for instance, the result of severe biochemical disturbances due to prolonged acute intestinal obstruction.

If the condition necessitating surgery is not of itself fatal, the patient may have other associated severe disease, notably ischaemic heart disease; in such cases surgery is obviously a calculated risk.

On occasions, however, the death is found to be due to a previously unsuspected natural disease, and it is in these instances, particularly, that the performance of autopsies on cases of post-operative deaths have value.

A middle-aged man, apparently healthy, was being operated upon for a torn cartilage in the knee. At the conclusion of the operation, as soon as the Esmarch bandage was removed from his leg, the patient suddenly collapsed, became pulseless and died. Autopsy revealed a massive pulmonary embolus, with thrombus also in the calf veins of the leg on which the operation was being performed. It was evident that the application of the bandage had loosened the clot and its removal allowed the embolus to escape into the circulation.

On another occasion, death immediately after operation was found to be due to haemopericardium resulting from rupture of a cardiac infarct caused by a coronary thrombosis. Histological examination demonstrated that this had probably occurred several days prior to the operation (F.M. 15,585 A).

Such unsuspected disease may produce unexpected emergencics during anaesthesia, which in turn may cause death. Griffiths (1958) describes, for instance, sudden collapse due to hypotension caused by adrenal hypoplasia; fulminant hypertension due to phaeochromocytomas; tension pneumothorax, which might occur from rupture of an emphysematous bulla, and cerebral thrombosis. Harrison (1968b) instances pontine haemorrhage, gross ischaemic heart disease, ruptured aortic aneurysm, etc.

(d) OBSTETRIC ANAESTHESIA

Anaesthesia in the course of childbirth has its own special risks. Thus reports on Confidential Enquiries into Maternal Deaths in England and Wales include anaesthetic fatalities as one of the major causes of maternal death (Moir, 1980). A survey of maternal deaths in Queen Charlotte's Hospital during a period of 20 years also showed that the greatest single cause was anaesthesia (Morgan, 1980).

Most authors indicate failed intubation, cardio-vascular failure, etc. as the cause but the one factor which seems to be more important in obstetric cases is inhalation of regurgitated stomach contents (Scott, 1978). This is presumably due, in part, to the fact that many obstetric anaesthetics are given in emergency situations, without time for adequate preparation of the patient. Mendelson's syndrome may result (Mendelson, 1946). Since it was thought that the damage is done by acidity the prophylactic use of antacids was advocated (Taylor and Pryse-Davies, 1966). It seems that inhalation may be particularly dangerous in pregnant women. In spite of prophylaxis the syndrome continues to form a large percentage of the admittedly small number of deaths due to anaesthesia.

FUNCTION OF THE PATHOLOGIST IN THE INVESTIGATION OF ANAESTHETIC DEATHS

It will be apparent from the foregoing that most of the hazards of anaesthesia are beyond detection by post-mortem examination and are out with the pathologist's sphere. None the less he has an important part to play in these investigations. He is an independent witness; he can detect or exclude evidence of instrumental damage, inhalation of foreign material, surgical mishaps and natural disease.

Although he may not be competent to perform, or have facilities for, toxicological analysis, he has the responsibility for the collection of the appropriate material for analysis. This must not only be of the right kind but in *adequate* amount. Therefore when in doubt he should consult the toxicologist so that a satisfactory analysis can be undertaken.

With regard to the other possible factors he should consult the anaesthetist or surgeon involved prior to the conduct of the autopsy on the patient. Such information should be given in evidence by them rather than at second hand by the pathologist. Questions might well arise which only they can answer. The pathologist's duty is to perform a thorough and competent autopsy and he should confine his evidence to his findings and their implications. It may be proper for the pathologist to adopt the factual report of the toxicologist if the latter is not required to give evidence.

References

ANNOTATION (1966) *Lancet*, **ii**, 628.
ANNOTATION (1966) *Lancet*, **ii**, 739.
BARLOW, M. B. and ISAACS, S. (1970) *Brit. J. Anaesthesia*, **42**, 1072.
BEECHER, H. K. and TODD, D. P. (1954) A Study of Deaths Associated with Anaesthesia and Surgery. Springfield, Illinois Charles C. Thomas.
BERGER, G. S. TYLER, C. W. and HARROD, E. K. (1974) *Am. J. Obstet. Gynec.*, **118**, 1142–43.
BLANKE, R. V. (1960) *J. Forens. Sci.*, **5**, 539.
BOBA, A. (1965) Death in the Operating Room. Springfield, Illinois: Charles C. Thomas.
BODLANDER, F. M. (1975) *Brit. J. Anaesthesia*, **47** (1), 408–411.
BOULTON, T. B. (1982) *Brit. Med. J.*, **285**, 730–31 (C).
BOURNE, J. G. (1973a) *Brit. Med. J.*, **i**, 293.
BOURNE, J. G. (1973b) *Brit. Med. J.*, **4**, 611–12.
BRIERLEY, J. B. and MILLER, A. A. (1966) *Lancet*, **ii**, 869.
CAMPBELL, J. E. (1960) *J. Forens. Sci.*, **5**, 501.
CAMPBELL, J. E., WEISS, W. A. and RIEDERS, F. (1961) *Anaesthesia and Analgesia*, **40**, 54.
CLUTTON-BROCK, J. (1967) *Brit. J. Anaesthesia*, **39**, 388.
CONWAY, C. M. and PAYNE, J. P. (1964) *Lancet*, **i**, 12.
COOPER, J. B., NEWBOWER, R. S., LONG, C. D. and McPEEK, B. (1978) *Anaesthesiol.*, **49**, 399–406.
COURVILLE, C. B. (1960) *Anaesthesia and Analgesia*, **39**, 361.
CRAWFORD v. Board of Governors, Charing Cross Hospital (1953) *The Times*, 23 Apr. 8 Dec.; *Lancet* (1953) **i**, 906.
CRAWFORD, J. S. (1974) *Proc. Roy. Soc. Med.*, **67** (9), 905–09.
CURSON, I. (1976) *Brit. Med. J.*, **1**, 957.
DINNICK, O. P. (1964) *Anaesthesia*, **19**, 536.
DRURY, P. M. E. and GILBERTSON, A. A. (1970) *Brit. J. Anaesthesia*, **42**, 1021.
Editorial (1982) *Brit. Med. J.*, **285**.
EDWARDS, G. MORTON, H. J. V., PASK, E. A. and WYLIE, W. D. (1956) *Anaesthesia*, **ii**, 194.
ELLIS, F. R. (1972) *Environ. Res.*, **5**, 1–58.
ELLIS, F. R. and HALSALL, P. J. (1980) *Brit. J. Hosp. Med.*, **24**, 318–21.
ENTICKNAP, J. B. (1961) *Med. Sci. Law*, **1**, 404.
GARNER v. MORREL and another (1953) *The Times*, 31 Oct.
GILLIES, A. L., ARTHUR, D. S., FORREST, A. L., LAWSON, J. I. M. and MASSON, A. H. B. (1979) *Brit. Med. J.* **i**, 1246–47.
GRIFFITHS, J. A. (1958) *J. Forens. Med.*, **15**, 131.
HARRIS, T. A. B. and HUTTON, A. M. (1956) *Lancet*, **ii**, 1024.
HARRISON, G. G. (1968a) *S. Afr. Med. J.*, **42** 513, 544.
HARRISON, G. G. (1968b) *J. Forens. Med.*, **14**, 71 (Classification).
HARRISON, G. G. (1978) *Brit. J. Anaesthesia*, **50** (10), 1041–46.
HEGGS, C. G. (1982) *Brit. Med. J.*, **285**, 731 (C).
HOVI-VIANDER, M. (1980) *Brit. J. Anaesthesia*, **52** (5), 483–89.
HUNT, A. C. (1958) *J. Forens. Med.*, **5**, 141.
ISAACS, H., and BARLOW, M. B. (1970) *Brit. Med. J.*, **1**, 275.
KEATING, V. J. (1966) Anaesthetic Accidents vol. 2. London: Lloyd Luke.
KEATS, A. S. (1979) *Anaesthesiology* **50**, 387–92.
Leading Article (1968) *Brit. Med. J.*, **3**, 69.
Leading Article (1982) *Brit. Med. J.*, **285**, 530.
LOVE, S. H. S. (1968) *Brit. J. Anaesthesia*, **40**, 188.
LUNN, J. N. and MUSHIN, W. W. (1982) Mortality associated with anaesthesia. London. Nuffield Provincial Hospitals Trust.
MACKINTOSH, R. R. (1948–9) *Brit. J. Anaesthesia*, **21**, 107.
MACRAE, W. A. MILLER, K. M. and WATSON, A. A. (1979) *Med. Sci. Law*, **19**, 261–4.
MANT, A. K. (1958) *J. Forens. Med.*, **5**, 137.

MARX, G. F., MATEO, C. V. and ORKIN, L. R. (1973) *Anaesthesiology*, **39,** 54–58.
MAZZIA, V. D. B. and SINION, A. (1978) *Leg. Med. Annu.*, 165–175.
MEDICO-LEGAL (1966) *Brit. Med. J.*, **2,** 1082.
MEDICO-LEGAL (1974) *Brit. Med. J.*, **i,** 207–208.
MEDICO-LEGAL (1974) *Brit. Med. J.*, **4,** 352–4.
MEDICO-LEGAL (1975) *Brit. Med. J.*, **i,** 341–342.
MEHTA, S. (1974) *Brit. Med. J.* **ii,** 224.
MENDELSON, C. J. (1946) *Am. J. Obstet. Gynec.*, **52,** 191.
Ministry of Health and Social Security (1972) Emergencies in Dental Practice, London: H.M.S.O.
MOIR, D. D. (1980) *Brit. J. Anaesthesia*, **52** (1), 1–3.
MORGAN, B. M. (1980) *Brit. J. Anaesthesia*, **35** (4), 334–8.
MORTON, H. J. V. and WYLIE, W. D. (1951) *Anaesthesia*, **6,** 190, 205.
MUSHIN, W. W. ROSEN, M., BOWEN, D. J. and CAMPBELL, H. (1964) *Brit. Med. J.*, **2,** 329.
PASK, E. A. (1964) *Lancet*, **i,** 165.
POLSON, C. J. (1955) The Essentials of Forensic Medicine. 1st ed., pp. 422, 426, 452. London: English
    Universities Press.
RIEDERS, F. (1969) *Legal Medicine Annual*, New York Appleton-Century-Crofts.
ROBERTSON, I. (1961) *J. Forens. Med.*, **8,** 157.
SCHAPIRA, M., KEPES, E. R. and HURWITT, E. S. (1960) *Anaesthesia and Analgesia* **39,** 49.
SCOTT, D. B. (1974) *Proc. Roy. Soc. Med.*, **67,** 909–910.
SCOTT, P. V. (1982) *Brit. Med. J.*, **285,** 731 (C).
SHARPSTONE, P., MEDLEY, D. R. K. and WILLIAMS, R. (1971) *Brit. Med. J.*, **1,** 448.
TATTERSALL, R. N. (1953) in *Medicine* vol. i, 1612, ed. H. G. Garland and W. Phillips, London: MacMillan.
TAYLOR, E. and PRYSE-DAVIES, J. (1966) *Lancet*, **i,** 288.
TYGSTRUP, N. (1963) *Lancet*, **ii,** 466 (Correspondence).
URRY and URRY v. BIERER and Another (1955) *The Times*, 15 July.

PART II

The Law Relating to the Practice of Medicine

CHAPTER 20

The General Medical Council

IN THE first half of the 19th century, the majority of persons claiming to practice medicine had no qualifications at all. In the 1841 census, only some 11,000 doctors held qualifications out of a total of 33,000 "practitioners". At least sixteen organisations dispensed medical qualifications and the ensuing chaos prevented the public from differentiating between properly-trained doctors and mere quacks.

Many attempts were made to introduce legislation to remedy this situation, no less than seventeen Bills being presented unsuccessfully to Parliament. In 1852, George Hastings, a Member of Parliament and son of Charles Hastings (the founder of the Provincial, Medical and Surgical Association that was to become the British Medical Association in 1855), drafted a Medical Bill that together with another 3 years later, also failed to become law.

However, support for these proposals had become so strong that the Government itself took up the matter and in 1858, the first Medical Act was passed, which established "The General Council of Medical Education and Registration of the United Kingdom".

This formal name was rarely used and the official body was known as the General Medical Council. This name was even cited in Statutes, though care was taken to include a definition that this was the body constituted by the Medical Act, 1858. However, by the Medical Act 1950, as from 23rd February 1951, it became known officially and unofficially by the title long-established by custom and universally abbreviated to "The G.M.C.".

The prime object of the General Medical Council, both in 1858 and subsequently, was to establish a Register of qualified doctors to enable the public to identify reputable medical practitioners.

The Council is responsible to the Privy Council which appoints some members and to which appeals lie in disciplinary decisions.

A series of many subsequent Acts has ensued, the most recent being that of 1978, which made radical changes in the composition and functions of the Council, following the Merison Report of 1975. The G.M.C. receives no grants from public funds and derives its income solely from registration fees, together with some profit from the sale of the Medical Register.

THE CONSTITUTION OF THE COUNCIL

Following considerable disquiet in the early 1970s about the introduction of a retention fee and the composition of the Council, the Merison Report of 1975 recommended sweeping changes, including the election of a majority of members directly by the medical profession. This report led to the Medical Act of 1978 from which stems the present composition and functions of the newly formed G.M.C.

As from September, 1979, the Council consists of 93 members made up as follows:

50 members elected by postal vote from the registered medical practitioners of the United Kingdom.

England has 39 members, Scotland 6 members, Wales 3 members and Northern Ireland 2 members.

21 members appointed by universities with medical faculties.

13 members appointed by Royal Colleges, Faculties and the Society of Apothecaries.

7 lay members and 2 medical members nominated by the Privy Council.

The Republic of Ireland is no longer represented, now having a Medical Council of its own.

The Council itself elects a President from amongst its members, the present President being Sir John Walton. All members must retire on reaching the age of 70 years.

The Council is administered by a Registrar who has a number of Assistant Registrars and a permanent staff, who reside at 44, Hallam Street, London W1N 6AE, the Registration Division being nearby in Gosfield Street.

FUNCTIONS OF THE GENERAL MEDICAL COUNCIL

The Medical Register

Since 1858, the Council's prime function has been the establishment and maintenance of the Medical Register which is the definitive list of doctors licensed to practice as "registered medical practitioners" in Britain. In this country, there is no necessity for any person to be either medically educated, qualified or registered with the G.M.C., in order to practice medicine. This is unlike the sister profession of veterinary surgery which has a legal monopoly to treat animals.

The Medical Register, which is published each year, contains the names and addresses of all persons who are fully or provisionally registered on 1 January of the year to which the register relates.

A copy of the Register, purporting to be printed and published by the direction of the General Medical Council, shall be accepted by the courts in evidence and the entry of a name in it is proof that that person is a registered or duly qualified medical practitioner.

Persons registered at a time between the issue of two editions of the Register can prove registration by production of a certified copy of the registration, issued by the Registrar of the Council.

Today the primary conditions are that the applicant has passed a qualifying examination in medicine, surgery and midwifery and that he holds a qualifying diploma or diplomas of one or more of the licensing bodies. Proof of qualification is sufficient if the person's name and address are included in a list of those who have been granted qualifications, as certified by an official of the licensing body and sent to the Registrar. Registration, and not qualification to be registered, is of paramount importance, because it is the entry and retention of his name on the Medical Register which confers upon him the privileges restricted by law to registered medical practitioners. If for any reason a practitioner's name has been erased from the Register, whether penally or otherwise, but he has not been deprived by the body (or bodies) which granted his qualifying diplomas, he loses the privileges of a registered practitioner, notwithstanding he is still a qualified practitioner.

Inclusion in the Register is legal proof of a doctor's professional status and confers upon him various legal benefits and responsibilities. Unless included in the Register he may not hold appointments within the National Health Service or Public Services, he may not prescribe dangerous drugs or treat certain classes of serious disease. Neither may he issue statutory certificates such as birth, death and cremation certificates. He is also subject to the code of ethics and behaviour as established by his professional colleagues acting through the Council.

A doctor remains on the Register until death (which is notified to the G.M.C. by the Registrar of Births and Deaths) unless:

1. He fails to reply within 6 months to the Registrar's enquiries. This is the most common cause of removal from the Register, due to the G.M.C. losing track of the doctor's address. In recent years, this has assumed greater importance, as there is now an annual fee payable for the retention of the doctor's name on the Register. Failure to pay the fee results in erasure from the Register, though reinstatement is automatic upon paying the arrears, together with an administration charge.

2. A practitioner may request removal from the Register, usually when he ceases to engage in medical practice.

3. On application for erasure on the ground that the practitioner does not wish to pay or continue to pay, the prescribed retention fee.

4. Erasure to correct error or an entry acquired by fraud.

5. Penal erasure, following conviction of serious professional misconduct. (Note that a practitioner who is sentenced to suspension, although deprived of the rights and privileges of a registered practitioner during the period of suspension, retains his name on the register but the entry is accompanied by a note of the fact of suspension).

Until 1970 a doctor was either on or off the Register. By the Medical Act of 1969, an intermediate state of suspended professional animation was instituted, whereby the Disciplinary Committee of the G.M.C. could suspend a doctor for a fixed period of time. Suspension may also be partial, in that certain functions such as the power to prescribe dangerous drugs may be forbidden the doctor in appropriate circumstances for a certain period of time (see below).

The Privileges of Registered Practitioners

The Medical Acts detail the statutory privileges of registered practitioners.

1. *Recovery of fees*: No person shall be entitled to recover any charge in any court of law for any medical or surgical advice or attendance, or for the performance of any operation, or for any medicine which he shall have both prescribed and supplied, unless he shall prove upon that trial that he is fully registered.

2. *Appointments open only to fully registered practitioners*: No person, not being fully registered, shall hold any medical appointment (a) in any of H.M. Services, the Navy, Army or Air Force, or (b) in any emigrant or other vessel, or (c) in any hospital not supported wholly by voluntary contributions, i.e. the National Health Service, or (d) in any prison, or (e) in any other public establishment, body or institution or to any friendly or other society for providing mutual relief in sickness, infirmity or old age.

3. *Medical certificates: the issue of valid certificates*: No certificate required by any enactment from a medical practitioner shall be valid, unless the person signing it is fully registered.

4. *Exemption from liability from certain offices*: A fully registered practitioner shall, if he so wishes, be exempt from serving any corporate or parochial office, and the name of such person shall not be returned in any list of persons liable to serve in any such office, e.g. of jurors. The foregoing privileges shall apply to *provisionally registered* persons in respect of their limited scope of practice, i.e. in resident employment.

5. *Authority to possess and supply controlled drugs*: Under the Misuse of Drugs Act, 1971, and the Regulations, registered medical practitioners are one of the classes granted authority to possess and supply these drugs. This is an important privilege, but the doctor is under an obligation to avoid its abuse e.g. by the use of these drugs for any improper purpose. The penalties for contravention of the Act and regulations are substantial and, upon conviction, there may be the added penalties of withdrawal of the general authority and erasure from the Medical Register.

Any person who wilfully and falsely pretends to be registered under any provision of the Medical Acts or that he is recognised by law as a registered practitioner shall be liable on summary conviction to a fine not exceeding £500.

He may not take or use the name or title of physician, doctor of medicine, licentiate in medicine and surgery, bachelor of medicine, surgeon, general practitioner or apothecary—or any description which would imply that he is a registered person.

Medical Education

Closely related to the original function of the Council in protecting the public from incompetent practitioners, the supervision of medical education is directed towards ensuring an adequate minimum level of competence of new medical graduates. Though the direction of the curriculum is less strictly controlled than in former years, the G.M.C. still maintains a primary interest in both undergraduate and postgraduate education, this being a major reason for the inclusion of appointed members from all the medical schools and Royal Colleges. The Council has the power to inspect qualifying examinations and the Medical Act of 1950 gave the additional power of visiting medical schools. They also issue a periodical booklet entitled *Recommendations on Basic Medical Education*, which though advisory rather than mandatory, is normally followed by teaching institutions in designing their curricula. Close monitoring of the examinations and the pass rates is carried out by the Education Committee of the G.M.C. An increasing role in postgraduate education is foreseen, under the provisions of the 1978 Medical Act. This Act charged the Council with overseeing the co-ordination of undergraduate and all stages of postgraduate education, a massive task which the G.M.C. is now undertaking.

The Medical Act of 1950 also introduced the compulsory pre-registration house-officer year and also laid down a minimum time for the medical course.

The Council also has the discretion to recognise many additional higher qualifications and a number of these are now included in the official description of doctors in the Medical Register.

Registration

At the outset, in 1858, the Council was required to appoint a Registrar, to whom it delegated the task of preparing a list, to be known as the Medical Register, of all persons who, at that time, were considered qualified to practice medicine. This first list included the names of some practitioners who, although they did not hold a registrable degree or diploma, were considered qualified by experience of actual practice in England (Medical Act 1858, section 17), or other specific experience of practice (*ibid.*, s. 46), to be registered practitioners.

The heaviest work-load of the Council is the registration of doctors, especially those from overseas. Radical changes in the procedure have occurred in the last few years and now registration consists only of the following categories, as "temporary registration" has been phased out.

1. Doctors qualifying in the United Kingdom obtain *provisional registration* on graduation and *full registration* after satisfactorily completing a pre-registration year. Applicants for full registration must have held resident posts of house officer in medicine and in surgery, each for 6 months. These posts include those which afford experience in any recognised special branch of medicine or surgery, e.g. dermatology and neurology or orthopaedic and thoracic surgery. Time spent as a house officer in midwifery may be counted as a period not exceeding 6 months, "and not more than 6 months in a health centre may be reckoned towards completion of this 12 month period". It was also decided that where a post affords a mixed medical practice the licensing body concerned will be required to determine its proportion of medicine, surgery and midwifery for the purpose of the Act. The term resident employment will apply not only to posts in which the holder is actually resident, but also to those where residence is conveniently near to the hospital or institution. Commonwealth and foreign practitioners, who desire to be registered in the United Kingdom, may either prove experience of the same kind or satisfy the Council that their experience is not less extensive. The licensing bodies have authority to approve resident posts in hospitals and institutions in their respective areas.

Provisional registration will permit the performance of all medical duties within the scope of a house officer as if he was fully registered, but these practitioners may not lawfully engage elsewhere in medical practice as registered persons, so long as they remain provisionally registered. When full registration is granted, the practitioner is entitled to engage in any form of medical employment including hospital work and general practice.

Nationals of any country within the European Economic Community holding registrable qualifications granted in a Member State are eligible either for full registration or for registration as a visiting E.E.C. practitioner, or for limited registration.

2. *Limited registration* was introduced in 1979 to supersede the former system of temporary registration. In order to be eligible for limited registration a doctor must hold a

qualification accepted by the Council for the purpose. Qualifications granted in 84 countries have been accepted for this purpose. Unless the doctor has previously held temporary registration, he must also pass a test of knowledge of English and of professional knowledge and competence (the PLAB test) conducted by the Professional and Linguistic Assessments Board. The PLAB test is financed by the Council, the Board consisting of members appointed by the non-university licensing bodies and certain other colleges, together with experts in linguistics.

Limited registration may be granted by the Council for specified appointments or for a range of practice, only in respect of supervised employment. It cannot be granted to any individual for a period exceeding an aggregate of 5 years. Thus limited registration is registration for either a particular appointment or a particular type of appointment and if the appointment lapses and the doctor wishes to work elsewhere, he must re-apply for an appropriate extension.

Doctors with limited registration may apply for transfer to full registration which may be granted if the Council thinks fit, having regard to the knowledge and skill shown and experience acquired by the doctor.

3. Visiting overseas specialists may be temporarily registered as fully registered medical practitioners for the purpose of spending time in the United Kingdom for some specialist purpose.

Full registration under reciprocal arrangements still applies to a number of overseas universities, mainly in Australia, New Zealand and South Africa.

Disciplinary Functions of the G.M.C.

Though the other functions mentioned above provide by far the largest part of the Council's workload, it is the disciplinary functions which are the most well-known from the point of view of the lay press.

The exercise of discipline over registered medical practitioners is a major duty delegated by Parliament to the General Medical Council. The jurisdiction of the Council does not extend to unqualified practitioners, whose professional misdeeds are dealt with by the courts. At the outset, under the Medical Act, 1858, the Council as a whole could sit in judgment and it was not until the Medical Act, 1950, that specific provisions were made to restrict the number of the defendant doctor's judges and to introduce procedure which approximates to that of a criminal court. A *Medical Disciplinary Committee* of the Council, whose membership was limited to the President and eighteen other members of the Council, was instituted by the Act.

The first Medical Act in 1858 empowered the Council to erase from the Register any doctor convicted of any felony, misdemeanour, crime or offence or judged after due enquiry by the Council to have been "guilty of infamous conduct in a professional respect". This last dramatic phrase persisted until the Medical Act of 1969, when it was replaced by the words "serious professional misconduct". This power of the G.M.C. is intended to protect the public and not to be a punitive measure against offending practitioners, though the deterrent value is obvious.

The phrase "infamous conduct in a professional respect" was defined in 1894 by Lord Justice Lopes as follows:

"If a medical man in the pursuit of his profession has done something with regard to it which will be reasonably regarded as disgraceful or dishonourable by his professional brethren of good repute and competency, then it is open to the General Medical Council, if that be shown, to say that he has been guilty of infamous conduct in a professional respect."

In another judgment in 1930 Lord Justice Scrutton stated that:

"Infamous conduct in a professional respect means no more than serious misconduct judged according to the rules, written or unwritten, governing the profession".

In proposing the substitution of the expression "serious professional misconduct" for the phrase "infamous conduct in a professional respect" the Council intended that both phrases should have the same significance.

The categories of "serious professional misconduct" are never closed, as with medical negligence, but fairly well-defined groups of offences are the usual cause of erasure or suspension from the Register. The removal of a doctor's name from the Register, either permanently or temporarily, is the greatest professional disaster that can overtake a medical practitioner, as he is then unable to carry on his profession in the usual sense of the word, as he cannot be employed by the N.H.S. or public services and cannot sign most certificates or prescriptions.

The G.M.C. cannot advise or discuss individual cases with practitioners (e.g. a doctor cannot obtain prior advice in respect of some professional course of action which he fears might be construed as professional misconduct) because the Council has a statutory disciplinary function. It therefore cannot be seen to be acting as both counsel and judge in the same case. However, the G.M.C. issues a "Blue Booklet" entitled *Professional Conduct and Discipline: Fitness to Practice* which gives detailed guidelines for standards of professional behaviour and outlines what might be construed as breaches of these standards, together with the details of the disciplinary machinery. Since 1980, this booklet also describes the new "Fitness to Practice" aspects, described later.

As erasure or suspension is the most serious professional disaster which can overtake a doctor, the disciplinary machinery of the G.M.C. should be fully understood by every practitioner.

The General Medical Council exercises its disciplinary powers only when cases are brought to their notice. Disciplinary enquiries may arise from two sources:

1. Accusations of serious professional misconduct may be made to the G.M.C. either from members of the public (including professional colleagues) or from certain public officials whose duty it is to communicate such accusations. This latter class includes various officials concerned with the administration of the National Health Service especially after committees of enquiry etc., at Health Authority level. Where the accusation is made by a member of the public or individual doctor, it must be in the form of a statutory declaration i.e. a legal document sworn before a Commissioner of Oaths.

2. There is statutory provision for the notification of the Council of the conviction of any registered practitioner of any crime or offence. The appropriate official of the court in the United Kingdom in which the conviction was recorded has a duty to send a certified copy of the record to the Registrar of the Council.

The term "conviction" means a determination by a Criminal Court in the United Kingdom. A conviction in itself gives the Professional Conduct Committee jurisdiction even if the criminal offence did not involve professional misconduct. The Committee is however particularly concerned with convictions for offences which affect a doctor's fitness to practice. In considering convictions the Council is bound to accept the determination of a court as conclusive evidence that the doctor was guilty of the offence of which he was convicted. Doctors who face a criminal charge should remember this if they are advised to plead guilty, or not to appeal against a conviction, in order to avoid publicity or a severe sentence. It is not open to a doctor who has been convicted of an offence to argue before the Professional Conduct Committee that he was in fact innocent. *It is therefore unwise for a doctor to plead guilty in a court of law to a charge to which he believes that he has a defence.*

A finding or a decision of a Medical Service Committee or other authority under the National Health Service does not amount to a conviction for these purposes. A charge of serious professional misconduct may however, if the facts warrant, be made in respect of conduct which has previously been the subject of proceedings within the National Health Service or before an overseas court or medical council: or in respect of conduct of which a doctor has been found guilty by a British Criminal Court but placed on probation or discharged conditionally or absolutely.

Until 1970, the Divorce Courts were obliged to notify the G.M.C. of any practitioner appearing as co-respondent in a divorce action, but now the G.M.C. only considers such cases if the injured party makes a direct claim to the Council of serious professional misconduct on the part of the doctor.

On receipt of the notification of complaints, they are scrutinized by the Registrar and the Council's Solicitor may be asked to make enquiries to establish the facts. Obviously, false, malicious or otherwise unfounded trivialities are rejected at this stage. The Registrar submits the remainder to the President, who decides whether any further action should be taken. He may direct that the doctor be contacted to clarify the circumstances, which may then result in the matter being closed. Where there appears to be some case to answer, the complaints are referred to a special committee, the Preliminary Proceedings Committee, whose function is similar to "examining magistrates" who decide whether a case be sent for trial. At this stage, the doctor is informed of the allegations made against him and is invited to submit a written explanation.

The Preliminary Proceedings Committee may decide either (a) to refer the case to the Professional Conduct Committee (b) to send the doctor a warning letter, (c) to take no further action. The second course is most commonly employed, the doctor being warned of the possible consequences of such conduct.

A minority of cases are referred by the Preliminary Proceedings Committee to the Professional Conduct Committee, which is conducted in a formal way, with barristers representing both the Council and usually the subject of the complaint, who is normally represented via his defence society.

The Professional Conduct Committee is elected annually by the Council and consists of 20 members, of whom only 10 sit on any case. Of the 20 members 12 are elected members of the Council and two are lay members. The Committee normally sits in public and its procedure is closely akin to that of a court of law. Witnesses may be subpoenaed and evidence is given on oath. Doctors who appear before the Committee may be, and usually are, legally represented.

The Preliminary Proceedings Committee consists of 11 members and is also elected annually. It sits in private and on the basis of written evidence and submissions determines which cases should be referred for inquiry by the Professional Conduct Committee. It may also refer cases to the Health Committee.

The Professional Conduct and Preliminary Proceedings Committees are advised on questions of law by a Legal Assessor, who is usually a Queen's Counsel and must be a barrister, advocate or solicitor of not less than 10 years standing.

When a registered medical practitioner is to be summoned before the Professional Conduct Committee he is entitled to have details of the complaint or information and due notice of the hearing. He has the right to be heard in person or to be represented by counsel or solicitor, or by an officer or member of any organisation of which he is a member or by a member of his family.

The Committee may administer oaths and now also has power to compel the attendance of witnesses and the production of documents. Any party to the proceedings may sue out writs of *subpoena ad testificicandum and duces tectum*, subject only to the same rules which apply to the Courts.

The Committee may receive as evidence any such oral, documentary or other matter as, after consultation with the Legal Assessor, they may think fit.

Provided that where any matter is tendered as evidence which would not be admissible as such if the proceedings were criminal proceedings in England, they shall not receive it unless, after consultation with the Legal Assessor, they are satisfied that their duty of making due inquiries into the case before them makes its reception desirable.

The Committee, therefore, has a wide discretion in this matter; it is not bound to accept the advice of its Legal Assessor. The rule does not have the same rigid character as those which apply to criminal proceedings. The Fox case (1950) evoked considerable criticism of the admission of certain evidence. *The British Medical Journal* (1959) took the view that it might be demanding too much to require the Committee to be subject to the rigid rules observed in criminal courts, but the degree of departure from them should be more clearly defined.

The matter proceeded to a debate in the House of Commons on a censure motion on 16 December, 1959. During the debate the Home Secretary indicated that the Government had decided to set up a committee, under Lord Simonds, to consider the powers of subpoena before disciplinary tribunals. This Departmental Committee issued its report in May, 1960. They stressed that "justice can only be done if material evidence is not withheld . . . it applies with particular force to tribunals having power to impose such formidable penalties as have the disciplinary tribunals of professional bodies . . ."
Their report provided a complete vindication of the Disciplinary Committee's action.

At the conclusion of the hearing, the Committee may take one of the following courses:
1. To admonish the doctor and conclude the case.
2. To place the doctor on probation by postponing judgment.
3. To direct the doctor's registration be conditional on his compliance (for a period not exceeding 3 years) with such requirements as the Committee think fit to impose for the protection of members of the public or in his own interests.
4. To direct that the doctor's registration shall be suspended for a period not exceeding one year.
5. To direct the erasure of the doctor's name from the Register.

Where judgment is postponed, the doctor is given an opportunity to conduct himself correctly during the period of postponement and to obtain references from professional colleagues as to his conduct. When next considered by the Council, the case will normally be concluded if the reports are satisfactory. If not, then the other disciplinary alternatives may proceed.

Conditional registration means that restrictions are imposed upon the doctor in certain specified areas, such that he may not, for example, be allowed to prescribe dangerous drugs or may only work under supervision.

Suspended registration means removal from the Register for a specific period not exceeding 12 months. During that time the doctor cannot practice as a registered medical practitioner. A further period of suspension or even erasure may be ordered during that time.

Where a doctor's name is erased from the Register, he cannot apply for restoration until at least 10 months have elapsed.

Where a doctor has suffered an erasure or suspension, he has a period of 28 days in which to give notice of appeal to the Judicial Committee of the Privy Council. During that period his registration is not affected unless the Professional Conduct Committee had made a separate order that it should be suspended forthwith, they being satisfied that it is necessary to do so for the protection of the members of the public or in the best interests of the doctor.

Fitness to Practice

Since 1980, as a result of the changes under the 1978 Medical Act, the Preliminary Proceedings Committee have an alternative course to referring cases to the Professional Conduct Committee. This is the new and somewhat controversial concept of "fitness to practice" which is supervised by the new Health Committee.

One of the complaints of the Merison Committee was that where a doctor by reason of physical or mental infirmity was unfit to practice, the only method of removing him from the Register was via the disciplinary machinery, which was inappropriate if the doctor's incapacity was due to sickness. The new machinery brings into being a means whereby a doctor can be prevented from practising if his physical or mental state makes him a risk either to his patients or himself. The procedure does not erase him from the Register, but suspends it or attaches conditions to it. The majority of these cases concern addiction to alcohol or other drugs or to mental illness. It is foreseen that many doctors unfit to practice will be persuaded voluntarily to cease practice, at local level, either by their own medical colleagues or possibly through the "Three Wise Men" procedure of the Health Authorities. Where such local measures are unsuccessful, then recourse may be made to the Health Committee of the G.M.C.

Where the Council receives information suggesting that the fitness to practice of the doctor is seriously impaired, it will first be considered by the President or other members of the Council appointed for the purpose. If he is satisfied that a case exists, the doctor will then be informed of this and invited to agree within 14 days to submit to examination by at least two medical examiners, who will be chosen by the President from panels of examiners nominated by professional bodies. It is then open to the doctor at this stage to nominate his own medical practitioners to examine him and send their own findings to the President.

The results of the medical examination will be communicated to the doctor, who will be asked to state within 28 days whether he is prepared voluntarily to accept the recommendations of the medical examiners as to the management of his case. If he does so, then no further action will be taken. If he refuses to be medically examined or to accept the recommendations, then the President with two other members of the Council may refer the case to the Health Committee, which may also be alerted by the Preliminary Proceedings Committee where complaints come via the disciplinary channel, until it becomes obvious that a health factor is involved.

The Health Committee may suspend the registration of a doctor for a period not exceeding 12 months, or impose conditions on his registration for a period not exceeding 3 years. These cases will be reviewed by the Health Committee from time to time.

Examples of Serious Professional Misconduct

The General Medical Council cannot indicate the limits of conduct or convictions which might be regarded as serious professional misconduct. Each case has to be decided on its specific facts and merits. The Council does not have a rigid code of offences nor can it speculate on hypothetical circumstances. The Council, however, includes in its pamphlet *Professional Conduct and Discipline* notes on certain offences which are likely to result in disciplinary inquiry. It is emphasised that the examples are not exhaustive. The precise order of gravity of the offences may have changed during the latter years but they all continue to be regarded as serious and likely to result in suspension, if not erasure.

Though the potential reasons for erasure or suspension from the Register is limitless, many of the cases arise from one of the so-called "six A's".

Abortion. The illegal termination of pregnancy, if notified as result of a conviction in the criminal court, is almost always an immediate cause for erasure, even on the first occasion. Even following the reform in the law brought about by the Abortion Act of 1967, criminal abortions are still performed by doctors. Lesser degrees of culpability in this connection may arise due to the letter of the Act not being followed, e.g. performing abortions in premises not officially recognised. It is imperative that all terminations of pregnancy be carried out in the prescribed manner, with more than one doctor assenting to the decision and the procedure being carried out only in a proper institution. This is discussed fully in a later chapter.

Alcohol. Abuse of alcohol is one of the most common causes for warning to doctors by the G.M.C. and if the offence is repeated, erasure or suspension from the Register. The most usual type of offence is drunken driving, though occasionally repeated convictions for other forms of drunkenness have led to erasure, especially when the doctor's ability to carry out his professional duties is impaired. Commonly the first offence for drunken driving is dealt with by the Preliminary Proceedings Committee with a warning letter, but further infringements lead to a grave risk of erasure. Occasionally, serious drunken driving offences, such as causing the death of a person by dangerous driving, have led to erasure on the first occasion.

Rarely, drunkenness has led to criminal proceedings for manslaughter, the classic case being R. V. Bateman, where a doctor attended a woman in childbirth when he was intoxicated, caused her death by avulsing part of the uterus and intestines during a forceps delivery. Such extreme cases are very rare, but serious professional misconduct with alcohol as the basic cause is increasingly common. It is an unfortunate fact that the medical profession has the highest rate of alcoholism in the country, a rate that is increasing annually.

Adultery. The professional consequences of a doctor's adultery with a patient have changed significantly in the past few years, mainly due to the advent of a more permissive society. The Merison Report recommended that such adulterous relationships with a patient should cease to be regarded automatically as serious professional misconduct, unless it was shown that the behaviour was likely to damage the crucial *professional relationship* between the doctor and patient.

This interpretation is now generally accepted by the disciplinary machinery of the G.M.C. though it is still possible for them to consider any case where a doctor has misused his professional privileges to gain entry to the woman's family.

It is obvious that a registered medical practitioner stands in a professional relationship to any person when he is attending that person for some current illness. It is reasonable to assume such a relationship also exists where, having personally attended a patient, it is to be expected that he would be again required to attend should some subsequent illness develop. It could be that if the introduction of the doctor to a person with whom he commits adultery arose out of medical attendance at any time, that is a professional relationship, notwithstanding that he had ceased, maybe for some time, to attend that person. In short, the test appears to be this: did the doctor come to know the person, with whom he commits adultery, as a result of personal medical attendance?

The emphasis is to be put on personal attendance since it is now clear that the mere inclusion of a person's name on the doctor's list of patients under the National Health Service is not normally, for this purpose, a professional relationship. The first indication on this point was given by a case before the Disciplinary Committee in 1950.

> The practitioner had been convicted by the Courts of an indecent offence, committed with a boy whose name was on his Health Service list but whom he had never attended professionally. Since the Council did not see fit to direct erasure, it would appear that the view which is likely to be taken is that mere inclusion of a name on the doctor's list does not constitute a professional relationship, for the purpose of disciplinary proceedings.

On a subsequent occasion the question arose in relation to adultery with an alleged patient. The doctor admitted adultery with a young woman whose name was on his N.H.S. list but denied that he stood in a professional relationship to her. He had never given her medical treatment. She was his domestic servant: the fact that she was on his list was wholly irrelevant. Such a person could be on his list and yet receive all medical treatment privately. The doctor's obligation to her only arose if she had requested treatment; there was no evidence that she had done so. The Disciplinary Committee appears to have accepted this argument since the doctor was found not guilty of infamous conduct, notwithstanding that he was the co-respondent in the divorce proceedings which arose out of this adultery (*Lancet*, 1956).

Actual adultery need not be proved, if it is shown that an improper relationship exists beyond the permitted range of professional contact. Formerly, clerks of Divorce Courts were obliged to report to the G.M.C. all doctors who had been cited as co-respondents, but this practice ceased in 1970. The G.M.C. only considers such cases if the injured party in a divorce action makes a complaint to them. Where adultery has been accepted by the court, the G.M.C. must accept this as a fact and only consider whether such adultery constituted professional misconduct.

Though disciplinary action is now relatively uncommon in this situation, the possibility still exists. A woman need not necessarily be a patient of the doctor, but if the acquaintance has been formed through his attending another person in the household, this may be deemed to be an abuse of professional privilege. Also, if a doctor ceases to attend the woman professionally before improper association takes place, this need not absolve him from misconduct, as the original association was gained through his professional position. Having said this, it is currently unusual for disciplinary action to be taken in such cases unless a florid breakdown of the doctor-patient relationship within the family has been facilitated by the doctor's professional advantages.

Addiction. Doctors, by virtue of their prescribing powers, have all too often fallen prey to addiction to therapeutic substances such as pethidine, morphine, heroin, barbiturates and amphetamines. Anaesthetists have also been prone to addiction to various substances such as cyclopropane or nitrous oxide. All these substances and many others have led to frequent appearances of doctors before the disciplinary machinery of the G.M.C. and in many cases to subsequent erasure or suspension. This is obviously a situation where suspension of the doctor from practice is necessary for both the protection of patients and for his own well being, so that he may be removed from access to the drug. Not infrequently, conditional suspension with restriction of his powers to prescribe may be proposed by the G.M.C. for a certain period.

Apart from personal addiction, offences against the Misuse of Drugs Act 1971 in respect of irregularities in prescriptions, supply and records may form grounds for referral to the G.M.C.

Advertising. The position of a doctor in regard to self-advertisement or allowing others to proclaim his skill, is one of the most confused aspects of professional misconduct. The very restrictive attitude of the past is no longer applied, due partly to the greatly increased impact of the media in the community. Advertising which draws attention to the professional skill etc. of one or more doctors for the purpose of obtaining patients or otherwise promoting professional advantage has resulted in disciplinary proceedings and, in one somewhat blatant case, erasure of the practitioner's name.

In May, 1960 the Disciplinary Committee heard the case of L.E.G., who was charged with having advertised for the purpose of obtaining patients or promoting his professional advantage. He had written and published a book in 1959 and had sanctioned or acquiesced in the publication of articles in non-professional journals, which contained matter directing attention to his professional skills, etc. The Committee acquitted him in respect of one of the articles, but found the facts proved in respect of his book and a series of articles, which had appeared in *Woman*! He was found guilty of infamous conduct and his name was ordered to be erased. Later, he gave notice of appeal (Minutes of the G.M.C., 1960, **97** pp. 38–41; *Lancet*, 1969).

The Privy Council began the hearing of the appeal on 11 April, 1961, which the applicant conducted in person (*Brit. Med. J.*, 1961a). In its essence, his submission was that "he had a proper message to deliver to the public and (therefore) it did not matter what language he used, to what extent he drew attention to his own skill or through what medium the message passed". The Disciplinary Committee had rejected this proposition. He also attacked the Committee because, in his submission, it had different standards; it had condoned articles in *Family Doctor*, but had condemned his publication as an advertisement. The appellant also contended that an opinion honestly held, even if wrong, could not amount to infamous conduct (Felix v. General Dental Council, 1960; *The Times*, 12 May). On 31 May, Lord Morris of Borth-y-Gest delivered the reserved judgment of the Judicial Committee, fully reported in the *British Medical Journal*, 1961, **i,** 1694–7. Their Lordships upheld the decision of the Disciplinary Committee. They considered there was ample material which warranted that decision and saw no error in it. The sentence of erasure was without any reason to show the Committee had erred in principle or that the decision was unjustifiable. Appeal dismissed: the appellant to pay the costs of the appeal.

The case was followed in November, 1961 by another in which seven plastic surgeons were charged with advertising for patients.

The complaint was based on the publication of articles in plastic surgery in certain women's journals. One invited its readers to apply for a pamphlet entitled *Operation Beauty*. This contained the advice to those who wished to consult a plastic surgeon to write to the British Association of Plastic Surgeons, 47 Lincoln's Inn Fields, London WC2. Mrs. G. (the wife of the cosmetic surgeon, whose name had been erased from the Register) wrote to the Association and received a list of names, which included those of seven persons now charged and that of one other surgeon. She caused a niece to write from Paris to these seven surgeons, asking for an operation on her nose and for information concerning their fees. All seven replied to her; only one of them had not seen her letter, the reply being made on his behalf by his secretary.

The Committee acquitted all seven of advertising and accordingly found none of them had combined to advertise. It was proved that they had been prepared to accept a patient, notwithstanding that they knew that the patient had been induced to seek their services in the alleged circumstances, i.e. articles in the lay press. The Committee, however, decided that this was insufficient to support a finding of infamous conduct in a professional respect.

Commenting on the circumstances, the Committee expressed serious misgiving over the state of affairs disclosed by this case. (1) Officers or members of the Association had, "wittingly or unwittingly, co-operated in the publication in the lay press of articles calculated to stimulate members of the public to apply to the Association for information about the services of plastic surgeons". (2) The Association had given applicants the names of a limited number of such surgeons (all being members of the Association). (3) Members of the Association had been prepared to accept patients who had applied in this manner. The Committee hoped that there will no recurrence of the events. (Reported at length in the *Lancet* (1961) and the *British Medical Journal* (1961b).

The advertisement which inevitably results from the publication of a book or article on any medical subject fortunately is amply justified, if the publication is intended to give information or to make a contribution to medical knowledge. It is not serious professional misconduct if at the same time the author thereby adds to his professional and pecuniary advantage. The Judicial Committee of the Privy Council was of the opinion that any reasonable practitioner could distinguish between objectionable and unobjectionable publications. A textbook written for the instruction of medical students and practitioners is permissible but a book or article, which praises the skill or abilities of the author and thus leads to increase in his practice, is not.

Since the more static patient lists of the National Health Service, there is far less likelihood of a mass migration of patients from one doctor to another following some publicity. Also, the greatly increased education and awareness of the community in medical matters has demanded far more public exposition of medical topics. Doctors are fully entitled to participate in this information transfer, so long as it does not confer personal professional advantages upon them. Gone are the days of early television, where doctors sat with their backs to the camera so that they would not be recognised!

There has been some complaint in past years that the attitude of the G.M.C. to this problem is inconstant and sometimes allegations are made that the risk of a doctor attracting censure from the G.M.C. is inversely proportional to his eminence in the profession. These complaints are largely ill-founded, but it is difficult to draw general guidelines, as each episode of alleged advertising must be judged on its own merits. It is obviously unethical for any practitioner to perform or condone any form of publicity which draws attention to his professional merits if thereby he stands to gain personally in a financial or professional manner.

In some classes of doctor, this is obviously impossible—the community physician or morbid anatomist for instance, could hardly be expected to gain patients or pecuniary advantage from any form of public notice. Yet it is difficult to draw distinctions between doctors and also doctor's circumstances may change—the community physician of today may be a general practitioner tomorrow. It remains a fact that compared to previous years when anonymity was absolute, the appearance of medically-qualified persons on radio, television and in newspaper articles is an everyday occurrence. The public have a right to be kept up to date with medical advances and opinions and especially in small communities, it is patently impossible to conceal identity. It is up to the individual practitioner to decide what is ethical and what is not.

The more obvious forms of advertising are now rare, such as overt publications drawing attention to some professional skill, either in newspapers, public places or upon the doctor's premises. The plate outside a doctor's premises should be unobtrusive and convey no more information than the name, qualifications and surgery hours. It has been held in the past that descriptions of specialities i.e. "Consultant Gynaecologist" are objectionable, but the practice is so widespread as to be accepted.

More recently, the attention of the G.M.C. has been directed to the use of notices such as "Middleton Health Centre" displayed outside a group practice. Fears have been expressed that this might suggest that this group practice has some official recognition over and above any other medical practices in Middleton to the possible professional detriment of other doctors. However, the appending of a geographical name to Health Centres is now so widespread as to be virtually beyond reversal.

Advertising also presents problems in relation to private clinics and specialist services, such as cosmetic surgery and hair transplantation etc. Here the organisation may be directed by lay persons, over whom the G.M.C. has no jurisdiction. Objectionable advertisements in newspapers cannot be controlled directly, but doctors who work for the lay directors of such organisations may themselves be censured by the G.M.C. for allowing themselves to be associated with undesirable advertising. Canvassing for patients (i.e. direct invitations to attend) is quite wrong, whether done by word of mouth or written means. It is also not correct for a doctor to advertise a change of surgery hours, for example in a public notice or newspaper. This should only be done by individual circulation of existing patients by private note, or a notice displayed in the interior of the surgery premises.

Association. This was a common offence in the last century and an important part of the
General Council's work in the early years. It is now very rare for such complaints to come
to the G.M.C.'s notice. They consist of "covering" unqualified assistants. This was once
particularly common in midwifery work, where unqualified women were employed as
midwives on behalf of the doctor. Association does not restrict proper employment of the
numerous types of medical auxiliary and technicians, nor the training of nurses and
medical students as long as the doctor retains personal responsibility and exercises
effective supervision. Naturally, in any emergency situation, including childbirth, the
assistance of an unqualified person would never be held to be "association".

Other Practices carrying the risk of Disciplinary Proceedings

An increasing cause for investigation, censure and possibly erasure by the G.M.C. is the
abuse or neglectful handling of the many forms of certification required by modern
community medicine. Serious inaccuracies in certification, either through oversight or
deliberate falsehood, may lead to removal from the Register.

These include the whole range of certification, especially those where some pecuniary
benefit is obtained by the doctor or by the patient. Though the pressures of both overwork
and persistent, vociferous patients in general practice may lead to careless or unwise
certification, this should be guarded against with the utmost care. Sick notes, cremation
certificates and certificates entitling patients to various grants are relatively frequent
causes for action by the G.M.C. The issue of untrue or misleading certificates and other
professional documents is a hazard to be avoided. The ever-increasing paper work in
practice can lead doctors to become careless in the issue of these documents. The
importance which is attached, to them, however, demands scrupulous care. The Council
emphasises the need for special care in relation to any statement that a patient has been
examined on a particular date. If he knows, or ought to know, that any of these
documents are untrue, misleading or otherwise improper, he may find himself the subject
of disciplinary proceedings. He may then be fortunate if their result is only a warning not
to repeat the offence.

Another common cause for the G.M.C.'s attention in relation to financial matters is the
improper behaviour of a doctor in respect of fees and expenses. Dichotomy or "fee-
splitting" was in former years a much more common offence than at present. This practice
rendered to the calling-in of a specialist by a practitioner, when the consultation fee would
be split between the two doctors. This provided an incentive for practitioners to consult
one particular specialist, who might not necessarily be the best person for the patient's
benefit. Other dubious activities include commercialisation of a patent medicine, the
financial or proprietary interest in a chemist's shop to which patients might be referred for
dispensing of prescriptions: prescribing drugs or surgical materials or appliances in which
a doctor had a commercial stake i.e. he is a partner or principal shareholder in some drug
company etc. The interest has to be direct and substantial and the mere holding of shares
in some large pharmaceutical company constitutes no offence. Breaches of professional
confidence i.e. medical secrecy, may also lead to disciplinary proceedings.

Failure to attend a patient is, in the isolated instance, a matter of complaint pursued
through the machinery of the N.H.S. or via a civil action for negligence. However, if
persistent or flagrant neglect of professional duties is alleged, then the G.M.C. may well

take notice in respect of professional misconduct. The G.M.C. is not concerned in matters of errors of diagnosis or treatment.

Last, but by no means least, an increasing cause for both N.H.S. enquiries, G.M.C. investigation and even criminal proceedings for fraud, is the deliberate falsification of claims by doctors for remuneration and expenses. An increasing number of allegations are being brought for obtaining money by deception and fraudulent claims in respect of all types of medical fees, extra-duty payments, subsistence allowances and travelling expenses.

Where such incorrect claims are shown to be deliberate and wilful, the doctor runs a grave risk of being found guilty of serious professional misconduct by the G.M.C. in addition to any other retribution that may be brought by the Health Authorities or the courts.

Republic of Ireland

A Medical Registration council of Ireland was set up in 1927, 5 years after setting up of the State. Representation on the British G.M.C. continued until 1979 when the recommendations of the Merison Committee brought about the exclusion of representatives from the Irish Republic. This coincided with recommendations from the E.E.C. with particular reference to registration of medical specialities. As a result, the Medical Practitioners Act, 1978, of the Irish Parliament (Dail Eireann) made several changes. It set up a Medical Council which took over the functions of the old Medical Registration Council.

The Council consists of 25 members comprising a person (usually the Dean) nominated by each of the five medical schools, two persons from the Royal College of Surgeons in Ireland, (one representing surgery and the other anaesthetics and radiology), two persons appointed by the Royal College of Physicians in Ireland (one presenting the medical specialities and the other jointly the specialities of Pathology, Obstetrics and Gynaecology), one person appointed by the Minister of Health to represent Psychiatry, one person to represent general medical practice, ten elected medical practitioners, representing the specialities, hospital doctors and general practitioners on different panels, and finally, four persons appointed by the Minister of Health, at least three of whom shall not be registered medical practitioners and shall in the opinion of the Minister represent the interests of the general public.

There are two statutory committees of the Council:

1. *The Fitness to Practice Committee*: This committee comprises only members of the Council, must contain a majority of elected members and must contain at least one of the laymen on the Council. It is the Fitness to Practice Committee which hears the complaints about medical practitioners and may find a doctor guilty of professional misconduct or unfit to engage in the practice of medicine because of physical or mental disability. The committee has the powers of a High Court judge to hear evidence under oath and to require the production of any medical records of that practitioner concerning a patient. If the committee finds the practitioner either guilty or unfit it reports him to the Council which then erases the name of the practitioner from the register or attaches such conditions as it thinks fit to the retention of that practitioner's name on the register. A doctor has the right to appeal to the High Court against his erasure. Unlike the U.K., the

Irish Republic has a written constitution, and this form of appeal is necessary because every citizen has a constitutional right to challenge any person or body which seeks to deprive him or her of his or her livelihood. As in Britain the Council may also erase from the register the name of any practitioner convicted, either inside the State or outside it, of an indictable offence. There is however a constitutional appeal against this decision to the High Court.

2. *The Educational Training Committee*: This has responsibility for the maintenance of standards in education and training, for the setting up of a post-graduate medical and dental board, and in pursuance of the E.E.C. directives, for the setting up of a specialist register. This matter of specialist registration has at present not been implemented.

References

EDITORIAL (1956) *Lancet*, **i,** 706.
EDITORIAL (1959) *Brit. Med. J.*, **ii,** supplement, **182**; 1316–17.
EDITORIAL (1960a) *Lancet*, **i,** 1243.
EDITORIAL (1960b) *Lancet*, **ii,** 309.
EDITORIAL (1961) *Lancet*, **ii,** 1251.
EDITORIAL (1961a) *Brit. Med. J.*, **i,** 1179.
EDITORIAL (1961b) *Brit. Med. J.*, **ii,** supplement, 223.
General Medical Council Minutes (1960) 97.

STATUTES

Medical Act 1858; 21 & 22 Vict., ch. 90.
Medical Act 1950; 14 Geo. 6, Ch. 29.
Medical Act 1956; (Amendment) Act, 1958; 6 & 7 Eliz. 2, ch. 58.
Medical Act 1969; Eliz. 2, ch. 40.
Medical Act 1978 Eliz. 2.
Medical Council Act (1862) 25 & 26 Vict., ch. 91.

STATUTORY INSTRUMENTS

General Medical Council Disciplinary Committee (Procedure) Rules, Order in Council, 1958; S.I., 1958, No. 1805.
Judicial Committee (Medical Rules) Order, 1958; S.I. 1958, No. 765.
Abortion Act 1967 Eliz. 2, ch. 87 Sheet 17.

CHAPTER 21

Consent to Medical Examination and Treatment

THE circumstances of medical practice do not ordinarily call for formal consent to medical examination because the patient conducts himself in a manner which implies consent. When he attends at a surgery, consulting room or out-patients' department, or when he agrees to be admitted to a hospital or nursing home, he thereby implies that he will submit to routine physical examination.

The conduct of the greater part of medical practice on the basis of implied consent, although entirely correct, is apt to lead medical practitioners to overlook the fact that medical examination is subject to consent, which, in the appropriate form, is necessary. Moreover, it is easily forgotten that any step beyond routine physical examination calls for express consent, oral or written, according to the circumstances.

Medical examination which is made without consent is at once an assault and a trespass upon the person of the patient and can be the source of criminal and civil proceedings. Today aggrieved patients may well institute proceedings.

> In 1950 a patient successfully sued a surgeon for technical assault. He had consulted the surgeon, who advised an operation for the repair of a hernia. The surgeon was alleged to have undertaken personally to perform the operation for a fee. The operation was in fact performed, in an entirely successful manner, by the house surgeon of that consultant. The patient complained that he had suffered damage because an apprentice had operated, whereas the patient had engaged a craftsman. The patient sued for breach of an alleged oral contract to operate and for procuring a trespass upon him by the house surgeon; the house surgeon was not sued. This agreement was denied and the plaintiff was said to have signed one under which he accepted the ministrations of the hospital staff (including the house surgeon); the operation was a part of those services. The patient occupied a bed in a public ward and the surgeon never charged a fee in such circumstances; there were no private wards in that hospital. It was held that there was no breach of contract. Although it was accepted that the surgeon had not said he would personally operate, he had not realised that the patient expected him to do so; the surgeon was not deemed to have led him to that belief. On the contrary, he contended he had made it clear that the patient would be in a public ward. The house surgeon, however, had operated without the patient's consent and there had been a trespass—"a highly technical trespass". In the circumstances only nominal damages, i.e. 20 shillings, were awarded. The judge observed that the action ought not to have been brought; the patient had received excellent treatment without fee. Although this was an unfortunate sequel to an entirely successful operation, "the case will serve to remind us all that any operation is an assault unless all proper consents have been obtained" (*Mitchell* v. *Molesworth*, 1950).

Following that case, the defence societies advised that the form of consent to operation should include a clause in which the patient agreed that no assurance had been given that the operation would be performed by a particular surgeon.

Attention must be paid also to this more serious case, which arose out of the injection of a boy, then aged 15, against his will and without appropriate consent.

> Through his father, he sued the doctor and the Regional Hospital Board, alleging assault, negligence and a breach of duty. The plaintiff had accompanied a younger brother, to look after him while he was subjected to a Mantoux test. It appears that when this was done the doctor, acting, as he believed in the best interests of the plaintiff, then proceeded to subject him also to this test. It was done against his will and without his parents' consent. Subsequently the plaintiff developed psoriasis. It was held that there had been no negligence in the giving of the injection. It had been given, however, without the consent of the parents, which would not have been given without the agreement of the family doctor, who said he would not have agreed. There had been an assault by the doctor and in assessing the damages at £25, the amount was intended to reflect the serious impropriety of forcing an injection on someone, in the absence of an emergency. It was moreover, something more than a mere pinprick. It was also held that psoriasis in this case was a result, although an unlikely and rare event, of the injection and flowed from the assault; for this, £200 damages were awarded. The case demonstrated that even in these days an individual cannot be forced to submit against his will to an injection because someone in authority thought it good for him to have it.

The National Health Service has not altered the fundamental principle that, except in an emergency, treatment requires appropriate consent; to act without it is an assault, irrespective of any question of negligence (*Odam* v. *Young and the East Anglian Regional Hospital Board* (1955)).

The right to refuse medical examination was upheld by the Court of Appeal in the case of *Pickett* v. *Bristol Aeroplane Company Ltd.* (1961).

> The plaintiff sued his employers alleging negligence, claiming that he had contracted dermatitis in the course of his employment. He submitted to a medical examination by two doctors acting on behalf of the company. Before the action came to trial, one of these doctors died and the company required the plaintiff to submit to an examination by a third doctor, chosen by them. He refused to be examined by that particular doctor. His employers then sought to have the proceedings stayed until he had submitted to this examination. The order was refused. On appeal, it was held that while his refusal was open to comment, he should certainly not be compelled to submit to this examination by a doctor to whom he objected; it was also doubtful whether the action should be stayed if he refused to be examined by any of the defendant's doctors. It appears there had grown up a practice for orders to be issued by Masters in Chambers, which stayed proceedings unless the plaintiffs submitted to examination by the defendant's doctors. This indirect compulsion was disapproved by the Court of Appeal. An inherent jurisdiction existed, but it was a power to be sparingly used, to prevent an abuse of the process of the Court.

Compulsory Medical Examination

There are a limited number of special circumstances, outside the scope of ordinary medical practice, in which an individual can be submitted to medical examination without his consent. Even in these circumstances, it appears that the doctor may not go beyond the limits of an ordinary physical (or mental) examination.

Persons admitted to any of H.M. Prisons must submit to routine physical examination for, otherwise, infection might be brought into a closed community with serious consequences to all concerned. This exception to the need for consent, however, does not extend to intimate examinations or the collection of body fluids for laboratory investigation. There must be consent, and express consent at that, before a blood sample may be taken from a prisoner to determine its Wassermann reaction or blood group; it may have an important bearing on the charge made against him, and he is not bound to incriminate himself.

Magistrates have certain powers to remand for medical examination. If on trial for an offence, which is punishable, on summary conviction, with imprisonment, and the court is satisfied that he is guilty, but is of the opinion that a medical report ought to be had, the case can be adjourned to enable an examination to be made and a report submitted, before the method of dealing with the case is determined. The court can make it a condition of release on bail that the accused undergoes a medical examination by a doctor and in such place as may be specified by the court (Magistrates Courts Act, 1952, section 26).

Probation orders requiring treatment for mental conditions may also be made. This method of dealing with an offender requires the evidence of a doctor approved for the purpose. It must be shown that the mental condition of the offender requires and is susceptible to treatment, but is not such as to warrant obligatory detention in hospital. The probation order will include a requirement that the offender shall submit to treatment for the period specified, not extending beyond one year from the date of the order. The order will specify the kind of treatment, i.e. as a resident or non-resident patient in a hospital or treatment by a doctor as specified in the order. Beyond this, the order may not specify the nature of the treatment. The probationer's consent is not entirely excluded. If it appears that part of the mental treatment by the specified doctor can be better given in or at a hospital not specified on the order, he may, with the consent of the probationer, make suitable arrangements for him to be treated accordingly. If the probationer is shown to have failed to comply with any of the requirements of the probation order, he will be dealt with in any manner open to the court, as if he had just been convicted before that court of an offence in respect of which the probation order had been made.

Persons who are believed to be suffering from a notifiable disease may be compelled to submit to medical examination. A magistrate has power to order the examination when satisfied by a certificate issued by a medical officer of health that there is reason to believe some person in the district is or has been suffering from a notifiable disease, that it is in his own interest or in the interest of his family or in the public interest that he should be medically examined and that he is not under the treatment of a registered medical practitioner or that that practitioner consents to the making of the order. The order may be combined with a warrant authorising the medical officer of health to enter any premises (Public Health Act, 1961, section 38; Public Health Act, 1936, section 287).

Compulsory medical treatment of tuberculosis is also provided for under section 172, Public Health Act, 1936. A magistrate can order the removal of the patient to a suitable hospital and his detention therein for a period not exceeding 3 months in the first instance. It is a section invoked with reluctance, but it became necessary on 4 February 1960 when a woman with open tuberculosis refused to take precautionary measures. Her promises to carry out home treatment were unreliable. She was infectious to other persons. The court issued an order to the Oxford City Council to have the patient removed to hospital and detained there for 3 months.

Port and airport medical officers can compel immigrants to submit to an examination in order to exclude infections. There is also provision for obligatory medical examination by a medical officer of health of any person whom he has cause to suspect may be suffering from a disease likely to cause infection of milk (Milk and Dairies (General) Regulations, 1959). The medical officer of health shall be given all reasonable assistance to make a medical examination of any person who is engaged in the commercial preparation and handling of food and drink and who may be a carrier of *salmonella* or *staphylococcal* infection (The Public Health (Infectious Diseases) Regulations, 1953).

The Education Act, 1944, section 49, made provision for medical inspection and treatment of pupils at any school or county college maintained by a local authority. The officer duly authorised by the local education authority "may require the parent of any pupil in attendance at any such school to submit the pupil for medical inspection in accordance with arrangements made by the authority".

These examinations are no longer obligatory but are available. The parents are invited to attend the examination of their children. If unable to attend, their written consent is required.

Although a school medical officer is apparently authorised by this section to inspect the children without consent, it may be prudent for him to defer such an examination if he has reason to believe that the parents of the child object to it. (This is an unusual event.) When this arises the parents should be referred to the education officer who will explain to them the purpose and desirability of the examination. This usually secures their cooperation. If the parents are still unwilling, they may agree to the pupil being examined by the family practitioner. Prosecution of the parents under the section should be a last resort.

In the matter of free medical treatment, of which the authority has a duty to encourage and assist pupils to take advantage (*Ibid.* section 48 (3) and (4)), there is specific provision for parental objection. Under the latter subsection it is provided that "if the parent of any pupil gives to the authority notice that he objects to the pupil availing himself of any medical treatment provided under this section, the pupil shall not be encouraged or assisted so to do".

THE DOCTRINE OF INFORMED CONSENT

To be valid, consent must be genuine and freely given, but in addition it must be given in the light of the patient's understanding. This concept of "informed consent" has acquired major importance in recent years—indeed, some doctors feel that it has assumed disproportionate importance in some instances.

The patient has two fundamental rights in connection with his condition, apart from the right to expect an adequate standard of care from his doctor. He is entitled to be confident that no other person learns of his condition without his permission, but also that he himself is informed of what is wrong with him and what is to be done about it.

Under this last heading, the right exists not only to be told details of what medical or surgical treatment is proposed, but also the nature and likelihood of any untoward complications.

In theory, this knowledge will allow him to decide whether or not to risk submitting to the procedure.

Unless the doctor fully explains the risks inherent in the treatment and offers some evaluation of the risk actually occurring the consent may not be "informed" and thus be invalid.

However, this rather simplistic concept, more subscribed to by lawyers than physicians, is by no means as straightforward as it sounds, yet can provide a minefield of medico-legal danger for the doctor, especially the surgeon and radiologist.

Though every patient is entitled to be told about his condition, this exposition must be modified—often drastically—by his or her ability to receive it, as measured by the doctor's clinical judgment. The doctor has to decide, after evaluating all aspects of the patient's personality, physical and mental state, how much can be safely revealed. For instance, the age, intelligence, education and mental awareness may all modify the amount of revelation and the way in which the doctor reveals it. The presence of a malignancy or an inevitably fatal lesion may be suppressed if the doctor feels the patient is not able to tolerate the knowledge. In a potentially suicidal patient, the medical attendant may well omit certain facts, either temporarily or permanently.

Similarly, where some potentially risky therapy is contemplated, which is to be offered in good faith with the intention of curing or improving the patient's condition, an adverse reaction to detailed information might either seriously upset the patient with perhaps the risk of a relapse—or more probably, cause the patient to refuse the operation or treatment, which may well have greatly improved his or her health.

Every doctor has to meet this dilemma, having to weigh up in every individual case the balance between providing legitimate information against the risk of prejudicing the patient's acceptance of treatment. The patient may decline the treatment either because the description of the procedure may be intimidating or because the risks appear out of proportion to the possible benefits. An example of the first instance might be the agitation and even terror invoked in markedly thyrotoxic patient who is given an over-detailed description of a proposed partial thyroidectomy; in the same circumstances, the surgeon's warning of the risks of laryngeal paralysis might also cause the patient to reject the operation. This in fact was the situation in the leading case on this topic, *Hatcher* v. *Black* (1954) when Lord Denning (then L.J.) gave his well-known opinion. The surgeon contemplating a partial thyroidectomy knew that there was some slight risk to the left recurrent laryngeal nerve, but admitted that he told the patient that there was none. He did it for her good, as he did not want her to worry. Lord Denning said "He told a lie, but he did it because in the circumstances, it was justifiable. This, however, is not a court of morals and the law left the question of the conscience of the doctor himself . . . though if doctors had too easy a conscience on this matter, they might in time lose the confidence of the patient which was the basis of all good medicine. But the law did not condemn the doctor when he only did what a wise doctor so placed would do. None of the doctors called as witnesses had condemned him—why should the jury?".

However, bearing in mind these very real limiting factors which are purely matters of clinical experience and judgment, there is a general duty to ensure that the patient receives an adequate explanation of the proposed procedure, whether it be diagnostic or therapeutic. Furthermore, it is the duty of the doctor who is in professional care of the patient to ensure that such explanation is given, either by himself or by a deputy and to assure himself that the patient actually *understands* that explanation. All too often, an explanation which the doctors think is adequate is given, but at a later date when a dispute arises, the patient swears that he either never received it or that it was couched such terms that he could not understand it.

The defence societies have advised that all such information should be in non-technical language and should be given by a medical practitioner, preferably the one who is to perform the procedure or his immediate assistant—and not by a para-medical person, such as a nurse or technician.

On the written consent form, the wording should include a phrase to confirm that the patient had indeed been informed of the nature of the procedure, before signing and witnessing takes place. The Medical Protection Society (1976) give a succinct summary of this problem in their Annual Report: "Clearly, if consent is sought from any person then it is essential to provide sufficient details and information so that the person consenting can form a proper decision and give informed consent. Thus the age and mental condition of the patient are relevant, for a child or a patient suffering from a mental disability may be unable sufficiently to comprehend the explanation. A misinformed consent or one given in ignorance of what is requested, is of no value. The extent of the explanation given must depend on all the circumstances of an individual case and considerations include the patient's physical state, mental capacity, intellectual attainment, standard of education etc. It will also depend on the questions put to the practitioner seeking consent, some patients wishing to know considerably more about side effects and complications than others. A considerable degree of judgment is required in knowing just how detailed the explanation should be, but there is—as yet—no legal requirement that every single complication, however rare or unlikely, should be explained to the patient. Clearly a balance must be struck between telling the patient sufficient to enable him to form a valid consent on the one hand and not so much as to frighten him needlessly on the other".

A recent judicial view of informed consent was given by Mr. Justice Bristow in *Chatterton* v. *Gerson* (1981), QB 432. "The duty of a doctor is to explain what he intends to do and its implications, in the way that a careful and responsible doctor in similar circumstances would have done. But he ought to warn of what may happen by misfortune however well the operation is done, if there is any real risk of a misfortune inherent in the procedure. In what he says, any good doctor has to take into account the personality of the patient, the likelihood of the misfortune and what in the way of a warning is good for the particular patient's benefit".

Two cases in the courts in 1982, described by the Medical Protection Society in their Annual Report for that year, concerned informed consent rather than technical negligence. In one where a spinal operation was complicated by infarction of the spinal cord with resulting paralysis, the court found that though the surgeon was meticulous in explaining the more common risks of the procedure, he did not give a complete list, omitting the one which actually occurred. Several expert witnesses agreed that his warning was consistent with accepted practice in 1974, when the mishap occurred. The plaintiff's counsel appealed to the judge to use a stricter criterion and cited some American cases in support, but the judge declined to accept these, preferring to adhere to previous English decisions in which there is no duty imposed of full disclosure. He adopted the standard accepted by Mr. Justice McNair in *Bolam* v. *Friern H. M. C.* (1957) I WLR 589, that a doctor is not guilty of negligence if he has acted in accordance with a practice accepted as proper by a responsible body of medical men skilled in that particular art. (Sidaway 1984)

The other case involved a patient who suffered brain damage after a carotid angiogram. Both the consultant and his senior house surgeon had explained the risks and obtained written consent, but the plaintiff's expert witness maintained that the word "stroke" should have been used as it would have been better understood by a layman. However, the defence claimed and the court upheld, that the use of this word was too frightening and would not have been used by the majority of surgeons placed in the same situation.

The recent reaction against the more absolute degrees of informed consent have come from radiologists, especially in the United States. Due to the higher rate of legal actions brought for real or alleged infringements of consent concerning radiological procedures (such as myelograms with their attendant risks of paraplegia and the other hazards of parenteral administration of various contrast media such as for excretion pyelography and choliangiography), a brisk debate has developed in the American medical press. Hinck & Wagner (1970) suggest that the magnitude of the risk should be defined in broad terms and the potential benefits and limitations of the examination should be described. They suggest that it is both unfair and unethical to tell, for example, a patient scheduled for cerebral angiography that "he is going down to the X-ray department where they will take a few pictures".

They further advise that no attempt is made to offer a complete list of possible dangers and complications, as this is inevitably incomplete; should the patient suffer one of the omitted complications, he can sue on the grounds that this risk was not mentioned.

Hinck & Wagner suggest the use of general terms such as "mild complications" and "serious complications" to avoid this situation. In 1976 another American radiologist, Robert Allen pointed out that he had performed 6000–8000 urograms over a 25-year period before having the first fatal reaction, upon which he was sued. He had not warned the patient of a possible reaction and never in fact made this his practice. As a deliberate policy, he felt it did no good, as if he had described the risks, the patient would have been distressed. But he knew that after having calmed down, further explanation would have obtained the necessary consent—but he had no doubt that the malpractice suit would still be brought; he therefore felt he had nothing to lose, but the thousands of other patients had much to gain. Further details of this controversy are given by Evans and Knight (1981).

Forms of Consent

Consent, as already indicated, may be *implied* or *express*, and the latter may be in the form of oral or written consent. Ordinarily, implied consent is sufficient authority for routine physical examination. It is otherwise when intimate examinations or the administration of anaesthetics or the performance of operations are contemplated. Even routine physical examination of an accused or suspected person is best undertaken only by express consent, in writing and given in the presence of a witness.

Although oral consent in the presence of a witness is good in law, the advantages of written consent, witnessed by a disinterested third party, are obvious. There should be no hesitation to secure written consent whenever the circumstances give rise even to the remote possibility of any subsequent allegations of assault or trespass.

Implied Consent

The nature and circumstances of implied consent to medical examination have already been indicated. It is sufficient only to repeat that the doctor should not allow himself to assume that consent in this form permits any step beyond an ordinary physical examination of the patient. It does not extend to the performance of intimate examinations, nor, in our opinion, to the collection of body fluids for the purpose of laboratory investigations. In both of these circumstances, express, oral consent is on all occasions necessary. When they are related to any legal proceedings, in which the results of the medical examination may be given in evidence, consent should preferably be in writing. (Maternity Cases are in a special category: see below.)

Legal considerations apart, medical examination is subject also to the demands of common courtesy. The fact that a patient is in hospital and it may be assumed he is prepared to submit to examinations, does not permit or excuse conduct of the kind which was once related in an imaginary story in the *Lancet*. A medical student was said to have walked into a ward and approached the bed of one of the women patients. Without a word to her, he threw back the bed-clothes, raised her nightgown and placed his hand on her abdomen. Remarking "Isn't it a beauty?" he then turned and left the ward. Whilst his enthusiasm over the successful palpation of an enlarged spleen is praiseworthy, it is no less understandable that he left behind an astonished and indignant patient. Conduct of this kind, it is hoped, is rare but lesser grades of offensive handling of patients can easily occur in ward classes and on other occasions in hospitals. Mistakes of this kind are unlikely to occur if the patient is approached in a manner which the examiner would wish to be shown to him, when he has to undergo medical examination. In these days, when patients are less ready to experience multiple examinations of the kind necessary for the instruction of medical students, attention to the manner of approach and questions of consent is imperative in order to secure the co-operation of the patient. Those in charge of the patients should, where necessary, explain the value of submission to this experience and should ensure that students make their examinations in a manner which avoids unnecessary distress or discomfort to the patient. If the patient has never previously received care and treatment in a teaching hospital, it is a wise precaution, to be taken by the doctor in charge of the patient or his deputy, to obtain permission to teach on the case, before students are brought to the bedside for clinical instruction.

Express Consent

Oral consent. Whenever the diagnosis and treatment of the patient call for steps beyond the limits of routine physical examination, it is necessary to obtain express consent.

On most occasions it is then sufficient to obtain oral consent, preferably in the presence of a disinterested third party, e.g. a ward sister, or the doctor's secretary or nurse. The several tests which entail the removal of body fluids, radiological examinations and, in particular, those which require the introduction of test substances into the air passages or the blood stream, and intimate examinations are all common procedures in hospitals; all of these call at least for oral consent before they are undertaken. Since the collection of body fluids, for example, blood samples, is not infrequently delegated to laboratory technicians, the doctor in charge of the patient should personally satisfy himself that consent is given either to him or to the person who is to take the samples.

The conduct of intimate examinations calls for the presence of a disinterested third party, as also does the administration of any general anaesthetic, to ensure that there can be no ground, real or imaginary, for allegations of indecent assault. The male doctor, who proposes to make an intimate examination of any woman patient, should always be attended by a nurse or other disinterested person. Indeed no kind of examination of a female patient, conducted behind screens, should be made except in these circumstances. It is unwise, also, to make any examination of schoolgirls at their school except in the presence of one of the mistresses or, where there is one, the school matron or nurse. When the school is one at which the pupils are submitted to routine medical inspection, the fact that the parents are aware of this and send their children to the school implies consent to routine medical examination. If, however, they raise objection, no examination should be made; the patient should be referred to her own doctor.

Insistence upon the presence of a disinterested third party may seem a counsel of perfection and, indeed, the risk entailed by omitting this protection is negligible with the majority of patients. At the same time it is not always possible to recognise the exceptional case, where a patient, either innocently or from one of several possible improper motives, misinterprets or misrepresents the procedure and alleges assault. The only safeguard is to observe the rule as strictly as the circumstances will permit.

In hospitals and nursing homes it is rarely, if ever, impracticable to arrange the examination so that it takes place in the presence of a member of the nursing staff or a female colleague. It is usual, also, for the consultant in private practice to be assisted by a nurse or secretary. In general practice it may well be otherwise; the practitioner must then use his discretion. If the patient is well known to him he may no doubt safely undertake an intimate examination without protection. Whenever he is in any doubt about this, his proper course is to explain its necessity and offer to arrange for its performance by a consultant, either in hospital or at his rooms.

Emphasis should be put upon the phrase "disinterested third party". No doubt on most occasions it is sufficient that a relative of the patient is present but it has happened that a husband, seated on the other side of a screen during an intimate examination of his wife, has joined with her in subsequent allegations of indecent assault by the doctor. Although the doctor is usually acquitted of these charges, he has to face the expense involved by his defence and the undesirable publicity of the criminal proceedings.

On one occasion a doctor was consulted by a woman because she was childless. She insisted upon an intimate examination, which, with reluctance, he made in the absence of a third party. The patient then sued him for trespass. Although the jury stopped the case and returned a verdict for the defendant, the incident cost him dearly in other ways (*Spicer* v. *Hall*, 1901).

Written consent. Written consent is necessary and should not be omitted in any of the following circumstances:

(a) The performance of surgical operations under general anaesthesia.
(b) The performance of dental operations under general anaesthesia.
(c) The administration of a general anaesthetic for any purpose, other than operative or manipulative procedures that are normally associated with childbirth.
(d) Any complex diagnostic or therapeutic procedure, whether radiological or by any invasive technique.
(e) The termination of pregnancy.
(f) The examination of persons in custody, at the request of the police.
(g) The examination of victims of alleged sexual assaults.
(h) The taking of blood samples from persons alleged to have an excess of alcohol in their bodies, when likely to be charged under the Road Traffic Act, 1972, requires the driver to supply a sample for analysis. The doctor must provide a certificate that consent had been given.

Before obtaining consent in any of these circumstances the doctor should give the person an explanation, in terms which the person can understand, of the nature and purpose of the operation, examination or test. And the doctor should personally satisfy himself that this is understood before consent is signed. The doctor should not act on the information of a police officer that the person had given consent; this should be confirmed by the doctor personally.

Written consent should be in proper form and suitably drafted for the circumstances. Such forms have been prepared by the defence societies and, having been drafted on legal advice, these, and no amateur forms, should be used. The form most often required is that for consent to a surgical operation under general anaesthesia and it will suffice to cite its contents: When completed this form of consent states that:

> I hereby consent to undergo the operation of (appendicectomy) the nature and purpose of which has been explained to me by Dr./Mr. (Jones). I also consent to such further or alternative operative measures as may be found necessary during the course of the operation and to the administration of a general, local or other anaesthetic for any of these purposes.
> No assurance has been given to me that the operation will be performed by any particular surgeon.
> Date: . . . .   Signed: . . . .
> (Patient)
> I confirm that I have explained to the patient the nature and purpose of his operation.
> Date: . . . .   Signed: . . . .
> (Medical Practitioner)

The Medical Defence Union strongly deprecate any form of consent which is drafted in general terms and doubt whether such forms give any protection to the surgeon or the hospital in the event of a claim for damages for assault.

(The foregoing form, and twelve others, are published by the Medical Defence Union in their "Consent to Treatment", revised issue, of July 1971. A copy of this authentic statement of the law relating to consent should be possessed and closely studied by all medical practitioners and hospital administrators.)

The Time for Obtaining Consent

It is no doubt convenient for the administrative staff to arrange that every patient admitted to hospital shall sign a form of consent to operation shortly after their admission to the hospital, irrespective of the reason for admission. This is no doubt satisfactory and proper when the patient is admitted for the specific purpose of the performance of an operation shortly afterwards. In other circumstances, e.g. admission for medical treatment or investigation, such consent is unsatisfactory. If given, fresh consent should be obtained when the doctor or surgeon has decided to advise an operation and consent should then be obtained shortly before the patient is due to undergo the operation.

Maternity Patients

It is the view of the Medical Defence Union that acceptance of admission to hospital for a confinement implies consent to any operative or manipulative procedures that are normally associated with childbirth and to administration of a local or general anaesthetic for these procedures. Written consent is not needed. If, however, it is decided to deliver the patient by caesarian section, this should be explained to the patient or, if she is unable at the time to give consent, the explanation should be given to a relative, preferably the husband. In circumstances where delay, in order to obtain consent, would endanger the life of the mother or child, the operation should be undertaken forthwith and consent assumed to have been given.

PERSONS WHO HAVE AUTHORITY TO GIVE CONSENT

(i) *The Patient, if of Full Age, which is now 18 years* (The age of majority was reduced from 21 years to 18 years by the Family Law Reform Act, 1969, section 1.)

Unless incapacitated by injury, disease, anaesthesia or other cause, so as to be unable to understand the nature and purpose of the operation and give valid consent, the consent of the patient is paramount. It cannot be overruled by a spouse or relative. In circumstances where the proposed operation interferes with marital rights it is necessary or advisable to consult the spouse and obtain agreement.

(ii) *Minors who have Attained the Age of 16 years* Until 1969 there was doubt as to whether these patients could give valid consent. The Family Law Reform Act, 1969, section 8, clarifies the matter precisely. These patients can give valid consent to any surgical, medical or dental treatment and it is not necessary to obtain the consent of the parent or guardian. The section also covers any procedure undertaken for the purpose of diagnosis, including the administration of an anaesthetic ancillary to any treatment. It does *not* sanction the validity of consent to the donation of blood by persons in this group.

(iii) *Minors Under the Age of 16 years* The above statutory right begins only at 16 years, but there is a common law right to give consent if the young person is sufficiently mature to appreciate the circumstances and significance of the procedure. Failing this, probably always below the age of about 12–13, then consent must be obtained (except in emergency) from a parent, guardian or person *in loco parentis*.

(iv) *Mentally Disordered Patients* Patients who are compulsorily detained, if capable of understanding the nature and purpose of the treatment or the administration of a general anaesthetic, should be asked if they are willing to undergo the treatment, and should sign a form of consent. In any event, whether their consent is or is not given, they can be compelled to submit to the treatment. The consent of the relatives has no legal validity and the consent form, if not signed by the patient, should be signed by the responsible medical officer (Medical Defence Union, 1971).

(v) *Consent in Emergencies* Consent to treatment in an emergency may be assumed to permit the performance of any operation or other treatment which is *immediately* necessary to save life or health. The circumstances include the treatment of persons injured in road or rail accidents, unconscious patients, or any other circumstances in which the patient is unable to give consent and it is not possible to delay treatment until a near relative is found to give consent.

As already stated, consent may be assumed for the delivery of a woman by caesarian section, if necessary as an emergency.

In the case of mentally disordered patients, compulsorily detained, consent is not required for treatment in any emergency due to a condition unrelated to his mental illness. The responsible medical officer can authorise it. On the other hand, if immediate treatment is not required, the valid consent of the patient is necessary. If unable to understand or unwilling to give consent, the treatment should be postponed until he has recovered from his mental illness to a sufficient degree so as to be able to give consent. If recovery fails to take place within a reasonable time, the condition may be deemed to have become an emergency and treatment can be authorised by the responsible medical officer. The Medical Defence Union is of the opinion that his decision, taken in good faith and in the interests of the patient, would not result in criticism by a court.

Informal mental patients stand in precisely the same position as any other patient in any other hospital. He alone can give valid consent to treatment of his mental or other illness. If he is incapable of giving consent or refuses treatment, it should not be given since this might constitute trespass to the person and be actionable in damages (Medical Defence Union, 1971). It is pointed out that the foregoing applies to patients over the age of 16 years.

The treatment of minors under the age of 16 requires the consent of a parent or guardian but the parent or guardian cannot refuse treatment for the mental disorder of a child who is compulsorily detained. The performance of electroplexy requires written consent. (An appropriate form is given in "Consent to Treatment" at p. 17.)

CONSENT TO THE TERMINATION OF PREGNANCY

Written consent by the patient is always obligatory.

Married Women

The consent of the husband should be obtained, even if it is not necessary in law.

When termination is necessary to save life or preserve health, the consent of the patient is sufficient and the husband cannot overrule her consent, even if it is his responsibility to pay the fee and expenses involved.

The husband should be consulted when the termination is proposed on "environmental" grounds or because there is the possibility that the child may be born with some physical or mental abnormality. In the event of his refusal of "environmental" termination, agreed to by his wife, the doctor is advised to consult at least one other doctor before terminating the pregnancy. Similarly, if he refuses termination to prevent the birth of an abnormal child. The Medical Defence Union was advised that if the doctor acted in good faith and there were reasons to anticipate that the child would have been abnormal, he is unlikely to be condemned by the courts.

Single Women

Their consent is sufficient. The putative father has no authority to consent to or refuse the termination of the pregnancy. It is advised, however, if the parties have a family outside marriage and the termination is proposed on "environmental" grounds, the father should be consulted.

The consent of parents of an unmarried girl, over the age of 16 years, is not required, *nor should the doctor disclose any information to them about the case without the girl's consent.* If the girl be under the age of 16 years the parents must be consulted, even if the patient forbids disclosure of information. Conversely, termination of her pregnancy must never be carried out against her wishes, even if her parents demand it (Medical Defence Union, 1971).

If the doctor considers the circumstances require disclosure without the girl's consent, i.e. that this is in her interests, he should *first* consult his defence society.

PRIMARY STERILISATION

If carried out with the valid consent of the patient, sterilisation by operation is considered by the legal advisers of the Union to be lawful not only on therapeutic but also eugenic or any other grounds.

If performed solely as a mode of birth control, the consent of the patient and the spouse, if they are living together, is necessary. Failure to get the consent of the husband might result in a successful claim for damages. If the parties are not living together, the patient's consent is sufficient; similarly, if the patient is unmarried.

Sterilisation on therapeutic grounds can be performed with the sanction of the patient alone; that of the spouse is not necessary in law.

Mentally disordered patients should not be subjected to sterilisation unless the patient is capable of understanding the nature and consequences of the operation.

The Medical Defence Union advises consultation with the doctor's defence society before undertaking the primary sterilisation of a minor.

Sterilisation of the male (vasectomy) is lawful under the N.H.S. (Family Planning) Amendment Act, 1972.

Disputes about consent are particularly prone to occur in relation to sterilisation. The defence societies record several such disputes in their reports. In one case, a woman undergoing her second caesarean section was sterilized by an assistant surgeon on the direction of his consultant, who considered the clinical indications sufficient, though no consent form had been signed. By the time the patient and her husband brought an action, the consultant had died. The woman, who had been wrongly assumed to have rheumatic heart disease, denied ever giving verbal consent or even having the matter discussed with her, maintaining that she would never have consented. A settlement was made in 1976 in excess of £4000.

The Medical Protection Society records the following case in their 1977 Annual Report, concerning informed consent in respect of the risks of failure of a sterilisation operation. A woman with a bad obstetric history underwent tubal ligation in 1968, histology confirming that parts of the fallopian tubes had been excised. Immediately after the operation, the patient asked "Have you done the operation so that I will have no more children? Does that mean that I don't come back (to hospital)"?. The registrar who had carried out the ligation replied "As far as I am concerned you won't come back". Neither the registrar nor his consultant had discussed the possibility of failure with the patient. In 1971, the patient became pregnant and required a hysterectomy. She then sued the doctors, claiming that they had failed to inform her that the failure rate in tubal ligation was 1 in 300 and that she had been wrongly informed that she could not again conceive.

At the trial, there was a marked difference of opinion amongst obstetric expert witnesses as to their practice in warning against failure and of the advisability of using other contraceptive methods.

The Judge held that the registrar had acted in accordance with a substantial body of accepted practice – i.e. the *Bolam v. Friern and Hatcher v. Black* principle—and dismissed the patient's claim.

CONTRACEPTIVE ADVICE AND TREATMENT

The propriety of giving contraceptive advice and prescriptions for contraceptives to girls under the age of 16 years was considered by the Medical Defence Union. Their legal advisers take the view that a prosecution is unlikely to succeed where a doctor in good faith provided contraceptive advice or fitted a contraceptive device to a girl who is under the age of 16. When it appears that the patient has informed neither her parents, nor her general practitioner, and does not wish them to know that she is receiving contraceptive advice and treatment the doctor should attempt to persuade her to inform them. She should be warned that in the event of her needing other medication, e.g., an antibiotic, she should then inform her general practitioner in order to avoid possible ill-effects of drug interaction. (Polson, 1984)

CONSENT TO SUBJECTION TO CLINICAL RESEARCH

Before subjecting any patient to clinical research, to experiments which are not necessarily part of a patient's treatment, the doctor is advised to consult his defence society for advice. (And that procedure should invariably be followed in any situation in which the question of the necessary consent presents difficulty.)

CONSENT TO THE TAKING OF BLOOD FOR DETERMINING PATERNITY

It is now recognised by the courts that the use of blood tests can be of assistance in determining the question of paternity in relation to divorce proceedings. No difficulty arises when the parties agree to submit to the tests. On the other hand, an adult party cannot be compelled to submit. Difficulties have arisen when consent to test of the child has been refused.

It was decided that a judge of the High Court had power to order the child to be tested when the subject of custody proceedings (In Re L., *The Times*, 16 Nov. 1967). On that occasion the Official Solicitor, the guardian *ad litem* of the child, refused his consent. It was held that he had no authority to give or withhold consent.

It was later decided by the Court of Appeal, in the case of *B.B.* (*The Times*, 28 May 1968), that a judge of the High Court, of whatever division, had jurisdiction to order that which he believed to be in the best interests of the child, including a blood test in divorce proceedings, and his authority was not limited to custody proceedings.

The power to direct the use of blood tests in cases of disputed paternity is given in the Part III of the Family Law Reform Act, 1969. The Act empowers civil courts, including county courts and magistrates courts, to give this direction on an application by any party to the proceedings.

The consent of an adult or of a person aged 16 or over will normally be required. A blood sample may be taken from a person under the age of 16, not being a person who is suffering from mental disorder, if the person who has care and control of him consents. If suffering from mental disorder and incapable of giving valid consent, a blood sample may be taken from a patient if the person who has the care and control of him consents and the medical practitioner in whose care he is has certified that the taking of a blood sample from him will not be prejudicial to his proper care and treatment.

Refusal to consent to give a blood sample, or failure to take any steps to give effect to the direction to submit to the test, entitles the court to draw such inferences, if any, from that fact as appear proper in the circumstances.

The Act, and regulations made under section 22, provide for the procedures to be adopted in carrying out the tests and the form in which the reports are given. These reports will be received in evidence.

It is an offence to impersonate another or proffer a child knowing that it is not the child named in the direction and the punishment, on conviction, is imprisonment for up to 2 years or a fine not exceeding £400.

The subject of Blood Test Law is considered in clear detail by Lenham in his articles, published in 1968 and 1969, in *Medicine, Science and Law.*

REFUSAL OF CONSENT TO BLOOD TRANSFUSION

(a) *Adults: aged 16 years or over* Members of the religious sect of Jehovah's Witnesses are adamant in their refusal of treatment by blood transfusion. They base this objection on the command "That ye abstain from meats offered to idols and from blood . . ." (The Acts XV, 29). They are entitled to their opinion and doctors are not always right in their judgment that transfusion is necessary. The sect may cite the case of a pregnant woman who was considered in immediate need of blood transfusion; this was refused and she proceeded to term and was delivered without any complication.

The doctor who, in good faith, believes transfusion is necessary, should explain the matter to the patient and leave him or her in no doubt as to the possible consequences of refusal. *This should be done in the presence of a witness.* If persuasion fails, the doctor should then require the patient to sign a form of refusal and it should be carefully drafted to suit the circumstances, i.e. transfusion for surgical or transfusion for medical cases. (The Medical Defence Union, 1971, provide examples.) The doctor must then continue to treat the patient under this limitation to the best of his ability but he must not administer a blood transfusion. The form of refusal exonerates him and the hospital from any of the consequences which might result from the omission of a blood transfusion.

(b) *Children: minors under the age of 16 years* The parents or guardians of these children (and the patients themselves, if capable of understanding the proposed treatment) will refuse blood transfusion of the patient even if needed to save life. This places the doctor in a particularly difficult position. It is his duty to explain the need for transfusion and the consequences of refusal; he should exhort the parents to accept the treatment. If they are adamant in their refusal, an application can be made to a magistrate for the removal of the child from the custody of the parents and the child is placed in the custody of a fit "person". In the event of the issue of a Fit Person Order, that person assumes the authority of the parents and can give consent to whatever treatment the doctors believe necessary. This procedure under the Children and Young Persons Act (1933) is not favoured by the medical defence societies and should be avoided.

If the child's life is in peril, it is a matter for the doctor's own professional conscience; the Medical Defence Union is of the opinion that despite the parents' opposition the blood transfusion should be given if the child's condition requires it. "Whatever course the member follows he may count upon the full support of the Union."

The decision to give blood in these circumstances should be supported by the written opinion of a colleague. The parents' refusal should be recorded in appropriate form. (An example is given by the Medical Defence Union, 1971.)

REFUSAL OF MEDICAL ADVICE AND A DEMAND FOR DISCHARGE FROM HOSPITAL (OR NURSING HOME)

Unless the patient is compulsorily detained in hospital under section 26 of the Mental Health Act, 1959, any patient who demands his discharge is free to leave and arrangements must be made for his discharge without delay. He should first be given an explanation of his condition and the possible consequences of his discharge and persuaded to remain until his treatment has been completed. If, however, he persists in demanding his discharge, he must be allowed to leave. "Detention" in hospital is not normally compulsory.

When medical advice is refused and the patient demands his discharge, that fact must be recorded in his case notes and it is imperative that, before he leaves the hospital, he has signed a form of refusal of medical advice and that he has taken his discharge against medical advice. (This should be in proper form and the defence societies have drafted one suitable for use on these occasions.)

If the patient refuses to sign such a form, this fact must also be entered into his case notes, preferably attested by the signatures of two doctors or a doctor and a senior nursing officer.

His relatives should be informed and requested to collect the patient; if no relative is available the aid of the local authority's social services should be sought.

If, in the opinion of the doctor, the patient is suffering from mental disorder and is temporarily unable to understand the situation, the matter should be referred to the local Mental Health Department; it may be necessary for the patient to be detained in a hospital under the Mental Health Acts, and their officer can make the arrangements.

References

ALLEN, R. (1976)

BOLAM v. FRIERN H. M. C. (1957) 1 WLR 589 (McNair, J.)

CHATTERTON v. GRIERSON (1981) Q B 432 (Bristow, J.)

EVANS, K. & KNIGHT, B. (1981) *Forensic Radiology*, Blackwell, Oxford.

HATCHER v. BLACK (1954) *The Times* 29, 30th June; July 1st, 2nd (Denning, L. J.).

HINCK v. WAGNER (1970)

LENHAM, D. (1968) *Med. Sci. Law*, **8**, 80.

LENHAM, D. (1969) *Med Sci. Law*, **9**, 172.

MEDICAL DEFENCE UNION (1971) Consent to Treatment, revised edition. London: Medical Defence Union.

MITCHELL v. MOLESWORTH (1950) *Lancet*, **i**, 1168; *Brit. Med. J.*, **ii**, 171; 370.

ODAM v. YOUNG AND THE EAST ANGLIAN REGIONAL HOSPITAL BOARD (1955) *Lancet*, **ii**, 1132; *Brit. Med. J.*, **ii**, 1453.

PICKETT v. BRISTOL AEROPLANE CO. LTD. (1961) *The Times*, 17 Mar.; *Lancet*, **i**, 764 (Barrington); *Brit. Med. J.*, **i**, 975.

POLSON, M. (1984). Personal communication.

SIDAWAY v. Bethlem Royal Hospital & Others (1984) Times Law Report Feb 24th.

SPICER v. HALL (1901) *Brit. Med. J.*, **ii**, 1787.

STATUTES AND REGULATIONS

Children and Young Persons Act, 1933; 23 and 24 Geo. 5, ch. 12.

Education Act, 1944; 7 and 8 Geo. 5, ch. 31.

Family Law Reform Act, 1969; Eliz. 2, ch. 46.

Magistrates Courts Act, 1952.

Milk and Dairies (General) Regulations, 1959; S.I. No. 277.

National Health Service (Family Planning) amendment Act, 1972. Eliz. 2, ch. 72.

Public Health Act, 1936; 26 Geo. 5 and 1 Edw. 8, ch. 49.

Public Health Act, 1961; 9 & 10 Eliz. 2, ch. 6.

Public Health (Infectious Diseases) Regulations, 1953; S.I. No. 299.

Road Traffic Act, 1972; Eliz. 2, ch. 20.

CHAPTER 22

Medical Negligence

IN PRESENT times doctors cannot be sure that they will never be threatened with an action for negligence. There are patients, now numerous, who seem ready to institute proceedings, notwithstanding they have had excellent treatment, with complete cure, and without cost. It may be that the transfer of hospitals to the State, thereby enabling them to pay substantial damages and costs out of the national funds, and the possibility of legal aid for the patient, play a part. The patient has nothing to lose and, perhaps, much to gain.

It is obviously difficult for a patient to appreciate that severe disability resulting from an accident in the course of his treatment is not necessarily negligence. Unfortunately, mishaps of this kind can cause grave injury to the patient. In such circumstances, it is understandable that the patient may allege negligence and seek compensation.

Doctors are rightly disturbed by the possibility of an action for negligence. Lord Denning, in *Hatcher* v. *Black and others* (1954), likened it to a dagger. The doctor's "professional reputation was as dear to him as his body—perhaps more so. And an action for negligence could wound his reputation as severely as a dagger could his body".

Actions for negligence are decided on the facts of each case; in all questions of negligence the circumstances condition the decision. In consequence, similar or apparently similar mishaps are not necessarily found negligent. The decision, moreover, may turn on the estimate given by the judge or a jury of the weight to be attached to the witnesses' evidence. The vivid stories of the witnesses for a plaintiff prevailed over the imperfect recollection of a defendant doctor who, unfortunately, had not made notes of the case at the time of his examination of the patient, a year prior to the trial (Medical Defence Union, 1961).

Grave though the results of mishaps in treatment may be, they are often entirely out of proportion to the nature of the mishap. A needle passed only a little too deeply, or a little more to the right or the left, can cause an injected fluid to enter the spinal canal instead of the paravertebral muscles. The result, however, can be a bilateral paralysis of the legs (an accident which did not result in litigation). Operative correction of squint resulted in injury to the retina and loss of an eye, yet the accident followed an incision only a fraction too deep into the wall of the eye, which, in the operation area, is of the order of about 1 mm thick (*White* v. *Board of Governors of the Westminster Hospital and another*, 1961).

It is not irrelevant to remind ourselves that accidents in treatment, regrettable though they are, occur but rarely; they form only a small proportion of the thousands of operations annually performed in our hospitals. Whenever they occur, no matter whether litigation results or is a possibility, a private inquiry should be held in the hospital in order to establish the cause and, whenever practicable, to introduce measures which will prevent a recurrence of the accident.

This survey of the subject, of course, is not a complete account; its full treatment requires a separate monograph written, preferably, by a practising advocate in conjunction with, or advised by, a competent medical practitioner.

Membership of a Medical Defence Society

The principal message of this chapter is to emphasise the importance to all registered medical practitioners in active practice, regardless of their field of practice, to belong to a medical defence society. And, whenever the possibility, however remote, of an action alleging negligence arises, they will consult their defence society without delay. If they then act in accordance with advice given, they can rely on full support. In no circumstances should they first take independent action, because they may then find that the defence society is unable to give assistance. Incidentally, this applies also to circumstances where the practitioner is required to appear before the General Medical Council.

Definition of Negligence

Negligence was defined by Baron Alderson in *Blyth* v. *Birmingham Waterworks Co.* (1856) as "the omission to do something which a reasonable man . . . would do, or doing something which a prudent and reasonable man would not do". It could be defined as a failure to perform the duty to exercise a reasonable degree of skill and care in the treatment of a patient.

Negligence, however, is a complex, as defined by Lord Wright in the *Lochgelly Iron and Coal Co.* v. *McMullan* (1934). There must be a duty owed; there has been a breach of that duty, either by an act of commission or of omission, and damage is suffered by the person to whom the duty was owing. It is something more than heedless, careless conduct; if there is no damage, there is then no ground for an action for negligence.

It was suggested that medical negligence was only an example of negligence at large, but the more modern view is likely to be that expressed by Lord Denning in *Hatcher* v. *Black and others* (1954). He declined to liken the case against a hospital to a motor-car accident or an accident in a factory. "On the road or in a factory there ought not to be any accidents if everyone used proper care. But in a hospital, when a person was ill and came in for treatment, no matter what care was used there was always a risk, and it would be wrong and bad law to say that simply because a mishap occurred the hospital and doctors were liable. Indeed it would be disastrous to the community. It would mean that a doctor examining a patient or a surgeon operating at the table, instead of getting on with his work, would be for ever looking over his shoulder to see if someone was coming up with a dagger; . . . " (i.e. an action for negligence). "The jury must therefore not find him negligent simply because one of the risks inherent in an operation (or anaesthetic) actually took place, or because in a matter of opinion he made an error of judgement. They should only find him guilty when he had fallen short of the standard of reasonable medical care, when he was deserving of censure."

See also Elewes, J. in *Williams* v. *North Liverpool H.M.C. and others* (1959): "There are risks inherent in most forms of medical treatment. All that one can ask is that he should keep these risks to a minimum. If he has done this, no injury which occurs, however serious, is actionable."

The Origin of the Duty to Exercise Skill and Care

A doctor is under a duty to exercise skill and care, independently of any contract for services, from the moment he assumes responsibility for giving advice or treatment to a patient. This duty arises not only when he accepts a fee, but whenever he gives advice or treatment gratuitously or when he treats a person without reward in any emergency, e.g. when he attends an injured or unconscious person involved in a road accident (Atkin, L. J., in *Everett* v. *Griffiths* (1920), at p. 213).

This duty is not peculiar to doctors, because it may be owed by anyone who undertakes the responsibility for care and treatment. It would not normally be a defence to plead lack of knowledge or skill as an excuse if, in consequence, something went wrong. A layman, however, could clear himself if, in an emergency, he did his best within the scope of his limited knowledge.

Even where the doctor is under a contract with an employer, e.g. the National Health Service, and not with the patient himself, there is a duty to the patient once the doctor assumes responsibility for advice and treatment. An action for negligence might then be brought against the doctor and his employer.

It is important to appreciate that negligent advice is just as actionable as negligent treatment. It must be something more than casual advice; there must be evidence of assumption of responsibility, e.g. the payment of a fee. The layman who gives casual advice is not liable. When a fireman had inhaled poisonous fumes a passer-by, a doctor of philosophy, was asked what antidote might be used. Believing the fumes to be of an acid, he suggested, by way of casual advice, the inhalation of ammonia, which in the circumstances was useless and, indeed, harmful. He did not assume responsibility for advice or treatment (Leeds City Coroner, No. 1040/56).

A doctor, merely because he is a registered medical practitioner, is under no legal obligation to accept a patient. He is at liberty to accept or refuse to treat private patients. He is under no legal obligation, but may regard it as a moral duty, to assist anyone in need of medical care in an emergency. In these circumstances he shares with any bystander a moral duty to help those in difficulties, e.g. someone in danger of drowning. He is not liable if he refuses to assist in an emergency if the victim is someone with whom he has not, nor ever has had, a professional relationship.

The Standard of Care and Skill

The person who professes to be a doctor implies that he is competent; " . . . every person who enters into a learned profession undertakes to bring to the exercise of it a reasonable degree of care . . . ". The standard is that of an ordinary, competent practitioner in the group or specialty to which the doctor belongs.

He is not required, in order to clear himself, to show that he possesses and exercised the maximum degree of skill and care. " . . . a surgeon (does not) undertake that he will perform a cure; nor does he undertake to use the highest possible degree of skill. There may be persons who have higher education and greater advantages than he has, but he undertakes to bring a fair, reasonable and competent degree of skill. . . . " This definition of the standard, by Lord Chief Justice Tindal in *Lanphier and wife* v. *Phipos* (1838), has since been generally adopted, if phrased in slightly different terms. Erle, C. J., in *Rich and Exor.* v. *Pierpont* (1862), said "It is not enough that there has been a less degree of skill than some other medical man might have shown . . . there must have been a want of competent and ordinary care and skill . . . ". Mr. Justice Streatfield, in *Patch* v. *the Board of Governors of the Bristol United Hospitals* (1959), gave this modern definition: "The liability of doctors is not unlimited; the standard of care required of them is not that standard shown by exceptional practitioners. Surgeons, doctors and nurses are not insurers. They are not guarantors of absolute safety. They are not liable in law merely because a thing goes wrong . . . the law requires them to exercise professionally that skill and knowledge that belongs to the ordinary practitioner". This confirms what was said by Lord Justice Scott in *Mahon* v. *Osborne* (1939) at p. 548: "If he (the doctor) professes an art, he must be reasonably skilled in it . . . He must also be careful, but the standard of care which the law requires is not insurance against accidental slips. It is such a degree of care as a normally skilful member of the profession may reasonably be expected to exercise in the actual circumstances of the case in question. It is not every slip or mistake which imports negligence . . . ".

The standard applied will differ according to the circumstances. Thus the performance of any operation normally undertaken by a specialist, fixes the standard as that of a competent member of that specialty. In the event that a doctor in some other group, e.g. a general practitioner, performs an abdominal operation he must show that he has at least the ordinary competence of a surgeon. Similarly, an unqualified doctor must show that he exercised the degree of skill and care which would have been shown by a qualified practitioner, or be liable for the consequences (*Ruddock* v. *Lowe* (1965)).

This is further conditioned by the actual circumstances of the case. A ship's doctor or a general practitioner, who finds himself compelled to undertake an abdominal operation in an emergency, would clear himself if he showed that he exercised reasonable care and skill, in so far as he was able, even though it was not that of a surgeon.

Reasonable care in circumstances of unreasonable fatigue was considered in *McCormack* v. *Redpath Brown and Co. and another* (1961).

The patient sued his employers and a Hospital Management Committee, claiming damages for a head injury and alleging negligent treatment. The employers maintained that the consequence of the accident flowed from a failure to X-ray the patient at the time or to perform an immediate operation. The Hospital Management Committee admitted failure to detect a skull fracture and that, had it been found, there would have been an immediate operation. Mr. Justice Paull assessed the damages at £5250 and then considered their apportionment. The doctor's failure to X-ray the skull or to find the fracture by physical examination was outside the limits of proper care. The learned judge, however, took a most sympathetic view of the doctor's conduct. This was a young and careful doctor. It was not surprising that a young doctor should fail on occasion to measure up to the standard of reasonable care. There was a heavy burden on him, he had had scanty sleep during a stretch of duty lasting some 33 hours. Such doctors should not be over-burdened. The deterrent effect of probable complaints by the X-ray department if a casualty officer sent too many cases for X-ray examination was also taken into consideration. The Hospital Management Committee was held responsible for any consequences of the accident flowing from failure to find that a piece of bone had been driven into the patient's brain. The damages awarded were apportioned as to £4675 against the employers and £575 against the Hospital Committee.

Who Sets the Standard?

In the ordinary course of events it seems reasonable to assume that the court will rely upon the evidence of competent practitioners in the relevant field of medical practice. The case of *Hucks* v. *Cole*, however, resulted in a disturbing decision. (The details are set out in the Annual Report of the Medical Defence Union, 1969.) The case was an allegation of negligence in the conduct of ante- and post-natal care. The patient complained (a) that the doctor failed to treat a septic finger when it was first brought to his notice; (b) that he failed to alter the antibiotic treatment he prescribed a week later; he then had a bacteriological report which indicated the presence of *S. aureus* and *S. pyogenes* for which an alternative antibiotic would have been more effective; (c) it was also complained that he suspended antibiotic treatment too soon; it was contended, by a bacteriologist, called by the plaintiff, that antibiotic treatment of this patient should have been continued until there was complete involution of the uterus. Unfortunately, the patient's delivery was complicated by fulminating streptococcal septicaemia. She recovered but suffered from neurological sequelae.

The expert witnesses for the defence included two consultant obstetricians and two general practitioners, who had experience of obstetrics; the witnesses for the plaintiff were a consultant obstetrician, a forensic pathologist and the consultant bacteriologist.

The trial judge exonerated the doctor in respect of the first two complaints but he considered the doctor to have been negligent in that he had failed to continue antibiotic treatment during the puerperium. It appears that this was based on the evidence of the bacteriologist alone. The witnesses for the defence, all of whom agreed that the doctor's conduct of the case was such as they would have adopted in similar circumstances, did not prevail, although they were described by the judge as "obviously very honest witnesses doing their best to help me in a very difficult case".

The judge found for the plaintiff and awarded her £2500 and costs. Appeal to the Court of Appeal was dismissed but a cross-appeal led to an increase in the damages to £4000. Leave to appeal to the House of Lords was refused. A petition for leave to appeal was also refused by the Appeals Committee of the House of Lords. In consequence, a ruling by their lordships as to when and in what circumstances a practice which would be followed by a substantial number of competent and careful professional men might properly be held to be a negligent practice was not obtained. Also a ruling was denied on the extent of precautions which would be necessary, however remote the risk, lest a practitioner might be held negligent. The decision is not a precedent for a change in the law. The *British Medical Journal* hoped that "this approach to the facts will not be indicated in other cases in the future. It need not be" (*Bri. Med. J.*, 1967).

Approved Practice as a Criterion of Reasonable Care

It is not infrequent that evidence is led to establish that reasonable care had been exercised by showing that what was done was in accordance with general, approved practice. The courts appear ready to attach considerable weight to the evidence of competent and experienced doctors on this matter. Lord Goddard, in *Mahon* v. *Osborne* (1939), said, "I cannot imagine anything more disastrous to the community than to leave it to a jury, or to a judge sitting alone, to lay down what it is proper to do in any particular case without the guidance of witnesses who are qualified to speak on the subject". "A doctor is not guilty of negligence if he acted in accordance with a practice accepted as proper by a responsible body of medical men skilled in that particular art" (McNair, J., cited with approval by Sellers, L. J., in *Landau* v. *Werner* (1961), who phrased the test thus: "Had he acted in accordance with a practice accepted as proper by fellow specialists?").

It by no means follows that such guidance is inflexible. The court, in considering the circumstances, will pronounce the practice negligent if it is apparent that it has inherent defects which ought to have been obvious to anyone giving the matter due consideration. It is not enough to refute negligence to say that what was done was precisely what everyone else did; this defence was of no avail in *Markland* v. *Manchester Corporation* (1934). A risky practice may well be held negligent, notwithstanding that it is widely followed; "when simple methods to avoid danger have been devised, are known, and are available, non-use with fatal results cannot be justified by saying that others have followed the same old, less careful practice . . . the existence of a practice which neglects them, even if the practice were general, cannot protect the defendant surgeon" (*Anderson* v. *Chasney*, 1949, 1950).

Failure to adopt generally approved methods of diagnosis or treatment in the appropriate circumstances is a perilous course. Thus, the omission of X-ray examination in circumstances where a fracture or dislocation was suspected, or ought to have been suspected, may be sufficient to establish lack of reasonable care. In the matter of treatment, failure to give anti-tetanic serum, in circumstances where this is generally recognised as a proper step, is to invite censure.

However, it should be noted that as medical practice evolves, so the criteria of "accepted practice" changes. In the context of the invariable necessity to X-ray head injuries, there has been something of a revolt amongst radiologists in recent years. Both on the grounds of unnecessary expense, harmful radiation but above all doubtful efficacy, it is no longer felt obligatory to submit all sufferers from a head injury to skull radiography. It has been pointed out that the presence or absence of a skull fracture is often irrelevant to both the severity of intracranial damage and the course of treatment. It is the clinical and especially neurological examination which is more important—and which of course can also provide the substrate for a negligence action. Usually the regime of treatment will be the same whether or not the X-rays reveal a fracture; careful analyses of large numbers of cases from Accident and Emergency Departments have shown that the practice of invariably X-raying head injuries has arisen from fears of medico-legal consequences, rather than from clinical necessity and now a doctor can more easily justify his decision not to insist upon skull radiography when challenged by an aggrieved patient (Evans and Knight, 1981).

A somewhat similar change has occurred in relation to automatic anti-tetanus injections following a dirty wound. Some serious reaction to the protein component of such injections and the diminishing prevalence of tetanus in the community make the procedure no longer as mandatory as in former years.

There could be circumstances in which failure to administer an antibiotic would be held negligent. In *Jones* v. *the Welsh Regional Hospital Board and Kemp* (1961), it was claimed that failure to administer penicillin had caused, or contributed to, the loss of an eye. By an oversight, the prescribed dose of penicillin was not administered until a delay of 5 days had elapsed. It was decided that, in the circumstances, the patient had only been deprived of the hope of the recovery of his eye. A foreign body had penetrated to the vitreous and virulent panophthalmitis ensued. This condition, however, had become established by the evening of the day of the accident and the prospect of saving the eye was then, at best, distinctly remote. Loss of hope could be sufficient damage to found an action, but it must be a measurable hope; in this case it was so remote that it did not justify a finding against a defendant.

Romer, L.J., in *Chapman* v. *Rix* (1958, 1960), in allowing the appeal, held that Doctor R. had not been negligent because it was not a usual and normal practice to communicate in the circumstances. He adopted the test applied by Lord Clyde in *Hunter* v. *Hanley* (1954), at p. 213. In order to establish liability by a doctor, where a departure from normal practice is alleged, it must be established: (a) that there is a usual and normal practice; (b) that practice was not adopted and, a crucial matter, (c) that the course adopted is one no professional man of ordinary skill would have taken, if acting with ordinary care. In the present case these three conditions were not satisfied. Usual practice could be negligent in some cases. Was the doctor aware, or ought he to have been aware, that the practice was inadequate?

The Duty to be Well-informed

A doctor is under no legal obligation to subscribe to any particular method of diagnosis or treatment. On the contrary, the Medical Act, 1956, section 14 prohibits the imposition upon any candidate offering himself for examination to adopt, or to refrain from adopting, the practice of any particular theory of medicine or surgery as a test or condition of admitting him to examination or of granting a certificate. It follows that the registered practitioner is free to exercise his judgement and discretion. At the same time, anyone who adopts a novel course of treatment or omits to use some form of diagnosis or treatment which has gained general approval, must be able to justify his action if anything goes wrong; success is the best justification (*Landau* v. *Werner* (1961)).

There is a duty to be well-informed of developments in medical practice and ignorance of them might lead to an action for negligence, as in the case of *Crawford* v. *Board of Governors of Charing Cross Hospital* (1953).

That action arose out of an accident in the course of blood transfusion and was based upon an alleged failure by the practitioner concerned to keep abreast with modern techniques.

The patient underwent an operation on his bladder, during the course of which he received a blood transfusion. He had lost the use of one arm, sometime prior to the operation, as a result of poliomyelitis. When he recovered from the anaesthetic he found that both of his arms were paralysed. Abduction of his sound arm during the blood transfusion had led to brachial paralysis.

The anaesthetist, who administered the blood, had not read and applied findings reported by Ewing (1950). That article drew attention to the dangers of abduction of the arm during transfusion; five cases, there described, demonstrated that this error could cause brachial paralysis. The anaesthetist admitted that he had not read the article, but he was aware of it. He had not troubled to read it because, in his long experience, he had never encountered this complication and he was satisfied that his own precautions were adequate. Gerrard, J., however, believed that "nice questions might arise as to how far a medical man could excuse his ignorance of a technical development he had not met in his reading of his professional journals . . ."; there was "a duty to follow up the writings on a subject which concerned him closely". The doctor was severely criticised for his failure to make himself aware of the opinions of distinguished men in an important subject so closely affecting his own work. There had been negligence and damages were assessed at £4000.

The Court of Appeal set aside the verdict because, in their view, if the evidence of negligence was no more than a failure to keep abreast of the professional journals, it was not enough. "It would be putting much too high a burden upon the medical men to say that they must read every article in the medical press." There was, also, evidence that abduction of the arm up to 90° during blood transfusion would do no harm; that "in only approximately one-third of 1 per cent of such operations did brachial palsy follow, and generally it was not permanent".

Notwithstanding this decision, it is prudent at least to glance at current journals at not too infrequent intervals and, if articles appear relating to matters within the doctor's range of practice, he should at least read the summary and conclusions. When it happens that a series of articles points to some current accident, it is surely worthwhile to take note of it and consider whether any modification of one's own methods is necessary. It is indeed too much to expect a busy practitioner to read each and every article, even when they concern only a specialty, but it is not too time-consuming to note the contents tables of a number of journals in a medical library and to select articles for more particular notice. The preliminary selection can be delegated to a competent secretary. It is also possible for members of one society to obtain information concerning recent articles.

The Duty to Make an Accurate Diagnosis

The doctor who accepts a patient does not overtly or by implication, promise to make an accurate diagnosis. His responsibility is fulfilled when he has exercised reasonable care and skill in making the diagnosis. He is not an insurer and therefore does not warrant a cure. Nor is he negligent by reason alone of errors in diagnosis. This is illustrated by the case of *Whiteford* v. *Hunter* (1948; 1950), on which the *Lancet* (1948) made the comment that when a wrong diagnosis is neither impossible nor unreasonable at the time and in the circumstances of the case, nothing but overwhelming evidence to the contrary should justify a finding of negligence.

Whiteford v. *Hunter and Gleed* (1950). In 1942 Mr. Whiteford consulted Dr. Gleed, a general practitioner, on account of retention of urine. In the belief that the illness required surgical treatment, Dr. Gleed referred the patient to Mr. Hunter, a consulting surgeon. As a result of his examination of the patient, which included a rectal examination, Mr. Hunter concluded that the cause was prostatic enlargement. He advised drainage of the bladder and prostatectomy. It appears that no cystoscopic examination was made prior to opening the bladder. Inspection of the interior of the bladder showed that there was an indurated mass, about the size of the palm of a man's hand, near its base. Its appearances led Mr. Hunter to the erroneous conclusion that this was an inoperable carcinoma. A biopsy was not performed.

After this operation Mr. Whiteford's wife was informed of the diagnosis of cancer and told that the probable expectation of the patient's life was only a matter of months. Mr. Whiteford, in this belief, gave up his post, sold his home in England and went to reside in America, where his wife's family lived. When he reached America Mr. Whiteford consulted another surgeon, a Dr. Barringer. Cystoscopy then detected what appeared to be the mouth of a diverticulum of the bladder. An operation was performed in September 1942 and a diverticulum, filled with calcareous material, was excised; a biopsy of the prostate gland was also taken. The prostate was small and fibrotic but no trace of cancer was found in it, nor in the bladder.

On his recovery, Mr. Whiteford returned to England and, in 1945, brought an action for damages against Dr. Gleed and Mr. Hunter, alleging negligence on their part and that he had suffered loss in consequence of their erroneous diagnosis.

At the trial Birkett, J., dismissed Dr. Gleed from the case because he was under no obligation to possess the special equipment required for the diagnosis of Mr. Whiteford's complaint and, although present at the operation, the patient was then in Mr. Hunter's care. Mr. Hunter, however, was found negligent because he had not used a cystoscope and had not made a biopsy. Having pronounced "a virtual sentence of death" he had done nothing afterwards to confirm or verify it, although the means of verification were available. This view was taken by the learned judge in spite of Mr. Hunter's explanation that he was sufficiently certain of the diagnosis by naked-eye inspection and palpation, and that it was not necessary or wise to perform a biopsy. Mr. Hunter believed that this step might have involved serious risk of perforating the bladder and, if the trouble had been cancer, biopsy might have left an ulcer, difficult to heal. The damages were assessed at £6300.

Mr. Hunter was successful in the Court of Appeal, where it was held that the law did not assume that medical practitioners guarantee accurate diagnosis and that not every slip or mistake constitutes negligence. The Court preferred the evidence of Mr. Hunter to that of Dr. Barringer, the American surgeon, whose evidence on behalf of Mr. Whiteford was given on commission; he had not been before the court as a witness.

Mr. Whiteford's appeal to the House of Lords was dismissed. Lord Porter followed Lord Maugham, L. J., in *Marshall* v. *Lindsey County Council* (1900) when it was held that "a defendant charged with negligence can clear himself if he shows that he acted in accord with general and approved practice". The defendant surgeon had given evidence that his action conformed with the approved practice of the profession and this had been supported by the evidence of two eminent surgeons.

In the event that the diagnosis was palpably wrong or inadequate steps were taken to make the diagnosis, the doctor may be found negligent. In the case of *Elder* v. *Greenwich and Deptford Hospital Management Committee* (1953) a casualty officer was held negligent because he failed to diagnose acute appendicitis in a child aged 11 years. She complained of severe abdominal pain and vomiting; on examination she winced when the right side of her abdomen was palpated. She was not admitted to hospital, but sent home with instructions to return if the pain continued. She died and an action alleging negligence was successful. Damages were assessed at £350. Again, in *Wood* v. *Thurston* (1951), failure to diagnose the occurrence of multiple fractures was held negligent. The patient was seen in a casualty department and deemed to be drunk. He was allowed to return home; he was later sent to a hospital where he died a few hours later. The post-mortem examination disclosed a fractured collar bone and fractures involving eighteen ribs, nine on each side. Failure to diagnose, and not failure to treat, the condition was held negligent.

Abdominal injuries are a potential source of litigation. There may be no external sign of injury and, at the time of the examination, no serious complaint or other indication of grave internal trouble; the lull, as it were, before the storm. Such cases, especially when there is a history of a substantial blow to the abdomen, and more so if the patient complains of pain, should be subject to guarded prognosis and the patient advised to remain under skilled observation for a reasonable period. A kick from a horse to a patient's abdomen ruptured the intestine and death occurred from peritonitis. At the time of the examination the grave internal injury was neither diagnosed nor suspected. Horses are becoming increasingly rare, but blows of appreciably less force than a kick from a horse can do grave internal intra-abdominal injury, e.g. rupture of liver or kidney (F.M. 8143 B).

Erroneous interpretation of a radiogram has been held negligent. On that occasion a casualty officer saw fit himself to interpret the appearances and failed to recognise a broken neck. He was held negligent, because he did not obtain the opinion of a radiologist who was available for consultation (*Fraser* v. *Vancouver Hosp.*, 1951–2; Canadian case). It is even clearer evidence of negligence if there is a failure to make, or arrange for, radiological examination in circumstances which call for one (*McCormack* v. *Redpath Brown and Co. and another* (1961)). This will be conditioned by the circumstances. The patient may be too ill to be subjected to X-ray examination or there may not be access to the apparatus. The doctor, however, is not negligent merely because he fails immediately to obtain X-ray examination. The timing of that examination depends on the circumstances. Providing the patient is under skilled observation, X-ray of the skull for a suspected fracture need not be immediate; indeed, it might be detrimental to the patient. (V. Supra, p. 643)

The Duty to Inform a Patient of the Risks attending Treatment

"In a hospital, when a person who was ill and came in for treatment, no matter what care was used there was always a risk . . ." (Lord Denning in *Hatcher* v. *Black* (1954)). There is always some risk involved in every operation under general anaesthesia. To what extent is a doctor obliged to inform his patient or his patient's relatives, of these risks?

Where there are special, known risks, the patient should be made aware of them before he consents to the treatment. If that has been done, then there is no liability for any injury of the kind which results from such risks. Electro-convulsion therapy provides an example. The patient was warned that fracture of the spine was a possible risk of this treatment, but he agreed to undergo it. He sustained a fracture of his eighth dorsal vertebra and later sued for negligence. Verdict for the defendants (*Davies* v. *Horton Road and Colney Hatch Hospital Management Committee and Logan* (1954)). It is now the practice to obtain written consent in terms which draw attention to the risk of injury.

The doctor is not required to bring to the notice of the patient each and every possible risk; he is not negligent because he failed to mention some remote risk. Otherwise patients might be faced with a formidable list and few would then consent to treatment which, for the majority, would be highly beneficial. To detail every possible risk might entail mention of such remote possibilities as collapse of the ceiling of the operating theatre. There is no negligence where the risk is negligible.

An example of a remote possibility is provided by the case of *Warren* v. *Grieg and White* (1935). Following the extraction of twenty-eight teeth, the patient suffered severe bleeding. It was subsequently found that he had a then rare blood disease, namely leukaemia. The patient alleged negligence because the dentist had failed to arrange for a blood examination prior to dental treatment. Although a dentist may well have the possibility of haemophilia in mind, and make suitable inquiry before attempting extraction, he cannot be expected to consider or warn the patient of the distinctly remote risk of severe bleeding due to leukaemia. It is impracticable to make a blood examination as a routine test before performing extractions. In this case the risk was deemed too remote for failure to draw attention to it to constitute negligence.

The position of the doctor who has to advise a nervous patient to undergo an operation may well be difficult. How much should he tell of the possible risks involved? Lord Denning (then L.J.) in *Hatcher* v. *Black* (1954) gave an indication. In that case the surgeon knew there was some slight risk and admitted that he had told the patient there was none. But he did it for her good, because he did not want her to worry. "He told a lie, but he did it because in the circumstances it was justifiable. . . . This, however, is not a court of morals and the law left the question to the conscience of the doctor himself—though if doctors had too easy a conscience on this matter, they might in time lose the confidence of the patient which was the basis of all good medicine. But the law did not condemn the doctor when he only did what a wise doctor so placed would do. None of the doctors called as witnesses had condemned him—why should the jury?" In this case, the patient suffered from toxic goitre and had accepted thyroidectomy. She had asked if the operation would affect her voice and it was deemed wise to reassure her, notwithstanding it was known there was a slight risk of injury to the recurrent laryngeal nerves. It was imperative that she should not worry. Unfortunately, the left recurrent laryngeal nerve was injured.

The Duty to Communicate with Other Doctors

When a patient has received treatment in an emergency, e.g. in a casualty department, and is then sent home, the doctor who gave the treatment has a duty to communicate with the patient's own doctor by telephone or by letter. It is not enough to tell the patient that on his return home he should consult his own doctor, and leave it to the patient to report the diagnosis and treatment.

This duty to communicate is not a legal obligation, but in view of the case of *Chapman* v. *Rix* (1958–60), it is clear that failure to communicate may result in litigation. Judicial opinion was almost evenly divided, 4:5, on whether this failure constituted negligence; on a subsequent occasion the opinion will probably incline yet further towards negligence. Be that as it may, the practical lesson of the case is clear.

Chapman, a butcher, while boning some meat, let his knife slip and he wounded his abdomen. A general practitioner, Dr. Rix, who was also on the staff of the local cottage hospital, was summoned and, after he had examined the patient in his shop, advised his transfer to the hospital so that a more extensive examination could be made and treatment given. There was no resident surgical staff at that hospital and the patient was re-examined by Dr. Rix. In his opinion, the wound extended to the deeper layers of the abdominal wall, but there had been no penetration of the peritoneum. The wound was stitched and the patient was sent home with the express instruction to consult his own doctor and inform him of what had been done. No letter was given by Dr. Rix, nor did he have any telephone conversation with the patient's doctor.

The patient summoned his own doctor, Dr. M., that evening, by which time he was complaining of abdominal pain and nausea. The patient said he had received treatment for an abdominal injury and that it had been deemed superficial. Dr. M. did not appear to have inquired further into the circumstances of the injury and was under the impression that the patient had been seen by a casualty officer; he had not realised that in fact the hospital was a cottage hospital without surgical staff and that the examination and treatment had been given by another general practitioner. In consequence he dismissed the abdominal injury as a factor and diagnosed a digestive upset, for which he prescribed liquid paraffin. General peritonitis set in and the patient died 5 days after the accident. Post-mortem examination showed that there had been penetration of the peritoneum and the small intestine had been perforated by the butcher's knife at the time of the accident.

The widow sued Dr. Rix alleging negligence on several grounds, but he was found negligent on one alone, namely failure to communicate directly by telephone or letter with the patient's own doctor. He was absolved from negligence on the ground that he had failed to make a correct diagnosis. Damages were assessed at £9050 by Barry, J., when he gave judgment for the plaintiff.

Dr. Rix appealed successfully. Romer and Wilman, L.JJ. allowed the appeal but Morris, L. J., in a dissenting judgment, absolved the patient's own doctor from negligence and held that he should have been made aware by Dr. Rix of the need for further observation. On the other hand, it was argued, if Dr. Rix was to be held negligent, why not Dr. M. also? That doctor knew the patient had stabbed himself and he should have considered the possible dangers. He also had the advantage of knowing what Dr. Rix could not know, that the patient was then complaining of abdominal pain and nausea.

The widow appealed to the House of Lords, where the decision of the Court of Appeal was upheld by a majority, 3:2. In dismissing the appeal, the view was taken that although the patient would be expected to pass on the reassuring part of Dr. Rix's message, that did not cancel out the main part, i.e. an emphatic warning that the patient's own doctor should be called in. If Dr. Rix had spoken to Dr. M. he would no doubt have told him that the patient needed watching. Was Dr. M. to know this without being told? Lord Keith and

Lord Denning, who dissented, held that he should have been told. A doctor might give the patient reassuring but misleading information. Some communication was necessary, but if the mode was inadequate it was negligent. In Lord Keith's view, the message was misleading. The second doctor should have had the information of what was observed and done by the first doctor, otherwise he was at a disadvantage in making his diagnosis. Non-communication was not really a medical question; it was scarcely in the category of professional negligence. Lord Denning also believed that Dr. M. had been misled. Misleading information was a dangerous thing. A doctor might give the patient misleading information to reassure him, but, in that event, true information should be given to the relatives and, most important of all, to his own doctor. This was not done. An elementary rule had been broken. He held Dr. Rix negligent. Lord Goddard, Lord Morton of Henryton and Lord Hodson, however, did not and, in consequence, the appeal was allowed.

Nine judges had considered the facts of this case; five absolved Dr. Rix and four condemned him. For future practice, however, it is prudent to heed the dissenting judgments, notably that of Lord Denning.

The Duty to Obey a Summons for Attendance

A private patient has the right to summon his doctor to attend him during the course of some current illness and the doctor fails to obey that summons at his peril. In one view, this right is extinguished when the patient recovers or dies or dismisses the doctor, but Lord Nathan (1955) considered that the right of summons to give attendance continues beyond a particular illness and remains so long as the patient may reasonably be regarded as the patient of that doctor.

Patients in the N.H.S. have a right to summon the doctor to give attendance, if they are on his list, and he is obliged by his contract with the N.H.S. to render all proper and necessary treatment. It may be that this right does not extend to times beyond his surgery hours, when the matter is not an emergency, but it is not always simple to determine, without seeing the patient, whether the circumstances are other than an emergency. Refusal, or failure, to attend might result in an action for breach of duty and negligence, a summons before the Health Authority and, perhaps, also before the Professional Conduct Committee of the G.M.C.

A general practitioner was censured by the London Executive Council, because he failed to visit a patient, on his list at that time, who died at home. This inquiry followed the coroner's verdict that death was due to acute pneumonia, aggravated by lack of care. In mitigation, it was claimed that the doctor had been misled by a letter about the patient from a hospital. The doctor decided there was no urgency and said he would call next morning. Another practitioner was summoned to make an emergency visit, but the patient died before he arrived. The first doctor had also issued a certificate of incapacity, unsupported by a medical examination (*Lancet*, 1962).

When any patient summons a doctor, then, according to the known requirements of the illness, he should be prompt to attend and should be regular in his attendance, he should show reasonable diligence. It is necessary to show that there was avoidable injury, or deterioration in the patient, before alleged inadequate attendance amounts to negligence.

The birth of a baby before the arrival of the doctor is not of itself evidence of negligence. It must be shown that the patient thereby suffered injury and the doctor's delay was unreasonable, e.g. due to forgetfulness or idleness on his part.

When the surgeon contracts personally to operate on a patient, he cannot delegate that duty to another without the consent of the patient. The surgeon, however, is not bound by such a contract personally to supervise any post-operative treatment normally delegated to the nursing staff. He would not be required personally to replace or shorten a drainage tube which he had inserted (*Morris* v. *Winsbury-White* (1937)).

Retention of Swabs, Packs, Instruments, Drains, etc.

The responsibility for the recovery of swabs used at an operation lies with the surgeon. "As it is the task of the surgeon to put the swabs in, so it is his task to take them out, and in that task he must use that degree of care which is reasonable in the circumstances and that must depend on the evidence. If on the whole of the evidence it is shown that he did not use that standard of care, he cannot absolve himself if a mistake be made, by saying 'I relied on the nurse' . . . ; unless there be evidence that the nature of the case be such that no search of any description—be it by eye, finger or mechanical means—was possible, a surgeon cannot show that he used reasonable care in that part of the operation which consisted of taking out the swabs by saying 'I relied on the nurse's count'" (Goddard, L. J. in *Mahon* v. *Osborne* (1939), at pp. 559, 560). Lord Goddard, however, considered the nurse's count important and failure by the surgeon to ask if the count was right would be an omission of a very necessary precaution. But the surgeon does not discharge his duty by merely asking and being told that the count is right. The circumstances, in which reliance on the nurse's count alone would be sufficient, must be such that the emergency was so great that the surgeon could not carry out an adequate search without endangering the patient's life.

The recurrence of these cases caused the *Lancet* (1961) to publish Mr. Clayton's report of the case of *Cooper* v. *Nevill* (1961) under the sub-head of "The eternal swab".

The Medical Defence Union (1960) summarised the surgeon's duty as follows: he must satisfy himself that (a) the current system for counting swabs is efficient and the persons on whom the duty falls are familiar with it and are competent to follow it; (b) that that system was followed during the operation and the count showed that all swabs used were accounted for; (c) he himself must take all reasonable precautions to verify that all the swabs used were recovered. He must recall the number and position of the swabs he inserted. Before concluding the operation he should make a visual and manual search of the operation field, in so far as that is compatible with the safety and welfare of his patient.

The desirability of having tapes attached to packs used in gynaecological surgery was considered in *Urry and Urry* v. *Bierer and others* (1955). Substantial damages, namely £3000, were awarded by Pearson, J. to the patient and £1146 to her husband, because a pack or swab had been left in the patient's body after a caesarian section. These packs, about 10 in. square, normally had tapes attached to them but this gynaecologist did not make use of tapes. Evidence was led to show the practice of other surgeons. The trial judge's view was that this evidence did not disclose any convincing reason why tapes should not generally be used; everyone seemed to agree they were an additional precaution. On appeal, Lord Justice Singleton, in agreeing with this view, considered that a surgeon who discarded or disregarded that safeguard could be said to place an additional burden on himself.

The sister's count of swabs had been wrong and responsibility for this was admitted by the sister and her employers. This count was an independent, additional check for the protection of the patient and the surgeon. The surgeon insisted that he was entitled to rely on the sister's count. His technique did not include any particular effort to remember or to have himself reminded of the location of particular packs. In the opinion of Hodson, L. J. the surgeon fell far short of the standard of care required of him and he was equally responsible with the sister. Appeal dismissed. Leave to appeal to the House of Lords refused.

In the case of *Garner* v. *Morrell and another* (1953) a patient died of asphyxia because he inhaled or swallowed a throat pack inserted prior to the extraction of teeth under general anaesthesia. Counsel for the defence had claimed that this was an unfortunate mishap which could not reasonably have been foreseen; that it happened was not proof of negligence. It appears that the throat pack used was too short. The defendants were called upon to explain the mishap, but their explanation had largely broken down (Somervell, L.J.). In the opinion of Denning (then L. J.) who agreed, the accident was one which could and should have been avoided; the facts of the case called loudly for an explanation by the defendants. Appeal dismissed; leave to appeal refused.

In 1961 and again in 1963 the Medical Defence Union, in conjunction with the Royal College of Nursing, prepared two memoranda; the first dealt with the possible causes of retention of swabs and instruments in the bodies of patients and suggested procedure to prevent these mishaps; the second was concerned with operations on the wrong patient, the wrong limb or digit. These were followed in 1965 by the well-known film "Make no Mistake", which has been widely circulated amongst the profession.

Despite the excellent propaganda, retention of swabs was reported again and again. Even in 1968 the society had had reports of forty-four cases of retained swabs. There is rarely any explanation and when the fact that a swab or instrument was retained is established, the plaintiff has only to prove that he had suffered damage; the onus is upon the surgeon to prove that he was not negligent. In consequence these claims are nearly always settled out of court and settlement can be expensive.

About the only defence to retention of a swab or instrument is that the circumstances were such that the operation had to be concluded with speed and delay; to search for a missing swab or instrument would have imperilled the life of the patient. This might serve to exonerate a surgeon in this country but not in America.

By 1979, the M.D.U. reported a slight decline in the number of retained swabs but the incidence of all foreign objects left behind at operation rose from 28 in 1970 to 115 by 1979.

Operations on the Wrong Patient or the Wrong Part of a Patient

These mistakes continue despite the advice on the safeguards freely available.

The range of possible mistakes is wide, ranging from an operation on the wrong digit to an operation on the wrong patient; sometimes it has been performed on the wrong side or the wrong limb. For examples, see the annual reports of the defence societies. These mistakes can be costly in disablement of the patient and in money to the defence society.

SAFEGUARDS

A memorandum was prepared jointly by the M.D.U., the Royal College of Nursing and the National Council of Nurses in the U.K.; its second revision was published in 1969 and the two principal safeguards recommended are:

(a) The side on which the operation is to be performed should be marked before the patient reaches the theatre and the mark should be made with an indelible skin pencil where it may be seen clearly by the surgeon before starting the operation. The mark should be made on or near the operation site and this is particularly important in the case of digits. The only exception would be the accident case with obvious wounds needing attention.

(b) In order to avoid ambiguity concerning the digit(s) on which the operation is to be performed, the following nomenclature should always be used:

The fingers should be described as thumb, index, middle, ring and little fingers and not as 1st, 2nd, 3rd, 4th and 5th and the toes as hallux (or big), 2nd, 3rd, 4th and 5th (or little).

Contamination of a Spinal Anaesthetic by Disinfectant

The cases of *Roe* v. *Ministry of Health* (1954) and *Woolley* v. *Ministry of Health* (1954) were the result of tragic accidents. Both patients received a spinal anaesthetic in 1947 for the treatment of relatively simple complaints. Unfortunately the ampoules of anaesthetic had been stored in a solution of phenol which had percolated the containers through invisible cracks or molecular flaws. In consequence both men sustained severe spastic paralysis due to the action of phenol and were permanently paralysed from the waist down. The trial judge, McNair, J., rejected the suggestion that the maxim *res ipsa loquitur* applied and gave judgment for the defendants. This decision was affirmed on appeal but the court disagreed on the application of the maxim. Denning, L. J. believed it applied. The facts did speak for themselves. They certainly called for an explanation. However, applying the standard of medical knowledge as it was in 1947, not that of 1954 at the time of the appeal, it was clear that neither the anaesthetist nor any member of the hospital staff could have known the danger of storing the ampoules in phenol and they were not negligent. In the unlikely event that the circumstances of these cases recurred, the defendant would have no cause for complaint if found negligent. Even if unaware of these cases, he should be familiar with Professor Mackintosh's textbook which contains a clear warning to avoid storage of ampoules of anaesthetic solutions in phenol or alcohol.

The case is also important for the dictum of Denning, L. J. While recognising the terrible consequences of these accidents he considered "it would be a disservice to the community at large if we were to impose liability on hospitals for everything that happens to go wrong. Doctors would be led to think more of their own safety than of the good of their patients. Initiative would be stifled and confidence shaken. A proper sense of proportion requires us to have regard to the conditions in which hospitals and doctors have to work. We must insist on due care for the patient at every point, but we must not condemn as negligence that which is only a misadventure".

Administration of the Wrong Substance

The allegation that a wrong substance has been administered is normally un-answerable, but it is not always a simple task to determine responsibility for the mistake.

A recurring error is the administration of a substance of the right kind, but in the wrong strength. The application to an eye of silver nitrate was in a strength of 20 per cent in error for a 2 per cent solution. Despite prompt irrigation of the eye with saline, the patient was deemed to be likely to suffer permanently some loss of vision and photophobia (M.D.U. 1960).

Local anaesthetics have also given rise to mistakes, because the solution used was in incorrect strength, a special risk when two preparations of rather similar name, but of very different strength, were on the market. Being colourless fluids, local anaesthetics can also be confused with other fluids, e.g. ether.

The cases of mishap show that it is not enough for the doctor to rely on the nursing staff, even on an experienced sister, to hand the correct solution in a small bowl or gallipot. If error is to be reduced to a minimum, the doctor should see the bottle or ampoule from which the solution is to be taken and personally verify the label. The eye injury mentioned above would have thus been avoided. In the second case, when ether was used instead of a local anaesthetic, the mistake would have been avoided if the contents of the gallipot had been smelt before, instead of after, the injection.

Doctors and nurses, having checked the label of the container, have discharged their responsibility. In the event that some dispensing error has occurred, it is imperative that the remainder of the fluid used and the stock bottle or ampoule are set aside for appropriate tests. These may be analytical or, as in one case, bacteriological; on the latter occasion gas gangrene followed the injection of an iron preparation into the buttock.

The possible defendants to an action for negligence on these occasions are the doctor and the hospital management committee. Failure by the doctor to take adequate precautions may result in the hospital management committee disclaiming responsibility, notwithstanding that a member of the nursing staff contributed to the mishap. It may be claimed that the absolute responsibility rests on the doctor. He should take care to verify the substance he is using; he cannot plead he had accepted the word of the nurse or sister. It is for him to see the bottle or ampoule before using any of the contents.

The Medical Defence Union (1960), however, considered that, having been handed a solution by an experienced sister as the right one, the surgeon had fulfilled his responsibilities. Although in that case the hospital authority eventually settled the claim, a personal check of the labelling by the doctor is a prudent, if not obligatory, step on all of these occasions.

A death occurred when cocaine was injected in error for procaine. On this occasion the surgeon had instructed his house surgeon by telephone. She misheard him and thought he had said cocaine. The hospital pharmacist was asked to prepare a solution of 100 ml of 1 per cent cocaine. Although 20 ml of it constituted a lethal dose he dispensed the solution without making further inquiry and, moreover, it was dispensed without written confirmation of the prescription by a doctor. At the operation the sister filled a syringe with the solution and handed it to the surgeon who then injected it. He maintained he had first asked if it was 1 per cent procaine and that the sister had replied, "Yes". This she denied. It was found that the inquiry was made after, rather than prior to, the injection. Judgment for the plaintiff and damages, £2500, were shared by the County Council and the surgeon (*Collins* v. *Herts. County Council and another* (1947)).

Paralysis of a Hand Due to Negligent Splinting

The patient had a Dupuytren's contracture of his left hand. This was treated by operation and the hand and forearm were bandaged to a splint. It remained so for some 14 days. During this time he complained of severe pain but apart from receiving sedatives nothing was done. Eventually, when the splint was removed, all four fingers of the hand were stiff and the hand was practically useless. The patient did not question the operative skill but alleged that the post-operative care was negligent. The facts showed a *prima facie* case of negligence and this was not rebutted. The importance of the case bears on the liability of hospital authorities in these circumstances. Much discussion in the past has been directed to the question of whether the doctor concerned was under a contract of service or a contract for services. Denning, L.J. made it clear that the liability for the negligence of a doctor depends upon who employs him. If the doctor has been selected and employed by the patient the hospital authority is not liable for his negligence but it is liable if the doctor is employed and paid by the hospital authority. Streatfield, J. had found for the defendants but the appeal succeeded (*Cassidy* v. *Ministry of Health* (*Fahrni, third party* (1951)).

Breakage of Needles

The breakage of a needle, causing part of it to lodge in the body of the patient, is not *prima facie* evidence of negligence and the maxim *res ipsa loquitur* does not apply to these cases. The decided cases tend to establish that this mishap is devoid of negligence. A patient may unexpectedly flinch violently, so as to cause the break. Failure to inform the patient or the patient's relatives or the patient's own doctor might be deemed negligent, as in *Gerber* v. *Pines* (1935). If extraction of the retained portion is impracticable at the time, arrangements must be made for this at a later date.

In *Hunter* v. *Hanley* (1954), S.L.T. 303 and (1955), S.L.T. 213 (Appeal), it was alleged that breakage of the needle was caused by its withdrawal at an angle different to that at which it was inserted. It was also alleged that the needle used was too thin for that purpose.

Another case arose out of the breakage of a needle, alleged to have been too short and pushed in too far; it was a No. 16 needle, 30/32 in. long, which broke close to the mount. The portion left in the patient had to be removed by an operation. It was held that the nurse had used a proper method correctly; although there was disagreement between the parties on the distance it had been inserted, the judge was not satisfied it had been pushed in too far. The accident could have been caused by an unexpected movement by the patient; something that could not reasonably be foreseen. Judgment for the defendants (*Marchant* v. *Eastham Borough Council* (1955)).

> It was alleged by a naval diver that personal injuries were due to the negligent injection of penicillin and breakage of the needle. McNair, J. held that the injection had not been given in the manner suggested; the injection had been properly given and, on the balance of probabilities, the breakage of the needle was due to an inherent defect. Judgment for the defendants (Brazier v. Admiralty; Law Report, The Times, 1964, Nov, 5th).

Fracture of Lower Jaw during Dental Extraction

In the case of *Fish* v. *Kapur* (1948), Lynskey, J. held that the fact of fracture of the jaw alone was not sufficient evidence of negligence on the part of the dentist and the doctrine of *res ipsa loquitur* did not apply in that case.

"Criminal Negligence"

The circumstances in which negligence is at one and the same time a crime are, happily, rare. The conduct of the doctor has been such that it caused, or contributed to, the death of the patient and resulted in a prosecution for manslaughter. It could be some gross mismanagement of the delivery of a woman, more especially by a doctor under the influence of drink or drugs, or grossly incompetent administration of a general anaesthetic by a doctor addicted to the inhalation of anaesthetics. " . . . In order to establish criminal liability the facts must be such that, in the opinion of the jury, the negligence of the accused went beyond a mere matter of compensation between subjects and showed such disregard for the life and safety of others as to amount to a crime against the State and conduct deserving punishment" (Lord Hewart, C. J., in *R.* v. *Bateman* (1925), at p. 11).

Illustrative Cases

R. v. *Bateman* (1925). In the case of Bateman, the death of a woman in childbirth was ascribed to gross negligence on the part of the doctor; it was accepted that he was not under the influence of drink at the time. The case was a difficult labour, which required the application of forceps, version of the child and manual removal of the placenta. A dead child was eventually delivered, but at the conclusion the patient was ill and in poor condition. The doctor did not decide to send her to hospital until the fifth day and she died there 2 days later. A post-mortem examination showed that part of the womb had been torn out, the bladder had been ruptured and the large intestine had been crushed against the spine.

Dr. Bateman was prosecuted for manslaughter, it being alleged that the death was due to criminal negligence because of faulty treatment and undue delay in sending the patient to hospital. He was found guilty and sentenced to 6 months' imprisonment, but his appeal was allowed.

R. v. *Gray* (1959). A child aged 2 years was submitted to general anaesthesia to permit an operation for the repair of a hernia. A critical situation arose during the operation, when the child's heart stopped beating. This was corrected, but the child remained unconscious until its death a month later. The post-mortem examination showed that death was due to cerebral softening and this could have been due to lack of oxygen (anoxia) during the operation. The anaesthetist was charged with manslaughter on the ground that his condition and the manner in which he administered the anaesthetic showed an utter disregard for the patient's safety. There had been a failure to change from an empty to a full cylinder of oxygen during the operation. This failure was due to the incapacity of the anaesthetist, brought about by addiction to anaesthetics. He had been told that the child's breathing was irregular and that the operation wound had become pale, but said there was nothing to worry about. He had been seen to suck the anaesthetic tube and had left the operating theatre for a brief period at a critical moment, thereby neglecting the patient. On his return he staggered: his speech was slurred. When told that the child's heart had stopped beating, he realised that the situation was grave and that cardiac massage was necessary. The surgeon then took charge. Another anaesthetist was summoned to take over the case.

The anaesthetist pleaded guilty. He was at the time under the influence of a general anaesthetic (nitrous oxide, fluothane or halothane and oxygen). In lesser doses it may give a feeling of well-being and, possibly, it clears the mind, but in larger amounts the effects resemble those of alcoholic intoxication. He had inhaled the anaesthetic before and during this operation and accepted responsibility for the patient's anoxia. In mitigation, he pleaded that his addiction was well known. Why were steps not taken earlier to replace him on this occasion? He was sentenced to 12 months imprisonment. (His name was erased from the medical Register but he was later successful in his application for its restoration.)

The Quantum of Damages

In recent times the amounts awarded tend to be astronomical. The amounts recorded in our last edition are now a nostalgic memory compared with the savage awards of recent times, running as they do into hundreds of thousands and even sizeable parts of a million pounds.

Medical Negligence versus Clinical Judgment

One of the most contentious and legally complex areas is the difficulty in differentiating between errors arising from the legitimate exercise of clinical judgment and negligent behaviour. Undoubtedly, the leading case in this issue was one extending over the whole decade of the 1970s, *Whitehouse* v. *Jordan*. This began in 1970 with an attempted forceps delivery and ended in 1981 in the House of Lords.

Mr. Jordan, an experienced obstetrician, was accused of causing cerebral palsy in an infant by pulling too hard and for too long during a forceps delivery of a high-risk pregnancy. The trial court found him negligent and the plaintiff was awarded damages of £100,000, but at the Court of Appeal, the appeal judges—by a majority of two to one—reversed the decision on the grounds that even if it had been proved that the forceps had been used too vigorously for too long a period, this was a matter of clinical judgment not amounting to negligence. The opinions of the three Appeal judges are of considerable interest to medical jurists and practitioners. Lord Justice Donaldson was the dissenting voice, in these terms:

"If a doctor fails to exercise the skill which he has or claims to have, he is in breach of his duty of care; he is negligent. But if he exercised that skill to the full but nevertheless takes what, with hindsight, can be shown to be the wrong course, he is not negligent and can be liable to no one. Both are errors of clinical judgment. The (trial) judge was solely concerned with whether or not the defendant's actions were negligent. If they were not, it was irrelevant whether or not they constituted an error of clinical judgment".

However, the Master of the Rolls, Lord Denning, disagreed:

"The judge required Mr. Jordan to come up to 'the very high standard of professional competence which the law requires'. That suggests that the law makes no allowance for error of judgment. This would be a mistake. Else there would be a danger, in all cases of professional men, of their being made liable when ever something happens to go wrong. If they are to be found liable whenever they do not effect a cure or when anything untoward happens, it would be a great disservice to the profession itself. Not only to the profession, but to society at large. We must say, and say firmly, that in a professional man, an error of judgment is not negligent". He was supported by the third Appeal judge, Lord Justice Lawton: "In my opinion allegations of negligence against medical practitioners should be considered as serious. First, the defendant's professional reputation is under attack. A finding of negligence against him may jeopardise his career and cause him serious financial loss over many years. Secondly, the public interest is put at risk. If courts make findings of negligence on flimsy evidence of regard failure to produce an expected result as strong evidence of negligence, doctors are likely to protect themselves by what has been known as defensive medicine: that is to say, adopting procedures which are not for the benefit of the patient, but safeguards against the possibility of the patient making a claim for negligence. Medical practice these days consists of the harmonious union of science with skill. Medicine has not yet got to the stage—and may be it never will—when the adoption of a particular procedure will produce a certain result".

The plaintiff then appealed to the House of Lords, where in 1981 the five Law Lords were unanimous in dismissing the appeal and upholding the majority decision of the Court of

Appeal. The Lords held that the appeal court was justified in reassessing the inferences of fact drawn by the trial judge and were entitled to reject his finding of negligence because the evidence did not justify the inference that the defendant had negligently pulled too hard and too long on the forceps.

Three of the Law Lords dissented with Lord Denning's distinction between an error of judgment and negligence, which they regarded as ambiguous. They were of the opinion that while some errors of clinical judgment were consistent with the due exercise of professional skill, other acts of omissions in the course of exercising clinical judgment may be so glaringly below proper standards as to make a finding of negligence inevitable. The Lords approved the well-known test of negligence stated by Mr. Justice McNair in 1957 as "the test is the standard of the ordinary skilled man exercising and professing to have that special skill".

The "No-fault" Concept in Medical Mishaps

One unfortunate aspect of a medical mishap under most systems of law is that the complainant has to show that the doctor was negligent before one penny of damages can be recovered. In the majority of mishaps, the line between clinical judgment and negligence is too blurred for a decision to be reached and as the onus of proof is upon the plaintiff, the action fails. Yet the physical harm suffered by the patient remains the same, as does the need for financial restitution.

To avoid this central issue of negligence, several countries—notably New Zealand and Sweden—have adopted a "no-fault" system, where a fund administered centrally by the government and contributed to from taxes, employers etc., forms a pool from which compensation is provided to damaged patients according to their clinical and social needs, rather than a retribution upon a doctor for his negligence.

Though in theory this is attractive, the practical difficulties are immense and it seems that the schemes already in operation are increasingly fraught with problems.

In Britain, this alternative was studied by the Royal Commission on Civil Liability and Compensation for Personal Injury, chaired by Lord Pearson. The Pearson Report, which appeared in 1977, had a wider brief than medical mishaps, being concerned with the whole range of transport, industrial and handicap disability, but was of considerable relevance to the medical profession.

The Report concluded that a "no-fault" system should not be introduced at present and that negligence must still be proved in medical malpractice claims.

References

CASES CITED

ANDERSON V. CHASNEY (1949) 4. D.L.R. 71; [1950] 4 D.L.R. 223.
BARNES V. CRABTREE (1953) *The Times*, 1 and 2 Nov.
BLYTH V. BIRMINGHAM WATERWORKS CO. (1856) 11 Exch. 781; 156 All E.R. 1047; 36 Digest (Repl.) 5, 1.
BREEN V. BAKER (1956) *The Times*, 27 Jan.
CASSIDY V. MINISTRY OF HEALTH (Fahrni, third party) [1951] 1 All E.R. 574 (C.A.).
CHAPMAN V. RIX (1958) *Lancet*, **ii**, 1118 (Wellwood, E. M.) (1959); *Lancet*, **ii**, 965 (Hill, M. M.) (1960); *Lancet*, **ii**, 1453 (Hill, M. M.) (1960); *The Times*, 22 Dec. (1961); *Brit. Med. J.*, **i**, 139.

CHASNEY V. ANDERSON (1950) 4 D.L.R. 223.
COLLINS V. HERTS. COUNTY COUNCIL AND ANOTHER [1947] 1 K.B. 598–625.
COOPER V. NEVILL AND ANOTHER (1961) *Lancet* (1962), **i,** 666 (Clayton, C.).
CRAWFORD V. BOARD OF GOVERNORS, CHARING CROSS HOSPITAL (1953) *The Times,* 23 April, 8 Dec.; *Lancet,* **i,** 906; *ibid.,* **ii,** 1320; *Brit. Med. J.,* **i,** 1011; *ibid.,* **ii,** 1329.
DAVIES V. HORTON ROAD AND COLNEY HILL HOSPITAL MANAGEMENT COMMITTEE AND LOGAN (1954) *Brit. Med. J.,* **i,** 883.
EDITORIAL (1948) *Lancet,* **ii,** 586.
EDITORIAL (1961) *Lancet,* **i,** 666.
ELDER V. GREENWICH AND DEPTFORD HOSPITAL MANAGEMENT COMMITTEE (1953) *The Times,* 7 Mar.; *Lancet,* **i,** 593.
EVANS, K. T. and KNIGHT, B. (1981) *Forensic Radiology,* Oxford: London: Edinburgh: Blackwell.
EVERETT V. GRIFFITHS AND ANOTHER [1920] 3 K. B. 163 (C.A.).
EWING, M. R. (1950) *Lancet,* **i,** 99–103.
FISH V. KAPUR AND ANOTHER [1948] 2 All E.R. 176.
FRASER V. VANCOUVER GENERAL HOSPITAL (1951) 4 D.L.R. 736; [1952] 3 D.L.R. 785.
GARNER V. MORELL AND ANOTHER (1953) *The Times,* 31 Oct.
GERBER V. PINES (1935) 79 Sol. J. 13.
HATCHER V. BLACK AND OTHERS (1954) *The Times,* 29 and 30 June, 1 and 2 July; *Lancet,* (1954) **ii,** 88–89.
HUCKS V. COLE (1967–9) see Med. Defence Union Ann. Report, 1969, p. 56; also *Brit. Med. J.* (1967) **3,** 624.
HUNTER V. HANLEY [1954] Scot. L.T. 303; [1955] Scot. L.T. 213; cited in *Chapman* v. *Rix* (1960).
JONES V. WELSH REGIONAL HOSPITAL BOARD AND KEMP (1961) Glamorgan Assizes, 20 Mar.; *Brit. Med. J.,* **i,** 1260; *Med. Sci. Law,* **1,** 449–50.
LANDAU V. WERNER 1(961) *Lancet,* **i,** 610 (Hill, M.M.); *ibid.,* **ii,** 1248 (Wellwood, E.M.); *The Times,* 8 Mar. 14 Nov.
LANPHIER AND WIFE V. PHIPOS (1838) 8 C. and P. 475.
LOCHGELLY IRON AND COAL CO. V. MCMULLAN (1934) A.C. 1 (at p. 25).
MCCORMACK V. REDPATH BROWN AND CO. AND ANOTHER (1961) *Lancet,* **i,** 736 (Wellwood, E. M.).
MAHON V. OSBORNE (1939) 2 K. B. 14 (at page 47); 1 All E.R. 53 (at pp. 548–59); *The Times,* 16, 17 and 18 Jan., 10 Feb.
MARCHANT V. EASTHAM BOROUGH COUNCIL (1955) *Lancet,* **ii,** 973 (Ellis, C.T.).
MARKLAND V. MANCHESTER CORPORATION (1934) 1 K.B. 566–90 (C.A.).
MARSHALL V. Lindsey County Council
MEDICAL DEFENCE UNION, The (1960) Annual Report, pp. 17–19, 43–44.
MEDICAL DEFENCE UNION, Annual Reports, 1962–79.
MORRIS V. WINSBURY WHITE (1937) 4 All E.R. 494.
NATHAN, LORD (1955) *Medical Negligence,* pp. 38, 40, London: Butterworth.
NICKOLLS V. MINISTRY OF HEALTH (1954) *The Times,* 3 July; *Lancet,* **ii,** 88; (1955) *The Times,* 4 Feb.; *Lancet,* **i,** 349; *Brit. Med. J.,* **i,** 426.
PATCH V. BOARD OF GOVERNORS, UNITED BRISTOL HOSPITALS (1959) *Brit. Med. J.,* **ii,** 701.
PEARSON REPORT (1977) Royal Commission on Civil Liability and Compensation for Personal Injury.
R. V. BATEMAN (1925) 19 Cr. App. R. 8 (at pp. 11–12); 41 T.L.R. 557; 133 L.T. 730.
R. V. GRAY (1959) C.C.C. Feb. 20; *The Times,* 21 Feb. *Lancet;* **i,** 464.
RICH and EXOR. V. PIERPONT (1862) 3 F. and F. 35; 22 Digest (Repl.) 506, 5609.
ROE V. MINISTRY OF HEALTH AND ANOTHER (Woolley v. Same) (1954) 2 Q.B. 66; 2 All E.R. (C.A.) 131.
RUDDOCK V. LOWE (1865) 4 F. and F. 519; Digest 547, 33.
URRY AND URRY V. BIERER AND ANOTHER (1955) *The Times,* 15 July.
WARREN V. GREIG AND WHITE (1935) *Lancet,* **i,** 330.
WHITE V. BOARD OF GOVERNORS, WESTMINSTER HOSPITAL AND ANOTHER (1961) *The Times,* 25 Oct.
WHITEFORD V. HUNTER AND GLEED (1948) *The Times,* 30 July; *Lancet,* **ii,** 232; (1949) *ibid.,* **i,** 586; (1950) *ibid.,* **ii,** 643; 94 Sol. J. 758 (H.L.) 2nd Digest Suppl.; W.N. 553.
WHITEHOUSE V. JORDAN (1970).
WILLIAMS V. NORTH LIVERPOOL H.M.C. [1959] *The Times,* 17 Jan.
WOOD V. THURSTON AND OTHERS (1951) *The Times,* 25 May.

STATUTES CITED

Medical Act, 1956; 4 & 5 Eliz. 2, ch. 76.
National Health Service Act, 1946; 9 & 10 Geo. 6, ch. 81.

CHAPTER 23

Trauma and Disease: Part 1
The Moment of Death: Part 2
Transplantation of Organs: Part 3

Part 1

The association of trauma and disease has profound medico-legal aspects, being important in two different ways. Firstly, the relative contribution to death of injuries and natural disease must often be evaluated, this having an important bearing upon criminal or civil liability. Secondly, it is often alleged that previous trauma gave rise to a debilitating or fatal disease, a situation which obviously has important consequences in terms of compensation.

Taking the first of these problems, the association between trauma and pre-existing disease is most often met in fatal cases, where an injury or alleged injury has been sustained by a person with substantial natural disease. The problem then is evaluate whether:

(a) death was due entirely to the injury and would have occurred whether or not the disease was present
(b) whether the death was due entirely to the disease and would have occurred at that time irrespective of the occurrence of the injury
(c) whether the two processes combined to cause death.

All manner of serious diseases can be implicated in this situation, but probably the most common are coronary artery disease, subarachnoid haemorrhage and pulmonary embolism.

The solution is least clear in the case of *coronary artery disease*. The disease process must have been present for many months and probably years before the application of the trauma. Unless there was a direct blow on the chest which can be shown morphologically to have damaged the heart and precipitated a worse coronary lesion (by dislodging an atheromatous plaque or causing a subintimal haemorrhage), there is no means of proving that other trauma caused the death from myocardial dysfunction. If the coronary disease is severe, then it can be justifiably claimed by the defence that death could have occurred at any time. The standard of proof in a criminal case is very high and must be "beyond reasonable doubt", in contrast to that in civil matters where only "a balance of probability" needs to be achieved. It is frequently an assessment of the circumstances rather than of post-mortem findings which decides the court's attitude to the association. If a man who, though subsequently autopsy reveals severe coronary disease, has had no symptoms whatsoever before an assault, drops dead immediately after a criminal injury, then the trial judge will decide whether the issue of the causation of death will be allowed to go to the jury for their decision. The average juror will be likely to assume that it would be far too much of a coincidence that a man's coronary artery disease happened to drop him in his tracks immediately after the assault, but much depends upon the individual circumstances, especially the interval between the assault and the death. The acid test is "Would death have occurred when it did, if the assault had not taken place?" The law says that an assailant must "take his victim as he finds him" and that if a sick man is assaulted and dies, whereas the same assault upon a fit man would not have killed him, this is the misfortune of the assailant as well as for the victim. However, this dictum is not always adhered to by the Director of Public Prosecutions: it is a matter of practical tactics that if an excellent medical defence can be put up to prove the parlous physical state of the deceased, the prosecution will not pursue the matter of the death, but only the lesser charge of assault.

However, no fixed rules can be stated for the legal consequences, as circumstances are so different from case to case and legal attitudes change, as will be mentioned below in connection with subarachnoid haemorrhage. The prevalence of coronary artery disease in the community is such that deaths are so commonplace from this cause that a close association in time must be present before the association can be given serious consideration. However, the actual death itself may not occur soon after the assault, if for instance, a period of hypotension occurs which may precipitate a myocardial infarct which later leads to death. The presence of the infarct must be proved to have occurred soon after the incident in order to retain the association between the two events. It is not only the actual trauma which could be held to have precipitated a coronary death, but even the emotional upset which accompanies the trauma: in fact, the blow may never be struck, but only threatened, for cardiovascular changes to occur such as a sudden increase in blood pressure which may rupture an atheromatous plaque or cause a subintimal haemorrhage and thus precipitate the coronary disaster. The endocrine "fight or flight" reactions due to adrenalin can themselves tip the scales of a critically balanced coronary circulation, in a similar way to the cerebral aneurysm described later. Although physiologically valid, such associations become even less acceptable as "beyond reasonable doubt" in a criminal court.

Any number of examples can be quoted to illustrate this situation. In one case (F.M. 15,803b) a man of 65 became incensed by lads playing football, who kicked their ball into his garden. He chased one of the youths across the village green. When returning to his house in a considerable state of excitement, he commenced to struggle with another youth and received a trivial blow on the jaw. He staggered back, went into his house and collapsed. He died almost at once. The only evidence of injury at autopsy was a single small bruise on the chin, but there was gross narrowing of all the coronary arteries. The precipitating factor in the death was obviously exertion associated with the incident and not the trivial injury received.

In another case, a man of 62 had a domestic argument with his younger son-in-law and received a blow of moderate severity upon the jaw. He collapsed dead upon the floor and the son-in-law was arrested by the police and charged with manslaughter. At autopsy, gross myocardial fibrosis and obliterated coronary arteries were found, upon which the charge of homicide was dropped.

A second important category concerns *subarachnoid haemorrhage*. Numerous cases are on record where a head injury, usually sustained in an assault or fight, has caused death from subarachnoid haemorrhage, usually due to the rupture of a berry aneurysm of the Circle of Willis. Sometimes no such aneurysm can be found, but this does not materially alter the situation, as 15 per cent of subarachnoid haemorrhages (unassociated with trauma) reveal no aneurysm.

Again the problem is the likelihood that the aneurysm would have ruptured spontaneously at the time when it did. Subarachnoid haemorrhage from such an aneurysm is a relatively common cause of death in younger and younger-middle-aged adults before the "coronary age" is reached—this particularly applies to women, who have their ischaemic heart disease later. As ruptured aneurysms can occur either without any previous exertion or on physical exertion such as sporting activities or sexual intercourse, the likelihood of such a potentially fatal event occurring before, during or immediately after a fight or assault is equally great. There has been much medical argument in the past about the role of trauma in causing the rupture of the aneurysm. Some authorities maintain that physical violence is unlikely to mechanically disturb the aneurysm, which is deep-seated and protected and that the rupture is more likely to be due to an acute rise of blood pressure and increase in circulation rate. Others, whilst acknowledging these factors, claim that the mechanical shock of an impact upon the head is a material cause of the rupture. Probably this last view must be accepted, though the role of sudden hypertension and increased pulse rate is probably the most important. It has also been noted for many years that berry aneurysms seem to rupture more often in intoxicated persons, but this observation must be tempered by the fact that many assault situations occur in an alcoholic environment, so to speak, and that the association may be parallel rather than causative.

Once again, the legal problem exists of the relationship of the trauma to the fatal bleed. The time interval is naturally extremely important, though in fact evidence of bleeding usually occurs either almost immediately or very soon after the injury. In a number of cases, death occurs so rapidly that it is difficult to understand the physiological mechanism. For instance, one author (B.K.) has had several cases in which the victim of an assault has fallen to the ground apparently dead, showing no subsequent signs of life. This very rapid death from bleeding around the brain can only be attributed to some brain stem affectation which causes immediate cardio-respiratory arrest. In the majority of cases, either severe headache or unconsciousness occurs very rapidly, death being delayed for minutes, hours or days.

Post-mortem examination is often not helpful in assessing the relative contribution of the assault and the pre-existing disease. Naturally, the demonstration of a recently-ruptured aneurysm is extremely helpful in elucidating the circumstances, but as mentioned, at least 15 per cent of subarachnoid haemorrhages do not escape from discrete aneurysms, but from apparently normal cerebral vessels. However, very small aneurysms may be destroyed by the bleeding process and not be recognisable at autopsy.

It was formerly the practice in England and Wales for no charge of homicide to be brought where an assault was associated with a demonstrably-ruptured berry aneurysm. However, in Scotland and on the continent of Europe, charges were usually pressed. The situation has perhaps been altered by a case which occurred in Gibraltar in 1978, as since then a number of similar cases have been prosecuted in England and Wales.

This involved a drunken fight between two British sailors, when one was kicked on the head. He went into coma and died several days later in brain death. Autopsy revealed a ruptured berry aneurysm on the Circle of Willis. The physical injuries were slight and the defence maintained that the rupture of the aneurysm was far more likely to have occurred from the raised pulse rate and blood pressure (including an increased pulse pressure between systolic and diastolic) in a drunken sailor, than from the actual blows. However, this view was not accepted by the court nor by the subsequent Appeal. (Knight, 1979).

It must be borne in mind that subarachnoid haemorrhage following trauma, in the absence of a berry aneurysm, may be due to rupture of a vertebral artery in the transverse process of the atlas vertebra, following a blow or kick on the side of the neck. This lesion has only been described in recent years, but is now fully documented (Cameron and Mant, 1972; Simonsen, 1976; Vanezis, 1979).

It is sometimes impossible to demonstrate the evidence of trauma at autopsy. For example, a man while unloading a lorry became involved in an altercation with one of the packers. The latter was seen to strike at the deceased—eye witnesses were uncertain where the blow had landed. The deceased stepped back and immediately collapsed and died: this was due to massive subarachnoid haemorrhage from a ruptured aneurysm. There was no sign of a blow to his head and it was possible that the deceased had violently jerked his head in dodging the blow. This could have precipitated rupture, but there was no other evidence to show that the rupture was due to any other cause other than raised blood pressure associated with the excitement of the altercation.

Another example is that of a middle-aged man who was struck a blow on the head by his son during an altercation. He had a definite, recent bruise on his jaw: he died of rupture of a berry aneurysm. While there was a probability that the blow precipitated rupture of the vessel, it could not be denied that the rupture was due to the deceased's own excitement rather than to the impact. In consequence, a criminal charge was dropped (F.M. 14033b).

The third important trauma-associated lesion is *pulmonary embolism*. This is almost always due to impaction of thrombus which has shifted from thrombosed leg veins, pelvic or axillary thrombosis being so rare as to be disregarded, except in special situations such as post-puerperal. Pulmonary embolism is an extremely common condition and is in fact the most under-diagnosed cause of death when clinical forecasts are compared with autopsy findings. It is a well-known complication of trauma, Virchow's triad of slowing of the circulation, local injury to the vessel walls and increase in the coaguability of the blood being factors which aid the formation of thrombus in the deep veins of the calves. Trauma (including surgical operation) and the subsequent immobility such as bedrest, are potent factors in leading to deep vein thrombosis. Where the leg is the site of the injury, it is more common for it to occur in this ipsi-lateral limb, though it can occur in the contra-lateral or both limbs. Where the injury is remote from the legs, then naturally the side affected is immaterial. However, it must be pointed out that the argument is not valid that because thrombus originated from the contralateral limb in leg injury, there could be no causative connection.

Pulmonary embolism classically occurs about 2 weeks after injury, but the range of time within which there can be said to be a cause-and-effect varies from 2 or 3 days up to several months, However, it is patently progressively more difficult to maintain a causative relationship when the time interval extends beyond a few weeks.

In medico-legal terms, the vital practical matter is to show that the initiation of the leg vein thrombosis occurred since the injury. For instance, if a man suffers a fatal pulmonary embolism 6 days after an injury, but histologically the thrombus in the leg veins reveal lesions of several weeks' duration, then the causative relationship is lost. The criteria for histological dating depends largely upon the interface between the thrombus and the vein wall in the deep vessels of the legs and it is essential when taking histological blocks to preserve sections of vessel with the thrombus still in place. Histological examination of the pulmonary emboli are far less useful in attempting to date the time of origin. It must also be appreciated that progressive thrombosis occurs in leg veins and therefore the most distal segments (often in the dorsum of the foot) will reveal the oldest parts of the thrombus. Thrombosis of the leg veins is naturally far more common than pulmonary embolism. In a hundred random coroner's autopsies studied by Knight and Zaini (1980) thirty two were found to have deep vein thrombosis, but only ten died of massive pulmonary embolism. The histological criteria were described in detail by Zaini (1981).

It is never possible to deny that venous thrombosis and pulmonary embolism can occur spontaneously from natural causes and therefore it cannot be said with certainty in any particular case that the death was without doubt related to a previous injury. In a series of hospital and coroner's autopsies studied by Knight (1966), 25 per cent of all fatal pulmonary emboli occurred "out of the blue" without any prior injury, surgical injury or confinement to bed. In a larger study of 38,000 post-mortem examinations (Knight and Zaini, 1980) only 10 per cent of cases of fatal pulmonary embolism were found to have no predisposing causes, but what ever statistical figure is obtained, it is apparent that a proportion of these deaths cannot be attributed to any prior injurious event. This provides a line of defence where it is alleged that a fatal pulmonary embolism is a direct consequence of some assault, as it can be shown that an appreciable proportion of pulmonary emboli can occur quite spontaneously. As with the previous lesions discussed, it is then a matter for the court to decide whether they feel that the burden of proof has been discharged "beyond reasonable doubt". In several road accident deaths, variable legal results have emerged from virtually the same medical situations. Where charged under Section 1 of the Road Traffic Acts, with "causing death by reckless driving" (a serious offence carrying a maximum penalty of 5 years imprisonment), the verdicts in at least two cases known to one of the authors were quite at variance. In both cases, a victim was struck by a motor vehicle and sustained a fractured leg. The injury in itself was not very serious, but after surgical treatment and confinement to bed, deep vein thrombosis and fatal pulmonary embolism occurred about 10 days after the incident. In one case, the judge accepted the chain of events as being a direct consequence of the injury and allowed the matter to go to the jury, who convicted. In the second case, the judge accepted a defence application that the possibility of a coincidental pulmonary embolism was strong enough to defeat the prosecution claim of direct causation and the judge directed that the standard of proof was not sufficient to be allowed to go to the jury.

Pulmonary infection is another well-recognised complication of injury: it occurs within the first few days or weeks after the injury. However, as with pulmonary embolism, infections such as bronchopneumonia may and commonly do, occur spontaneously in persons who have not suffered any predisposing injury. When the infection occurs relatively soon after the injury and during the intervening period, the patient has been immobilised or for any other reason has suffered impairment of respiratory function, then a connection between the trauma and the infection is a probability. In all of these cases the relationship between injury can only be assessed in relation to the facts of each case. They are not open to precise mathematical evaluation nor are there precise rules for guidance.

Many other instances can be found and are seen every day by coroner's pathologists. In fact, this is one of the most constant problems for the pathologist, both following injuries and surgical operations, which are an elective form of injury. A severe blow to the abdomen can sometimes be followed by the development of acute pancreatitis. Such an effect on the pancreas appears to be more liable to occur if the injury is sustained shortly after the victim has eaten a large meal or taken a substantial amount of alcohol. Meningitis may follow a head injury. If the injury is a penetrating wound, then obviously infection may enter via the wound track, but even in a closed head injury if a fracture of the skull crosses the ethmoid plates or the temporal bones over the roof of the middle ear, then a route is open to permit the entry of infection. A tiny crack in the frontal bone beneath an insignificant wound was the pathway on one occasion (Polson and Gee, 1973; F.M. 5393).

Ulceration of the gastrointestinal tract is another well-recognised late complication of injury. Acute ulceration of the oesophagus following head injury is described by Dalgaard (1957). Ulceration of the stomach and oxyntic cell necrosis are also recognised as following head injury. Acute gastric erosions are a common cause of gastric bleeding, sometimes massive in volume. These are frequently seen after the stress of injuries and appear to be mediated by the parasympathetic nervous system. Similar erosions are seen in hypothermia. Adrenal haemorrhage is also not uncommon as a stress lesion following acute infections or severe injuries. The Waterhouse-Fredrichsen haemorrhage in the adrenals, classically in meningococcal septicaemia, is due to the systemic effects of a severe infection rather than to a local infective lesion. Adrenal haemorrhage following injury is often unrecognised by clinicians and only discovered at autopsy (Knight, 1980).

The second matter concerns the causation of chronic diseases by a previous injury or other insult, as opposed to the more closely associated causation of death by a substantial injury in the immediate past, as has just been discussed. Once again, the probability of an injury giving rise to disease varies greatly according to the type of disease under discussion and the nature of the injury—there can be no generalisation possible.

In this context, injury may be held to include certain toxic or irritative states, as well as direct trauma which widens the field of positive causation. For example, this then includes such things as chemical and physical carcinogenesis, including the well-established connection between asbestos and mesothelioma or the malignant diseases caused by radiation. Confining the discussion to mechanical injury, the probability of the effects of this upon human tissues in causing natural disease at a later date has been much overstated, especially by those involved in civil litigation. The prospect of financial compensation not unnaturally leads to unjustifiable connections being drawn between injurious events and later disease. Though there are certain diseases where a connection, on the balance of probabilities, is thought to exist, such a connection is incapable of absolute proof, as all these diseases are well known to occur spontaneously. For example, although the association of asbestos exposure and mesothelioma is well recognised, it must be appreciated that 15 per cent of all such tumours occur without any discoverable asbestos exposure. Similarly, the tumours of the bladder in certain chemical workers, naso-pharyngeal cancers in nickel workers and leukaemias in workers exposed to ionising radiation can all occur quite independently of any such exposure. Although statistically an association can clearly be detected, it can never be absolutely proved in any individual case that the condition was due to the statistically-likely cause, though where the association is probable, the legal outcome is usually favourable to the victim.

One of the most common claims for an association between injury and disease is in coronary artery disease and the Appeals machinery of the Department of Health and Social Security have to process hundreds of such claims each year. In many instances, they are obviously untenable at first glance, such as cases where a widow or trade union claims that death from a myocardial infarct in a diabetic of 65 years was caused by a broken ankle at work 22 years previously! More sensible claims relate to the acute onset of a coronary episode soon after some over-exertion in an industrial situation. These claims must be carefully analysed, as there is no evidence whatsover that injury or exertion can cause the underlying disease i.e. trauma and effort played no part in the aetiology of coronary atheroma. However, it must be allowed that in a person who already had severe coronary artery disease, over-exertion may on occasions precipitate an acute episode in the natural history of the disease, usually myocardial infarction or death from ventricular fibrillation or cardiac arrest. Even so, this association, even if it is close in time, must be viewed in the light of the fact that at least 180,000 deaths per year occur from coronary artery disease in the United Kingdom. It then becomes a matter of the balance of probabilities to successfully maintain that any trauma or overexertion caused an exacerbation of the disease at that particular time. Where the sudden onset of chest pain, collapse, myocardial infarction or death is very closely related in time to severe exertion, then it is reasonable to assume that the death was precipitated or accelerated by that exertion, though death in the absence of such exertion may have occurred on the next day or next week. Direct trauma very rarely causes a coronary occlusion, unless there is substantial direct injury to the front of the chest which causes bruising or other mechanical damage to the structures of the heart. Sudden over-exertion such as the lifting of a heavy weight or sudden stress beyond the usual physical capabilities of the person, may precipitate some new episode in the cardiac condition, though claims are often exaggerated and are allowed on the principle of "giving the benefit of the doubt".

The same tenets apply in other types of heart disease, such as hypertension, valvular disease and ruptured aortic aneurysm. Each case must be examined on its particular merits.

Tumours have already been mentioned and again are fertile ground for litigation. In recent years, cases are appearing in relation to ionising radiation from Servicemen present at nuclear weapon tests many years ago and from workers in the nuclear power industry.

The relationship between malignant disease and injury is a frequent source of controversy, but in general there is very little evidence to allow such a causal connection to be made except where chemical, irradiation or long-standing irritative states exist. The examples quoted above, especially asbestos and mesothelioma are ones with a far greater chance of acceptance, sometimes being accepted statutorily due to statistical evidence.

Physical trauma is much less likely to lead to tumours, except in a direct manner such as the classical jagged tooth acting for years upon a tongue. It is inconceivable that a single act of mechanical injury could give rise to a tumour, though this is often alleged. Most allegations arise because the existence of a tumour appears to date from the time of the traumatic incident. In almost all these cases, the attention drawn to the injured part is instrumental in bringing to light the presence of the tumour which must have pre-existed in all cases. A blow on a part of the body may draw attention to a previously unnoticed lump or the temporary signs of the injury may render the first signs of the tumour apparent.

To definitely relate trauma to a malignant growth, certain criteria known as "Ewing's postulates" must be satisfied. These are:

(a) the tumour must arise exactly at the site injured.

(b) definite and substantial trauma must be proved.

(c) the tumour must be confirmed pathologically.

(d) the tissue at the site must have been healthy before the trauma.

(e) a reasonable interval (neither too long nor too short) must elapse between the time of the trauma and the appearance of the tumour.

(f) though not one of Ewing's original postulates, there should be some good scientific reason for ascribing the tumour formation to the injury—and this is rarely possible.

The postulate concerning the timing is also less definite than stated by Ewing. There is really no interval which can be too long, as the appearance of a mesothelioma may be 15 to 20 years after the cessation of exposure to asbestos: there may also be an extremely long interval between irradiation and the appearance of the tumour.

Intra-cerebral tumours present a particular problem in relation to head injury, but there is no good evidence that a causal relationship exists. Courville, one of the best authorities on the subject, has stated his invariable conclusion that in no case, evaluated from a clinical or pathological viewpoint, has a glioma ever been proved to be of traumatic origin. As head injuries are so common in the general population (over 10 per cent of a non-tumour-suffering population can recall a significant head injury) it is inevitable that tumour formation and a history of trauma must frequently coincide. Once again, the coincidence is understandable in that when a serious lesion develops, there is naturally a search for causative events and the ubiquitous head injury is all too easy to cast in the role of the instigator. This statement must be modified according to the type of tumour, as meningiomata may have a slightly better chance of establishing a cause-and-effect relationship than tumours of the brain substance itself.

A more likely relationship between head injury and disease exists in epilepsy, especially where this begins later in life and is of a focal nature which may be localised to an injured part of the brain, such as the temporal lobe. Post-traumatic epilepsy is a well-known neurological condition but direct evidence of a local area of injury in the site that neurologically can be related to the fits must be produced, as well as an assurance that no fits were suffered before the head injury. It is difficult or impossible to differentiate the usual types of idiopathic epilepsy from post-traumatic epilepsy unless there are these localising signs. The use of electroencephalography may be vital in strengthening the association, as would any anatomical or surgical data indicating that there had been a depressed fracture, meningeal adhesions or cortical damage at a site consistent with the focal origin of the fits.

References

CAMERON, J. M. and MANT, A. K. (1972) *Med. Sci. & Law,* **12,** 66–70.
COURVILLE, C. B. (1950) *Pathology of the Nervous System,* 3rd ed. Pacific Press Associates.

DALGAARD, J. B. (1957) *J. Forensic Med.*, **4**, 1l0.
KNIGHT, B. (1966) *Med. Sci & Law*, **6**, 3, 150.
KNIGHT, B. (1979) *Brit. Med. J.* **i**, 1430: Medico-Legal.
KNIGHT, B. (1980), *Forensic Sci. Internat.*, **16**, 227–229.
KNIGHT, B. and ZAINI, M. R. S. (1980) *Amer. J. Foren. Med & Path.*, **1**, 3.
POLSON, C. J. and GEE, D. J. (1973) *The Essentials of Forensic Medicine*, 3rd ed. p. 158.
SIMONSEN, J. (1976) *Med. Sci. & Law*, **16**, 13–16.
VANEZIS, P. (1979) *Foren. Sci. Internat.*, **13**, 2, 159.
ZAINI, M. R. S. (1981) MD Thesis, University of Wales.

Part 2

The Moment of Death

Considerable discussion, controversy and even acrimony has occurred during the past few years about what constitutes the death of a human being. Much of the escalation of this debate has been prompted by problems of obtaining organs for transplantation surgery, but it must be emphasised that this is by no means the only issue. The difficulties over the definition of death would still exist if transplantation became obsolete tomorrow due to other means of treatment—the basic factor in causing the dilemma is the advent of mechanical cardio-pulmonary support devices.

Until a couple of decades ago, a person was considered to be dead when his heart, lungs and brain permanently ceased functioning. When the heart stopped, breathing and cerebration ceased within minutes due to ischaemia and anoxia. Less commonly, failure to respirate caused cardiac and cerebral death from hypoxia. When the brain failed, as in severe head injuries, hanging or decapitation, breathing ceased immediately and the heart stopped after a few minutes.

This inevitable interaction between the three major systems was broken when methods became available to support respiration almost indefinitely by mechanical ventilation. Also, greatly improved methods of treating cardiac arrest may allow a stopped heart to begin beating once more, after a period of circulatory stagnation sufficient to cause irreversible brain damage. Thus the old criteria of death, though still applicable to over 99 per cent of individuals, are no longer inevitably correct.

In Britain and many other countries, there is no legal definition of death. A person is dead when his doctors say he is dead. This places an onerous responsibility upon the medical attendants, both from a medical, legal, ethical, philosophical and even religious standpoint.

The whole body does not die simultaneously, except in the rare event of cataclysmic incineration. Therefore *somatic* death must be differentiated from *cellular* death. If this were not so, tissues and organs would be of no use for transplantation.

Most cultures now accept that irreversible failure of the organism *as an integrated mechanism* is the point of somatic death, notwithstanding that some or even most of the individual cells are still alive. More and more in recent years, the concept of "brain death" has been accepted and more recently still, the further refinement of "brain-stem death". There are three types of brain death:

(a) *Cortical or cerebral death* with an intact brain-stem. This leads to a vegetative state in which respiration survives, but there is total loss of sentient activity. Cerebral hypoxia, toxic conditions (such as the Karen Quinlan case) or widespread brain injury can lead to this state.

(b) *Brain-stem death*, where the cerebrum may be intact, though cut off functionally by the stem lesion. Raised intracranial pressure, cerebral oedema, intracranial haemorrhage, etc., may lead to this state. In Britain, head injury and subarachnoid haemorrhage account for the majority of cases. Cranial nerve function is lost, including the respiratory outflow.

(c) *Whole brain death*, combining the two above, is also common.

In the context of determining death it is now generally accepted within the medical profession that *brain-stem* death is sufficient to establish that somatic death has occurred. It is not necessary to prove whole brain death—and cortical death cannot be accepted as a criterion of death, though some tentative suggestions in the United States are moving in that direction.

The practical need is for a scheme of examination which will establish the existence of irreversible brain-stem death beyond any doubt raised by critics, of whom there is no lack. This was the issue which caused the notorious BBC television programme "Panorama" to wreak such damage to renal transplantation when it was screened in November, 1980. Patients (almost exclusively in the U.S.A.) were portrayed who allegedly had been declared "dead" by various neurological tests, but who subsequently recovered. Following an outcry from the medical profession in Britain, it was shown that the criteria applied were not those used in this country.

Following two conferences of the Royal Colleges and Faculties of the United Kingdom in 1976 and 1979, a Code of Practice was recommended and later incorporated into a booklet issued by the Department of Health and Social Security—*The Removal of Cadaveric Organs for Transplantation–A Code of Practice (1979—revised 1983)*.

This set out the criteria for the establishment of brain-stem death as given below. The decision should be taken by two doctors, one being the consultant (or his deputy) in charge of the patient, who should have been registered for at least 5 years and be experienced in such cases, together with another suitably experienced doctor who is clinically independent of the first. Neither should be part of a team wishing to transplant any donor organ or tissue. The result of the examination should be recorded in the case notes—in Britain, a model checklist is available to ensure that all the recommended procedures are carried out. This is then signed by the two doctors, who in practice—though not of necessity—are usually neurologists, anaesthetists or intensive-care physicians.

The battery of tests is carried out twice, the interval between them being decided upon by the attending doctors. If the second set confirms absent brain-stem function, then the disconnection of mechanical ventilation (which is the final part of the tests) is made permanent, unless organ donation is to be carried out. The time of death is recorded as the moment of this final diagnosis of brain-stem death, so that it becomes obvious that where donation of tissues is made, it is being carried out on a ventilated, but certified-dead body.

The Clinical Criteria of Brain-stem Death

The diagnosis of brain-stem death is that recommended by the 1976 and 1979 Conferences of the Royal Colleges and Faculties of the United Kingdom and is now widely accepted. These criteria are:

1. The Patient is Deeply Comatose

(a) There should be no suspicion that this state is due to depressant drugs. Narcotics, hypnotics and tranquillisers may have a prolonged duration of action, particularly where some hypothermia exists. The benzodiazepines are markedly cumulative in their action and are commonly used as anticonvulsants or to assist synchronisation with mechanical ventilators.

(b) Primary hypothermia as a cause of coma must be excluded.

(c) Metabolic and endocrine disturbances which can be responsible for, or can contribute to, coma should have been excluded. There should be no profound abnormality of the serum electrolytes, acid-base balance or blood glucose.

2. The Patient is Being Maintained on a Ventilator

This is because spontaneous respiration had previously become inadequate or ceased altogether.

Relaxants (neuromuscular blocking agents) and other drugs should have been excluded as a cause of respiratory inadequacy or failure.

3. Irremediable Structural Brain Damage

There should be no doubt that the patient's condition is due to the above. The diagnosis of a disorder which led to brain death should have been fully established.

Diagnostic Tests for the Confirmation of Brain-stem Death

(a) All brain-stem reflexes are absent.

  (i) The pupils are fixed in diameter and do not respond to sharp changes in the intensity of incident light.

  (ii) There is no corneal reflex.

  (iii) The vestibulo-ocular reflexes are absent.

  (iv) No motor responses within the cranial nerve distribution can be elicited by adequate stimulation of any somatic area.

  (v) There is no gag reflex or reflex response to bronchial stimulation by a suction catheter passed down the trachea.

  (vi) No respiratory movements occur when the patient is disconnected from the mechanical ventilator for long enough to ensure that the arterial carbon dioxide level rises above the threshold for stimulation of respiration.

(b) There should be repetition of these tests, especially if any give equivocal results. The interval between the tests depends upon the particular patient and may be as long as 24 hours.

(c) It is well established that spinal-cord function can persist after insults which irretrievably destroy brain-stem function. Reflexes of spinal origin may persist or return after an initial absence in brain-dead patients.

(d) It is now widely accepted that electro-encephalography is not necessary for the diagnosis of brain-stem death, neither are other investigations such as cerebral angiography or cerebral blood flow measurements. However, in some countries, such as Germany, such ancillary investigations are legally required before death certification in these circumstances.

(e) Hypothermia is sometimes present due to depression of central temperature regulation by drugs or brain-stem depression. It is recommended that the body temperature should be raised to not less than 35°C before these diagnostic tests are performed.

For further practical details and safeguards, the original publications should be consulted, especially the British *Code of Practice*.

Medico-legal Implications of Brain-stem Death

From the purely medical point of view, brain-death is of importance for the following reasons, as the diagnosis limits:

(a) The period of distress to relatives.
(b) The futile utilisation of limited facilities, which may be of more use to potentially recoverable patients.
(c) Demoralisation of nursing staff in caring for brain-dead victims.
(d) The cost of expert care and equipment in hopeless cases.

The provision of organs for transplantation is a separate, though important issue, dealt with in another section of this chapter.

There are profound legal considerations, especially when the brain death is due to criminal injuries.

A number of cases have arisen where, as a result of a criminal assault, the victim has been placed upon mechanical ventilation, where in theory, he might have survived for a long period, if not indefinitely. When irreversible brain-death was diagnosed, the support was withdrawn and the victim died in every accepted sense of the word.

The original charge of criminal assault now becomes homicide and an appropriate charge is brought by the prosecution. However, the defence has been raised that it was the doctors who caused the "death" by switching off the respirator. In English law, an assailant cannot be held responsible for the death of another if survival lasted for at least one year and a day. It could therefore be argued that if support had been maintained for that period, no charge of homicide could arise.

With the wider acceptance of "death" being equated with brain-stem death, this argument loses credence, as once the diagnosis and declaration of death is made by the medical attendants, any further mechanical support is merely the ventilation of a heart-beating corpse.

The following cases are of interest in this context:

The case of John David Potter, who died in 1963, indicated that modification in the determination of the occurrence of death was necessary where a patient is receiving treatment in an artificial respirator. This patient sustained head injuries when he was knocked down during a brawl on 15 June 1963. He lost consciousness and so remained until he died. On admission to hospital an emergency operation was performed and a sub-dural haematoma was removed. Although very ill next morning he was not deemed to be moribund. At 1.50 p.m. on 16 June he had respiratory collapse. A tracheostomy was performed and resuscitation then permitted a second exploration of the interior of the skull; the brain was under pressure. His breathing ceased at 3.15 p.m. and he was then placed in an artificial respirator, but it was assumed that "technically" he was dead. It was proposed to transplant one of his kidneys to another patient and the consent of several persons was sought and obtained. That of the widow was given at about 7 p.m. after she had been informed that "offically and medically her husband was really dead and to all intents and purposes the machine was keeping him alive". At 11.30 a.m. on 17 June he was moved in the respirator to the operating theatre and the transplantation operation was performed. The donor patient "died" at 2.22 p.m. when the respirator was switched off and his heart stopped beating.

At the inquest held on 25 July the jury decided that the transplantation of the kidney had nothing to do with Potter's death: this they accepted as due to his head injuries and, in consequence, a verdict of manslaughter was returned against his assailant, who was then committed for trial. He had admitted in a statement that he had butted Potter in the face, causing him to fall backwards on to his head, but the defence was that the operation was a *novus actus*, which shifted the responsibility for the patient's death.

Several pertinent questions arose out of this case but the present one related to the time of the death. In the view of the casualty officer he died at 1.50 p.m. on 16 June. The neurosurgeon agreed that his heart and respiration were thereafter maintained artificially. The urologist and anaesthetist considered the patient to have been dead at 11.30 a.m., circulation and breathing being wholly and artificially maintained. (The hospital records, it appears, gave the time of death at 11.40 a.m. on 17 June). The pathologist, although also of the opinion that the transplantation did not play any part in the death, considered that death did not take place until the patient's heart ceased to beat at 2.22 p.m. on 17 June. Obviously, in the circumstances of this case, the precise moment of death was important.

More recently, two further cases were heard together in the Court of Appeal (March 1981). Both were appeals against convictions for murder, where the trial judges had prevented the jury from considering the issue of whether the original injuries or the discontinuation of mechanical ventilators had caused death.

In the first case, Richard Malcherek had stabbed his wife, who had later had a pulmonary embolus, which though it had been removed surgically, had resulted in about half an hour of impaired cerebral circulation. Three days later, she was still unconscious and next day, five of the six "Royal Colleges" tests were carried out and found to indicate brain-stem death. The gag reflex test was omitted. After consultation with relatives, the ventilator was withdrawn and though oxygen was continued, spontaneous respiration did not commence. The appellant's counsel maintained that the discontinuance of ventilation was a "*novus actus interveniens*" and was the cause of death, and that not all the criteria for brain-stem death were used.

In the second case, heard simultaneously, Anthony Steele had been convicted of murdering Carol Wilkinson, in a savage attack with a stone, in which she suffered severe head injuries. All motor and other cerebral activity ceased almost immediately and she was ventilated straight away. Twelve hours later, a neurosurgeon concluded that there had been devastating impact injury to the brain. The next day it was demonstrated that there was no cerebral blood flow and two days later, the ventilation was discontinued. An autopsy conducted less than an hour later showed that the brain was already autolysing.

Again, Steele's counsel appealed against the trial judge's decision that the cause of death was not a matter for the jury. Counsel complained that two of the tests for brain-stem death had not been performed, as the corneal reflex test and the vestibulo-ocular test could not be carried out due to the state of the eyes. He complained that the chain of causation had been broken by the switching-off of the ventilator and that the jury should have been allowed to decide upon the cause of death—a curious claim in the presence of a demonstrably disintegrating brain.

The Appeal Court, through the Lord Chief Justice, Lord Lane, dismissed the appeals, saying that there was no need to lay down a legal definition of death—which many observers had expected as the outcome to these cases. Lord Lane said that the issue was whether the trial judges had been correct in withholding the matter of causation from the injury. He quoted two previous cases—not involving respirators, but where later medical events had followed the initial injuries and contributed to death (*R. v. Smith* and *R. v. Jordan*). Lord Lane also quoted *R. v. Blaue*, where a stab victim, who was a Jehovah's Witness, died because she refused blood transfusion. In all these cases, as well as those now being considered by the Court of Appeal, it was held that the original wounds were still a *"continuing operation and substantial"* cause of death at the time when death occurred and therefore secondary factors such as the discontinuance of ventilation did not remove the responsibility of the appellants.

"Where a medical practitioner, using generally acceptable methods, came to a *bona fide* conclusion that the patient was for all intents and purposes dead and that such vital functions as remained were being maintained solely by mechanical means, and accordingly discontinued the treatment, that did not break the chain of causation between the initial injury and the death."

Thus the English courts have still declined to define the moment of death, though it is acknowledged that this might in certain circumstances become necessary; for example, if brain-stem activity ceased on the 365th day after injury, but the patient was ventilated until the 366th day.

References

Point of death; no judicial definition. (1981) *Brit. Med. J.*, **282**, 1083–84
R. v. SMITH (1959) 2 QB 35
R. v. JORDAN (1956) 40 Cr App Rep 152
R. v. BLAUE (1975) 3 All ER 446
PALLIS, C. "ABC of Brain-Stem Death", series of nine articles. *Brit. Med. J.*, (November 1982–January 1983) **285**, 6354, 1558.)
Conference of Medical Royal Colleges and their Faculties in the UK. (1976) Diagnosis of Death. *Brit. Med. J.*, ii, 1187–8
Conference of Medical Royal Colleges and their Faculties in the UK. (1979) Diagnosis of Death. *Brit. Med. J.*, i, 3320
The Removal of Cadaveric Organs for Transplantation. (1979 and 1983) *A Code of Practice*, DHSS/HMSO.

Part 3

The Transplantation of Tissues and Organs

Though some forms of tissue transplantation have been employed for many years—blood transfusions, for example—the topic has expanded almost explosively in both the medical and public eye in recent times, mainly due to the emotive introduction of cadaver donation of whole organs. Even this was not in itself the cause of the unprecedented attention given by the media, but the associated problem of the *definition of death* in relation to the harvesting of donor organs. This is dealt with in the previous section of the chapter.

Ethical and Legal Aspects

The nature of the tissue to be transplanted makes a great difference to the legal and ethical considerations. Where a procedure such as blood transfusion is concerned, there are few problems, as the donation is harmless where the tissue regenerates quickly. Marrow transplantation is similar, though where the donor (for genetic reasons) has to be a child, some care has to be taken in defining the ethics of consent.

More problems are likely to occur on the part of the recipient, as some religious sects, notably Jehovah's Witnesses, have a steadfast objection to receiving any blood or tissue containing blood. This objection must be upheld in relation to adult patients, even if they are *in extremis*, but difficulties arise when parents refuse to allow transfusion to be given to their children.

In these instances, it was formerly the practice to convene a court at the bedside, when a magistrate would transfer the custody of the child from the parents to an official of the Local Authority, who then immediately gave consent. However, this practice has been discontinued, due to the lack of opportunity for appeal against a legal decision. It is now the responsibility of the doctor in charge of the infant patient to decide upon the treatment, even in the face of parental objection. When carried out for good clinical reasons in an urgent medical situation, it seems highly unlikely that the parents would succeed in any legal action against the doctor, except perhaps to gain derisory damages.

Corneal grafting is another type of tissue transplantation that has been established for many years—indeed, the first legislation in Britain, the forerunner of the Human Tissue Act, was the Corneal Grafting Act of 1952, arising from the pioneer work of Sir Tudor Thomas, a Cardiff ophthalmic surgeon.

With corneal grafting (and the now almost defunct use of arterial grafts for vascular repairs) the legal problems are relatively slight, because these tissues may be removed up to many hours after the cardiac arrest of conventional death, when there is no problem about determining the moment of death or of maintaining oxygenated perfusion by the circulation up to the time of tissue removal.

It is the recent technical advances in *organ* transplantation that have caused such profound problems in the ethical and legal considerations surrounding the donation of tissues. The most common organ to be transplanted—and the one with the best record of long-term success—is the kidney, but the same questions arise with other organs, notably the heart.

These problems have led to much controversy—and indeed acrimony—in the medical press and in the general media. The most controversial episode was a B.B.C. "Panorama" television programme in November 1980, where because of misguided and ill-informed statements about the reliability of the diagnosis of brain death, the British kidney transplant programme was decimated for many months because of unjustified public concern.

The legal aspects of organ donation also depend to a large extent upon whether the donation originates from the living or the dead:

(a) The use of kidney transplants from live donors has a higher success rate than with cadaver organs. The former offers a 93 per cent chance of surviving for one year, compared with 82 per cent for cadaver donation. However, live donation is extremely rare in Britain and throughout Europe only 4 per cent are obtained in this way, contrasted with the United States, where the rate is 35 per cent.

When live donation is contemplated, the potential donor must be given a full explanation of the consequences and risks. If they are accepted, written and witnessed consent must be obtained. No donation can be accepted which would cause any significant risk to the life of the donor, no matter how willing that person might be to sacrifice the organ.

(b) The great majority of transplant material is obtained from cadavers—and where an unpaired organ, such as heart or liver is required, then naturally there can be no alternative.

Taking renal transplantation as the most common and most successful technique, it must be noted that there is a marked shortfall of donor material compared to the number of patients in end-stage renal failure who need a transplant. Due to the origin of renal donations, they must be obtained from brain-dead victims on mechanical life support. Most of this category of donor patient will have had severe brain damage, due either to a head injury or to a cerebral vascular accident, primarily sub-arachnoid haemorrhage. Though in Britain there are over 6000 fatal road accidents a year (a large number of them head injuries who theoretically could each donate two kidneys) the number of renal transplants is less than a thousand—and due to the unfavourable publicity following the 1980 B.B.C. television programme, this number declined sharply for a long period.

The reason for the shortfall is partly the reluctance or apathy of doctors to request permission for donation—it is rare for relatives to refuse such a request for kidneys, though curiously, the refusal rate for corneal transplants is appreciable.

In former years, the removal of kidneys for transplantation was only carried out after the heart had stopped following the termination of mechanical respiration. As any "warm ischaemic time" – i.e. anoxia of the organs whilst still in the body – significantly reduced the success rate of transplantation, kidneys are now removed with a beating heart, but after death has been certified on the grounds of brain-stem death. This results in a better chance of the renal graft "taking", which is medically and ethically a justification for the removal during cardiac activity, as otherwise the recipient has a greater risk from two surgical operations, one to install the graft and the other to remove it.

The Human Tissue Act (1961) is the statute which regulates the donation of tissues in Britain. Although imperfect in its drafting, which has resulted in some ambiguities in interpretation, it serves the purpose of transplantation well.

Section 1 (1) of the Act states that if a person during his lifetime expresses in writing (or orally in the presence of two witnesses) a request to donate tissue for therapeutic purposes, the person lawfully in possession of the body after death may authorise removal for that purpose. This is what is termed a "contracting-in" situation, where a person makes a positive act of donation. It is usually mediated through the official Donor Cards, which are obtainable through doctors, Post Offices etc., and are carried upon the person so that in the event of a mortal accident, authority is readily available for donation of any or specified organs.

In some countries, there is a "contracting-out" system, whereby donor organs can be taken from any victim, unless he has left instructions to the contrary. In yet other countries, such as East Germany, there is statutory power for organs or tissues to be taken from any dead person.

Section 1(2) of the Human Tissue Act indicates that where no ante-mortem permission was given by the donor, the person *lawfully in possession of the body* may authorise removal of the required tissues *if having made such enquiry as may be practicable*, he has no reason to believe that:

(a) the deceased had expressed his objection to donation, or

(b) that the surviving spouse or *any surviving relative* objects to the procedure.

Though these provisions appear simple, there are some difficulties in interpretation. For instance, *reasonable enquiry as may be practicable* has never been defined. The circumstances of obtaining suitable donor organs are often urgent and may even occur in the middle of the night, so how extensive, both numerically and geographically, need these enquiries be? *The Code of Practice* issued by the Department of Health in 1979 comments as follows upon this point:

"In most instances it will be sufficient to discuss the matter with any one relative who had been in close contact with the deceased, asking him his own views, the views of the deceased, and also if he has any reason to believe that any other relative would be likely to object. There is no need actually to establish a lack of objection before authorising the removal of organs or to make enquiries which are unreasonable or impracticable. If a donor's relatives are inaccessible, it would be impracticable to ask them; and if they were, for example, young children, or seriously ill it would be generally unreasonable to do so".

The person giving authority for the removal of organs is the person lawfully in possession of the body, almost always the relevant Health Authority or District etc., in whose institution the body died. It remains lawfully in his possession until claimed by the person with the right to possession, such as the next-of-kin, coroner, Procurator Fiscal etc.

The person originally in possession need not make the enquiries under the Act himself, but only satisfy himself that they have been carried out, before authorising removal of tissues. The Health Authority delegates this power to an appropriate person—usually a senior doctor. The tissues must be removed by a fully registered medical practitioner, and not a provisionally-registered house officer.

Permission for donation of tissues is thus an *absence of objection* and where sought from relatives, is not normally recorded on a written permission form, as is the practice for autopsy permission. The permission is obtained orally by conversation between the doctor of the treatment team and the relatives. The lack of objection thus obtained is noted in the patient's case record.

As the majority of subjects from organs are taken will be the victims of head injuries, these cases will of necessity be reported to the coroner or Procurator Fiscal. No organ donation can be performed in such cases without the permission of these law officers, as it is possible that the medico-legal investigation of the death may be hampered by such operative interference. In fact, this is rarely a valid objection, as removal of the kidneys is unlikely to interfere with a forensic autopsy concerned mainly with the head injuries. When heart transplantation is involved, it is possible that a previous heart condition may have contributed to a fatal accident. However, it is also unlikely that a potential donor with a history of heart disease would be used.

The permission of the coroner is usually prior "blanket" consent, rather than an individual discussion on every occasion, but there are some coroners who desire to be telephoned in the early hours of the morning to provide their consent.

Where death has been caused by criminal action, the effect of organ removal prior to a forensic autopsy must be carefully considered. The coroner's pathologist may also be consulted as to the possible effect of donation upon the subsequent autopsy.

The booklet *The Removal of Cadaveric Organs for Transplantation: A Code of Practice* (DHSS/HMSO 1979 & 1983) is a most valuable and comprehensive guide to all aspects of organ donation, diagnosis of brain-stem death, corneal transplantation etc.

CHAPTER 24

Disposal of the Dead

In England and Wales—and in most other jurisdictions—it is unlawful to dispose of a dead body until that death has been officially certified, either through the usual registration procedures or after medico-legal investigation has been initiated. This is not quite the same as saying that disposal is unlawful until the *cause of death* and the *identity* of the deceased has been satisfactorily determined, as a small but significant proportion of bodies remain unidentified and have no satisfactory cause of death ascertained. About 5 per cent of autopsies reveal no convincing cause of death. This is more common in infants and young adults, where there is no overlay of arterial degenerative disease to provide a convenient, though not necessarily true cause of death.

In England and Wales, there are about 600,000 deaths each year, of which about two-thirds are disposed of through the medical attendant's certificate and subsequent registration pathway, the remainder being investigated by the coroner.

The formalities surrounding death are designed to provide mortality statistics for the public health (through the Registrar-General and the Office of Population Censuses and Statistics –OPCS) and to prevent concealment of criminal and other unnatural deaths.

The Duty to Dispose of the Dead

Where one has been appointed, the duty to dispose of the body of the deceased falls upon his executor, who has the right of custody of the body for the purpose of disposal. The executor is personally responsible for the charges incurred and it is prudent therefore, before accepting probate of a will, to ensure that there are assets sufficient for this purpose; if there are not, probate should be renounced, unless the executor is prepared to meet the charges personally.

The remains of an intestate are, by custom, disposed of by the surviving spouse or next of kin, failing whom it might be the duty of the person under whose roof the death took place. The local authority within whose area the death occurred, or where the body was found, has the duty to dispose of the remains if it appears no one else has arranged, or is going to arrange, for disposal.

In 1946 it was decided that normally a husband is no longer responsible for the funeral expenses of his deceased wife, when her estate is sufficient to bear them (Rees v. Hughes, 1946). It was not then decided whether he is still responsible in the event that she had left no estate. He may be entitled to a Death Grant.

The Duty to Give Information of a Death

The law is precise on the duty to give information of a death and provision is made to ensure that in all circumstances and on all occasions there will always be some person upon whom this duty shall fall. A succession of persons upon whom the liability falls, as indicated on the back of the "Notice to informant", is prescribed for deaths which occur in a house, in an institution or elsewhere. When the death occurs in a house, the duty falls first upon any relative present at the death. In the last resort, on all occasions, the duty is that of the person causing the body to be buried or cremated.

The informant is required to attend at the office of the registrar of births and deaths to give information and to surrender the personal documents of the deceased, i.e. his medical card and any documents relating to pensions derived from the national funds. The informant must take with him the "Notice to informant" which he receives from the certifying medical practitioner. A medical certificate of cause of death must also be delivered to the registrar, either by post or by the hand of the informant, before the death can be registered. When this has been done the registrar issues his certificate for disposal after registry.

Provision is also made for circumstances in which it is required to dispose of the body before registry. Providing the registrar has notice in writing of the death and receives a satisfactory death certificate, he may issue a certificate for disposal before registry, but only when disposal is to be by burial. The informant must in due course attend at the office of the registrar in order that the death be registered.

Report of a Death to the Coroner

At common law, "It is the duty of every person who is about the deceased to give immediate notice to the coroner or to his officer, or to the appropriate officer of police, of circumstances requiring the holding of an inquest" (Jervis, 1957, p. 56). There is however, no means open to a coroner to enforce the performance of this duty.

It has become a widely adopted practice by doctors to report such deaths to the coroner and to withhold the medical certificate of cause of death. This procedure has no legal sanction, since the practitioner who is in attendance during the last illness has a statutory duty to issue a medical certificate. However, it has been the convention for very many years for a doctor who intends to report a death to the coroner, to abstain from issuing a death certificate. In 1979, the Registrar-General of Births and Deaths requested that the strict requirements should be more closely adhered to, though the British Medical Association protested that this was impracticable in many cases. In the event, a compromise has been reached:

(a) It is for the doctor to decide whether he was "in attendance during the last illness". If the mode of death is one which reasonably could be expected to arise from the illness for which the doctor was attending, then the Registrar General wishes the doctor to issue a certificate, even with a speculative cause of death. The fact that such a certificate is issued by no means inhibits the doctor from reporting to the coroner, in order that a coroner's autopsy might more exactly arrive at the cause of death.

(b) If the doctor honestly has no idea as to the cause of death, even though he attended during the last illness, then there is obviously no point in him attempting to issue a certificate.

(c) If he does issue a certificate in a case which he wishes to report to the coroner, he should initial "Box A" on the back of the certificate, but also contact the coroner by telephone in the usual way. He should not rely upon the delivery of the certificate to the Registrar of Births and Deaths as a means of notifying the coroner.

(d) Irrespective of whether the doctor attended the patient in his last illness (which has no particular time scale), if his last visit to the patient was more than 14 days before death and he has not seen the body after death, then the local Registrar of Births and Deaths has instructions to report the case to the coroner. The doctor should anticipate this and if he realises that he had not seen the patient in the last fortnight before death, he should spontaneously report the case to the coroner, whether or not he sees fit to give a certificate. The alternative allowed by the Registrar of seeing the body after death is most unsatisfactory, as it merely excludes obvious trauma and is virtually useless as an aid to determining the cause of a natural death.

The paramount consideration of the doctor is in reporting to the coroner all those cases which should come under his jurisdiction.

The office of coroner is one of the most ancient in the English legal system and one which retains a considerable amount of power, though this has lessened over the years. The name derives from *custos placitorum coronas*—Keeper of the Crown Pleas, and possibly dates as far back as Saxon times. The office was certainly in existence at the end of the 12th century.

The coroner investigated unnatural deaths, treasure trove, wrecks, fires and so on, all of which had a financial aspect. Over the years most of these responsibilities have been shed, until the coroner of the present day is involved almost totally with the investigation of death, though some vestigial interests such as treasure trove still remain.

There are about 180 coroners in England and Wales, the vast majority being practicing solicitors who carry out coroner's work on a part-time basis. A few large cities, including the area of Greater London Council, have full-time coroners who are both medical practitioners and barristers. It has always been a matter of some controversy as to whether a medical or legal qualification is the more important requisite for a coroner, but the Brodrick Report (1971) made recommendations in favour of lawyers. The coroners are employed by the local authority, but once appointed, enjoy a large degree of autonomy and cannot be dismissed except for a grave breach of behaviour. The ultimate authority over coroners is the Lord Chancellor, who himself has the powers of a coroner, as do all High Court Judges.

Following the partial implementation of the Brodrick Report (1971), a number of changes in coroner's procedure were made in the period 1977–1980. The major changes were the abolition of the coroner's power to commit a person for trial on a charge of criminally causing a death (Criminal Law Act, 1977): the abolition of the need for the coroner to himself view the body before inquest (Coroner's Act, 1980): the acceptance of written, instead of oral, evidence, which is of great advantage to doctors as they now attend the coroner's court much less frequently (Coroner's Rules, 1980): the referral of criminal deaths to the Director of Public Prosecutions (Coroner's Rules, 1977): and the dispensing with the need for a jury in many inquests (Criminal Law Act, 1977).

According to the Coroner's Rules 1953–1980 (Consolidated), the following deaths should be reported to the coroner:

1. When no doctor has treated the deceased in his or her last illness.
2. When the doctor attending the patient did not see him or her within 14 days before the death or after death.
3. When the death occurred during an operation or before recovery from an anaesthetic.
4. When the death was sudden and unexplained or attended by suspicious circumstances.
5. When the death might be due to an industrial injury or disease or to accident, violence, neglect or abortion or to any kind of poisoning.

This "official" list does not specifically mention other types of death which should invariably be reported, such as deaths in legal custody or any allegation of negligence, medical or otherwise.

It is broadly similar to the list of situations in which a Registrar of Births and Deaths must himself report cases to the coroner: in the latter instance, the Registrar reporting is mandatory whilst that above referring to doctors is advisory, though as the Registrar will query any doubtful death certificate sent by the doctor, the difference is largely academic, apart from the delay involved.

Numerically, by far the largest group of cases reportable to the coroner are those natural deaths (or presumed natural deaths) which have occurred either suddenly and/or unexpectedly. Though a patient may be under the care of the medical attendant for a long period, the nature of his disease may not be such as to give to an expectation of sudden death.

Death should be reported to the coroner if:

(a) The doctor has not been in attendance during the last illness, which for the purposes of reporting to the coroner means during the last 14 days. Though legally he can provide the Registrar with a certificate if he sees the body after death, this is a most unsatisfactory alternative, and one which the Registrar may well reject.
(b) Even if he has attended recently, if he does not know the cause of death, then he must report to the coroner.
(c) If he has any doubts about the natural causation, again he must report.

In passing, it may be mentioned that though the doctor may be satisfied in his own mind as to the cause of death, he is frequently incorrect. Several surveys have been carried out, one as recently as 1980, in which the cause of death as given by the clinician was compared with the cause of death obtained after autopsy. In several of these series the error was of the order of 50 per cent—that is, the clinician was as often wrong as he was correct! It must be admitted that the difference between the clinical and pathological diagnoses was often trivial e.g. coronary thrombosis as opposed to myocardial fibrosis, but in 25 per cent of the cases, the disparity was marked, often laying in a totally different anatomical system. These errors may sometimes be of considerable medico-legal importance, especially in relation to insurance and compensation aspects: they also introduce a great error in mortality statistics.

The coroner's routine work is carried out by his "coroner's officer", usually a police officer of considerable experience. In rural areas, this function is performed by the first police officer attending the death, though this is not such a satisfactory method.

The doctor, as well as the general public, usually contacts the coroner's officer for routine matters associated with deaths. The coroner studies the papers supplied by the officer and decides whether he wishes to dispose of it without ordering a post-mortem examination. This is uncommon in large cities, where the autopsy rate may approach 100 per cent, but if the coroner is satisfied that the medical attendant is confident that he knows the cause of death, he may dispose of the case on his Form A. This may be done for instance, when a case is reported because of the "24-hour rule" after emergency admission to hospital, but the doctor is satisfied that he knows the cause of death. Form A notifies the Registrar that the coroner is taking no further action: the doctor must then issue a death certificate in the usual way.

Most commonly—almost invariably in large jurisdictions—a post-mortem examination will be ordered. Formerly, this could be done by any practitioner, but the coroner is now strongly recommended by his Rules only to employ a pathologist with access to laboratory facilities.

In criminal or suspicious cases, the coroner is advised by the Coroner's Rules to accept the advice of the Chief Constable in choosing a pathologist of special experience, i.e. a forensic pathologist with experience in criminal matters.

When the post-mortem has been completed, the disposal of the case will depend partly on the determined cause of death and partly on the surrounding circumstances of the death. The great majority of the cases are due to natural death and can be signed up on the coroner's pink Form B, which notifies the Registrar of the medical cause of death and allows disposal without the necessity for an inquest.

Certain types of cases cannot be disposed of without an inquest. These comprise criminal cases (murder, manslaughter and infanticide), suicides, road, aviation, rail, domestic and other accidents, industrial accidents and diseases, deaths in prison or police custody, deaths where negligent medical treatment is alleged, deaths from neglect and any other case where the coroner feels that a public hearing would be beneficial.

The relatives of the deceased may not take kindly to the suggestion that the coroner should be informed and pressure may be brought to bear upon the doctor to issue a medical certificate which ascribes the death to natural causes. It is then an invidious situation but the doctor's duty is clear. He issues a false or dishonest certificate at his peril.

Disposal by Burial

The first step is the issue of a medical certificate of cause of death and the notice to informant. This is followed by registration of the death. When the death is registered, the informant receives a certificate for disposal after registry from the Registrar of Births and Deaths. Disposal by burial then takes place and the formalities are completed by the return to the registrar of a certificate of disposal. If there are no grounds for reporting the case to the coroner, the death certificate must be issued by a registered medical practitioner (which in hospital practice, includes a provisionally registered doctor working under supervision of his seniors) and as cannot be too often repeated, may only be issued if the doctor was in attendance upon the deceased during his last illness, though no time limit is laid down for this attendance. The "14 day rule" refers to reporting to the coroner, not to the issue of a death certificate, though formerly the two were interdependent. The doctor must also be satisfied as to the cause of death.

The books in which death certificates are issued to the doctor contain a wealth of information and directions as to the proper method of completion; unfortunately this advice is all too often ignored. Improper completion of certificates so frequently causes delays and further distress to the relatives, that considerable care should be employed by the doctor when writing them. The local Registrar is obliged to reject any certificate which shows facts incompatible with registration.

The information to be given on the face of the certificate, firstly, relates the particulars of the deceased and details of the doctor's attendance. The name and age of the deceased and place and date of death are entered. The doctor must then state when he last saw the deceased alive, whether the body was seen or not seen after death, and whether the cause of death has or has not been confirmed by post-mortem.

The second part of the certificate states the cause of death. The completion of this part may sometimes create difficulty but the examples given in the books of forms are a valuable guide. It is desired to state the disease or condition directly leading to death i.e. 1(a), and the antecedent cause in 1(b). Under II, the doctor will insert any other significant conditions which contributed to but were not related to the cause given in 1(a) and 1(b). On most occasions an entry under 1(a) is alone necessary, e.g. lobar pneumonia, pulmonary tuberculosis or cancer of the stomach. Post-operative deaths provide greater difficulty in the arrangement of the certified causes, but useful examples are given by the Registrar-General.

Due care is necessary to avoid indefinite or unsatisfactory terms and the book of forms includes a list, arranged in alphabetical order, of those terms which should not be used. If they appear on the certificate a registrar is obliged to make further inquiries or to suspend registration of the death and to refer the death to the coroner. This may interfere with the funeral arrangements.

Since 1951, it is also necessary to state in the space next to that provided for the cause of death, the duration of the illness. This is to bring the certificates into line with those used elsewhere in the world.

The third and last part of the certificate contains the certifying clause, by which the doctor certifies (1) that he was in medical attendance upon the deceased during the last illness, and (2) that the particulars and cause of death above written are true to the best of his knowledge and belief.

His signature is accompanied by his qualifications as registered by the Medical Council. It is well to ensure that this detail is correct. A doctor of medicine, who has not registered his higher degree, should sign only M.B., Ch.B., when that is his only registered qualification.

At the back of the certificate there are two spaces (or statements) which may have to be initialled. In space "A" the insertion of doctor's initials shows the registrar that the coroner has been informed of the death and this at once suspends registration until the coroner's decision be made known to the registrar.

When space "B" is initialled the Registrar-General is informed that, at a later date, the doctor may be able to give more precise or additional information, as may be obtained by microscopy for example, concerning the cause of death. This is for the purpose of statistical classification. When space "B" is initialled, the Registrar-General, in due course, sends an application for further information concerning the death.

A doctor is still under no legal obligation to see the body after death, but prudence dictates that an inspection of the body be made. The possibility of an accident sustained by the deceased e.g. a fall out of bed, capable of accelerating the death, has to be excluded. Nor is it beyond the bounds of possibility that homicidal violence has been inflicted on the deceased, or that the patient is not, in fact, yet dead. The importance of seeing the body after death is increasingly appreciated and is now apparently undertaken after over 95 per cent of all deaths; it should be made obligatory.

Attendance upon the deceased should have been by way of more than one visit, since it is not usually possible, especially if a patient be *in extremis*, accurately to diagnose his condition by one examination alone. Unfortunately there is, as yet, no statutory definition of attendance.

The certificate when completed is to be sent to the registrar. It may be sent by post in a franked envelope, or it may be delivered by hand. The notice to informant, the right-hand portion of the form, is also signed and handed to the relative or other person who is to act as the informant. It may be more convenient also to hand the death certificate to this person; the doctor is required to ensure its safe delivery to the registrar forthwith, but the mode of delivery is at his discretion.

Upon the informant attending the Registrar, (when in addition to the Notice to Informant, he must give up certain other documents such as the Medical Card, Pensions certificates etc.) death will be registered and the Registrar will issue a certificate for disposal. This is delivered to the undertaker and after burial formalities have been completed the Registrar is further notified that burial has been completed. It is a criminal offence to dispose of a body otherwise than via this Statutory procedure. The person responsible for seeing that the procedure is carried out is the executor or if the deceased was intestate, the next of kin. If no relatives can be traced, the local authority is obliged to both organise and pay for disposal of the body.

Disposal by Cremation

The first step is the issue of the medical certificate of cause of death and registration of the death as already described. The only difference in this part of the procedure is that a registrar may not issue a certificate for disposal, before registry, when he has reason to believe that disposal is to be by cremation.

Due to the almost complete destruction of the body following cremation, there were natural fears that all medico-legal evidence would be lost. About the only post-cremation evidence that has ever been obtained concerns thallium poisoning! In consequence, the regulations governing cremation are much more stringent than for burial, though in fact this is now rather an anachronism, as over 70 per cent of dead bodies are cremated, leaving burial to be the minority procedure. The legislation concerning cremation is thus archaic and overdue for radical reform. This has been discussed in the Brodrick Report but attempts to modify the procedure have not yet materialised.

Cremation in Great Britain became legal at the end of the last century, mainly due to the somewhat bizarre activities of a South Wales general practitioner, Dr. William Price of Llantrisant. This eccentric family doctor, towards the end of a colourful career, became the father of a small son named Jesus Christ Price. When the infant died, his father publically cremated him in a field in full view of a departing chapel congregation. The public outrage caused him to be arrested, but he conducted his own defence at Cardiff

Assizes and was acquitted. This became a precedent for cremation and the first Cremation Act was passed in 1902. The current outdated procedure basically stems from that time.

The cremation formalities are set out on no less than seven forms, distinguished by the letters, A, B, C, D, E, F, and G. Only two of these need concern the medical practitioner.

The Application for Cremation: Form "A"

The executor, or other person responsible for the disposal, must apply to the Cremation Authority for cremation. This is done on Form "A", which contains a number of questions to which the applicant must give true answers. The applicant must disclose his authority to apply for cremation; he or she should be either the executor or the nearest surviving relative. Any other person must give satisfactory reasons for assuming this duty. The applicant must state whether the deceased left any written instructions as to the mode of disposal of his remains. Opposition to cremation, expressed by any near relative, must be disclosed. The date and place of the death are stated. The applicant is also required to disclose any reason he may have to suspect that the death was due directly or indirectly to violence, poison, privation or neglect. He must also say whether there is any reason to suppose that an examination of the remains may be desirable. The name of the ordinary medical attendant and the names of the doctors who attended during the last illness are to be given.

Formerly this application had to be supported by a statutory declaration, but under the Cremation Act, 1952, amending the Cremation Act, 1902, a statutory declaration has been replaced by the countersigning of the application by a responsible person to whom the applicant is known. Provision is made by the Cremation Regulations, 1952 for persons in one or other of twelve groups to be competent to verify these applications. They include members of parliament, justices of the peace, professional men and women, permanent civil servants, officers of H. M. Forces, police officers, not below the rank of sergeant, and trade union officials. It is therefore possible for any applicant promptly to obtain verification.

Certificate of Medical Attendant: Form "B"

This is a lengthy document which must be completed by the medical practitioner in attendance during the last illness. The form itself should be examined carefully and due note taken not only of the eighteen questions, but also the instructions.

The practitioner must answer all the questions. He must see and identify the body after death. If he is a relative or if he has any pecuniary interest in the death of the deceased, this must be disclosed.

Details of the cause of death are required, as in the ordinary certificate, but in addition the mode of death, e.g. syncope, coma, exhaustion or convulsions, is stated, and also its duration. This answer may depend upon his own observations or on statements made by others. If not based on his own observations, the name of his informant is to be stated. In the event of any operation upon the deceased during the final illness, particulars of it are given, including the name of the surgeon. The names of those who nursed the deceased are required and it must be shown whether they were professional nurses or relatives. The names of the persons (if any) present at the death are given.

The doctor must state whether he has any doubts about the character of the disease or the cause of death. Has he any reason to suspect it was due, directly or indirectly, to violence, poison, privation or neglect? Is there any reason to suppose a further examination of the body is desirable?

The certifying clause certifies that the answers are true and accurate to the best of belief and knowledge. Also, that there is no reason to suspect that the death was due to a violent or an unnatural cause or that it was sudden, of which the cause is unknown, or occurred in any place or circumstances as to require an inquest.

Confirmatory Medical Certificate: Form "C"

This second medical certificate may be signed only by a registered medical practitioner of not less than 5 years since *full* registration and one who is not related to the deceased, nor a relative or partner of the doctor who has issued certificate "B".

This doctor should see the body of the deceased and should have made personal inquiry, as stated in his answers to the questions. He must answer all of eight questions. Special attention is drawn to the fourth, namely, "Have you *seen* and questioned the medical practitioner who issued Certificate "B"? (The rubric says he must see the body, and the certifier in Form B.)

He is asked also if he has seen and questioned any other doctor in attendance, any person who nursed the deceased during the last illness or was present at the death, or any of the relatives of the deceased. If he did so, their names must be given and he must say whether he saw them alone.

He must certify that he is satisfied that the cause of death is that stated in his certificate and that he has no reason to suspect the death was either a violent or unnatural one or a sudden death of which the cause is unknown or that it occurred in a place or circumstance such as to require an inquest.

Authority to Cremate: Form "F"

The final document necessary in the normal procedure for cremation is issued by the medical practitioner appointed by the cremation authority as their medical referee. This is usually a Community Physician often the District Medical Officer.

Before granting his authority to cremate, it is his duty to satisfy himself that all the requirements of the Cremation Act and Regulations have been complied with, that the cause of death has been *definitely ascertained* and that there exists no reason for any further inquiry or examination.

He must therefore scrutinise the documents with care. He must also be satisfied as to the manner in which the cause of death, and the identity of the deceased were ascertained.

When the official in charge of the crematorium has received Form "F", the authority to cremate, from the funeral director, he will give instructions for the cremation to proceed. It is also reasonable for this step to be taken when the crematorium superintendent receives verbal information from the Medical Referee or his representative, that "Form F" has been issued, but is not immediately available.

After the cremation the notification of disposal is completed and returned to the registrar of births and deaths. This will have been furnished by the registrar or by the coroner as a detachable portion, either of the certificate for disposal, or the coroner's Form "E".

Comment on the Procedure

Medical practitioners must give due attention to the questions and answer them truthfully. The confirming practitioner should not omit to see and question the doctor who issued certificate "B". The failure of a practitioner to observe this rule led to his prosecution and conviction. This practitioner, who had otherwise punctiliously fulfilled all the other requirements, stated that he had seen the doctor who issued certificate "B", when in fact, on each of nine occasions, he had not done so. His conviction subsequently brought him before the General Medical Council who, however, after administering a reprimand decided, in view of his excellent character, not to direct erasure of his name.

It is unlawful, also, for a confirming practitioner to issue certificate "C", when in fact he is himself confined to bed and unable to see the body or those persons he should see and question before he issues the certificate. We have reason to believe this reminder is not superfluous.

Cremation After Report of the Death to a Coroner: Form "E"

When a death has been reported to the coroner and he has dealt with it either by ordering a post-mortem and without holding an inquest, or by holding an inquest, certification of cause of death is by his Form "E". This replaces the usual certificates "B" and "C", but it is not the authority to cremate. The medical referee must also issue his Form "F" before cremation can take place.

In these circumstances then, the necessary documents will include the application in Form "A", the coroner's certificate in Form "E" and the authority to cremate, Form "F". After cremation has taken place, the notification of disposal, which is a part of the coroner's Form "E", is completed and returned to the registrar.

Inquiry by the Medical Referee: Form "D"

The medical referee has power to order, or himself to make, a post-mortem examination before he authorises cremation. It is an unusual procedure in England since a medical referee is more likely to notify the coroner when he has reason to believe a post-mortem examination may be necessary. If, however, he orders or makes this investigation, certification of the cause of death is by Form "D", which replaces the usual medical certificates, namely "B" and "C".

The medical referee is in a unique position in relation to cremation since he can, if also a coroner, issue at one time or another certificates "B", "C", "D", "E" and "F", although when he is the medical attendant of the deceased and has issued Form "B", he cannot then issue any of the other certificates required for that cremation.

A recent addition to cremation procedure (though not part of the statutory requirements) is to safeguard crematoria and their employees from the risk of explosion and contamination from cardiac pacemakers. Pacemakers frequently have mercury-containing batteries and some modern types are even powered by nuclear fuel. The cremation of a body containing such a pacemaker may be hazardous, as mercury batteries explode.

Therefore most cremation medical forms have an addition requesting notification of whether a pacemaker is fitted and whether it has been removed. The procedure for removal is at present a matter of some doubt, but where there is an autopsy, it is removed by the pathologist. Where no post-mortem takes place, it may be removed by any doctor or possibly by an embalmer or funeral director, though the exact legal position of non-medically qualified removers is yet to be clarified.

Still-births

A still-birth must be registered before it is lawful to dispose of the body. Forms for this purpose are to be obtained from the registrar of births and deaths.

The statutory definition of a still-born child is "a child which has issued forth from its mother after the 28th week of pregnancy and which did not, at any time after being completely expelled from its mother, breathe or show any other signs of life".

The certifier, who may be either a registered medical practitioner or a certified midwife, is competent to issue these certificates either when in attendance at the birth or, if absent at that time, when they have examined the body of the child. (Where a doctor and midwife are both in attendance, the certificate should be issued by the doctor.)

The upper portion of the certificate indicates the circumstances, i.e. present at the birth or that the body was examined, and includes the certifying clause. There follows a statement of the "cause of death" together with an estimate of the duration of the pregnancy and, if known, the weight of the foetus. (This addition to certificates of still-birth was introduced by an amendment of the Births and Deaths Registration Act, 1953, Section 11, by Section 2 of the Population (Statistics) Act, 1960). In the lower third of the certificate an indication is given as to whether the certified cause of death was, or was not, confirmed by post-mortem. The certifier then signs and dates the certificate and inserts his or her registered qualification and address. The books of forms issued by the Registrar-General include examples of the method of using these forms and a list of indefinite or undesirable terms to be avoided.

These certificates, at the reverse, indicate the persons who are qualified as informants. It is emphasised that the certificates are not an authority for burial or cremation.

The issue of these certificates is now a statutory duty. No fee is prescribed or prohibited but, in the case of National Health Service patients, medical practitioners and midwives have been advised to waive a fee.

Certification based solely on external examination of the body and by persons unskilled in forensic pathology is most unsatisfactory, and should cease to be lawful. The pathologist has sufficient difficulty in ascertaining the cause of death in newly-born infants, even when he has opportunity to apply the full range of investigations open to him. Furthermore, killing the newly-born, without leaving obvious traces, is only too easy to accomplish.

The certificate is handed to the informant, who may be the father, if of a legitimate child, the mother, the occupier of the house in which the birth took place or, if in an institution, the chief resident officer, or any person present at the birth. The informant must attend at the office of the registrar of births and deaths for the purpose of registration.

When the procedure for registration of still-births was revised in 1960 no change was made in the law which allows registration of still-birth, in the absence of one of these certificates, when the informant makes a statutory declaration of still-birth and states why a certificate cannot be obtained.

Disposal Procedure in Scotland

The Registration of Births, Deaths and Marriages (Scotland) Act 1965 provides that either the doctor in attendance upon the deceased (or if there was no such doctor, any other doctor) is able to issue a certificate. As in England and Wales, the doctor does not have to see the body after death in order to issue a certificate. Due to geographical difficulties, such as in the remote islands, it was necessary to provide for registration without viewing by a doctor, though in fact few deaths are not actually seen by the certifying doctor.

Unlike England, it is possible for a body to be buried before the death has been registered, though in such a case, the Registrar must be notified of such an event. Cremation can only be carried out after registration: similar documentation exists in the English system.

In Scotland, the Act requires the doctor to "transmit (the certificate) to any person who is a qualified informant in relation to the death, or to the Registrar". This is official recognition of the usual practice in both England and Scotland of the relative personally conveying the certificate to the Registrar.

The Scottish certificate is very similar to that in England and Wales, but has no separate "Notice to Informant". It has an extra box requesting notification if the deceased was a married woman and death occurred during pregnancy or within 6 weeks thereafter.

Unlike the English certificate, it does not require the doctor to state when the deceased was last seen alive and the back of the certificate does not carry the boxes "A" and "B", which indicate whether the death was reported to the coroner nor whether further clinical information (other than that from a post-mortem) is likely to be available.

Still-birth Procedure in Scotland

The procedure differs only in detail from that for England and Wales. A registered medical practitioner, or a certified midwife, is qualified to certify a still-birth when present (formerly when "in attendance") at the birth or after examining the body of the child, but when not present at the birth. The Certificate of Still-birth requires the cause of death to be stated and an estimate made of the duration of pregnancy. Differences in detail from the English Certificate include these omissions: the name of the mother; the weight of foetus, if known; an indication of confirmation, or lack of confirmation, of cause of death by post-mortem.

Those who are qualified and liable to act as informants in Scotland are as for England and Wales, with the addition of the nurse present at the still-birth. It is provided that a registered medical practitioner or certified midwife, present at the birth or who has examined the body of the still-born child, shall, on request, give a Certificate of Still-birth to any person who is required to give information of the still-birth.

It is lawful in Scotland, as in England and Wales, for a person to declare a still-birth in circumstances where the normal certificate has not been obtained.

The registrar, on receiving a satisfactory Certificate of Still-birth, and information touching the birth, registers the still-birth in the presence of the informant. The informant is required to verify the particulars entered in the register and any necessary correction must be made in the presence of the informant. A certificate of registration is then issued.

When the birth has been brought to the notice of the procurator fiscal, he sends a schedule of result of his precognition to the registrar. If the still-birth has not already been registered, the registrar shall register the still-birth and the entry will show that it is on the confirmation of the procurator fiscal (or his deputy).

Burial of a still-born infant in Scotland must be notified to the registrar. This notice is issued by the keeper or other person in charge of the burial ground. No notice of disposal by cremation is as yet required.

Scottish Procurator Fiscal

There is a Procurator Fiscal for each Sheriff Court District and his main responsibility is the initiation of prosecutions of criminal offences. Procurators Fiscal are appointed by the Lord Advocate and most of them are full-time officers, though in a few areas local Solicitors act as Fiscals on a part-time basis.

Apart from his main function in initiating prosecutions, the Fiscal has the duty to investigate any sudden, violent, suspicious, accidental deaths or deaths from unknown causes, which are reported to him.

His interest in these deaths is closely linked with his criminal responsibility, in that his main concern is to establish whether or not there has been any criminality or possible negligence involved in the death. He is not obliged to establish the precise cause of death in the medical sense, once the possibility of criminal proceedings have been ruled out.

The duties of the Procurator Fiscal in the investigation of sudden or suspicious deaths, differ from the English system in that there is no public inquest, though public enquiries take place in certain circumstances. The Fiscal's enquiry takes the form of "precognition" of witnesses, both lay and medical. A precognition is an informal statement, not on oath, which could form the basis of the oral testimony to which a witness would give at any subsequent trial. This precognition is taken in person by a Procurator Fiscal or a Deputy at a private sitting and a person who fails to attend for the taking of such a precognition may be fined or imprisoned for contempt of court.

The main difference between the English and Scots system of reporting deaths is that in Scotland, any doctor can certify a death if he feels competent to do so, whereas in England only a doctor who was in attendance during the last illness can do so. As in England and Wales, the Registrar of Births and Deaths is the only person with a statutory obligation to report deaths to the Procurator Fiscal or coroner, though in fact, as in England and Wales, most cases are voluntarily reported by doctors and the police.

The Registrar of Births and Deaths and Marriages is obliged to notify the Procurator Fiscal of all deaths which fall into any one of nineteen categories. The types of death which the Registrar must report are as follows:-

1. Any uncertified death.
2. Any death which was caused by an accident arising out of the use of a vehicle, or which was caused by an aircraft or rail accident.

3. Any death arising out of industrial employment, by accident, industrial disease or industrial poisoning.
4. Any death due to poisoning (coal gas, barbiturate, etc.)
5. Any death where the circumstances would seem to indicate suicide.
6. Any death where there are indications that it occurred under an anaesthetic.
7. Any death resulting from an accident in the home, hospital, or institution or any public place.
8. Any death following abortion.
9. Any death apparently caused by neglect (malnutrition).
10. Any death occurring in prison or a police cell where the deceased was in custody at the time of death.
11. Any death of a newborn child whose body is found.
12. Any death (occurring not in a house) where deceased's residence is unknown.
13. Death by drowning.
14. Death of a child from suffocation (including overlaying).
15. Where the death occurred as a result of smallpox or typhoid.
16. Any death as a result of a fire or explosion.
17. Any sudden death.
18. Any other death due to violent, suspicious or unexplained cause.
19. Deaths of foster children.

These provisions are currently under review to bring them up to date e.g. the references to smallpox, typhoid, coal-gas, overlaying etc.

When apprised of a death, the Procurator Fiscal makes further enquiries via the police, his only form of investigative agency. There is no exact parallel to the English "coroner's officer" but investigations are carried out on the Fiscal's behalf by uniformed or plain clothes officers, seconded for duty as "sudden death officers". The C.I.D. may be involved where necessary. The police make investigations in all cases except those concerning anaesthetic deaths, for which there is a special procedure.

When the available information is to hand, the Fiscal will decide whether or not an autopsy is necessary. The autopsy rate in Scotland is far lower than in England and Wales and again is often directed at the main necessity for confirming or excluding criminality or negligence. The police surgeons are more involved in the system than in England. The Fiscal will normally invite a police surgeon to make an external examination of the body. The police surgeon will, if he feels able after having seen the police report, certify the cause of death. If the Fiscal requires an autopsy or if the police surgeon cannot certify, the pathologist will issue a death certificate based on his findings. The Procurator Fiscal cannot himself issue a death certificate as can the English coroner, but he will issue a cremation certificate if required.

The Fiscal may also ask another doctor who has not previously seen the deceased to examine the body and if this doctor is willing to give a certificate, the investigation may go no further.

If the Fiscal considers that an autopsy is necessary, he must apply for authority for this from the Sheriff. This is almost invariably granted by the Sheriff, on the grounds of one of the following four reasons:

(a) That his enquiries cannot be completed unless the cause of death is fully established.
(b) That there are circumstances of suspicion.
(c) That there are allegations of criminal conduct.

(d) That death was associated with anaesthesia in connection with a surgical operation and the fact that all precautions were taken must be established.

Certain categories of death are reportable by the Procurator Fiscal to the Crown Office, to whom he must communicate the result of the investigation. Outside these categories, the Fiscal can conclude the investigation with or without autopsy, without reference to other authorities.

Deaths which must be reported to the Crown Office are as follows:

1. Where there are any suspicious circumstances.
2. Where death was caused by an accident arising out of the use of a vehicle.
3. Where the circumstances point to suicide.
4. Where the death was caused by an accident, poison or disease, notice of which is required to be given to any government department or to any Inspector or other officer of a government department under or in pursuance of any Act.
5. Where the death occurs in circumstances continuance of which or possible recurrence of which is prejudicial to the health and safety of the public.
6. Where the death occurred in industrial employment.
7. Where the death occurred in any prison or police cell or where the deceased was in custody at the time of his death.
8. Where death occurred under an anaesthetic or in unusual circumstances or if there are features which suggest negligence.
9. Where death was due to gas poisoning.
10. Where death was directly or indirectly connected with the actions of a third party whether or not criminal responsibility rests on any person.
11. Where any desire has been expressed that a public enquiry should be held into the circumstances of the death or where the Procurator Fiscal is of the opinion that a public enquiry should be held under the Fatal Accidents and Sudden Deaths Enquiry (Scotland) Act, 1976.

The Crown Office may order further enquiries to be made if they are not satisfied with the conclusiveness of the Procurator Fiscal's investigation. Otherwise the Lord Advocate, acting through Crown counsel, may decide that no further action is necessary or he may initiate criminal proceedings against a third party or may order a Fatal Accident Inquiry to be made in public. The latter is about the only parallel to the English inquest that exists in Scotland. A public enquiry must be held on deaths occurring due to industrial accidents or deaths occurring in legal custody. The Lord Advocate also has discretionary powers to order a public enquiry into the death if he considers it to be in the public interest or if the relatives request it.

Such accidents at places of employment are investigated under the Fatal Accidents Enquiries (Scotland) Act 1976 and no reference to the Crown Office need be made until the enquiry has been concluded. Such an enquiry, must be preceded by a petition to the Sheriff, who appoints a date for the enquiry which is held in public after being advertised in the press. Since the 1976 Act, there is now no jury.

Witnesses can be compelled to attend and evidence is given on oath. Legal representation of the parties is allowed and questioning of the witnesses is permissible. There is no "verdict" as in English inquests, the outcome being the "Sheriff's determination" which may attribute the cause of the accident to negligent persons and defects in the systems of working may be pointed out.

The Lord Advocate can instruct the Procurator Fiscal to apply to the Sheriff for the holding of an enquiry in any case where he considers it expedient to do so in the public interest. Any type of death may form the basis for such an enquiry, and medical mishaps are included in this category.

It is a fundamental principle of Scots law that evidence in criminal cases must be corroborated. Therefore, where medical evidence upon a death is given to the courts, two doctors must have conducted an autopsy, again a parallel with certain European continental countries. There is no necessity for their opinions to be identical, but both are giving evidence on behalf of the Prosecution and should be distinguished from any other medical evidence called for the defence. The new Criminal Justice (Scotland) Act 1980 requires that only one of the two doctors need attend the trial unless the defence request that both be present.

Disposal Procedure in Northern Ireland

Death certification in Northern Ireland is broadly similar to that in England. The doctor is statutorily obliged to issue a certificate of the cause of death. Like the Scottish certificate there is no Notice to Informant. The Informant, the categories of which are listed on the back of the certificate, must deliver the form within 5 days to the Registrar of Births and Deaths. The certificate does not require the age of the deceased to be stated nor whether a post-mortem examination was held. On the reverse there are spaces "A" and "B" as on the English certificate, but "B" does *not* refer to notification to the coroner, but to whether the deceased was a married woman whose death occurred during pregnancy or within 4 weeks of delivery, similar to the Scottish certificate. It is lawful to dispose of a body by burial without obtaining a death certificate or registration of death certificate provided the Registrar of Births and Deaths is notified within the next seven days. It is unlikely that a burial would be permitted in an urban cemetery without the prior production of a registrar's certificate, or coroner's order.

Unlike England and Wales, especially since the 1979 instructions of the Registrar General, a doctor has a statutory obligation not to issue a death certificate and to refer the death to the coroner when the cause of death is unknown, whenever he has reason to believe that the death was due to unnatural causes, negligence or malpractice on the part of others or the administration of an anaesthetic and, where "natural" deaths are concerned, whenever he has not seen and treated the patient for the fatal condition within 28 days of death.

The Coroner's system is very similar to that in England and Wales. Once again coroners are virtually all lawyers rather than doctors and in future only lawyers will be appointed to vacancies.

There is a statutory duty on doctors and funeral directors (amongst others) to report unnatural or suspicious deaths to the coroner. A disposal certificate for burial of a body can be issued without the necessity for opening an inquest, as has to be done under English coroner's practice.

Still-birth Procedure in Northern Ireland

Still-births in Northern Ireland shall now be registered in accordance with the provisions of the Births and Deaths Registration Act (Northern Ireland), 1967, as amended by regulation in 1973. The general procedure now to be followed resembles that in England and Wales and in Scotland, differing only in detail.

It is the duty of an informant to furnish the registrar with particulars for the purpose of registration and the informant must either (a) deliver a Certificate of Still-birth in prescribed form, signed by a registered medical practitioner or a midwife, who was either present at the birth or, if not present, has examined the body, or (b) the informant makes a declaration in prescribed form to the effect that neither a registered medical practitioner nor a midwife were present at the birth, nor has examined the body, or that for some other reason a Certificate of Still-birth cannot be obtained. The declarant must also state that the child was not born alive.

The Certificate of Still-birth will state, to the best of knowledge and belief, the cause of still-birth (note: not as in England and Wales "the cause of death"), the weight of the foetus and the estimated duration of the pregnancy.

In Northern Ireland every registered medical practitioner or midwife present at a still-birth, or who examines the body of a still-born child, shall, without any request being made in that behalf, give a Certificate of Still-birth to the informant.

The registrar, upon registering the still-birth, shall, if so required, give a certificate of registration of the still-birth, to the informant or to the person who has control over, or who ordinarily effects the disposal of bodies at any burial ground or other place where it is intended to dispose of the body of the still-born child. Alternatively, on receiving a written notice of still-birth, accompanied by a Certificate of Still-birth, the registrar, before registering the still-birth, may give a certificate that he has received notice of the still-birth to the person sending that notice. There is no charge for any of these certificates given by a registrar.

The person who lawfully permits disposal of the body of a still-born child shall notify the registrar in prescribed form within 7 days after the date of the disposal, unless he has received a registrar's certificate of notification, or Registry of Still-birth, or an order or authority of a coroner in respect of the still-birth.

Where a coroner at an inquest has found the body to be one of a still-born child, he shall send the registrar, within 5 days after the inquest, a certificate concerning the still-birth, and, where possible, state the cause of the still-birth and give the weight of the foetus and the estimated duration of the pregnancy.

With a view to the compilation of statistics, the informant is required to furnish the same confidential particulars, as is required in England and Scotland, already detailed, with regard to the parentage of the still-born child.

No still-birth shall be registered after the expiration of 3 months from the date of the still-birth.

Definition of still-birth: "the complete expulsion or extraction from its mother after the 28th week of pregnancy of a child which did not at any time after being completely expelled or extracted from its mother breathe or show any other evidence of life". In Northern Ireland, therefore, the statutory definition of still-birth makes specific provision for delivery by Caesarian section, as well as natural delivery.

Procedure in the Republic of Ireland

In the Republic of Ireland, certification is very similar to that of the English procedure.

However, a certificate of the cause of death is not statutorily required for registration and 3 per cent of registered deaths are uncertified as to the medical cause. No disposal note is required to the superintendent of cemeteries and in theory, relatives may bury without registration or certification. If a doctor refuses to issue a certificate to the relatives he should refer to the coroner and the Coroner's Act requires doctors and undertakes to report any suspicious circumstances to the Gardai Siochana (police) or to the coroner.

Still-births are notifiable but do not require still-birth certificates.

A crematorium was opened in Dublin in late 1981 without any specific disposal legislation. A voluntary code of certification has been drafted by the City Coroner and State Pathologist pending legislation on this matter.

The Medical Certificate of the Cause of Death in the Republic of Ireland is very similar to the English counterpart, except that there is no Notice to Informant. As in Scotland, and Northern Ireland, there is provision to record whether the deceased was a married woman and the death was known to òccur during pregnancy or within four weeks thereafter. The approximate interval between the onset of the fatal disease and death is also recorded, if known. The date of last attendance must be recorded, but not the fact that the body was seen after death or that a post-mortem examination was held.

In the Republic of Ireland, the Coroner's Act places a statutory duty on doctors to report any suspicious circumstances to the Gardai or the coroner himself. He cannot return any verdict at an inquest which imputes any crime or civil liability against a third party. The coroner has powers to subpoena a witness to give evidence on oath and failure to comply renders the witness liable to referral by the coroner to the High Court on a charge of contempt of court. The coroner, like the English official, can dispense with the jury in some cases but must summon a panel of between 6 and 12 persons in cases of (a) suspicious death or poisoning (b) traffic accidents (c) in matters prejudicial to public health or safety and in various other statutory circumstances, for example industrial deaths. The coroner does not have the overriding power of the English coroner to nominate a pathologist to carry out a particular post-mortem. The Minister of Justice has the power to do this in suspicious cases, a power which is vested in a Garda (Police) Officer of the rank of Inspector upwards, whereas the English coroner need only be "advised" by the Chief Constable as to the choice of the most suitable pathologist. Relatives or other parties dissatisfied with a Coroner's verdict may appeal to the High Court to have it quashed.

References

BRODRICK COMMITTEE (1971) Report on Death Certification and Coroners. Cmd. 4810. H.M.S.O.
DAVIES, M. R. R. (1982) *The Law of Burial, Cremation and Exhumation*. 5th. ed. London. Shaw and Sons.
JERVIS (1957) *The Office and Duties of Coroners*. 9th. ed., Purchase, B. and Wollaston, H. W. Editors. London. Sweet and Maxwell.
KNIGHT, B. (1982) *Legal Aspects of Medical Practice*. 3rd. ed. London and Edinburgh. Churchill-Livingstone.
POLSON, C. J. and MARSHALL, T. K. (1975) *The Disposal of the Dead*. 3rd. ed. London. English Universities Press.
REES V. HUGHES (1946) 1 K.B. 517; [1946] All E.R. 47.

STATUTES AND REGULATIONS

Births and Deaths Registration Act, 1953; 1 & 2 Eliz. 2 ch. 20.
Coroners Act, 1980; 1980, c. 38.

Coroners Rules, 1953–80; consolidated 1953: S.I. 205; 1956: S.I. 169, 1970: S.I. 1403.
Coroners Amendment Rules, 1977; S.I. 1977, No. 1881.
Coroners Amendment Rules, 1980; S.I. 1980, No. 557.
Cremation Act, 1902; 2 Edw. 7, ch. 8.
Cremation Act, 1952; 15 & 16 Geo. 6; 1 Eliz. 2, ch. 31.
Cremation Regulations, 1952; S.I. 1952, No. 1568.
Criminal Law Act, 1977; 1977, ch. 45.
Criminal Justice (Scotland) Act, 1980. 1980, ch. 62.
Fatal Accidents and Sudden Deaths Inquiry (Scotland) Act, 1976; 1976; ch. 14.
Population (Statistics) Act, 1960; 8 & 9 Eliz. 2 ch. 32.
Registration of Births, Deaths and Marriages (Scotland) Act, 1965; 1965, ch. 49.

CHAPTER 25

The Medical Witness

THOSE who are liable to give evidence, and few doctors are never called upon to give evidence in one or other of the courts, may be assisted by the comments below, especially those on the keeping of records and preparation of evidence.

Impartiality

Procedure demands that the witness will be called by one side or the other. It is, however, the duty of a medical witness at all times to avoid partisanship and to give his evidence impartially. His accurate account of the facts and honest opinion thereon should omit nothing which is relevant, whether it favours or harms the party who calls him. The whole value of his testimony may be lost if any sign of partisanship be apparent.

Records

Since the liability to give evidence cannot always be foretold, a practitioner's only protection is *to make detailed records at the time of his examination of a patient* whenever there is the slightest possibility that the case may become the subject of legal proceedings. To omit this when it is obvious that a criminal prosecution will arise is to court disaster. No detail can then be too trivial to record because, when the case comes to trial, much may depend upon a detail which, at the time of the medical examination, may have seemed insignificant. It is essential to record negative as well as positive findings. It is never satisfactory to assume that absence of mention of a finding implies that it was negative; *mention of it is much more convincing than oral* recollection, which may be vague or faulty.

Accurate, detailed records are invaluable when preparing to give evidence, because this may take place weeks or even months after the examination of the patient. Furthermore, a medical witness has the privilege of refreshing his memory, by reference in court to any record which he had made *at the time of his examination*. Not infrequently the original records require rearrangement and amplification before they are intelligible to others; it is also necessary for them to be reproduced in typescript. In the event that counsel challenges the typescript as happened at one Assizes, the witness has a complete answer if he has with him his original notes and explains that the typed document is a transcription and amplification in order to make it intelligible to the court. If, however, he does not have the original notes to hand, he may not be allowed to refresh his memory from the transcript.

Preparation

No medical witness should give evidence in any court, including the coroner's court, without due preparation. He should refresh his memory of the facts and consider with care the opinion he proposes to express on them. Some thought must be given to the arrangement and presentation of the facts so that his evidence is precise and also intelligible to a lay audience. Fact and opinion should be kept separate in any report. He should also inform himself of the subject in general and thus be better placed to answer questions put in cross-examination by counsel, who has read the books and probably has had advice from competent medical persons.

Precision, especially in respect of dates, dimensions, and quantities, is essential. Testimony which refers to hen's eggs instead of inches or centimetres as a measure of size is wholly unsatisfactory.

Professional Privilege

A medical witness has no professional privilege and, therefore, he must answer any question, unless the answer would incriminate him, although it may disclose matters learnt in professional consultation. He should first obtain a ruling from the judge and, if directed to answer, he must do so without further delay; he may be allowed to write down his answer. Persistent refusal constitutes contempt of court for which the witness will be punished.

Doubt or Ignorance

Honest doubt or ignorance need be no disgrace because the most expert cannot know everything. Ignorance of some matter with which the witness ought to be familiar permits only one course, namely, to say at once he does not know. Prevarication, evasion and, certainly, deliberate lying will bring prompt and condign punishment by way of stern cross-examination and, maybe, rebuke. The witness cannot then complain if, in consequence, he finds himself discredited.

Explanation

A medical witness is unlikely to be refused permission to explain on those occasions when he finds a short answer is inappropriate. Pressure to reply "yes" or "no" to any question which will not admit of it may be countered by the reply, "If I say yes, that would be the truth, but not the whole truth, which I have sworn to tell".

Authorities Cited by Counsel

Not rarely counsel may cite passages from medical books or other publications and invite the opinion of the witness on them. Before making reply it is advisable to ask to see the reference. Check the title, author, *date* and *context*. Time to allow the witness to examine the reference, when it needs close study, should always be granted by the judge.

A witness may adopt the views of any authority as his own, providing he has an honest belief in them. In England he is not permitted to cite living authorities since they could be present as witnesses; he may do so in Scotland.

Conduct in the Witness Box

Clarity of speech and slow delivery are essential. A note of the evidence is being taken, usually in longhand, by judge and by counsel. The jury must hear the evidence and understand it, since the prisoner's fate is in their hands.

Let it be clear that the gravity of the occasion and personal responsibility are well appreciated.

It is not for the witness to argue but simply to answer all questions properly put; the judge will be prompt to rule on their propriety.

Give close attention to the questions and think before making a reply. If the question is not clear or there is doubt about its import, the witness should not hesitate to say so. A courteous request to have it repeated, or restated in some other form, will normally be granted. If the question is of importance to counsel he will want it to be clearly understood by the witness, in order to produce the answer he requires and expects. Counsel's questions are not idle inquiries but are the result of thorough preparation; the witness, therefore, must consider each of them with care.

The Role of the Advocate

Medical practitioners will get a better understanding of the role of the advocate if they read Richard du Cann's *The Art of the Advocate* (1964).

Attendance to give evidence in the Coroner's Court and in the Criminal Courts is required in response to a Summons to attend. This must be obeyed and only in exceptional circumstances, e.g. illness certified by another registered medical practitioner, is the witness likely to be excused. Personal or professional inconvenience is not an excuse; the practitioner must make adequate arrangements for his duties elsewhere to be undertaken by another doctor.

Fees for Medical Witnesses

Fees and expenses for attendance in the Coroner's Court and in the criminal courts are fixed by statute (and the Coroner's schedule). These are revised from time to time.

In civil cases the practitioner should agree, *in advance*, his fee and expenses with the solicitor who proposes to call him as a witness. The solicitor is then entitled to a proof of evidence, i.e. a statement of the doctor's findings and opinion; this forms the basis of instructions to counsel, on which the latter will base his examination of the witness.

If the doctor declines to give evidence in a civil case he can be compelled to attend and produce relevant reports, X-ray films, etc., by writ of subpoena. In these circumstances the solicitor is not entitled to a proof of evidence; he must wait until the doctor gives evidence in order to know what he will say and the solicitor is not entitled to a sight of the documents, etc., until they are produced in court.

Failure on the part of the solicitor to pay the agreed fee and expenses should be reported to the doctor's defence society or to the Law Society. The mere threat of a report is normally effective.

Expert and Ordinary Witnesses

In the past it was customary to teach that when the doctor gave evidence as to fact, including medical facts, he was an ordinary witness but when required to express an opinion on the facts he became an expert witness and thus entitled to a higher fee. The Medical Defence Union (1971) was advised by counsel "that the taxing master has authority to determine the fee payable after considering the whole circumstances. A medical witness giving his opinions on facts would not necessarily become an expert witness; this can be decided only on the facts of the case. A professional witness to fact could not refuse to express an opinion on the facts, unless he felt unqualified by training and experience to do so, in which case he should tell the court that he does not consider himself qualified to express an opinion" (Medical Defence Union, Annual Report, 1971).

Conclusion

It must be stressed that the two principal rules for all medical witnesses are:

1. Keep detailed records, made at the time of the examination of the patient. If impracticable to follow this rule in all cases, it should be kept whenever the circumstances might be the subject of litigation or criminal proceedings at a later date.

Remember that the interval between the date of the examination and the date of the trial may be inordinately long, months, even years. Note the case of "Fall from a helicopter". The medical examinations were made in 1963–4 but the case did not come to trial until December, 1970. Judgment for the defendants turned in no small way on the excellent case notes and letters to the consultant (Medical Defence Union, Annual Report, 1971, p. 49). In the same report, at p. 47, attention is drawn to another case in which 3 years elapsed between examination and the trial. Judgment was given for the defendant doctor, who was also awarded costs. The judge expressed his appreciation of the excellent clinical notes, which he described as "quite out of the ordinary"; they led him to consider the doctor as "intelligent, knowledgeable and concerned for his patients". Remember "Ogden v. Bell", the M.D.U. film.

2. When warned that he is required to give evidence the doctor must make time to prepare himself by a thorough refreshment of his memory of the case and the relevant field of medical practice.

Privileged Occasions and Documents in Relation to the Law of Defamation

In general, a person is responsible for all the consequences which flow from his statements. On occasion, however, it is necessary in the public interest that he shall speak or write the truth without fear of the consequences, i.e. by way of legal proceedings for defamation of character.

Absolute privilege therefore attaches to statements made in either House of Parliament or in a court of law, where the protection extends to all participants, including judge, counsel, the parties and witnesses.

Qualified privilege confers protection of limited extent on those who make oral or written statements in the course of the discharge of any duty, whether it be imposed by law or is a moral or social duty. Qualified privilege attaches to a statement made to protect an interest, which may be one's own or another's. Strict observance of the rules, however, is necessary to secure protection.

The statement must not be malicious, that is, it must not arise from an improper motive, nor be deliberately, unfairly, recklessly or carelessly made. There must be an honest sense of duty.

The statement must be made only to those who have an interest or duty to receive it; wider publication destroys protection.

Common examples of written statements which are covered by qualified privilege are provided by medical certificates of cause of death, and notifications of infectious disease, which a doctor has a statutory duty to issue. In order to secure protection, such documents must be issued only to the proper authority, for example the registrar of births and deaths or the medical officer of health. Their circulation elsewhere, without consent of those entitled to give it, would be a breach of the rules which apply to qualified privilege.

Communications which contain defamatory information, e.g. letters concerning patients, "should be sealed in an envelope, marked confidential and addressed (correctly) to the intended recipient" (Editorial, *Brit. Med. J.,* 1962).

Doctors, being responsible and trusted persons, are not infrequently asked to speak of the character of others. It is important that due care is exercised on these occasions to observe the rules, otherwise there is liability to legal proceedings for defamation of character.

Particular care should be exercised by doctors to refrain from disclosure, even to their wives, of the fact that a recent delivery or abortion has occurred, when the patient is an unmarried woman, widow, or a married woman, separated from her husband. Careless disclosure of such information by Dr. Playfair to his wife resulted in a successful action brought by the patient, his sister-in-law, and the award of exemplary damages; the mistake cost him several thousand pounds (*Kitson* v. *Playfair and wife, The Times,* 21–30 Mar. 1896).

A doctor, as a citizen, has a duty to assist the police but he is under no obligation whatsoever to supply them, at their request, with a list, e.g. of the names of all patients then under his care after recent delivery. Such requests have been made in the past, if made again they should be ignored.

The whole relationship of the doctor to the police has undergone some changes in recent years and the British Medical Association have attempted to reach agreement with police authorities on a Code of Practice, though this is applied inconstantly.

In general, doctors should co-operate with the police to the best of their ability, until their willingness to assist begins to conflict with the ethical duty of professional confidentiality.

This voluntary code had been eroded progressively in recent years; one such example is the Road Traffic Act, 1972 (Section 168) which statutorily obliges members of the public, not excluding doctors, to give information leading to the identification of a driver in a traffic accident.

A leading case in 1974 (Hunter v. Mann) involved a general practitioner who treated two people for minor injuries after they had crashed a stolen car. Police requested the doctor to give them the names and addresses of these patients and when he declined, he was fined £5 at the local magistrates court. The case was taken through the whole of the appeal machinery to the House of Lords, where the conviction was upheld.

The view of Avory, J., expressed in his charge to the grand jury at the Birmingham Autumn Assizes, December, 1914, was otherwise. His remarks were *obiter dicta* and, valuable though the opinion of a learned judge is, these constituted only his opinion.

Following this case the Royal College of Physicians (1916), having obtained counsel's opinion, passed the following resolutions concerning the duties of medical practitioners in relation to abortion:

The College is of opinion:

1. That a moral obligation rests upon every medical practitioner to respect the confidence of his patient; and that without her consent he is not justified in disclosing information obtained in the course of his professional attendance on her.

2. That every medical practitioner who is convinced that criminal abortion has been practised on his patient, should urge her, especially when she is likely to die, to make a statement which may be taken as evidence against the person who has performed the operation, provided always that her chances of recovery are not thereby prejudiced.

3. That in the event of her refusal to make such a statement, he is under no legal obligation (so the College is advised) to take further action, but he should continue to attend the patient to the best of his ability.

4. That before taking any action which may lead to legal proceedings, a medical practitioner will be wise to obtain the best medical and legal advice available, both to ensure that the patient's statement may have value as legal evidence, and to safeguard his own interest, since in the present state of the law there is no certainty that he will be protected against subsequent litigation.

5. That if the patient should die, he should refuse to give a certificate of the cause of death, and should communicate with the coroner.

Although these resolutions are not the law, any medical practitioner who acts in accordance with them would be supported by the College and his medical defence society.

In the event of inquiries which relate to a specific patient, in circumstances which are those of felony, the doctor should first refer the matter to his defence society.

Disclosure of the fact that a patient suffers from syphilis is a breach of professional secrecy. There are, however, occasions on which the doctor may feel it his moral duty to disclose this knowledge; if he does so, he must be careful to observe the rules which apply to qualified privilege. Two examples will suffice to illustrate the right and wrong course of action. In the first case a doctor found himself in the same public swimming-pool as a patient whom he knew to have syphilis. The doctor informed the manager of the baths, who requested the patient to leave. The patient was unsuccessful when he sued the doctor for damages for defamation of character. The doctor had acted in good faith, it was in the public interest for the matter to be disclosed and he had restricted publication to a person who had an interest to receive the information. The occasion, therefore, was privileged; the verdict was for the defendant.

In *Guy* v. *Green* (Leeds Assizes, 1903) the plaintiff was awarded damages against the defendant doctor. On this occasion, a doctor who knew that a barmaid, one of his patients, suffered from syphilis, informed her employer and the housekeeper of the hotel.

Unfortunately he did so in the hearing of one of the other barmaids. It was held that the occasion was privileged as to the employer and the housekeeper but the question of privilege in respect of the other barmaid was left to the jury. They returned a verdict for the plaintiff and awarded £75 in damages.

Disclosure of infection by syphilis to a husband or wife, or to an employer is today a less difficult problem since, it appears, modern treatment can speedily render the patient innocuous to others. The patient should be advised to conduct himself in a manner which will prevent harm to others, so long as he is a danger to them. If the nature of his disease, e.g. general paralysis, renders him unsafe to follow his employment, e.g. that of an engine driver, he should be advised to change his employment. It is only when the patient refuses to co-operate that the doctor may find that he has a moral, social or public duty to disclose his knowledge. Before he takes this step he should obtain the opinion of his medical defence society and act upon their instructions. It is impossible to lay down general rules, since each occasion must be considered separately in the light of its particular circumstances.

The doctor has no duty to inform anyone if he finds that a girl aged 16 years or over is pregnant. It is no doubt in her interests that her parents should be informed, but the doctor should not do so without the consent of the patient. It is not unlawful for a doctor to prescribe or supply contraceptives to a girl under 16, even though this is condoning or assisting an illegal act. It is otherwise if the patient is a mental defective, since intercourse, even with her consent, is unlawful, irrespective of her age. In the latter circumstances it is again for the parent or guardian, in the first instance, to inform the police.

When a homicidal poisoning is suspected the doctor must exercise particular care. In such circumstances, as soon as he has reasonable grounds to suspect this crime, the doctor's best course is to obtain a second opinion without delay. It may then be thought advisable to consult his defence society for guidance. Meantime, specimens should be obtained for toxicological analysis, although the precise purpose of their collection should not be disclosed to the patient or his relatives, lest the suspicions prove groundless.

Disclosure of insanity may be privileged when a third person communicates with the patient's doctor. It may be that the doctor will impart the information to an employer or, as in the case of *Phelps* v. *Kemsley* (1943), the employer imparted the information to the patient's doctor.

It became apparent to Lord Kemsley that his secretary, Mr. Phelps, was mentally deranged. He telephoned the man's doctor to suggest he should be seen because he needed medical attention. Lord Kemsley had terminated the man's employment and, when paying 3 months' salary, Lord Kemsley wished to have advice from the doctor on the way the money should be divided between Mr. and Mrs. Phelps. This communication led Mr. Phelps to bring an action for slander. Mr. Justice Macnaghten ruled that the occasion was privileged, and this was confirmed by the Court of Appeal. The Court believed Lord Kemsley ought to have communicated his fears to the man's doctor, who had an interest to receive the information. In addition, the employer required advice about the payment of money to Mr. Phelps and he had an interest to learn whether the patient was fit to receive it.

The case also illustrates the reciprocal element in privilege.

The doctor's position is relatively simple when, as a matter of *legal* duty, he has to disclose defamatory information. *Before he acts in the belief he has a moral or social duty, he should on all of these occasions, at once report the facts to his defence society and act upon their instructions.*

Reports on Mishaps: Privileged Communications

The Department of Health and Social Security, instructs hospital authorities to require all concerned in any untoward incident which occurs during treatment in hospital, to prepare a report which would be sent to the hospital's solicitors in anticipation of possible litigation. The Medical Defence Union (1961) approved this prompt preparation of reports on untoward incidents.

When a Mr. Patch developed gas gangrene following operative treatment, the consultant and others prepared reports within 10 days, which were sent to the hospital's solicitors. Two years later the Board of Governors of the hospital were sued for negligence. It was unsuccessfully claimed that gangrene was due to overtight bandaging and failure of post-operative care, following treatment of contracture of a finger. Counsel for the plaintiff contended that the reports prepared at the time of the incident were not privileged documents, but Mr. Justice Streatfeild held that they were privileged, although made in anticipation of litigation. They " . . . were privileged from disclosure as if they had been made for the purpose of litigation already begun" (*Patch* v. *Board of Governors of the Bristol United Hospitals*, 1959).

In any circumstances it is wise to keep contemporary records of treatment. The Medical Defence Union (1961) instance the experience of a doctor who lost his case because, a year after the incident, he had to rely on his recollection, not too clear, and he had kept no notes. (In their film of the hypothetical case of "Ogden v. Bell", the Union lay emphasis on the value of good notes made at the time of an examination or treatment. Respectfully, we wholeheartedly concur.)

Unfitness to Drive a Motor Vehicle

Any patient who is subject to fainting or other fits or whose ability to drive a motor vehicle is for any other reason impaired should be told by his doctor to notify the licensing authority of his disability. If he does not do so, the doctor should make it clear that he will have to consider doing so himself.

Child Abuse

It is clear that the doctor is implicitly criticising the parents in reporting to a third person, who has a statutory right to investigate the parents' treatment of the child. The Community Physicians, the Children's Officer of the local authority and the officers of the N.S.P.C.C. are all appropriate persons to whom a doctor can impart information (Medical Defence Union, Annual Report, 1968).

Privilege in Relation to Evidence

The foregoing must not be confused with the matter of privilege in relation to the giving of evidence in court. On these occasions the doctor stands in the same position as any other person who is not specially privileged in this respect. "He may be asked to disclose on oath information which came to him through his professional relationship with a patient, and if the question is not inadmissible on other grounds, he may be committed for contempt of court if he refuses to answer or if he fails to attend on sub-poena" (Halsbury, 1959).

The doctor should respectfully demur on the ground that the answer would involve a breach of professional secrecy. He could offer, if ordered to answer, to write it down and hand it to the court. But when ordered to give oral reply he must obey or suffer the consequences.

A judge has power to prevent any improper line of cross-examination; it is for him to decide to what extent disclosure is to be made by the doctor. This will depend on the circumstances of the case. (The subject is discussed, with a review of the case law, by Lindsay (1960).)

The position of spiritual advisers in relation to disclosure of information received in confidence was also discussed by Lindsay (1959). There has been general acceptance of the observation of Jessel, M. R., in *Wheeler* v. *Le Marchant* (1881), that communications to the priest in the confessional . . . are not protected. There is reason to believe that if this question is again raised in a court, that court would decide it in favour of the inviolability of the confession.

References

AVORY, MR. JUSTICE (1914) Birmingham Autumn Assizes, *Brit. Med. J.*, 1916, i, 206.
DU CANN, R. (1964) *She Act of The Advocate*, A 665, Penguin, Book. Harmondsworth; Penguin Books.
Editorial (1962) *Brit. Med. J.*, i, 1422 (Medico-Legal).
HALSBURY (1959) *Laws of England*, ed. Lord Symonds; 3rd ed., vol. 26. Medicine and Pharmacy, Part 1, pp. 6–73, London: Butterworth.
HUNTER V. MANN (1974), QB 767.
KITSON V. PLAYFAIR and WIFE (1896) *She Jimes*, Mar. 21–30.
LINDSAY, J. R. (1959) *Northern Ireland Legal Quarterly*, **12**, 160–72.
LINDSAY, J. R. (1960) *Northern Ireland Legal Quarterly*, **13**, 284–306.
Medical Defence Union (1961) Annual Report, p. 8. *ibid.*, 1968 and 1971.
PATCH V. BOARD OF GOVERNORS OF THE BRISTOL UNITED HOSPITALS (1959), *Brit. Med. J.*, i, 426.
PHELPS V. KEMSLEY (1943) *Lancet*, i, 59.
PHYSICIANS, ROYAL COLLEGE OF, Resolutions (1916) *Brit. Med. J.*, i, 207.
WHEELER V. LE MARCHANT (1881) L. R. 17 Ch.D. 675; 50 L.J. Ch. 793; 44 L.T. 632.

CHAPTER 26

The Abortion Act, 1967, and other Statutes which Relate to the Practice of Medicine

EVER since the decision in *R. v. Bourne* (1939) the legality of the termination of pregnancy on medical grounds has been unsatisfactory. It was assumed that it had then become lawful to undertake therapeutic abortion in order to preserve the life of the pregnant woman or to preserve her physical or mental health. It is true that no subsequent prosecution had been instituted but the Bourne decision related to the circumstances of that case alone.

In order to amend and clarify the law relating to the termination of pregnancy by registered medical practitioners the Abortion Act, 1967 was enacted and provision was made for the making of regulations under the Act. The Abortion Act, 1967 did not repeal sections 58 and 59 of the Offences of the Person Act, 1861; the termination of a pregnancy, except in accordance with the Abortion Act and Regulations, continues to be a major crime.

The Abortion Act, 1967

It is lawful for a registered medical practitioner (apparently any registered practitioner) to terminate a pregnancy if two registered medical practitioners, *any* two such practitioners, are of the opinion, formed in good faith, (a) that the continuance of the pregnancy would involve risk to the life of the pregnant woman, or of injury to the physical and mental health of the pregnant woman *or any existing children of her family*, greater than if the pregnancy were terminated, or (b) that there is a substantial risk that if the child were born it would suffer from such physical or mental abnormalities as to be severely handicapped (Abortion Act, 1967, section 1).

It was further provided in section 1 (2) that in determining whether the continuance of a pregnancy would involve such risk of injury to health . . . account may be taken of the pregnant woman's actual or reasonably foreseeable environment.

These provisions not only confirm the decision in *R. v. Bourne* but appreciably extend the scope of therapeutic abortion.

The Abortion Bill was severely criticised by the medical defence societies and others in respect of the proposed sanction of abortion based on the opinion of *any* two registered medical practitioners. This had been approved by the House of Commons and, only after a long debate the House of Lords deleted the amendment to the effect that one of the doctors should be either a N.H.S. consultant or a doctor approved for this purpose by the Ministry of Health or the Secretary for Scotland. The Act, therefore, retains the provision that the opinion of any two registered medical practitioners is sufficient. Not infrequently the opinion of a psychiatrist is sought.

The termination must be carried out either in a State hospital or in places specifically approved by the Secretary of State for Health (Section 1 (3)). Where the termination is immediately necessary as an emergency to save the life or prevent grave permanent injury to the mother, it may be carried out anywhere and no second medical opinion is required. The actual *termination* must be carried out in an N.H.S. or approved nursing home, but this does not apply to the mere *examination* to decide upon the need for the abortion. Abortions under the Act must be notified in accordance with the Abortion Regulations to the Chief Medical Officers of the D.H.S.S., the Scottish Home and Health Department or the Welsh Office respectively.

As stated above, the Act does not specify the doctors involved but they are almost always the pregnant woman's general practitioner or a psychiatrist and a gynaecologist. The latter may be the doctor who will perform the termination, but this is by no means invariable.

Where a practitioner has religious or ethical objections to abortion, either in general or to any particular case, he is at liberty to refuse to participate in the matter, even though he may have a contractual obligation under the N.H.S. to offer treatment of other types. Where a doctor had such conscientious objections, usually because of religious convictions especially within the Roman Catholic faith, he still has an ethical duty to his patient and should refer her without delay to another doctor if he thinks that either were it not for his own conscientious objection, it might be lawful to recommend or perform termination or if he feels that his conscientious objection makes it impossible for him to form an opinion on the question in good faith.

Some of the provisions of the Act have acquired certain interpretations since the law came into force. "Children of the family" must be interpreted in a broad sense, to include all those dependent upon the women, such as illegitimate, adopted, step-children and children over the age of 18 dependent because of some mental or physical defect. Even brothers and sisters of an unmarried pregnant woman living with the applicant might be brought within the definition. The test is whether in the broad sense, the children are members of the family and are dependent upon the pregnant woman for their health, care and well being.

Similarly, the "actual or reasonably foreseeable environment" includes substandard housing, overcrowding, the husband's circumstances (i.e. whether he is chronically sick, an alcoholic, drug addict or in prison), the number of other children living in accommodation and a variety of social factors which vary greatly from case to case. Verification of these matters may require the service of health visitors, probation officers and other social service workers.

Another controversial aspect is the substantial risk of serious handicap. The degree of both the risk and the extent of the handicap are not defined in the Act, but left to clinical judgment. Unwelcome publicity has occasionally occurred when it has become known that the aborted foetus was in fact free of the deformity for which the abortion was performed. The risk of serious foetal abnormality must be more than a mere possibility, but the common example of maternal rubella in the trimester constitutes a degree of risk that is certainly sufficient. The definition of "serious handicap" is also undefined, but it can probably be established if the child would be unlikely to be able to live an independent life when of an age normally to do so.

Consent to therapeutic abortion is rather complex. Where the woman is married and living with her husband, her written consent is necessary and the matter should be discussed with the husband, though his permission is not strictly needed, especially if the grounds are for the preservation of the life or prevention of injury to the woman. Where the abortion is performed for grounds including the health of the woman or any existing children, then naturally her husband's views are part of the environment which must be taken into account.

The decision is very difficult where the abortion is performed because of the risk of a seriously-handicapped child being born, and the husband refuses his consent. However, if the doctors both believe in good faith that the termination is the right course, they do not legally require the husband's consent and it seems likely that the husband would not succeed in a civil action based upon the loss of a potential heir.

No consent is necessary from the father or putative father of an illegitimate pregnancy nor from a common-law husband. However, if the grounds are the environment, then his situation may well be relevant.

No consent is needed from the parents of an unmarried girl between 16 and 18, though it would be advisable to discuss the matter with them (if the girl consents), especially if she is living at home with them. Where a girl is below the age of 16, the parents should be informed whether the girl wishes it or not. In the case of such young girls, consent for such termination should be obtained from the parents, but if they refuse and the girl is of sufficient maturity to understand the issues, her own desires should be upheld, and parental refusal not be accepted. If the parents of a girl under sixteen wish for her pregnancy to be aborted, but she herself is unwilling, her wishes are to be dominant.

The Abortion Regulations 1968 came into effect simultaneously with the Act. Its main provisions:

(a) The forms to be used by the certifying practitioners are set out (Certificate A and Certificate B) the latter is the one to be used in an emergency. Certificate A must be completed before the operation and Certificate B must be completed not later than 24 hours afterwards. These certificates must be retained for 3 years.

(b) Notification of all abortions must be made to the Chief Medical Officer at the Ministry of Health or his counterpart in Scotland within 7 days of the operation.

(c) The following exceptions are made to the strict confidentiality of the documents:
 i. to authorise the officials of the D.H.S.S. or of the Registrar General for statistical purposes.
 ii. to the Director of Public Prosecution in relation to offences against the Act.
 iii. to a police officer not below the rank of Superintendent in relation to offences against the Act.
 iv. for the purpose of criminal proceedings which have begun.
 v. for *bona fide* scientific reasons.
 vi. to the practitioner who terminated the pregnancy, or to any other practitioner with the patient's consent.

Divorce and Nullity of Marriage

*Divorce Reform Act, 1969: Matrimonial Causes Act, 1965
and the Matrimonial Causes Rules, 1968*

The Divorce Reform Act, 1969 enacted that the sole ground for divorce shall be irretrievable breakdown of the marriage. The court will require proof of this on one or more of the following facts:

(a) that the respondent has committed adultery and the petitioner finds it intolerable to live with the respondent;

(b) that the respondent has behaved in such a way that the petitioner cannot reasonably be expected to live with the respondent;

(c) that the respondent has deserted the petitioner for a continuous period of at least 2 years immediately preceding the presentation of the petition;

(d) that the parties to the marriage have lived apart for a continuous period of at least 2 years immediately preceding the presentation of the petition and the respondent consents to a decree being granted;

(e) that the parties to the marriage have lived apart for a continuous period of at least 5 years immediately preceding the presentation of the petition.

Adultery is normally proved without the aid of medical evidence but on occasions when the disputed paternity of a child is relevant, the court will receive evidence of the results of blood tests. Provision for these was made under the Family Law Reform Act, 1969, in its Third Part (see below, p. 709).

The doctor may be called upon to give evidence of cruelty, which, of course is not restricted to physical cruelty. He may also give evidence of the ill effects on the health of the petitioner arising out of refusal to permit intercourse or the use of unnatural or repugnant sexual practices. There may be medical evidence of intercourse per anum. Mental illness may be a factor leading to behaviour which makes life intolerable for the petitioner; it may be the cause of the parties being obliged to live apart. In respect of (d), when the consent of the respondent if suffering from mental illness, is required, the doctor in charge of the patient will have to determine whether the respondent is capable of understanding the consequences to him of his consenting to a decree being granted and the steps which he must take to indicate that he consents to the grant of a decree. There may be occasions when the respondent contests the grant of a decree on the ground that his ill health made it necessary for him to live apart. In the event that the parties require medical evidence its nature will depend on the circumstances of that case.

Nullity

The grant of a decree of nullity is governed by the provisions of the Matrimonial Causes Act, 1965 and the Matrimonial Causes Rules, 1968.

In addition to any other grounds on which a marriage is by law void or voidable, a marriage shall be voidable on the ground

(a) that the marriage has not been consummated owing to the wilful refusal of the respondent to consummate it; or

(b) that at the time of the marriage either party to the marriage was of unsound mind, or was suffering from mental disorder within the meaning of the Mental Health Act, 1959 of such a kind or to such an extent as to be unfitted for marriage and the procreation of children, or was subject to recurrent attacks of insanity or epilepsy; or

(c) that the respondent was at the time of the marriage suffering from venereal disease in a communicable form; or

(d) that the respondent was at the time of the marriage pregnant by some person other than the petitioner.

A decree of nullity shall not be granted in respect of petitions which are based on grounds (b), (c) or (d) unless the court is satisfied that: the petitioner was at the time of the marriage ignorant of the facts alleged; and proceedings were instituted within a year from the date of the marriage; and marital intercourse with the consent of the petitioner has not taken place since the petitioner discovered existence of the grounds for a decree. It is further provided that where a decree of nullity is granted, any child of the parties, who would have been legitimate if the marriage had been dissolved instead of being annulled, shall be deemed to be their legitimate child.

The medical evidence in these cases is governed by Rules 30 and 31 of the Matrimonial Causes Rules, 1968. When the ground for a petition of nullity is impotence or incapacity, the petitioner makes application to the registrar to determine whether medical inspectors shall be appointed to examine the parties. He may appoint a medical inspector, or if he thinks it necessary, two medical inspectors, to examine the parties. They will report to the court the result of the examination.

The conduct of the examination is prescribed by Rule 31. Every medical examination under Rule 30 shall be held at the consulting room of the medical inspector or, as the case may be, of one of the medical inspectors. The registrar may direct, on the application of a party, that the examination of that party shall be held at the court office or at such other place as the registrar thinks convenient.

Every party presenting himself for examination shall sign, in the presence of the inspector or inspectors, a statement that he is the person referred to as the petitioner or respondent, as the case may be, in the order for examination, and at the conclusion of the examination the inspector or inspectors shall certify on the statement that it was signed in his or their presence by the person who has been examined.

Family Law Reform Act, 1959

This statute amended the law relating to the age of majority. Under section 1 a person shall attain full age on attaining the age of EIGHTEEN instead of on attaining the age of 21. The necessary changes substituting 18 for 21 in extant statutes are listed in Schedule 1 of the Act. Although the alteration was made in relation to section 38 of the Sexual Offences Act, 1956 with regard to the power of the court where a person convicted of incest with a girl under 21, the minimum age at which certain forms of buggery and gross indecency are no longer offences remains at 21 years.

Section 8 of the Act is of special importance to the medical profession because it removed doubt about the validity of consent of persons aged 16, but under 21 years of age, to medical treatment. It is now the law that:

The consent of a minor who has attained the age of SIXTEEN years to any surgical, medical or dental treatment which, in the absence of consent, would constitute a trespass to his person, shall be as effective as it would be if he were of full age; and where a minor has by virtue of this section given effective consent to any treatment it shall not be necessary to obtain any consent for it from his parent or guardian.

Section 9 expressly includes any procedure undertaken for the purpose of diagnosis, including the administration of an anaesthetic.

It follows that patients aged 16 and under 21 are entitled to the benefits of professional secrecy.

PATERNITY TESTS

Provisions for use of blood tests in determining paternity are made in Part III of the Act. Under section 20 (1) in any civil proceedings in which the paternity of any person falls to be determined by the court hearing the proceedings, the court may, on an application by any party to the proceedings, give a direction for the use of blood tests to ascertain whether such tests show that a party to the proceedings is or is not thereby excluded from being the father of that person and for the taking . . . of blood samples from that person, the mother of that person and any party alleged to be the father of that person or from any, or any two, of those persons.

A report will be made by the person carrying out the tests in which he will state: (a) the results, (b) whether or not they exclude the party to whom the report relates from being the father of the person whose paternity is to be determined and, (c) if that party is not so excluded, the value, if any, of the results in determining whether that party is that person's father. This report will be received in evidence but provision is made for circumstances in which a written statement may be required to explain or amplify the report (section 20 (4)).

The need for consent is detailed in section 21. If the person is of full age of sample shall not be taken without consent. If aged 16, that person's consent is effective and it shall not be necessary to obtain consent from any other person for it. If under the age of 16, it will be necessary (unless a person suffering from mental disorder and is incapable of understanding the nature and purpose of the blood tests) to obtain the consent of the person who has the care and control of that person. If mentally disordered this consent will have to be supported by that of the medical practitioner in whose care the mental patient is. The doctor will then be required to certify that the taking of a blood sample will not be prejudicial to the proper care and treatment of the patient.

Failure to comply with a direction for taking blood samples will permit the court to draw such inferences, if any, from that fact as appear proper in the circumstances (section 23).

Regulations for Blood Tests to Determine Paternity

On and after 1 March, 1972, when Part III of the Family Law Reform Act came into force, the performance of blood tests for the purpose of ascertaining the paternity will be carried out in accordance with the Blood Tests (Evidence of Paternity) Regulations, 1971 (S.I. 1971, No. 1861).

Direction Form (Regulation 3)

A sampler, i.e. a registered medical practitioner or nominated tester, shall not take a sample from a subject unless Parts I and II of the direction form have been completed and the direction form purports to be signed by the proper officer of the court or some person on his behalf.

Subjects under Disability to be Accompanied to Sampler (Regulation 4)

A subject who is under a disability who attends a sampler for the taking of a sample shall be accompanied by a person of full age who shall identify him to the sampler.

Taking of Samples (Regulation 5)

1. Without prejudice to the provisions of rules of court, a sampler may make arrangements for the taking of samples from the subjects or may change any arrangements already made and make other arrangements.

2. Subject to the provisions of these Regulations, where a subject attends a sampler in accordance with arrangements made under a direction, the sampler shall take a sample from him on that occasion.

3. A sampler shall not take a sample from a subject if
    (i) he has reason to believe that the subject has been transfused with blood within the 3 months immediately preceding the day on which the sample is to be taken; or
    (ii) in his opinion, tests on a sample taken at that time from that subject could not effectively be carried out for the purposes of and in accordance with the direction; or
    (iii) in his opinion, the taking of a sample might have an adverse effect on the health of the subject.

4. A sampler may take a sample from a subject who has been injected with a blood product or blood plasma if, in his opinion, the value of any tests done on that sample would not be thereby affected, but shall inform the tester that the subject was so injected. (A tester is a person appointed by the Secretary of State to carry out blood tests.)

5. Where a sampler does not take a sample from a subject in accordance with arrangements made for the taking of that sample and no other arrangements are made, he shall return the direction form relating to that subject to the court, having stated on the form his reason for not taking the sample and any reason given by the subject (or the person having the care and control of the subject) for any failure to attend in accordance with those arrangements.

6. A subject who attends a sampler for the taking of a sample may be accompanied by his legal representative.

Sampling Procedure (Regulation 6)

1. A sampler shall comply with the provisions of this Regulation, all of which shall be complied with in respect of one subject before any are complied with in respect of any

other subject; so however that a report made in accordance with the provisions of section 20 (2) of the Act or any other evidence relating to the samples or the tests made on the samples shall not be challenged solely on the grounds that a sampler has not acted in accordance with the provisions of this Regulation.

2. Before a sample is taken from any subject who has attained the age of 12 months by the date of the direction, the sampler shall ensure that a photograph of that subject is affixed to the direction form relating to that subject unless the direction form is accompanied by a certificate from a medical practitioner that the subject is suffering from a mental disorder and that a photograph of him cannot or should not be taken.

3. Before a sample is taken from a subject, he, or where he is under a disability the person of full age accompanying him, shall complete the declaration in Part V of the direction form (that that subject is the subject to whom the direction form relates and, where a photograph is affixed to the direction form, that the photograph is a photograph of that subject) which shall be signed in the presence of and witnessed by the sampler.

4. Where a subject is suffering from a mental disorder, the sampler shall not take a sample from him unless the sampler is in possession of a certificate from a medical practitioner that the taking of a blood sample from the subject will not be prejudicial to his proper care and treatment.

5. A sample shall not be taken from any subject unless
   (a) he or, where he is under a disability, the person having the care and control of him, has signed a statement on the direction form that he consents to the sample being taken; or
   (b) where he is under a disability and is not accompanied by the person having the care and control of him, the sampler is in possession of a statement in writing, purporting to be signed by that person that he consents to the sample being taken.

6. The sampler shall affix to the direction form any statement referred to in sub-paragraph (b) of the preceding paragraph.

7. If a subject or, where he is under a disability, the person having the care and control of him, does not consent to the taking of a sample, he may record on the direction form his reasons for withholding his consent.

8. When the sampler has taken a sample he shall place it in a suitable container and shall affix to the container a label giving the full name, age and sex of the subject from whom it was taken and the label shall be signed by the sampler and by that subject or, if he is under a disability, the person accompanying him.

9. The sampler shall state in Part VII of the direction form that he has taken the sample and the date on which he did so.

Dispatch of Samples to Tester (Regulation 7)

1. When a sampler has taken samples, he shall, where he is not himself the tester, pack the containers together with the relevant direction forms and shall dispatch them forthwith to the tester by post by special delivery service or shall deliver them or cause them to be delivered to the tester by some person other than a subject or a person who has accompanied a subject to the sampler.

2. If at any time a sampler dispatches to a tester samples from some only of the subjects and has not previously despatched samples taken from the other subjects, he shall inform the tester whether he is expecting to take any samples from those other subjects and, if so, from whom and on what date.

Procedure where Sampler Nominated is Unable to take the Samples (Regulation 8)

1. Where a sampler is unable himself to take samples from all or any of the subjects, he may nominate another medical practitioner or tester to take the samples which he is unable to take.

2. The sampler shall record the nomination of the other sampler on the relevant direction forms and shall forward them to the sampler nominated by him.

Testing of Samples (Regulation 9)

1. Samples taken for the purpose of giving effect to a direction shall (so far as practicable) all be tested by the same tester.

2. A tester shall not make tests on any samples for the purpose of a direction unless he will, in his opinion, be able to show from the results of those tests (whether alone or together with the results of tests on any samples which he has received and tested or expects to receive subsequently) that a subject is or is not excluded from being the father of a subject whose paternity is in dispute.

Report by Tester (Regulation 10)

On completion of the tests in compliance with the direction, the tester shall forward to the court a report in Form 2 in Schedule 1 to these Regulations, together with the appropriate direction forms.

Procedure where Tests not made (Regulation 11)

If at any time it appears to a tester that he will be unable to make tests in accordance with the direction, he shall inform the court, giving his reasons, and shall return the direction forms in his possession to the court.

Fees (Regulation 12)

The fees payable to samplers and testers shall be those specified in Schedule 2 to these Regulations.

Prescribed Forms

The prescribed forms are set out in Schedule 1, and the prescribed Fees are given in Schedule 2 of the Regulations. The fee for a report and testing four or less samples is £25.

Misuse of Drugs

Misuse of Drugs Act, 1971

Legislation controlling dangerous or otherwise harmful drugs was revised by the Misuse of Drugs Act, 1971, which consolidated and amended the law in an endeavour to check the rise in drug addiction in this country. The Dangerous Drugs Act, 1965 and the Dangerous Drugs Act, 1967, together with the Drugs (Prevention of Misuse) Act, 1964, were repealed and their provisions in amended form were re-enacted. The statute controls a wider range of drugs than the previous Acts and the term "Dangerous Drug" is replaced by "Controlled Drug".

The Advisory Council

The Act set up an Advisory Council whose duty is to keep under review the situation in the United Kingdom with respect to drugs which are being or appear to them likely to be misused and of which the misuse is having or appears to them capable of having harmful effects sufficient to constitute a social problem and to advise on measures for preventing the misuse of such drugs. The first members of this council were appointed in December 1971; they included eleven doctors and sixteen laymen, under the Chairmanship of Professor Hugh Robson, Vice-Chancellor of the University of Sheffield (*Brit. Med. J.,* 1971, **4**, 124; *ibid.,* p. 693).

The terms of reference of the Council include the giving of advice on the restriction of the availability of drugs and arrangements for their supply; enabling persons affected by the misuse of drugs to obtain proper advice and the provision of proper facilities and services for the treatment and rehabilitation and after-care of these addicts; the promotion of cooperation between the various professional and community services in dealing with social problems connected with the misuse of drugs; educating the public (and in particular the young) in the dangers of misusing drugs and for giving publicity to those dangers and the promotion of research into matters relevant to the prevention of the misuse of drugs or any social problem connected with their misuse.

"Controlled Drugs"

The drugs to which the Act relates are those which are for the time being included in one or other of three categories specified in Schedule 2 of the Act. They will be known as Class A, Class B and Class C drugs. The Schedule can be amended, by Order in Council, so as to add or remove drugs to the list. Class A drugs include those drugs formerly designated "Dangerous Drugs", e.g. the morphine group and cocaine, but there is the notable and imperative addition of the Lysergamide group and Mescaline. Class B drugs are a much smaller group of which amphetamine is one as, also, is cannabis and cannabis resin (Cannabinol, except where contained in cannabis or cannabis resin, is allocated to Class A). The third Class, "C", includes Pemoline, Benzphetamine and Methaqualone.

Since changes will take place from time to time in the Schedule, it will be necessary for those who have authority to supply or prescribe drugs to have access to the current list.

Restrictions on Controlled Drugs

Importation and exportation requires a licence issued by the Secretary of State and it may embody conditions limiting the scope of the licence.

Regulations will prescribe the production and supply of controlled drugs. The possession of controlled drugs are also subject to regulations. It is unlawful to cultivate any plant of the genus *Cannabis*.

It is lawful for a doctor, dentist, or veterinary practitioner to prescribe, administer, manufacture, compound or supply a controlled drug. A pharmacist or a person lawfully conducting a retail pharmacy business can manufacture, compound or supply a controlled drug. It is not unlawful for any of these persons to have a controlled drug in his possession for the purpose of his professional needs. The relief from restriction permitted to these persons is the subject of regulations. The Secretary of State has power to make it unlawful, if of the opinion that it is in the public interest to restrict the production, supply and possession of any controlled drug except for the purposes of research or other special purposes. Any drug thus designated, while the order is in force, may not be possessed, prescribed or administered, etc., except under licence granted by the Secretary of State.

It is an offence for a person, the occupier or manager of any premises, knowingly to permit the use of those premises for the production of a controlled drug in contravention of the regulations: to allow the premises to be used for the preparation of opium for smoking or the smoking of cannabis, cannabis resin or prepared opium. It is an offence to smoke or otherwise use prepared opium or to frequent a place used for the purpose of opium smoking or to have in one's possession any pipes or other utensils connected with the smoking of opium.

The Secretary of State has power to make regulations for preventing the misuse of drugs. These will include regulations concerning their safe custody, the keeping of records, the inspection of precautions taken and records kept. Regulations also relate to the issue of prescriptions, the supply and the dispensing of controlled drugs. Those issuing or dispensing prescriptions will be required to furnish to the prescribed authority such information as may be prescribed in the regulations.

Any doctor who attends a person whom he considers, or has reasonable grounds to suspect, is addicted to controlled drugs of any description will be required to furnish to the prescribed authority such particulars with respect to that person as may be prescribed.

Doctors are prohibited from administering, supplying and authorising the administration and supply to addicts and from prescribing for such persons, controlled drugs except in accordance with a licence issued by the Secretary of State.

Prohibiting Directions

Practitioners or pharmacists convicted of certain offences under the Act will have their authority to prescribe, administer or supply controlled drugs withdrawn by direction of the Secretary of State. If he considers that there are grounds for giving this direction he may refer the matter to a tribunal who will consider the case and report to the Secretary of State. They can find that the respondent has not committed any offence, or, if an offence has been committed, they may not recommend a direction. On the other hand, if they recommend a direction, their report shall include a recommendation indicating which drugs should be specified in the direction or indicating that the direction should include all controlled drugs. The doctor (or other practitioner) has the right to make any representations he wishes to be considered by the Secretary of State; these must be made in writing within 28 days of service of the notice of a direction. If any representations are made, the Secretary of State shall refer the case to an advisory body; they will consider the case and advise the Secretary of State as to the exercise of his powers.

After the expiration of 28 days, in the absence of any representations or after reference of the case to the advisory body, the Secretary of State may issue a direction prohibiting the person from the use of controlled drugs in his practice, specifying which, or all, of the drugs are prohibited, as recommended by the tribunal. The case may be referred back to the tribunal, or to another tribunal, or the Secretary of State may decide that no further proceedings shall be taken.

Temporary Prohibition

If the Secretary of State considers the circumstances require the issue of a prohibiting direction with the minimum of delay he will refer the case to a professional panel constituted for the purpose. The respondent will have the right of an opportunity of appearing before and being heard by the panel. The panel will report to the Secretary of State who shall not issue a direction unless the panel reports that there are reasonable grounds for its issue. A direction in these circumstances will operate only for a period of 6 weeks. If it has not already occurred, the case will be referred to a tribunal for its consideration of what further action should be taken. (The Secretary of State has power to cancel or suspend any direction given by him.)

The constitution of tribunals, advisory bodies and professional panels is prescribed in Schedule 3 of the Act. The chairman of a tribunal shall be a lawyer of not less than 7 years standing and the other members will be persons appointed by the Secretary of State on the nomination of the relevant bodies, according to the respondent's profession. The Schedule also prescribes the procedure. The hearing will be in private unless the respondent requests otherwise and the tribunal accedes to the request.

Power to Obtain Information

If it appears to the Secretary of State that there exists in any area in Great Britain a social problem caused by the misuse of drugs in that area, he may, by notice in writing served on any doctor or pharmacist practising in that area, require him to furnish to the Secretary of State information with respect to any drugs specified and to supply particulars concerning those drugs. *In the case of a doctor*: the quantities, the number and frequency of the occasions on which they were prescribed, administered or supplied by him, and *in the case of a pharmacist*: the quantities and the number and frequency of the occasions on which those drugs were supplied by him. The pharmacist may be required also to furnish the names and addresses of the doctors on whose prescriptions for controlled drugs he supplied the drugs but he will not be required to give details relating to the identity of the patients. It will be an offence to give any of this information which the person knows to be false in a material particular or he recklessly gives any information which is so false.

Offences and Penalties

The offences under the Act, mode of prosecution and punishment upon conviction, are prescribed in Schedule 4 of the Act. Having possession of a controlled drug with intent to supply it to another can, on conviction or indictment, result in imprisonment for 14 years or a fine or both. Similarly, if a doctor contravenes a prohibiting direction and the drug belongs either to Class A or Class B.

Road Safety

Road Traffic Act, 1972

A series of statutes over many years has been designed to protect the population against the drinking driver. Although successive Acts superseded its predecessors, since 1960 all the Acts have remained in force and are still available for use when necessary.

The Road Traffic Act 1960, is still employed when the driver is suspected of being under the influence of drugs other than alcohol, as later legislation was solely designed to detect alcohol. The 1960 Act required a doctor to determine whether the driver was unfit to drive through drink or drugs. This involves a thorough clinical examination which must take into account natural disease and injury as the possible explanation of the driver's condition. It should be undertaken only by those who have the requisite experience of these examinations. The disadvantages of the procedures under this Act were that the doctor's assessment of ability to drive was subjective and provided fertile grounds for clinical disagreement with the result that many undoubtedly incapable drivers were acquitted. In order to avoid this ever-increasing evasion, the law was amended by the Road Traffic Act 1972, which made it an offence to drive a vehicle with more than a certain amount of alcohol in the blood or urine, irrespective of the effect of such alcohol upon the driver's behaviour.

The 1972 Act was itself overtaken by amendments brought in by the Road Transport Act of 1981, which allowed for the use of breath analysis as the definitive test for the offence. However, the 1981 Act has not repealed the provisions relating to alcohol in the 1972 Act, which may be used when no breath testing apparatus is available or where the results of breath testing are only marginally positive (see below).

Procedure under the Road Traffic Act, 1972

A constable in uniform may require the driver of a motor vehicle, who is driving or attempting to drive it, to take a breath test. He is required to blow up a plastic bag which is fitted with a device containing a chemical, potassium dichromate, which turns green if the amount of alcohol in the driver's breath is in excess of 80 mg per cent.

The driver has the right to refuse to take the test but if he does so, without reasonable excuse, he renders himself liable to a fine not exceeding £50. The officer must have reasonable cause to suspect that the driver has alcohol in his body or to have committed a traffic offence while the vehicle was in motion. In the latter case, the breath test must be applied as soon as is reasonably practicable after the commission of the offence. (The circumstances in regard to drivers who have been admitted to hospital are considered separately.)

If the breath test be positive the officer may arrest the driver without a warrant and take him to a police station. The driver is then requested to provide another sample of his breath not less than 20 minutes after the first test to allow any alcohol in the mouth to dissipate. If that test be positive, he may be required to provide a specimen for a laboratory test. The constable, when making this request, must warn the driver that failure to provide a specimen of blood or urine may make him liable to imprisonment, a fine and disqualification. If the constable fails to give this warning the court may direct an acquittal or dismiss the charge.

The driver is first requested to provide a specimen of blood but if he refuses to do so he is then requested to provide two specimens of urine, within an hour of the request. If he fails or refuses to do this he is again requested to provide a specimen of blood.

The first specimen of urine shall be disregarded. If the alcohol content of the second is 107 mg/100 ml, the result will be treated as equivalent to a blood content of 80 mg/100 ml.

The driver is entitled to one of two specimens taken at the same time or half of a single specimen divided at the time it was taken. The amount supplied must be adequate for analysis by a competent person using ordinary skill and equipment.

Refusal to give a specimen of blood or urine, without reasonable excuse, is an offence and he may be dealt with as if it had been shown that he had excess of alcohol in his blood above the prescribed limit.

Samples of blood for laboratory test must be taken by a medical practitioner. He is not required to express any opinion on the condition of the driver. His duty is to secure the consent of the driver to the taking of a blood sample and to provide a certificate that consent had been given. (Obviously, if it appears to the doctor that the driver is injured or is suffering from illness he will seek consent to treatment, or, if the driver is unable to give consent, the case may be regarded as an emergency and the patient is transferred to hospital or given whatever treatment is deemed immediately necessary.) The doctor must be given reasonable co-operation by the driver who consents to the taking of a blood sample. Insistence of its collection from the penis has been held to constitute refusal, since the doctor rightly refused to attempt this mode of collection. On another occasion the driver consented to allow blood to be taken from one of his toes but kept wriggling them thereby preventing the collection of blood. The results of the laboratory tests are in the form of a certificate which states the amount of alcohol in the specimen in terms of mg/100 ml. These certificates are admissible in evidence.

Road Transport Act 1981

Following the Blennerhasset Report, British practice was brought into line with many other countries in using breath analysis in place of blood or urine testing. One advantage of this system, from the point of view of the police, was that the trouble and expense of calling a police surgeon or other medical practitioner was avoided, as the apparatus could be used by trained police officers. However, there are some potential defects in this system, especially where the driver's condition may be due to injury or disease, recognition of which cannot be expected to be made by a police officer.

The new Act states that it is an offence to drive a motor vehicle if the concentration of alcohol in a sample of breath exceeds 35 micrograms per 100 ml.

The procedure is as follows:-

A motorist may be stopped at the roadside by a police officer for a moving traffic offence or if the officer has reason to suspect that he has been drinking. As in the previous legislation, a breath test is taken to screen the motorist, but instead of the more crude dichromate tube equipment, the Lion Laboratories *Alcolometer* is used. This is a quantitative test in which the apparatus when perfused with a sample of deep expiratory breath, gives a result displayed by coloured lights. There are three lights on the apparatus, green, amber and red. A green light indicates that the breath is below the limit, amber alone is a warning but still negative, red and amber is also a warning but not a positive test. Only if the red light alone is illuminated (which may take several seconds to proceed from amber to red) is the screening test accepted as positive.

When this occurs, there is a roadside arrest and the motorist is taken to the nearest police station possessing more sophisticated apparatus. At the station, there is no further screening test as in the 1972 procedure, but a pair of definitive tests are made using a larger apparatus called the Lion *Intoximeter 3000*. Of these two tests, taken in sequence, the lowest result must be utilised by the police. Although the official limit is 35 micrograms per 100 ml. of alcohol in the breath, no action is taken if the result (produced on a paper ribbon as in a computer or supermarket till output) is between 35–39 micrograms per 100 ml.

If the written result is 40 micrograms or more, this is a positive test which will lead to conviction unless some cogent defence is successful. The Intoximeter produces two sets of printed results, one of which is given to the driver as evidence of his breath level. It will be noted that there is no defence sample available, as with blood and urine tests.

As an additional safeguard, if the Intoximeter 3000 result is between 40–50 micrograms per 100 ml, the driver may be given the option to provide a blood or urine sample, but the final decision is that of the police officer and not the driver. If such a sample is given, then the procedure is identical to that of the 1972 legislation and no conviction will result if the blood analysis reveals less than 80 mg. per 100 ml. or the urine sample less than 109 mg. per 100 ml.

Some disquiet has been voiced since the introduction of the breath testing in May 1983, because of allegations that other substances in the breath such as acetone and a variety of volatile products in food-stuffs, may give a positive result. This has been energetically denied by the manufacturers of the apparatus and to date, no substantiation of these claims has been produced.

It will be noted that the new legislation does not attempt to equate breath alcohol with blood or urine alcohol and the 1981 Act states merely that it is an offence to drive with more than 35 micrograms of alcohol per 100 millilitres of breath. However, there must obviously be a theoretical relationship between body fluids and gases and an unofficial chart used by magistrates indicates that, for example, 52 micrograms per 100 millilitres of breath is equivalent to 120 milligrams per 100 millilitres of blood or 160 milligrams per 100 millilitres of urine. As a useful working rule, it can be assumed that 1 milligram of alcohol per 100 ml. of blood is equivalent to 0.43 micrograms of alcohol per 100 millilitres of breath.

Hospital Cases

In the past an astute driver, involved in an accident and aware that he might be found under the influence of drink, would conduct himself in a manner which would lead him to be taken forthwith to hospital, although only slightly injured. Under the Road Traffic Act he will not be required to take the breath test at the scene but he may be required to do so at the hospital. He shall not be so required if the medical practitioner in immediate charge of the patient is not first notified of the proposal to make the requirement or objects to the provision of a specimen on the ground that its provision or the requirement to provide it would be prejudicial to the proper care or treatment of the patient. It should be noted that the doctor's sanction is needed not only for the taking of blood but also the collection of urine; sanction to take a blood sample does not cover the latter; a specific request is required for each.

Seat Belt Legislation

From 31st January, 1983, legislation made the wearing of seat belts obligatory for the front-seat occupants of motor cars in Britain. It is also the driver's responsibility to ensure that passengers under 14 years of age are wearing seat belts or restraints while travelling in the front seat. Infants under 1 year of age travelling in the front passenger seat must be in an approved restraint, specifically designed for their weight, such as a carry-cot harness or child safety seat. The law allows children over 1 year to wear an adult seat belt or approved child restraint. This seems an unsatisfactory alternative for children under 10 years of age, as the diagonal seat belt cannot be positioned across the chest where it is most effective. Indeed, even small adults may find that the diagonal component of the harness crosses their throat, due to the non-adjustable anchorage point on the door pillar being too high.

The problem of the diminutive person was solved by the issue of extension brackets, e.g. by Kangol and Britax., at under £2. The motorist could fit them but the public were advised to have this done by professionals.

Reference

R. v. BOURNE [1939] 1, K. B. 687; *Brit. Med. J.* 1938, **2**, 97; *ibid.*, 185., 185: *ibid.*, 199: *Lancet* 1938, **2**, 280; Med.-leg. Rev., **6**, 379.

STATUTES AND REGULATIONS

Abortion Act, 1967: Eliz. 2, ch. 87.
Abortion Regulations, 1968: S.I. 1968, No. 390.
Abortion (Amendment) Regulations, 1969: S.I. 1969, No. 636.
Abortion (Scotland) Regulations, 1968: S. I. No. 505 (S. 49).
Blood Tests (Evidence of Paternity) Regulations, 1971: S. I. 1971, No. 1861.
Divorce Law Reform Act, 1969: Eliz. 2, ch. 55.
Family Law Reform Act, 1959: Eliz. 2, ch. 46.
Matrimonial Causes Act, 1965: Eliz. 2, ch. 72.
Matrimonial Causes Rules, 1968: S. I. 1968, No. 219.
Ministry of Health Memorandum: H. M. (68) 21.
Ministry of Health Memorandum: ECN 656 (ECL 39/68).
Misuse of Drugs Act, 1971: Eliz. 2, ch. 38.
Road Traffic Act, 1972: Eliz. 2, ch. 20.

Index

Abdomen injury 187–8
  by firearms 267
  by shotgun 218
  in child abuse 538
Abortion 496–513, 613
  air embolism 503–7
  and medical practitioner 509–10
  by digital interference 501
  by drugs 507–8, 510
  by general violence 498
  by local violence 499
  by syringing 501–3, 506–7, 510–11
  case reports 505–7
  cause of death following 497–8
  consent in 707
  criminal 496–7
  definition 496
  duties of medical practitioners in 701
  fabricated 512
  instrumental 500–1, 510
  methods used in procuring 498
  pastes 507
  post-mortem evidence 510
  religious or ethical objections 706
  septic 511
  simulation 512
Abortion Act 1967 496, 613, 705–19
Abortion Regulations 1968 707
Abrasions 93
  differential diagnosis 97
  due to criminal violence 97
  inflicted after death 97
  parallel drag 95
  patterned 94
  sustained at or about moment of death 96
Accident injuries 132
  penetrating 132
Accidental stabbing 134–6
Acid, dilution and neutralisation 332
Acroreaction test 290–1
Adenosine triphosphate (ATP) 16
Adipocere formation 21, 23–6
Adrenal gland injury 189
Adrenal haemorrhage 664
Adrenaline 594
Adreno-genital syndrome 43
Adultery by doctors 614
Advertising by doctors 615–18

Age determination 49–54
  adults over 30 years 52
  by inspection of individual teeth 67
  by jaw bone 70
  children and adults under 30 51
  dental 66
  foetus and neonatal infant 66
  new born infant 50
Air in gastro-intestinal tract 523–4
Air embolism 179, 498, 503–5, 556
Air guns 196–7
  injury 197
Air Guns and Shot Guns, Etc., Act 1962 196
Air way obstruction 351
  by foreign bodies 464
Aircraft crashes 184
Alcohol abuse 613
  and firearm injuries 268
  driving offence 717
  manslaughter 136–7
  suicide 131
Alimentary system 562–4
Alkali injury 333–5
Alveolar duct membrane 522
Ammonia injuries 333
Ammonia poisoning 566
Ammonia throwing 340
Ammunition 198, 200–2, 208, 210
Amnesia after head injury 177
Amniocentesis 511–12
Amniotic fluid embolism 556–7
Amniotic sac, asphyxia by 458
Amphetamines 319
Anaesthesia
  cause of death from 592
  childbirth 598
  classification of deaths associated with 591
  clinical hazards 594
  deaths associated with 591
  deaths attributable to 592
  deaths due to disease 597–8
  deaths due to inexperience 592
  deaths during or shortly after 592
  deaths occurring during 590–600
  dental 595
  drug use in 593
  emergencies during 598
  investigation of death during 598

Anaesthesia (*contd.*)
  maternal death due to 592
  nitrous oxide 593
  obstetric 592, 598
  technical mishaps 595
Anaesthetics, contamination 652
Anatomy Act, 1832 61
Anderson v. Chasney 643
Aneurysms 560
Animal injury to dead body 36
Ante-mortem digestion 186
Aorta 183
Aortic arch syndrome 556
Approved practice as criterion of reasonable
  care 642–4
Aqueous humour 5
Arc eye 293
Arsenic poisoning 22
Arson, death by 336
Arterial damage in electrical injury 292
Arterial diseases 555–6
Artificial respiration 97, 307, 390, 596
Asbestos exposure 664
Asphyxia
  and strangulation 408
  by amniotic sac 458
  by smothering 449–50
  by throttling 415–16
  classical 352
  traumatic or crush 351, 468–72
  case reports 470–2
  See also Mechanical asphyxia; Suffocation
Association by doctors 618
Asymmetrical cardiomyopathy 554
Atheromatous aneurysms 555
Atropine 319, 594
Auscultation 8
Auto-erotic practices 455
Automatic pistol 199–200, 205, 207
Automatic pistol injuries 244–5, 247, 248, 254–5,
  258
Automatism 266
Autopsy 548, 598–9

Ballistics 196
Barberio's test 492
Barbiturate anaesthesia 595
Barbiturate poisoning 559
Basilar arteries 180
  bone disease in 539
Battered child 515
  case reports 532–4, 540–5
  examination of 532
  natural disease in 539
  pathological diagnosis of 539
  records 539
  sub-dural haemorrhage in 537–8
  syndrome manifestations 538
  See also Child abuse
Bestiality 489

Birth concealment 529
Birth re-registration 43
Births and Deaths Registration Act, 1953 687
Births and Deaths Registration Act (Northern
  Ireland), 1967 692
Bite marks 94, 95, 101, 352
  identification by 68–70
Bladder rupture 191
Bleeding, ante-mortem and post-mortem 140
Blister formation 20
Blood
  cadaver 32
  carbon monoxide in 254
Blood group substances in teeth 71
Blood incompatibility 595
Blood loss 141
Blood pigment tests 59
Blood stains 577–80
Blood tests 634, 718
  determination paternity 710–13
Blood transfusion 635–6, 672, 673
Blood vessels, rupture 141
Blyth v. Birmingham Waterworks Co. 639
Body cooling 8
Body cooling curves 11
Body examination 577
Body temperature 5, 9
  at death 12
Bolam v. Friern H.M.C. 626
Bolam v. Friern and Hatcher v. Black 634
Bone disease in battered child 539
Bone injuries 289
Bone measurement 54
Bones
  amino-acid content 59
  ancient or modern 57
  dating 57–60
  immunological activity 59
  laboratory tests 59
  nitrogen content 59
  See also Long bones
Bowel rupture 191
Boxing injuries 172–4
  retinal detachment 174
Brain, bruising 170
Brain damage 669
  after head injury 178
Brain death 667, 668
Brain injury 291
Brain-stem death 668
  clinical criteria of 668–70
  confirmation of 669–70
  medico-legal implications of 670–2
Brain-stem injury 171
Breath test 717–19
Brodrick Report 679, 683
Bronchial asthma 558
Bronchiolitis 558
Bronchitis 558
Bronchopneumonia 552, 663
Bronchus, swab in 596

Brown house moth 35
Bruises and bruising 14, 15, 97, 98
  age of 104–5
  ante-mortem 102–4, 141, 142
  as measure of degree of violence 102
  brain 170
  by flexible agents 100–1
  by metal-studded belt 100
  child abuse 534–5
  circular 100
  elliptical 100
  medico-legal significance 97–8
  multiple 112
  neck 98
  patterned 98–101, 112, 574
  post-mortem 102–4, 141, 142
  proof of 105
  situations of special importance 98
  tram lines 100
Bulbar palsy 464
Burial, disposal of dead by 681–3
Burking 474
Burning buildings, deaths in 322–4
Burns 320
  acid 331
  alkali 333–5
  ante-mortem 324
  appearances of 321
  by corrosive poisons 331
  circumstances of 335
  due to dry heat 320
  electrical 329
  fatalities due to 322
  first degree 321
  in child abuse 535
  medico-legal aspect of 322
  post-mortem 325
  received before or after death 322
  second degree 322
  self-immolation 335–6
  third degree 322
  ultraviolet light 329–30

Cadaver blood 32
Café-coronary 351, 461
Candle effect 339
Carbon dioxide 323
Carbon monoxide 14, 323
  in blood 254
  poisoning 17, 104, 190
Cardiac arrest 8, 351, 355, 466–7, 563, 667
Cardiac conducting tissue 557
Cardiac contusion, heart 181–3
Cardiac disease 278
  See alo Heart
Cardiac hypertrophy 553–4
Cardiac infarction 553
Cardiomyopathies 554–5
Cardio-respiratory arrest 661
Cardio-vascular system 549–59

Carotid artery, thrombosis of 179
Cartridge case 207
Cataract in electrical injury 293
Caustic soda injuries 334–5
Central nervous system 559–71
Centres of ossification 517
Cerebral infarction 561
Cerebral ischaemia 561
Cerebral thrombosis 560
Cerebral tumours 561
Cerebro-spinal fluid 5
  chemical analysis 31
Cerumen, dust in 85
Cervical spine accidents 180
Chapman v. Rix 644
Chatterton v. Gerson 626
Chest cage fractures 537
Chest injuries
  shotgun 218
  See also Lungs; Ribs; Thorax
Child abuse 534, 703
  abdomen injury 187–8
  bruises 534–5
  burns 535
  external appearances 534
  fractures 536
  investigation of 540
  lacerations 535–6
  miscellaneous varieties 538
  scalds 535
  spinal injury 191
  wounds 535–6
  See also Battered child
Child destruction 514–31
Child homicide 486–7, 533
Child injury 533
Childhood, sudden death in 567–8
Children, stature of 57
Children and Young Persons Act, 1933 320, 473
Children and Young Persons (Amendment) Act, 1952 320
Chloral narcosis 457
Choking
  accidental 461–4, 466
  by external causes 464
  death by 461–4
  due to disease 462
  homicidal 465–6
  infanticide 465–6, 525
  laryngeal spasm 467–8
  suicide 465
  vagal inhibition 466–7
Circle of Willis 661, 662
Circulation cessation 8
Clostridium welchii 497, 498
Clothing
  dust on 85
  examination of 43, 211–12
  ignition of 320
Cocaine 594

Cold injury 340–8
  clinical appearance 347
  general effects of 341
  local 348
  neo-natal 345
  post-mortem examination 347
  prevention 347
  prognosis 342
  treatment 343, 347
Cold stiffening 32
Collins v. Herts. County Council and another 653
Concussion 175–7, 266
Congenital malformations 43
Consent to medical examination and treatment
    621–37, 709–10
  abortion 707
  blood tests 634, 718
  blood transfusion 635–6
  circumstances not requiring 622
  clinical research 634
  contraceptive advice and treatment 634
  doctrine of informed consent 624–31
  emergencies 631–2
  express consent 628–31
  form of 621, 625, 627
  implied consent 621, 627–8
  legal proceedings 621–2
  maternity cases 630–1
  oral consent 628
  persons authorised to give consent 631–2
  refusal of medical advice 636
  requirements of 621
  sterilisation 633–4
  termination of pregnancy 632–3
  time for obtaining consent 630
  written consent 629, 632
Consumer Protection Act (1980) Regulations 321
Contact flattening 13
Contraceptive advice and treatment 634
Contre-coup haemorrhage 170
Cooper v. Nevill 650
Corneal clouding 7
Corneal grafting 673
Corneal Grafting Act, 1952 673
Coronary artery damage 182
Coronary artery disease 549–53, 659–60, 665
Coronary atheroma 549–53
Coronary thrombosis 551, 598
Coroner, report of death to 678–81
Coroner's Act 694
Coroner's Rules 679–81
Corrosive acids 331–3
Corrosive alkalis 333–5
Corrosive injuries, prevention of 333
Corrosive poisons 331
Cot or crib death 568
*Crawford v. Board of Governors of Charing Cross
    Hospital* 644
Cremation
  disposal by 683–7
  formalities 684–6

Cremation Act, 1902 684
Cremation Act, 1952 684
Criminal Justice (Scotland) Act, 1980 692
Criminal Law Act, 1977 679
Criminal negligence 654–5
Crown-heel length 50, 517
Crown Office 691
Crucifixion 473–4
Cruelty to children 532
Cut-throat, pseudo 117–19
Cut-throat wounds 113–17
Cyanide fumes 324
Cyanide poisoning 566
Cyanosis 352

Dangerous Drugs Act, 1965 714
Dangerous Drugs Act, 1967 714
Dating of human bones 57–60
*Davies v. Horton Road and Colney Hatch Hospital
    Management Committee and Logan* 647
Dead body, animal injury to 36
Death
  asphyxial 12
  body temperature at 12
  cause of 117, 582–3, 677
  cellular 667
  cerebral 6, 667
  definition of 667, 673
  diagnosis of 4
  duty to give information of 678
  establishing time since 3, 5–6, 10, 12, 26, 31, 32,
      583–4
  identification after 25–7
  in burning buildings 322–4
  molecular 3, 8
  moment of 667–8
  multiple 140
  phases of 3
  reporting to coroner 678
  signs of 3–39
  somatic 3, 8, 13, 667
  stiffening after 15
  stomach contents after 32–4
  traditional signs of 6
  see also Brain-stem death
Death certification 4, 7, 677, 681–3, 687, 688, 692–4
Defamation of character 700–2
Delayed air embolism 503
Dental anaesthesia 595–6
Dental characteristics 22
Dental charts 64–5
Dental extraction, negligence in 654
Dental identification 28, 60–71
  historical note 60–4
  modes of 64–71
Dental records 40
Dentition
  first 66
  in age determination 49
  second 66

Dentures, identification by 65–6
Desquamation of bronchial epithelium 522
Devastator bullets 201
Diabetes mellitus 563
Diagnosis, errors in 645
Diaphragm rupture 186–7
Dinitro-ortho-cresol (DNOC) 19, 319
Disposal of body
    by fire 339
    by submersion 526
Disposal of the dead 677–95
    by burial 681–3
    by cremation 683–7
    executor's duty 677
    in Ireland 693–4
    in Northern Ireland 692
    in Scotland 688
Disseminated intravascular coagulation (D.I.C.)
    145
Divorce 708
Divorce Reform Act, 1969 708
Drowning 18, 421–48
    atypical 438–40
    chemical tests of 432–3
    circumstances of 441–2
    death by 30
    diagnosis of death 441
    diatom analyses 433–5
    disposal by submersion 440–1
    dry lung 351
    extent and duration of submersion 422–4
    external signs of 427–31
    homicidal 95, 442–4
    infanticide by 526, 440
    internal signs of 431–2
    laryngeal spasm due to submersion 438
    mechanism of 424–5
    medium of submersion 421–2
    post-immersion syndrome 436–7
    prognosis of 436
    secondary 436–7
    signs of 426–7
    signs of submersion and duration 444–6
    stomach contents in 435–6
    submersion when unconscious 440
    suicide by 442
    symptoms of 425–6
    treatment of 437–8
    vagal inhibition due to submersion 438
Drug abuse 559, 714–17
    by doctors 615
    in sudden death 567
    offences and penalties 717
    power to obtain information on 716
Drug effects 319
Drug interaction 560
Drug overdose 3, 21, 22, 558
Drug prohibition, temporary 716
Drug use in anaesthesia 593
Drugs
    controlled 714–16

    dangerous 714
    prohibiting directions 715–16
Duodenal injury 190
Dust
    in cerumen 85
    in nail scrapings 85
    on clothing 85

Earth-leak circuit breaker 273
Ecbolics in abortion 509
ECG 3, 8, 342
Education Act, 1944 623
EEG 3, 666
Elder v. Greenwich and Deptford Hospital Management Committee 646
Electric blankets 295–6, 319–20
Electric earthing 294
Electric marks 282–7, 290, 299
Electric shock 3
Electric wiring 294, 295
Electrical injury
    case report 275, 300, 301, 304–7
    cataract in 293
    classification of deaths due to 272
    contact with supply 277–80
    danger of imported appliance 272–3
    delayed effect on 292–4
    diagnosis: post mortem 291–2
    domestic 294
    electrical equipment 302
    factors influencing effects of 274–5
    fatalities due to 294
    hedgeclippers 300
    high-tension 288–94, 300–2
    hold on 277
    important factors in 279
    incidence of fatalities 272
    industrial accidents 279, 300
    literature on 273
    low and medium-tension circuits 282–8, 298
    mechanism of death by 279–80
    mortality from 279–80
    overhead cables 301
    patient monitoring 301, 303
    photographic flash unit 298
    pregnancy 311–12
    prognosis 293
    pylons 301
    repair of 293–4
    television 300
    underground cables 302
    see also Electrocution
Electrical insulation 277
Electricity
    historical note 271
    scientific study of 271
Electrocardiograph insulation 302
Electro-convulsive treatment 303
Electrocution
    accidental 294–7

Electrocution (*contd.*)
    auto-erotic 304
    circumstances of 294
    deaths due to 272, 303
    electric blanket 296
    homicidal 306–7
    iatrogenic 302–3
    in bath 296–7
    manslaughter by 307
    pathognomonic features 291
    recognition of 291
    signs of death by 282
    suicide 286, 304
    See also Electrical injury
Electronic thermometer 9
Embolism of missiles 266
Emmenagogue action on uterus 508–9
Encephalitis 561
Endocrine system 565
Endogenous burn 287–8
Entomology of the dead 34
Entrance marks 289
Enzyme activity in relation to wounds 143–4
Epilepsy 177, 666
    accidental smothering in 452
    in sudden death 561–2
European Economic Community 607
Everett v. Griffiths 640
Ewing's postulates 666
Excoriation of skin by excreta 97
Exhumation procedure 587
Exit marks 289
Exogenous burns 288–94
Explosions 184, 192–3, 243, 246
Explosive bullets 201
Express consent 628–31
Extra-dural haemorrhage 164–6, 325
Extra-uterine pregnancy 512
Eye injury 293, 332, 334
Eye wounds 93
Eyebrow laceration 109
Eyes
    in identification 85
    in mechanical asphyxia 353

Factory Act, 1837 60
Faecal stains 494
Falls from heights 192
Family Law Reform Act, 1959 709
Family Law Reform Act, 1969 631, 635
Fat embolism 145
Fatal Accidents Enquiries (Scotland) Act, 1976 691
Fatty change in liver 564
Features, reconstruction of 83–5
Femoral fracture 192
Financial compensation 664
Fingerprints 22, 40, 42, 77–8
    and medical practitioner 81
    forgery of 79
    mutilation of 79

    on firearms 206
    practical application of 79–80
    practical importance of 81
Fire, disposal of bodies by 336
Fire hazards 320
Firearm injuries 98, 208–65
    accidental 260, 265
    alcohol effects 268
    circumstances of 263
    entrance wound behind right ear 260
    homicidal 262, 264–5
    in the living 210–11
    investigation of 209
    mobility after 266–7
    multiple contact entrance wounds 267–9
    near wound behind right ear 261
    penetrating wounds 184
    pregnant uterus 262
    rifled wounds 243–60
        case reports 246–53
        contact wounds 243–53
        direction of aim 259
        distant wounds 257–8
        entrance wounds 243–58
        exit wounds 258–9
        near wounds – within about 1 yard 253–7
        odd and even rule 259
    sites of 260–5
    tandem-bullets 268
    see also Shotgun injury
Firearms 196–208
    handling rules 208
    identification 205–8
    rifled 199–202
    smooth bore 197–9
    unusual 202–5
Firearms Act, 1968 196
Fires
    in buildings 322–4
    removal of bodies 588
Flaccidity 8
Flash over burns 289
Florence test 492
Fluorescence tests 59
Foetal abnormality 706
Foetal age and weight relationship 517
Footprints 77–8
    practical application of 79–80
Foreign bodies
    in airways 464
    swallowing of 185
Forensic Odontology 71
Fractures 144–5
    à la signature 153
    chest cage 537
    comminuted 159
    cricoid cartilage 406
    depressed 154
    femoral 192
    fissured 153
    gutter 161

hyoid bone 179, 375, 377, 405, 407
in child abuse 536
localised depressed 150, 153, 155–8
long bones 536
pelvis 192
pond or indented 161
ribs 184, 191
ring or foramen 161
skull 152–7, 162–64, 526, 536
'Spider web' or 'mosaic' 160
thyroid cartilage 179, 406
Fraser v. Vancouver Hospital 646
Freezing 32
Frostbite 348

Gangrene in electrical injury 292
Garrotting 394
Gas formation 20
Gastrointestinal tract
air in 523–4
ulceration 664
General Medical Council (G.M.C.) 603–20
Constitution of Council 604
disciplinary functions 608–12
disciplinary proceedings 618–19
fitness to practise 612–13
functions of 604–20
registration procedure 607–8
serious professional misconduct 613–18
Genitalia 191
Genito-urinary system 564
Gerber v. Pines 654
Giant cell arteritis 556
Glass wounds 119–22
Guy v. Green 701
Gyrojet weapon 205

Hadlum v. Hadlum 524
Haemopericardium 598
Haemophilia 539
Haemopoietic system 564
Haemorrhage 559
Contre-coup 170
extra-dural 164–6
in boxers 173
in electrical injury 292
intra-cranial 164, 177
massive traumatic 171
traumatic cerebral 170–9
traumatic pontine 171
traumatic sub-arachnoid 169
Haemorrhagic leuco-encephalopathy 558
Haemorrhagic pneumonitis 185
Hair
examination procedure 72–3
in identification 71–3
Halothane 319, 593
Handwriting, identification by 41
Hanging 357–88

accidental 359, 377–9, 381–3
and interference 387
and murder 357, 383–5
and suicide 357, 368, 370, 383–7
auto-erotic 379–80
death by 29
differential diagnosis of mark 374
experimental 371
external signs of 373, 374
homicidal 383
internal signs of 375–7
ligature in 357–8
mechanism of 368–9
mode of application of ligature 358
modification by position of knot 369–70
neck structures 375–7
point of suspension 364
position of knot 358
posture and clothing of victim 367–8
recovery from 371
scene of 357
symptoms of 370–2
typical 369
without fixed or running noose 358–67
Hatcher v. Black and others 638, 639, 647
Head injury 138, 148, 182, 184, 675
and disease 666
brain damage after 178
in boxers 172–4
mechanism of 150–3
mobility of victim after 178–9
self-inflicted 157–64
stud gun 205
unusual complications of 175
Heart
contact wounds over 252
firearm injury 262
Heart contusion 180–1
Heart failure 593
Heart injuries 180–3
Heart lacerations 181
Heart muscle damage 552
Heart rupture 553
Heart transfixion 182
Heat contractures 327
Heat exhaustion 318
Heat haematoma 325–7
Heat hyperpyrexia 318–19
Heat ill-effects 318–40
Heat ruptures 325
Heat stiffening 32
Heat stroke 319
Heating Appliances (Fireguards) Act, 1952 321
Heating Appliances (Fireguards) Regulations, 1953 321
Hinck v. Wagner 627
Histamine detection in wounded tissue 142
Histological examination 547
sex determination 48
Homosexuality 76, 487
Hospital discharge demand 636

Hucks v. Cole 642
Human Tissue Act (1961) 673–5
Humane killers 202–4
Hunter v. Hanley 644, 654, 701
Hyaline membrane 185, 522
Hydrocephalus 175
Hydrostatic test 520
Hyoid bone fracture 179, 375, 377, 405, 407
Hyperglycaemic coma 563–4
Hyperpyrexia 296
Hypertension 661
Hypertensive heart disease 553–4
Hypoglycaemic coma 566
Hypostasis 13
Hypotension 660
Hypothalamic injuries 174–5
Hypothermia 340
    accidental 341–5
    due to exposure 344
    fatal 345
    in long-distance swimmers or shipwrecked 344
    post-mortem findings 342

Identification 40–90
    after death 26, 27
    by bite marks 68–70
    by dental examination 28
    by extraneous means 85
    by eyes 85
    by hair 71–3
    by handwriting 41
    by impressions 78–9
    by malocclusion 71
    by manufacturers marks 86
    by occupational marking 81–3
    by personal impressions 40
    by photography 42
    by pulse rate 42
    by radiography 84
    by reconstruction of features 83–5
    by scars 73–5
    by spectacles 86
    by tattooing 75–7
    of bodies 43–57, 588
    of living 40–2
    of typescript 41–2
    See also Dental identification
Identification parades 40
Immersion foot 348
Impressions, persistence of 81
Incisions, tentative 114–16
Indecency with Children Act, 1960 480
Indecent assault 487
Infanticide 514–31
    as result of fracture 525
    autopsy procedures 516
    by burning 526
    by choking 465–6, 525
    by drowning 440
    by poisoning 528

    by smothering 450, 473
    by starvation and exposure 528
    by strangulation 390
    by suffocation 451
    by wounding 527
    case history 522
    exsanguination 527
    injuries suggestive of 515
    lung inspection in 520
    modes of 524–8
    overlying asphyxia 472–3
    psychological basis of 515
    respiratory system 519
    viability 516, 518
    See also Live-birth; Separate existence; Still-birth
Infanticide Act, 1922 514
Infanticide Act, 1938 514
Inflammatory reaction 140–1
Influenzal pneumonia 557
Informed consent doctrine 624–31
Inhalation pneumonia 557
Injuries
    accidental penetrating 132
    ante-mortem 140, 141
    from firearms 98
    general features 91–147
    internal 137
    multiple 192
    non-fatal 93
    of specific regions 148–95
    penetrating 158
    permanent 93
    post-mortem 141
    superficial 93
    sustained before or after death 140
    See also Head injury; Lacerations; Wounds
Inquest 678, 686
Insanity disclosure 702
Insect infestation of dead body 34–6
Insect succession on corpses 36
Instant rigor mortis 17–19
Intestinal injury 190
Intestinal rupture 191
Intra-cerebral haemorrhage 559, 560
Intra-cerebral tumour 666
Intra-cranial haemorrhage 164, 177
Intra-cranial meningioma 138
Intra-ocular tension 7
Ireland
    disposal of dead 693–4
    medical registration council of 619
Ischaemic heart disease 661

Jawbone in age determination 70
Jehovah's Witnesses 635, 673
Jones v. the Welsh Regional Hospital Board and Kemp 643
Joule burn 285, 287–8, 291, 296, 301
Jugular vein injury 179

Kicking 111
Kidney injury 188–9
Kidney transplant 673
Kitson v. Playfair and wife 700

Laboratory tests 718
Lacerations 105–12
  agents producing 105–7
  by contact with sea bed 112
  by shod foot 111
  features of 107–8
  following street brawl 112
  heart 181
  in child abuse 535–6
  inflicted before and after death 111–12
  margins of 112
  of eyebrow 109
  of gums 112
  of neck 118–20
  of scalp by blows with shovel 108
  of tissue applied to bone 108–9
Landau v. Werner 643
Lanphier and wife v. Phipos 641
Larder beetles 35
Laryngeal spasm 467–8
  in choking 467–8
Larynx, rupture of 474–8
Laundry marks 86
Lightning conductors 315
Lightning stroke 307–15
  diagnosis of death by 312
  examples of 308–10
  flash over 310–11, 315
  historical note 271–2
  in pregnancy 311–12
  prognosis 315
  protection from 315
  recoveries from 313–14
  resuscitation 314
  side flash 310
Lip prints 71
Live-birth 518, 520, 523, 529
Liver, fatty change in 564
Liver biopsy 188
Liver injury 187–8
Liver necrosis 188
Lividity 13
Lochgelly Iron and Coal Co. v. McMullan 639
Long bones
  fractures of 536
  in age determination 52
  in sex determination 47
  in stature determination 54–7
Luminescence 21
Lungs 183–5
  carcinoma of 558
  contusion of 522
  inspection in infanticide 520
  microscopical changes in 521
  microscopical examination 520–2

naked-eye inspection 520
oedema of 521

Maceration 31
McCormack v. Redpath Brown and Co. and another 641, 647
Mahon v. Osborne 641, 642
Mallory-Weiss syndrome 186
Malocclusion as identification aid 71
Manslaughter
  by electrocution 307
  by stabbing 136–7
Manufacturer's marks in identification 86
Marchant v. Eastham Borough Council 654
Markland v. Manchester Corporation 643
Marriage, nullity of 708
Marshall-Hoare formula 12
Marshall v. Lindsey County Council 646
Massive traumatic haemorrhage 171
Mastoid process in sex determination 47
Maternal rubella 707
Maternity cases 630–1
Matrimonial Causes Act, 1965 708
Matrimonial Causes Rules, 1968 708
Mechanical asphyxia 351–6
  death by 351
  internal examination 354
  signs of 352
  use of term 351
Mechanical cardio-pulmonary support devices 667
Medical Act, 1858 603, 608
Medical Act, 1950 603, 606, 607
Medical Act, 1956 644
Medical Act, 1969 608
Medical Act, 1978 606, 612
Medical advice refusal 636
Medical defence society 639
Medical Defence Union 703
Medical education 606–7
Medical examination, compulsory 622
Medical Register 604, 607
Medical treatment
  compulsory 623
  risks involved 647
Medical witness 696–704
  absolute privilege 699
  authorities cited by counsel 697
  conduct in the witness box 698
  defamation of character 700–2
  doubt or ignorance 697
  expert witness 699
  explanation 697
  fees 698
  impartiality 696
  ordinary witness 699
  preparation 697
  principal rules for 699
  privilege in relation to evidence 703–4
  professional privilege 697
  qualified privilege 700

Medical witness (*contd.*)
  records 696
  role of advocate 698
Mendelson's syndrome 598
Mental Health Act, 1929 637
Mental Health Act, 1959 636
Mesothelioma 664
Metacarpal bones in sex determination 47
Metallisation 289–90
Miliary plaques 22–23
Milk and Dairies (General) Regulations, 1959 623
Mishaps, reports on 703
Missiles
  embolism of 266
  preservation and examination 206–7
  surgical removal 206
Mistaken identity 41
Misuse of Drugs Act, 1971 606, 714
Mono-amine oxidase inhibitors 560
Moribund state 10
Morris v. Winsbury-White 649
Motor vehicle, unfitness to drive 703
Mountaineering 344
Mouth-to-mouth respiration 437
Mugging 394
Mummification 26–30, 34
Murder
  and hanging 357, 383–5
  and homosexuality 487
  by burning 337–9
  by drowning 95, 442–4
  by electrocution 306–7
  child cases 486–7
  false charge of attempted 139
  sexually-orientated 485–7
Muscle biopsy 593
Muscle shortening 17
Myocardial infarction 552, 553
Myocardium 182

Nail marks 95, 96, 141
Nail scraping, dust in 85
Narcolepsy in electrical injury 292
Narcotic addiction 457
National Health Service 609, 614, 622, 649, 687
National Health Service (Family Planning) Amendment Act, 1972 633
Neck bruising 98
Neck structures 179–80
Neck transfixion 130
Negligence 638–58, 703
  administration of wrong substance 652
  and approved practice 642–4
  breakage of needles 654
  case reports 655
  communication with other doctors 648
  contamination of anaesthetic 652
  criminal 654–5
  damages awarded 656
  definition of 639–40

  dental 654
  diagnosis 645–7
  duty to be well-informed 644–5
  'no-fault' concept 657
  operations mistakes 651
  retention of swabs, packs, instruments, drains, etc 650
  risks attending treatment 647
  safeguards against 651–7
  splinting 653
  standard of skill and care 640–2
  summons for attendance 649
  versus clinical judgment 656
Neurological changes in electrical injury 292
Nightdresses (Safety) Regulations, 1967 321
Nitric acid, injuries 332
Nitrous oxide anaesthesia 593
Nitrous oxide poisoning 594
Notifiable diseases 623
Nuclear weapon tests 665
Nullity of marriage 708

Occupational marking, identification by 81–3
Oesophagus injuries 185–6
Offences against the Person Act, 1861 339, 496, 529, 705
Ogden v. Bell 699
Ophthalmoscopic examination 7
Organ donation 674, 675
Organ removal 676
Organ transplantation 672–6
Oscillometer 8
Oscilloscope 3, 4
Ossification centres 50–1, 517
Overheating
  by electric blanket 296
  of cots 319–20
Overlying 472–3
Oxyntic cell necrosis 175

Pacemakers 686–7
Pachymeningitis interna haemorrhagica 167
Paederasty 488
Palmprints 42, 77–8
  practical application of 79–80
Pancreas diseases 563
Pancreas injury 189–90
Parathion 17
Patch v. Board of Governors of the Bristol United Hospitals 641, 703
Paternity determination 634
Paternity tests 710–13
Peat bog preservation 29–30
Pelvis
  fracture of 192
  in sex determination 45
Peripheral vasoneuropathy after chilling 348
Peritonitis 562–3
Petechial haemorrhages 353

Phagocytosis of meconium 522
Pharmacy and Medicines Act, 1941 496
Phelps v. Kemsley 702
Phosphotungstic acid haematoxylin 552
Photography in identification 42
Picket v. Bristol Aeroplane Company Ltd 622
Pituitary injuries 174–5
Plastic bag suffocation 452–9
Pneumothorax following tracheal rupture 477
Poisons 14
Poisoning 22, 547, 578
  and sudden death 566–7
  by arsenic 22
  by carbon monoxide 17, 104, 190
  by dinitro-ortho-cresol (DNOC) 19
  by seconal 34
  death from 588
  homicidal 702
  infanticide 528
  nitrous oxide 594
  wounds sustained in 138
Polar explorations 344
Police, relationships with 700
Poliomyelitis 464
Pontine haemorrhage 559
Population (Statistics) Act, 1960 687
Post-contusional (post-concussional) states 177–8
Post-mortem biochemistry 565–6
Post-mortem examination 661, 686
Post-mortem hypostasis 13
Post-traumatic automatism 178
Potency determination 489, 490
Pot-holing 344
Pregnancy
  ectopic 512
  electrical injury 311–12
  extra-uterine 512
  lightning stroke 311–12
  termination of 632, 705
Pregnant uterus, firearm injury of 262
Prematurity 524
Pressure sores 97
Pseudo-cyst formation 190
Public Health Act, 1936 623
Public Health (Infectious Diseases) Regulations, 1953 623
Pulmonary embolism 556, 558, 662–3
Pulmonary infection 663
Pulmonary oedema 553, 559
  in mechanical asphyxia 355
Pulmonary tuberculosis 462
Pulse rate, identification by 42
Punch-drunk condition 173
Putrefaction 20–3

R. v. Barney 81
R. v. Bateman 655
R. v. Blaue 672
R. v. Bourne 705
R. v. Briggs 126

R. v. Butterworth 179
R. v. Christie 62
R. v. Crippen 73
R. v. Dobkin 22, 44, 62
R. v. Donald 72, 390, 466, 483
R. v. Ellison 18
R. v. Gardner 18
R. v. Gray 655
R. v. Greenwood 43
R. v. Haigh 62, 65
R. v. Handley 72
R. v. Heath 98
R. v. Hoyle 42
R. v. Humphreys 134
R. v. Jordan 672
R. v. Kemp 526
R. v. Lee 336
R. v. M'Loughlin 92
R. v. Manton 22, 42, 440
R. v. Nodder 440
R. v. Orton 74
R. v. Podmore 72
R. v. Rouse 72, 325, 336, 337
R. v. Ruxton 22, 43, 44
R. v. Sangret 154
R. v. Sheldon 460
R. v. Smith 92, 672
R. v. Teague 72
R. v. Thorne 97
R. v. Warman 92
R. v. Whiteway 579
R. v. Wood 92
Radiation injuries 330–1
Radio-active substances 331
Radiographic identification 84
Radiographic measurements 57
Rail-roading 6, 7
Rape cases 97, 480–5
  case history 481
  definition 480
  examination of accused 484–5
  examination of victim of 480, 481–4
  injuries 482
  male 487
Reasonable care criterion 642–4
Record Traffic Act, 1972 701
Records
  battered child 539
  legal proceedings 696
Rectal temperature 5, 8, 9, 341
  and time since death 10
  as sign of death 10
Rees v. Hughes 677
Registered medical practitioners 604–6
  privileges of 605–6
Registration of Births, Deaths and Marriages (Scotland) Act, 1965 688
Renal transplantation 674
Respiration cessation 8
Respirator lung 185
Respiratory arrest 314

Respiratory system 557
Resuscitation 3, 5, 7, 595
Retinal blood columns, segmentation of 6, 7
Retinal detachment in boxers 174
Revolver injuries 246, 248–9, 256
Revolvers 199, 200, 207, 208
Ribs, broken 184, 191
Rich and Exor. v. Pierpont 641
Rifles 199
Rigor mortis 15
Road accidents 94, 121, 180, 190–2
Road safety 717–20
Road Traffic Act, 1972 663, 717, 718
Roe v. Ministry of Health 652
Ruptured aneurysms 661–2

Saliva in stomach 523
Scalds 328–9
  in child abuse 535
Scalp injuries 148–50
Scanning electron microscope (SEM) techniques 71
Scapula in sex determination 47
Scars
  age of 75
  and identification 73–5
  disappearance of 74
  erasure of 75
  examination of 74
  medico-legal aspect 75
Scenes of crime 574–89
  approach to body 576
  blood and blood stains 578–80
  case reports 580–2
  concealed bodies 585–8
  initial inspection 578
  location by means of general search 586
  observation of body 577
  protection of body 575–6
  removal of body 584–5
  retrospective visit to 588–9
  use of animals 586
Scottish Procurator Fiscal 689–92
Seat belt legislation 720
Seconal poisoning 34
Segmentation of retinal blood columns 6, 7
Seminal fluid
  analysis of 490, 492–3
  collection of 489–90
  grouping of 494
  histo-chemical tests for 492–4
  medico-legal aspects 489–94
  nature of 490
  stains 491–3
Separate existence 518
  external signs of 518–20
  internal examination 519
  tests of 523
  use of term 518
Sex determination 43–9
  histological 48–9

of skeletons 44
  pelvis in 45
  skull in 46
  sternum in 47
Sexual deviation 304, 357, 377, 378, 556
Sexual intercourse 486
  death during 486
Sexual interference 389
Sexual offences 480–95
  between males 488
  See also Rape cases
Sexual Offences Act, 1956 480, 709
Sexual Offences Act, 1967 488
Sexual Offences (Amendment) Act, 1976 480
Sexual Offences (Scotland) Act, 1976 480
Sexually-orientated homicide 485–7
Shock effects 185
Shooting, death from 588
Shotgun injuries 140, 184, 211–43
  abdomen or chest 218–23
  back of head 214
  blast 240–1
  case report 214–40
  contact wounds 212
  entrance wounds 212
  exit wounds 241
  forehead 213
  mouth 213
  near wounds 223–33
  ranges of over 1 yard 234–40
  ranges of up to 1 yard 223–33
  tangential, non-fatal 243
Shotgun pellets, balling of 198–9
Shotguns 197–8, 205, 207
  ammunition 198
  rifled slugs 199
Skeletal system, injuries to 191–3
Skeleton
  age determination 22, 49
  examination of 44
  sex determination 44
  stature determination 54
Skill and care
  duty to exercise 640
  standard of 640–2
Skin injuries 332
Skull
  in age determination 52
  in sex determination 46
Skull comminution 159–60
Skull fractures 152–7, 162–4, 526, 536
Skull injuries, penetrating 158
Smothering
  accidental 450–2
  asphyxia 449–50
  external signs of 460
  homicidal 459–60
  infants 450, 473
  suicide by 450
Sodomy 488
Soil samples 587

Soleprints 42
Somatic death 3, 8, 667
Sommer's Movements 17
Spectacles in identification 86
Spermatozoa morphology 493–4
Spheno-occipital joint 51
Spicer v. Hall 629
Spinal cord injury 180
Spinal injury 191
  in child abuse 537
Spleen, diseases of 564
Spleen injury 188
Spontaneous combustion 339
Stab wounds. *See* Wounds
Stabbing with hay fork 133–4
Stasis haemorrhages 354
Stature of children 57
Stature determination 54–7
Sterilisation 633–4
Sternum in sex determination 47
Stiffening after death 15
Still-birth 31, 515, 516, 518, 520–2, 529, 687–8
  diagnosis of 522–3
  procedure in Northern Ireland 692–3
  procedure in Scotland 688–9
Stomach
  saliva in 523
  tablets in 33–4
Stomach contents after death 32–4
Stomach injury 190
Str. basalis 290
Str. germinatorum 290
Strangulation 389–420
  accidental 400–1
  after death from other causes 408
  and asphyxia 408
  circumstances of 389
  external signs of 402
  homicidal 389–95, 403
  infanticide by 390, 525
  internal examination 405–8
  ligature 402
  manual 409–20, 525
  mark on neck 404
  neck structures 405
  palmar 393
  pseudo- 408
  self- 395–400
Stud gun 204–5
Subarachnoid haemorrhage 558–62
Subcutaneous ruptures of trachea 179
Sub-dural haematoma 168
Sub-dural haemorrhage 166–70, 539
  in battered child 537–8
Succinodehydrogenase activity 5
Sudden death 181, 547–73
  drug abuse 567
  in abortion 500, 502
  in childhood 567–8
  misdiagnosis of cause 547
  natural causes 547, 548

  unnatural causes 547, 549
  See also under specific diseases
Sudden Infant Death Syndrome (S.I.D.S.) 568–71
  cases 515
  theories of causation of 570
Suffocation 449–79
  accidental 454
  due to subcutaneous rupture of larynx and
    trachea 474–8
  general considerations 449–52
  homicidal 458
  in refrigerator 453
  of infant 451
  plastic bag 452–9
  suicide by 458
  See also Smothering
Suggilation 13
Suicide 18, 19, 138, 351
  alcohol effects 268
  and hanging 357, 368, 370, 383–7
  by burning 336
  by choking 465
  by drowning 442
  by electrocution 286, 304
  by head injury 157–64
  by smothering 450
  by suffocation 458
  by throttling 409
  case reports 246–52, 260
  cut-throat 114–17
  electrocution 286, 295, 299, 304–6
  firearm 263–4
  humane killer 203–4
  injury inflicted on 387
  multiple contact entrance wounds 267
  site of firearm injury 260
  stab wounds 127
  suggesting homicide 138
  transfixion of neck 130
  See also Strangulation, self-
Suicide Act, 1962 383
Sulphuric acid 332, 333
Sunburn 329
Surgical mishaps 597
Suspended animation 3
Suxamethonium 319, 593
Swab in bronchus 596
Swallowing of foreign bodies 185
Syphilis, disclosure of infection by 701–2

Tablets in stomach 33–4
Tache noire de la sclérotique 7
Takyashu's disease 556
Tardieu's spots 521, 523
Tattooing
  erasure of 76
  fading of 76
  identification by 75–7
Teeth. *See* Dental identification
Temporal arteritis 556

Thallium poisoning 683
Thermal burns 296
Thermal injuries 318–56
Thermometers 9
Thorax injuries 114, 180–5
Throat wounds 113
Thrombosis of carotid artery 179
Throttling 409–20
  accidental 409
  asphyxia in 415–16
  case reports 417–20
  circumstances of 409
  duration of 417
  external signs of 410–13
  force used in 417
  homicidal 410
  in death from other causes 416
  infanticide 525
  internal signs 413–15
  suicidal 409
  survival after 416
Thyroid cartilage, fracture of 179
Tibia measurement 57
Tissue donation 675
Tissue transplantation 672–6
Toeprints 42
Trachea rupture 179, 474–8
Tracheotomy 596
Transfixion
  of heart 182
  of neck 130
Transplantation of tissues and organs 672–6
Trauma and disease 659–76
  incidence of 138–39
  medico-legal aspects 659
  pre-existing disease 659
Traumatic cerebral haemorrhage 170–9
Traumatic encephalopathy 173
Traumatic myocarditis 182
Traumatic pontine haemorrhage 171
Traumatic sub-arachnoid haemorrhage 169
Trichloroethylene 593
Triple-X syndrome 49
Tumours 664–6
Typescript identification 41–2
Tyre marks 94

Umbilical cord 515, 527
Urine tests 718
Urry and Urry v. Bierer and others 650

Vagal inhibition in choking 466–7
Vaginal douching 498
Valvular heart disease 554
Varicose veins 556
Vasectomy 633
Venereal disease 487–8
Venous thrombosis 663
Ventricular fibrillation 6, 273, 291, 302, 303, 552

Vertebral arteries 180
Vertebral bodies in age determination 52
Vital reaction 140, 142
Vitreous fluid 563
Vitreous humour 5
Vitriol throwing 339
von Recklinghausen's disease 562

Warren v. Grieg and White 647
Waterhouse-Fredrichsen haemorrhage 664
Weight determination 50
Wheeler v. Le Marchant 704
Whiteford v. Hunter 645
Whiteford v. Hunter and Gleed 645
Williams v. North Liverpool H. M. C. and others 640
Winchester rifle injury 247, 248, 251
Wood v. Thurston 646
Woolley v. Ministry of Health 652
Wounds
  age estimation 142–4
  by glass 119–22
  causation of 91
  cut-throat 113–17
  enzyme activity in relation to 143–4
  eyes 93
  fatal 93
  homicidal 115
  in child abuse 535–6
  incised 112–14
  legal definition 91–2
  main features of 92–3
  medical reports on 92
  multiple 92, 127, 138
  obscure penetrating 159
  opinion on 93
  penetrating 184, 188, 190
  rate of healing of 142–4
  self-inflicted 114–17, 139, 157–64
  special aspects of 137–40
  stab 112, 122–37, 159, 180, 182, 190
    accidental 134–6
    direction of wound 125–6
    external appearances 123–32
    homicidal 134
    manslaughter 136–7
    number of 126–7
    site of wound 126
    with hay fork 133–4
  stab-like 121
  surgical intervention with 137
  sustained in presence of pre-existing disease or poisoning 138
  unusual 137
  See also Injuries
Wrist wounds 115
Wrongful conviction 41

X-ray examination 259, 268
X-ray injuries 330–1